Mason & McCall Smith's

LAW &
MEDICAL ETHICS

Twelfth Edition

A. M. FARRELL
BA LLB BLITT MA PHD

Chair of Medical Jurisprudence at the University of Edinburgh

E. S. DOVE
BA BCL LLB LLM PHD

Reader in Health Law and Regulation at the University of Edinburgh

T0202370

OXFORD
UNIVERSITY PRESS

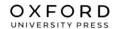

Great Clarendon Street, Oxford, OX2 6DP,
United Kingdom

Oxford University Press is a department of the University of Oxford.
It furthers the University's objective of excellence in research, scholarship,
and education by publishing worldwide. Oxford is a registered trade mark of
Oxford University Press in the UK and in certain other countries

Ninth Edition 2013
Tenth Edition 2016
Eleventh Edition 2019

Published in the United States of America by Oxford University Press
198 Madison Avenue, New York, NY 10016, United States of America

British Library Cataloguing in Publication Data
Data available

Library of Congress Control Number: 2023932754

ISBN 978–0–19–286622–6

Printed in the UK by
Bell & Bain Ltd., Glasgow

Mason & McCall Smith's
LAW & MEDICAL ETHICS

'It would not be correct to say that every moral obligation involves a legal duty; but every legal duty is founded on a moral obligation.'

LORD CHIEF JUSTICE COLERIDGE
in *R v Instan* [1893] 1 QB at 453

PREFACE

It is now forty years since the first edition of *Mason and McCall Smith's Law and Medical Ethics* was published and this marks the 12th edition of what has become a classic and enduring textbook in the field. Marking this milestone, it is important to acknowledge, with some melancholy, a passing of the guard from one group of authors to the next. Just as Graeme Laurie has noted in his Foreword to this edition, the textbook has changed hands over time, although we hasten to add, thankfully relatively infrequently: from Ken Mason and Alexander (Sandy) McCall Smith to Graeme (with Ken Mason), and then over to the trio of Graeme, Gerard Porter, and Shawn Harmon, through to this edition, with the two of us now at the helm with considerable contributions from our wonderful colleagues at Edinburgh Law School. We express our deep gratitude to Graeme and Shawn, as authors of recent past editions, as well as Ken and Sandy. Their pioneering work in crafting a textbook in what was once a niche area of the law helped to establish what has today become a mainstream and highly popular area of academic study in law schools across the UK and beyond. This edition carries on the *Mason and McCall Smith* tradition of providing a comprehensive overview and analysis of core topics within medical law and ethics, in addition to offering a diversity of views that encourages students to explore and form their own opinions on contested issues in the field.

Since the previous edition was published in 2019, a number of important legal and regulatory developments have taken place, which we have incorporated into our analysis into this edition. This has also led to some reorganising and streamlining of the textbook's chapters to enhance the clarity and focus on current issues in the field, with reference made to the UK's four jurisdictions where relevant. We have included developments that have emerged post-Brexit and during the course of the Covid-19 pandemic, in addition to substantially updating chapters covering the governance of the UK health system, public health, the regulation of health and social care professionals, and mental health. We have included analysis of critical policy and legal developments involving, for example, the National Health Service (e.g. Health and Social Care Act 2022), patient safety (e.g. Medicines and Medical Devices Act 2021), public health (e.g. Coronavirus Act 2020), mental health laws (e.g. the Mental Health Bill 2022), data protection laws (e.g. Data Protection and Digital Information Bill 2022), and new deemed consent regimes for deceased organ donation. We have also included coverage of key new cases in the area, such as *Bell* v *Tavistock*, *ABC* v *St George's Healthcare NHS Trust*, *A Local Authority* v *JB*, *Khan* v *Meadows*, *Toombes* v *Mitchell*, and *McCulloch* v *Forth Valley Health Board*. Recognising the importance of the inter-relationship between law and ethics in this field of study, we have also added two new ethics chapters ('Introduction to Bioethics') and 'Critical Frameworks in Bioethics') at the start of the edition. These chapters introduce students to concepts, theories, and tools that frame interpretation and analysis of medical law which we hope aid understanding and analysis of legal issues covered in later chapters. We have also added a new chapter on the regulation of health and social care professionals, reflecting the increasing importance and visibility of this layer of medical law and ethics.

Forty years after the first edition was published, the *Mason and McCall Smith's Law and Medical Ethics* textbook continues to carry on with pride the ground-breaking work started by Ken Mason and Sandy McCall Smith, with new paths charted along the way and with enormous support from those in our growing subject area at Edinburgh Law School. Indeed, this edition could not have been completed without the wonderful contributions from many of our colleagues in the Health, Medical Law, and Ethics subject area. We are indebted to their expertise in a number of domains that far exceed our own, and for their willingness to spend significant amounts of their time on researching and writing for this edition. Our sincere thanks to our colleagues Murray Earle (chapters on 'Withdrawal and Withholding of Medical Treatment' and 'Euthanasia and Assisted Suicide'), Agomoni Ganguli-Mitra and Emily Postan (chapters on 'Introduction to Bioethics' and 'Critical Frameworks in Bioethics'), Catriona McMillan (chapters on 'Contraception and Abortion' and 'Assisted Conception'), Ruby Reed-Berendt (chapters on 'Mental Health Law' and 'Consent to Medical Treatment'), and Annie Sorbie (chapter on 'Health and Social Care Professionals').

Last but not least, our particular thanks go to Rhiannon Frowde and Ruby Reed-Berendt for their excellent and diligent research assistance throughout this past year, to Christopher Long for his adroit copyediting, and to Emily Cunningham, Liana Green, and Hayden Merrick at Oxford University Press for their patience and stewardship in helping to bring this 12th edition to publication. Although this is a fast-moving field of study, we have endeavoured to ensure the accuracy of coverage of legal and regulatory developments up to January 2023.

Anne-Maree Farrell and Edward Dove
Edinburgh, January 2023

LIST OF CONTRIBUTORS

Dr Edward Dove Reader in Health Law and Regulation, University of Edinburgh

Dr Murray Earle Lecturer in Medical Law, University of Edinburgh

Professor Anne-Maree Farrell Chair of Medical Jurisprudence, University of Edinburgh

Dr Agomoni Ganguli-Mitra Senior Lecturer in Bioethics and Global Health Ethics, University of Edinburgh

Dr Catriona McMillan Lecturer in Medical Law, University of Edinburgh

Dr Emily Postan Chancellor's Fellow in Bioethics, University of Edinburgh

Ms Ruby Reed-Berendt PhD Candidate and Research Associate, University of Edinburgh

Dr Annie Sorbie Senior Lecturer in Health, Medical Law and Ethics, University of Edinburgh

FOREWORD

It will be a source of unending pride for me to have been involved in the authorship of *Mason and McCall Smith's Law and Medical Ethics*. This was the textbook that I used in my own studies in the mid-to-late 1980s under the watchful eye of Sheila McLean at the University of Glasgow (3rd and 4th editions), and it was a milestone in my career when I was asked by Ken and Sandy to contribute two new chapters to the 5th edition to reflect the rapid changes in the field. It was then an honour to steward the 6th to 11th editions with Ken and other colleagues, as the Edinburgh team grew and inevitable changes came to us all, including the loss of Ken in 2017.

While it is trite to observe that change is the only constant in life, it is our attitude towards change that defines us. I am immensely proud to see the changes that have happened in medical law and ethics at Edinburgh over the years, and these are represented incredibly well in this new edition of the textbook. The range and depth of new expertise is reflected throughout this latest edition, particularly with respect to the *medical ethics* dimensions. This, in turn, crystallises a core aspect of the original vision of Ken and Sandy when they set out to write the first edition in the early 1980s and when 'medical law' was often viewed as merely an offshoot of other areas of law, such as family law or criminal law. That vision was to communicate the essential symbiotic nature of law and medical ethics in education and in informing policy and practice in medicine and associated professions. Now, more than ever before, the original vision is being realised.

I congratulate my colleagues on the 12th edition of *Law and Medical Ethics*. It is a wonderful example of why we should all embrace change. It reflects the changes in the team in Edinburgh and it captures the wealth of never-ending changes in the field of medical law and ethics. There is no growth without change. Long may this textbook continue to grow and change those who read it and those who have the privilege to be involved with it.

Graeme Laurie

Sri Lanka, January 2023

CONTENTS

DETAILED CONTENTS

TABLE OF CASES

TABLE OF UK STATUTES

TABLE OF STATUTORY INSTRUMENTS

TABLE OF LEGISLATION FROM OTHER JURISDICTIONS

TABLE OF EUROPEAN UNION LEGISLATION

TABLE OF INTERNATIONAL TREATIES
AND CONVENTIONS

1
INTRODUCTION TO
BIOETHICS

1.1 INTRODUCTION

This chapter is the first of two in this textbook that focus on bioethics. This chapter introduces the aims, scope, and methods of the applied field of bioethics, and of the wider discipline of ethics in which it is located. It explains why (bio)ethical analysis is an essential companion to legal scholarship when it comes to thinking about 'what should be done' in health and medical contexts. This chapter takes the first steps in equipping the reader with the tools to engage in bioethical debate.

Medicine and health give rise to many kinds of ethical concerns. While this may not initially be apparent if you have not given it much thought, these first two chapters are dedicated to making precisely this point, and to give you some tools to think about such concerns. Medicine, while strongly informed by scientific evidence, is inherently a social endeavour. In other words, it is practised and accessed by human beings, within specific social structures and relationships. As such, medicine is also strongly influenced by history, politics, economics, social, and cultural values, as well as the values and interests of those engaged in the practice and governance of medicine. The clinical encounter itself is constructed through and influenced by historical and current social forces and factors, and the imprint of these can be seen in bodies and in the very conceptualisation of health and illness. Often, when we think about ethical issues arising in the context of health and medicine, we tend to think about those that pertain to the physician-patient relationship. Questions arising from medical progress and emerging healthcare technologies might also come to mind. However, moral questions related to medicine go far beyond these matters and include the best use of social resources, social and health inequalities, the realities of living in different types of bodies, with different types of abilities and well-being, and the best ways of organising society and its institutions in ways that reduce inequality and allow people to live flourishing lives.

It will not come as a surprise that health and medicine involve many different actors and institutions, each with their own histories, interests, and values, some of which might be, at times, in conflict with each other. Bioethics is concerned both with identifying and evaluating such issues and with developing well-reasoned arguments, concepts, framings, and other tools to address such issues. This chapter provides an introduction to bioethics and its various sub-topics, as well as outlining significant features of ethical thought. We discuss key aspects of good reasoning, the language and concepts encountered in ethical discussions, as well as some of the tools and lenses appropriate to bioethical deliberation and writing. The first section of this chapter examines how we should understand the relationship between ethics and law, and how the tools of one can be used to critique and develop the other. The second section explores the defining features of ethics and bioethics, as well as the ways in which ethics as a discipline can be distinguished from other types of thinking. This allows us to consider the ways in which a systematic approach to considering moral questions differs from intuitive or gut reactions. Here we also consider the possibility and the limitation of the universal nature of ethical thinking and the challenge from relativism. The third section offers an overview of the sub-topics within bioethics and the ways in which they are similar to or differ from each other. In the final section, we provide an overview of methodology, that is, the defining features of good bio(ethical) work. This does not purport to be an exhaustive methodology, but rather provides an overview of methods, tools, and skills readers might encounter and should be kept in mind in the context of the specific topics covered in the textbook.

1.2 THE RELATIONSHIP BETWEEN ETHICS AND THE LAW IN HEALTH AND MEDICINE

In this textbook, we are explicitly concerned with *both* law and ethics. However, at several points in this chapter we note that ethics and law are not the same thing. Why are these seemingly distinct disciplines paired together in this textbook, and how do they interact in the contexts of health and medicine?

We can start by noting some clear similarities between law and ethics (including bio-ethics). Perhaps most obvious is that they are both normative systems. They each lay claim to tell us what we ought or ought not to do in particular situations. They are both concerned with directing us towards 'the right thing to do', albeit with somewhat different meanings of 'right'. They are also both broadly concerned with the proper application of more general principles, rules, or frameworks to specific facts and circumstances.

However, despite both being normative systems, they are markedly different in several significant respects.[1] Most importantly, obligations and prohibitions in law and ethics may neither perfectly overlap, nor share the same underlying justification. An action or practice could be lawful but unethical, or ethical but unlawful. For example, knowing that contractually binding commercial reproductive surrogacy arrangements are against the law in the United Kingdom does not yet tell us whether such arrangements are morally wrong. Conversely, just because it may be lawful for a healthcare provider to share anonymised patient data with a pharmaceutical company without patients' consent, this does not tell us that they are ethically justified in doing so.

A further distinction is that the law is usually set out in statute, regulations, or case law, whereas ethical judgements are not always recorded in a similar way. Even where ethical guidelines, such as those of a professional body like the General Medical Council, are published, these guidelines are not exhaustive of all defensible ethical perspectives.[2] Nor do they mark an end to legitimate ethical debates about the topics at hand. Similarly, the procedures and priorities prescribed by research ethics review may not always reflect the full scope of relevant ethical concerns.

It is sometimes assumed that ethics is more context responsive than the law, and should perhaps be seen as more loosely action-guiding rather than tightly prescriptive. It is true that there is comparatively wide scope for diverse perspectives and debate when it comes

---

[1] Raymond Wacks, *Understanding Jurisprudence: An Introduction to Legal Theory* (OUP 2020).
[2] See, for example, GMC, 'Decision Making and Consent – Ethical Guidance' (2020) available at <https://www.gmc-uk.org/ethical-guidance/ethical-guidance-for-doctors/decision-making-and-consent> accessed 08 December 2022.

to ethical judgements. Nevertheless, as will be seen, robust ethical judgements must be supported by reasoned argumentation; they are not merely the expression of subjective preferences. Ethical reasons can provide strong motives to act in one way rather than another. These motives may be no less powerful than those supplied by legal obligations, even if the incentives and penalties differ. Given all these differences, it is reasonable to ask what the connection *is* between law and ethics and why this warrants their pairing in this textbook. Why would a student wishing to write an essay, a lawyer wanting to develop a strong case, or a healthcare professional or research scientist wanting to do the right thing by patients and participants, need to concern themselves with arguments and reasons based in ethics? Why can they not simply refer to what the law says about what should or should not be done?

The first answer to these questions is that ethical reasoning provides the means of working out what the morally right thing to do is, independently of what the law says. As such, ethical analysis is instructive in its own right. It is also a vital tool for analysing and critiquing the focus and operation of the law. Ethical arguments can be presented as appropriate grounds for law reform. For example, we can use ethical analysis to interrogate whether the existing law governing lawful human embryo research is striking the right balance in supporting or restricting worthwhile activities and whether it is achieving valuable outcomes for society, science, and health care.[3] Ethical arguments may also give us reasons to go beyond the bare minimum required by law. For example, feeding back and explaining individual research findings to participants, even when this is not legally mandated, could demonstrate respect for research participants and promote their interests in making sense of and governing their own lives.[4]

A second way in which ethical reasoning can usefully complement legal analysis occurs when ethics helps to fill gaps or introduce nuance in circumstances when the law alone does not, or cannot, tell us what to do.[5] It can also help us work out what is the right or best thing to do when decisions need to be made in an area where there are not yet any established legal rules. For example, researchers may wish to know what should guide the choices they make in conducting research using a new technology that is not yet subject to regulation. Even when an activity is regulated, these regulations may be framed in broad terms that leave room for interpreting their applicability in specific cases. Leaving space for further interpretation, specification, and evolution is often a necessary feature of laws and regulations that govern practices arising from the contested use of emerging and innovative health technologies.[6] Subsequent chapters in this book will provide examples of instances where health and medical law leaves space for this kind of interpretation.

A third way in which law and ethics are closely entwined is in the foundation and development of law. Some areas of law are particularly intimately connected to ethical reasoning. Human rights law is one such example. It seeks to codify entitlements, protections, and liberties that are widely held to be minimally necessary for a good human life.[7] Questions about what such a life looks like and what is needed for such a life are ethical

[3] For discussion of this debate, see Giulia Cavaliere, 'A 14-day Limit for Bioethics: The Debate Over Human Embryo Research' (2017) 18(1) BMC Medical Ethics 1.

[4] For discussion of this debate, see Emily Postan, 'Identities in Disclosure of Research Findings' in Graeme Laurie et al. (eds.), *The Cambridge Handbook of Health Research Regulation* (CUP 2021).

[5] Charles Foster and José Miola, 'Who's in Charge? The Relationship Between Medical Law, Medical Ethics, and Medical Morality?' (2015) 23(4) Medical Law Review 505.

[6] See, for example, Kathy Liddell, 'Purposive Interpretation and the March of Genetic Technology' (2003) 62(3) The Cambridge Law Journal 563.

[7] For further discussion of the nature and origins of human rights, see James Griffin, *On Human Rights* (OUP 2009).

questions, not legal ones. Human rights law is not unique in this respect. Conduct related to, for example, assisted reproduction, public health emergencies, the donation and supply of organs, end of life care, or processing of sensitive personal data all have profound implications for our well-being, sense of who we are, and our deeply held values. In recognition of this, ethical deliberations by legislators and regulators, and consultation with wider stakeholders and publics, often play a key role in the development of laws and policies governing activities in these fields.

In common law jurisdictions such as those that operate in the UK, judges do not simply apply the law, they also make the law through their judgments.[8] Ethical reasoning is often integral to these judgments, particularly in the appellate courts. The wording of these judgments may not always explicitly use the words 'ethical' or 'moral'. Nevertheless, it is possible to identify where ethical reasoning is doing some of the work when we see references to evaluative concepts such as fairness, interests, well-being, or harm. Ethically informed laws, judicial opinions, and policies do not provide the last word on what is ethically defensible. We might judge that some of them fail to get the ethics right. It is always possible to stand back and critique the law from an ethical perspective. It is worth noting that even in areas of law closely informed by ethical reasons, the resulting legislation or statutory instruments do not usually reflect the pure, direct transposition of moral argument into practical directions. Pragmatic, social, economic, and political considerations will also play key parts in the mix, alongside the need for consistency with other laws.

A fourth way in which law and ethics are connected is via the ethical guidelines and frameworks that are developed and adopted by public or professional bodies at state, regional, and international levels. These may aim to embed ethical practices, for example around patient confidentiality.[9] When published by bodies with statutory remits and high-profile standing, these ethical guidelines can acquire the status of soft law. For example, the Declaration of Helsinki, produced by the World Medical Association,[10] sets out international principles for the ethical conduct of health research involving human participants. While the Declaration is not itself legally binding, it has had significant influence in the development of regional and national laws and policies in the area.

The relationship between ethics and law is not all one-way as the preceding paragraphs might imply. Aspects of the law can inform our ethical reasoning. For example, reading legal judgments can present us with vivid examples of challenging circumstances faced by patients, populations, and healthcare professionals and thus with new ethical dilemmas and perspectives. This can lead us to revisit our ethical positions. And looking at the ways in which particular areas of the law have evolved or how they operate in different jurisdictions can also provide instructive insights into ways that societal values and priorities vary between times and places.

As students and practitioners working in law, bioethics, medicine, health sciences, public health, and related fields, it may sometimes be necessary to focus solely on what the law requires, or conversely on just what ethical reasoning suggests is the good or right thing to do. However, we will usually have reasons to look to the normative frameworks,

[8] Raymond Wacks, *Law: A Very Short Introduction* (2nd edn, OUP 2016).

[9] See for example, GMC, 'Confidentiality: Good Practice in Handling Patient Information' (2016) available at <https://www.gmc-uk.org/ethical-guidance/ethical-guidance-for-doctors/confidentiality> accessed 08 December 2022.

[10] World Medical Association, 'Declaration of Helsinki: Ethical Principles for Medical Research Involving Human Subjects' (2013) available at <https://jamanetwork.com/journals/jama/fullarticle/1760 318> accessed 08 December 2022.

analytical tools, and arguments of law and ethics in combination. Indeed, we may often need to go further than this and view these alongside the methods and materials from yet other disciplines—such as the biomedical and social sciences—to work out what is required, what is permissible, or what is forbidden in different circumstances. So close and pervasive is the entanglement of ethics and law in health and medical practice, that a combined interdisciplinary area of teaching, study and research has emerged in recent decades. This is identified under various labels, including 'medical law and ethics', 'medical jurisprudence', and 'health law and ethics'.[11] The practical rules and principles governing health and medicine that are subsumed within the scope of these combined disciplines are not limited to statute and case law. They include also regulations, policies, professional standards, guidelines, and codes of practice. Therefore, when we talk of law, ethics, and bioethics in this space, we are often actually talking of a wider family of interconnected normative frameworks and tools that seek in diverse ways to govern conduct in relation to health and medicine. This textbook is concerned with all aspects of this broad family.

1.3 WHAT IS ETHICS?

1.3.1 DEFINING ETHICS

Consider the following example:

Ms Ahmad and her 15-year-old daughter Maryam are meeting with a gynaecological surgeon to discuss a surgery to remove a cyst from Maryam's left ovary that is causing her a great deal of pain, as well as damage to the ovary. The surgeon advises surgery as soon as possible, as the effect on blood supply might result in Maryam losing her ovary. Ms Ahmad agrees. However, Maryam is a competitive swimmer who is training for a national championship. She insists that she would prefer to manage the pain and wait to have the surgery until after the competition.

Various ethical questions might arise in this context:

- What is the right thing to do?
- Who gets to decide?
- Whose values and interests should be part of the decision-making process?
- In what ways is the age of the patient ethically relevant?
- What is the appropriate role of medical expertise in this decision?

Ethics can be described as a systematic approach to conceptualising, developing, and defending moral ideas and concepts. These include ideas of right and wrong, good or bad, permissible or impermissible, obligatory, supererogatory, virtuous, fair, just, and so on. These judgements are made not on the basis of what the law says, but on the basis of

---

[11] Richard Ashcroft, 'A Philosopher Looks at "Law and Medical Ethics"' in Edward Dove and Niamh Nic Shuibhne (eds.), *Law and Legacy in Medical Jurisprudence: Essays in Honour of Graeme Laurie* (CUP 2022); Sharon Cowan, Emily Postan, and Nayha Sethi, '"Doing" Medical Law and Ethics' in Edward Dove and Niamh Nic Shuibhne (eds.), *Law and Legacy in Medical Jurisprudence: Essays in Honour of Graeme Laurie* (CUP 2022).

moral reasons. Developing these reasons involves thinking about questions concerned with value. These might include, for example, thinking about what kinds of experiences and goals matter to us, what a good life involves, what a fair, safe, and non-oppressive society looks like, what kinds of bonds and responsibilities we have to other people, what kinds of character traits it is desirable to have and to enact, and what it means to conduct ourselves well.

'Right' and 'wrong', 'good' and 'bad' are perhaps the most straightforward and familiar terms in which ethical judgements are expressed. When we are asking whether an action is right, ethically speaking, we are in fact asking whether it is moral or not. In some contexts, people prefer to make a distinction between ethics and morality, referring to morality as everyday values and principles, or those closely aligned with family, culture, and upbringing, and to ethics as the more academic or systematic study of morality. It is common, however, to use the terms synonymously, and we will do so for the purpose of this book.

In ethics we are—implicitly or explicitly—asking questions such as:

- What is the right thing to do?
- Is X good or bad?
- Is X right or wrong?
- What matters here?
- Who matters?
- What do we owe to each other?
- How should we treat each other?
- How should we distribute goods and benefits in society? How should we distribute its burdens?
- What counts as harm?
- What is a good life?
- Is doing X permissible/impermissible/obligatory?

The answers to these questions can be varied and at times conflicting, as there are diverse ways of living and world views. Nevertheless, there are systematic ways of talking about morality as well as some common conceptions that can provide the basis of dialogue in this area. Bioethics is also influenced and informed by the methods, practices, and findings of the natural and physical sciences, social sciences, and law, among other disciplines, each of which can provide important insights to thinking about moral aspects of the world.

In Maryam's case, for example, there might also be legal questions related to the age of capacity in the relevant jurisdiction, political issues arising in the context of allowing a minor to make certain decisions about their own bodies, and various gendered dimensions to questions related to reproductive choices, all of which will be relevant to thinking about the ethics of the case. Bioethics is concerned with raising and helping to answer such questions and can be defined as the discipline applied those questions to topics in health and (bio)medicine. The tools explored in this chapter are most closely related to the philosophical foundations of bioethics. In this sense, bioethics can be described as a sub-topic of applied moral and political philosophy and is an 'overtly critical and reflective exercise'.[12]

[12] Helga Kuhse and Peter Singer, 'What is Bioethics? A Historical Introduction' in Helga Kuhse and Peter Singer (eds.), *A Companion to Bioethics* (2nd edn, Blackwell Publishing 2009).

1.3.2 RECOGNISING ETHICAL QUESTIONS

An important aspect of doing bioethics is the ability to recognise an ethical question and equally importantly, to distinguish those concerns or questions that are indeed moral ones, as opposed to those that are not. Let us take, for example, a contentious topic in this field, the ethics of abortion. Abortion is both a compelling and difficult topic, due to the many historical, religious, cultural, political, and legal complexities associated with the issue. It is a morally complex area, which can at times challenge the deepest values and world views that people hold.

Consider the following case:

Sasha and Mae are debating various aspects of the morality and legality of abortion. Both Sasha and Mae agree that abortion is morally permissible under certain conditions, but they do not agree on whether it is permissible for health professionals to decline to participate in abortion care on the grounds of conscience, that is, based on personal, value-based commitments not to terminate a viable pregnancy. In other words, they disagree on whether the law should allow health professionals with such objections to choose not to participate. Sasha believes that the current UK legislation, which allows for conscientious objection under certain conditions, is justified, but Mae disagrees and argues that the law should be reformed to remove such an option.

Mae and Sasha appear to be engaged in an ethical debate: that is to say, it seems they are discussing whether there is a place for deeply held moral beliefs such as freedom of conscience, within professional contexts. As the conversation develops, it appears that they disagree on a very specific matter. Sasha believes that if legislation does not allow for conscientious objection, some of the best students in medicine and nursing will avoid specialising in obstetrics and gynaecology. Mae does not believe that this would happen. She agrees that if this were to happen, then indeed it would be problematic, but she does not think that such a talent drain would be the result of a legal reform removing conscientious objection as a right of health professionals. Note that what originally appeared to be a significant moral disagreement—about whether freedom of conscience is the kind of value that warrants protection—is in fact not an ethical debate at all, but a speculative empirical debate about the potential practical effects of legal reform.

Drawing on the previous example, consider the following additional scenario:

Mae and Sasha's colleague Jo joins their conversation and agrees that the law on abortion should be reformed. Jo believes that abortion should be available on demand because someone who is pregnant should have full control over their body and pregnancy. Moreover, Jo also believes that personal beliefs have no role in the workplace, and that health professionals should not be entitled to exercise conscientious objection on this matter. Mae agrees but Sasha still disagrees because he thinks that professional contexts should make space for some deeply held moral positions.

The previous example should now be viewed as an ethical disagreement about the potential conflict between professional responsibilities and protection of conscience, and the extent to which freedom of conscience should be legally protected.[13] One of the first things

---

[13] For a similar treatment on the difference between ethical and non-ethical disagreement see: Stephen Darwall, *Philosophical Ethics* (Westview Press 1998) p 5.

ethicists do when considering what appears to be a moral disagreement is to consider which aspects of the debate are in fact about ethics, rather than about facts, evidence, or speculation about what might happen. Note that it is not that empirical evidence and facts about the world are irrelevant to ethical debate—we return to discuss their potential relevance later in this chapter—rather, it is about recognising which questions are moral questions.

1.3.3 NORMATIVITY

Let us return to the example provided in relation to the medical treatment being offered to Maryam. Consider the following additional information:

> The surgeon tells Maryam and her mother that without immediate surgery, there is an 80% risk of Maryam losing her ovary. In the surgeon's opinion, that risk is relatively high. Ms Ahmad agrees and attempts to convince her daughter accordingly. However, Maryam is willing to take the risk, as the alternative risk—being unable to perform at the championship—is too high in her opinion.

Note here that the 80% risk presented (however tentative that actual figure may be), is factual or empirical. Whether the risk is too high, on the other hand, is a value judgement or a normative claim. Similarly, an oncologist might discuss various treatments with a cancer patient according to their likely efficacy, and might even recommend a course of action, one that is based on the likelihood of success, or increased lifespan. However, the patient might balance other kinds of values and priorities, such as how much time they would have to spend in hospital, or how much pain they might experience with each of the options. They will make a value-based judgement that might differ from the value that the physician is focusing on, such as success rates, for example. This is an important distinction to keep in mind in ethics, and sometimes the distinction can be difficult to spot.

Ethics is normative in two ways:

- It *evaluates* the rightness or wrongness of actions and states of affairs; and
- It *prescribes* attitudes, actions, practices and processes to achieve good or better states of affairs.

This means that ethical statements can be:

- *Evaluative* (e.g. 'keeping your promise is good'), or
- *Prescriptive* (e.g. 'you should always keep a promise').

Note that either statement might imply the other: keeping promises is good and therefore you should always keep a promise, or you should always keep a promise because promise-keeping is a good thing. Ethics and law are both normative enterprises in that they aim to tell people what to do, how to be, or behave in the world.

In some disciplines, 'normative' is used to mean something different from the sense described above. It is used to refer to widespread social standards ('norms') of conduct. In essence, the term is used in a way that is roughly synonymous with 'according to the norm', 'normal', 'prevalent', or 'widely endorsed'. That use of normative does not on its own carry the value implications with which it is associated in ethics. At other times, 'normative' may be used in a way that combines these two senses, that is, to critique or make a value judgement about prevalent or predominant attitudes and behaviours. Consider, for example, the statement, 'the representation of families in children's books are far too heteronormative.' Here the term heteronormative captures both the imagined default of cis-gendered, heterosexual parents and their children, and critiques its lack of inclusivity.

1.3.4 DISTINGUISHING ETHICS FROM PERSONAL PREFERENCES

When we make ethical statements, we often express these in the language of opinion or points of view. This might suggest that ethical judgements are just matters of preference or perspective. What is the difference between an ethical position or conviction, and a preference, or taste? Consider the following example:

> Eamon and Tashira have a strong disagreement about the merits of kale. Eamon enjoys all dishes involving this particular vegetable, from kale stew to kale chips. Tashira on the other hand, cannot stand it. They are not allergic, nor do they have any childhood memories associated with being forced to eat kale. Tashira only discovered kale as an adult and never took to it. Eamon then spends some time discussing mouth-watering dishes that contain kale. Tashira remains unconvinced, and in the end, they eventually agree to disagree. Some food preferences might appear strange to those unfamiliar with them, but in the end, we agree that it is a matter of taste.

We might be tempted to think that all ethical disagreements are similar to disagreements about kale. There are indeed real and significant disagreements about the morally right thing to do, as is often the case with abortion and conscientious objection. Coming across such strong disagreements sometimes lead to subjectivism and scepticism about ethics. The first of these refers to the idea that ethical positions are a little bit like matters of taste, entirely subjective and therefore only subject to personal, inner scrutiny. The second holds that because no consensus can be reached, ethical discussion is ultimately pointless and we will always have to agree to disagree. However, this assumption is misplaced. Drawing on the previous example, consider the following:

> Eamon and Tashira are instead discussing an event in the news involving the incarceration of migrant children at the US border with Mexico. Eamon strongly believes that the incarceration of migrant children is always wrong. Tashira's position is that such measures can sometimes be justified.

Unlike Sasha and Mae in our earlier example, it is important to note here that Eamon and Tashira are not in disagreement about facts: it is not the definition of incarceration that they disagree on, nor do they disagree about the factual circumstances, why they are detained, or what conditions they are detained in. What they disagree about is whether such an act can ever be morally justified. In this case, should they swiftly agree to disagree in the same way as they did for kale and consider this just a matter of preference? A more accurate explanation of what is going on here is that each of them thinks that they are right. They consider their own moral position is the correct one and that the other person is wrong.

At the very least, we might think that there are good reasons for arguing that the incarceration of migrant children is morally wrong, and that a reasonable person should be able to recognise and accept those reasons. Eamon might ask Tashira to justify their position and then use their reasons to challenge this position, in a manner that is fundamentally different from debating the culinary merits of kale. It is not just that the fate of migrant children is far more important than whether people like or dislike kale. The reasons or grounds given to justify one's position and to change the other person's mind will be of a very different nature. In giving his reasons, Eamon might of course use empirical facts. Eamon might show Tashira the conditions under which children are detained and they might in turn say: 'Yes, I agree, the conditions are terrible and children should never be detained under those conditions. However, there might be better conditions under which migrant children can justifiably be detained.' In other words, Eamon and Tashira might still have a moral disagreement about whether it is *ever* right to detain migrant children.[14]

Ethics is less subjective than it might initially appear. While we might disagree, there may in fact be a right or wrong position, unlike questions of pure taste or preference. Similarly, scepticism about ethics is based on a false assumption: that because it is often difficult to achieve consensus about difficult moral problems, there is no point in reasoning and arguing about them. The fact that sometimes we cannot reach an agreement does not mean that there are no good or bad ways of thinking about and discussing ethical issues. The point of engaging in reasoning is to find the proper justification and the correct standards, in addition to providing coherent reasons for holding certain positions or values. Many ethical questions are particularly compelling and worthy of debate because they do not have an obvious solution. What we need to do is equip ourselves with the ability to recognise and use reasons and reasoning so as to build clear and consistent arguments for holding a particular ethical position.

1.3.5 RELATIVISM

The existence of different value systems and disagreements about 'the right thing to do', or 'the right way to behave', both between and within different social contexts, might—at first sight—be taken to indicate that ethical values and principles do not apply universally. It is indeed the case that different values and moral outlooks coexist in many contemporary societies and that some of these might conflict. This coexistence is commonly referred to as 'value pluralism' and it presents particular challenges for policymakers when it comes to developing laws and guidance around issues that raise different ethical concerns for different sections of the population—around end of life decision-making or reproductive care, for example.[15] One particular theoretical position—one that focuses on the nature of moral claims and judgements and what makes these true—goes much further than acknowledging the undeniable fact of the existence of value pluralism and divergence between moral norms in different social contexts. This position, known as moral relativism, makes the much stronger conceptual claim that there simply are no universal or objective truths in ethics.[16] Instead, morality simply consists in the codes

---

[14] For a similar treatment on the difference between ethical opinion and matters of taste see ibid pp 17–18.

[15] For more on pluralism, see for example Elinor Mason, 'Value Pluralism' (Stanford Encyclopedia of Philosophy 2018) available at <https://plato.stanford.edu/entries/value-pluralism/> accessed 08 December 2022; and Leigh Turner, 'Bioethics in Pluralistic Societies' (2004) 7(2) Medicine, Health Care and Philosophy 201.

[16] Chris Gowans, 'Moral Relativism' (Stanford Encyclopedia of Philosophy, 2021) available at <https://plato.stanford.edu/entries/moral-relativism/> accessed 08 December 2022; Neil Levy, *Moral Relativism* (Simon & Schuster 2001).

and norms that exist among communities and peoples in specific historical and cultural contexts. To say that something is morally right simply means 'believed to be right in this context'. Therefore, the truth and defensibility of ethical positions can only be judged relative to the norms of the context concerned.

Adopting a relativist approach might initially appear attractive and appropriate. After all, who are we to judge other people's values, especially ones that appear to be strongly entrenched within family, community, or social contexts? A progressive moral attitude might suggest 'to each their own'. However, there are two reasons to question the underlying claims of relativism (as contrasted with respect for pluralism). Firstly, the starting point for moral relativism may seem to overstate the nature and depth of disagreement. Of course, some of our morality and many of the ethical positions we hold are initially derived from the standards and norms we learn at a young age from the contexts in which we grow up. But this does not mean that there are no shared roots and common ground between these contexts. Consider for example, the universal prohibition against murdering innocent people without justification, the universal value of truth-telling, promise-keeping, or the idea that parents may have certain special moral responsibilities in relation to their children. Some values or norms can be correctly characterised as being shared across context and time. Additionally, what may at first appear to be very different values might in fact be different expressions or interpretations of similar values. We may observe different practices around child-rearing, caring for the elderly or respect for the dead across societies, but we will also usually observe a common core thread across such practices, that of care and respect, rather than negligence and indifference, for example.

Secondly, according to a strongly relativist position, any attempt to assess or critique different values and different moral codes is not only problematic, because it could appear arrogant or intolerant, it is also fundamentally incoherent to do so. The strength of this position gives rise to several critical and practical challenges. It means that someone who adheres to moral relativism cannot claim that the moral norms of their own social context are superior to those of detractors. Furthermore, the relativist does not have the means to critique moral positions—whether those of their own society or those of other societies—because they can appeal neither to their own local moral standards nor to an independent moral framework in order to do so. Relativism holds that to do the former would be inappropriate, and the latter framework simply does not exist. A relativist would, therefore, have to accept, for example, that enslaving people was actually morally acceptable in times and cultures when it was widely morally condoned, even when judged from a perspective that recognises the horrors and profound moral wrongs of slavery. Relativism removes the means to say that those fighting for emancipation had better moral principles than those engaging in enslavement. Strong moral relativism removes the tools and space both for dissent within a social contexts and debates between contexts, because a relativist must accept that every moral position is right provided it accords with widespread and dominant social norms.

Rejecting relativism and the idea that the truth and reasonableness of moral beliefs can only ever be judged relative to 'local' norms does not mean that there cannot be disagreement about values and ideas. While there may strong grounds to think that showing respect for other people is universally a good thing, there may well be variations across contexts regarding what kinds of behaviours are considered respectful, for example. That is the very nature of accepting that different world views and values can coexist, and we generally believe that it is right to hold on to diverse worldviews and societies. Additionally, refuting moral relativism does not mean that we should not be attentive to how values, concepts, and ideas are mediated by social, political, and other contexts, or the ways in which historical events such as colonialism and imperialism have shaped what might at first glance appear to apply to all moral and social contexts.

1.4 WHAT IS BIOETHICS?

As mentioned in the previous sections, bioethics is a sub-discipline of ethics. Specifically, it is an applied sub-discipline. It applies ethical concepts, theories, and methods of reasoning to practical questions and dilemmas.[17] The practical matters with which bioethics is concerned are those relating to health, medicine, health care, health research, public health, and the biomedical sciences, including biotechnologies. Bioethics itself can also itself be divided into further specialised branches that correspond to these fields. Some of these overlap but might have a slightly different focus; some might have core ethical concerns that are different and therefore pull our moral attention and ethical deliberations in different directions. Each of these areas also speak to governance differently, given rise to their own dedicated policies, guidelines, and regulatory mechanisms. This section provides an overview of these various branches.

1.4.1 MEDICAL ETHICS

Medical ethics usually refers to ethical concerns that arise within (although not exclusively from) the clinical encounter, of which Maryam's case which was highlighted at the beginning would be an example. Similarly, medical ethics deals with concerns related to patient interest and autonomy, the ethical foundations of confidentiality and negligence, questions related to the harms and benefits for patients, ethical obligations of health professionals towards their patients, patients' relatives, the medical institutions, and each other, as well as the responsibilities of hospitals, for example.

Some questions we might ask in relation to medical ethics include:

- To what extent should patient autonomy be respected?
- What kind of reproductive technology should be made available to patients?
- What are the limits of parental autonomy when it comes to the treatment of children?
- Should individuals be allowed to sell their organs?
- How should we address abuses of power, racism, sexism, or ableism in the medical context?
- Should conscientious objection to providing some kinds of care be permissible?
- How should we respect the interests and rights of patients with dementia?
- Which types of medical interventions can be described as treatment, and which are enhancement, and what are the moral implications of such labelling?
- Do physicians have a moral responsibility to disclose relevant genetic information or sexual health status to relatives of patients under any circumstance?

---

[17] According to some views the relationship between theory and practical challenges works in both directions. That is, our ethical thinking about specific practical challenges may also inform and reshape our theoretical frameworks. For further discussion, see John Arras, *Methods in Bioethics: The Way We Reason Now* (OUP 2017).

- What are the ethical issues arising in the care of children versus adults, or of people who do not have capacity?
- How do we best allocate ventilators in contexts of public health emergencies?

1.4.2 HEALTH CARE AND HEALTH ETHICS

In some contexts, the phrases 'healthcare ethics' and 'ethics in health care' are considered more or less synonymous with medical ethics. In other contexts, healthcare ethics suggests a focus on those moral issues that arise beyond the clinical encounter. These might be related to the allocation of scarce resources, such as ventilators, organs, or hospital beds. Broader questions around healthcare coverage, such as universal health care, insurance-based systems, or payment-based care, might all also be addressed in the context of healthcare ethics. Another term in use, 'health ethics', often aims at addressing questions that reach beyond access and distribution of health care, or are particularly informed by considerations beyond medicine, such as the social determinants of health.

Questions we might ask in this context include:

- Should we establish an opt-out system in order to increase the availability of organs?
- Should undocumented migrants have access to the same level of health care as citizens?
- How do we address health inequalities in a fair manner?
- How can we ensure better health for everyone knowing what we know about social determinants of health?
- How can different kinds of institutions (health, education, housing, employment) work together so that people can live healthier and more flourishing lives?
- How does systematic racism or sexism affect the ways in which people can access health and health care and how can policies and practice be improved to address discrimination and oppression in the context of health?
- What do we owe to more vulnerable members of society when it comes to health?

1.4.3 PUBLIC HEALTH ETHICS

Public health ethics is the study of ethical issues arising from the policies and practices related to public health, that is, the promotion and protection of health of populations. An important characteristic of public health ethics is that there is a shift in emphasis away from the individual patient or citizen at the core of our moral consideration to greater attention to collective action, interests, and benefit. Ethical issues in public health could be said to arise in the following areas. The first relates to the tension arising between individual liberty and the legitimate coercive measures that the state might implement in order to improve the health of the population, for example through policies related to water or air safety. The second relates to tensions and responsibilities arising from the fact that collective action in public health requires contributions. This could include the potential sacrifice on the part of individuals in order to achieve collective benefit, such as mask-wearing in the context of infectious diseases. A third important area of public health arises from inequalities and considerations of social justice. The health of populations depends not only on health care but also on social determinants of health—including gender, education, disability, and income—as well as commercial and political determinants of health. In other words, public health is concerned with not only people's encounter with the healthcare or public health system but how social processes, structures and institutions beyond those directly associated with health affect the well-being of a population. These give rise to various types of ethical concerns and considerations of moral obligations on the part of individuals, collectives, and institutions. We return to the importance of social (and other) determinants of health in Chapter 2.

Public health ethics questions might include:

- Is the state ethically justified in implementing sugar taxes and limits on salt or calorie intake?
- To what extent are nudges justified as tools of public health?
- What is the role of solidarity in collective public health action?
- What are our ethical obligations beyond borders when it comes to pandemics?
- What are ethical obligations of health professionals and public health actors as opposed to health care actors?
- Which social inequalities must be addressed in order to also achieve the aims of public health?
- What type of coercive measures can the state implement when it comes to controlling an epidemic?
- Should vaccines be compulsory?
- How might we justify a ban on smoking in public?

1.4.4 RESEARCH ETHICS

Bioethics has evolved as much as a response to ethical issues arising from research with human participants as it has from concerns in medical ethics. Research ethics (in this context research ethics mostly refers to biomedical research) has a long history, often developing in response to historical abuses and exploitation of vulnerable individuals and populations such as prisoners of war, children and adults living institutions, and minoritised populations, and giving rise to ethical guidelines such as the Declaration of Helsinki,[18] the Belmont Report,[19] and the CIOMS guidelines,[20] and procedural ethics such as institutional ethics approval and ethics review committees.

Research ethics now covers a wide range of endeavours, some of which bear little resemblance to clinical research with human participants. Although there remains a focus in the literature on clinical research, covering issues such as participant consent and voluntariness,

---

[18] World Medical Association, Declaration of Helsinki—Ethical Principles for Medical Research Involving Human Subjects, as at 6 September 2022 <https://www.wma.net/policies-post/wma-declaration-of-helsinki-ethical-principles-for-medical-research-involving-human-subjects/#:~:text=The%20World%20Medical%20Association%20(WMA,identifiable%20human%20material%20and%20data> accessed 29 March 2023.

[19] HHS.gov, Office for Human Research Protections, The Belmont Report: Ethical Principles and Guidelines for the Protection of Human Subjects of Research <https://www.hhs.gov/ohrp/regulations-and-policy/belmont-report/index.html> accessed 29 March 2023.

[20] Council for International Organizations of Medical Sciences (CIOMS), International Ethical Guidelines for Health-related Research Involving Humans (Geneva, 2016) <https://cioms.ch/publications/> accessed 29 March 2023.

risk-benefit consideration, and fair participant selection, this is changing. Similar to public health ethics, there is a growing shift away from the individual to broader considerations of burdens and benefits, for example in populations or across countries. There is a further important shift in that the aim of research is to produce generalisable knowledge, as well as new drugs, devices, or interventions that will benefit future patients, not current participants. In other words, there is an inherent ethical tension between protecting the interests of the participants and supporting the social value of research.

In research ethics, we ask questions such as:

- What counts as valid consent for participation?
- What is an acceptable risk-benefit ratio for clinical trials?
- Is it exploitative to offshore clinical research to low-income contexts?
- Should pregnant women be included as research participants as a matter of justice?
- What counts as responsible and ethical innovation?
- Should patients be able to access experimental and unapproved treatments as a last recourse for conditions that are otherwise untreatable?

1.4.5 ADDITIONAL AND EMERGING AREAS IN BIOETHICS

Other areas of bioethics have their own labels such as neuroethics, genethics, data ethics, and AI ethics, which often link into the emergence of new technologies in health and medicine. For this reason, the prominence of such sub-disciplines may rise and recede alongside views about the novelty and exceptional features of the technology. These sub-disciplines often share longstanding bioethical concerns. However, some fields of innovation and research may introduce a new focus or relevantly new moral concerns. Examples include the ways in which machine learning algorithms have shown to reproduce existing social biases that require renewed attention or novel ethical approaches. Such areas also bring into focus actors and sectors, for example, technology industries, engineers, and social media, whose actions affect health but would have otherwise not been considered part of the health landscape.

Questions in this area might include:

- How should we update our thinking about research ethics to take account of research that does not directly involve human participants, but does make use of large quantities of data about their lives, health, and behaviours?
- Is attention to individual consent adequate to address ethical issues arising from the inherently shared nature of genetic information?
- How should we address the risk that algorithms used in health AI build-in and exacerbate social biases such as racism, ableism, and sexism?
- How should we understand the boundaries human agency and integrity of the body as the use of networked assistive devices become increasingly common in health care?

In the remainder of this textbook when we talk about 'bioethics', we will predominantly be concerned with features of the wider applied discipline that captures all of the specialised branches. When our aim is instead to highlight the distinctive features of one of these branches, or to emphasise that the ideas and methods discussed owe their source to the broader parent discipline of ethics, we will make this clear.

1.4.6 PROCEDURAL ETHICS

Before leaving the topic of the branches of bioethics, it is useful to draw attention here to an important distinction between bioethics as a discipline and a way of understanding and defining questions of value, on one hand, and what might be referred to as 'procedural ethics', on the other. The latter, which we might also think of as 'ethical review', refers to the formal guidelines and approval processes that are used to make sure that health research (and other kinds of scientific and social science studies) is conducted in responsible ways and contribute useful knowledge, without posing disproportionate risks to anyone involved. The principles applied in procedural ethics will, ideally, be richly informed by the bioethical analysis, particularly that of research ethics. However, they will usually be more narrowly prescriptive and process-focused. Procedural ethics is not chiefly concerned with debating, for example, the meaning of confidentiality or the reasons for valuing and respecting it. Rather, its function is to ensure that, where confidentiality has been raised as a priority, likely risks to confidentiality are identified, weighed against other considerations, and appropriately averted or mitigated. Procedural ethics is also concerned to see that research studies comply with relevant laws, such as data protection regimes, some elements of which may be driven by procedural or pragmatic considerations, rather than ethical ones. Procedural ethics, therefore, should be seen as a route by which some kinds of bioethical thinking are operationalised, but not strictly as a branch of bioethics itself.[21]

1.5 HOW TO DO BIOETHICS

This section provides an introduction to some of the basic tools for conducting bioethical analysis—for thinking about bioethical problems, and for developing and justifying our responses to these problems. It starts by reviewing some of the language we can use when thinking or writing about bioethics and making the kinds of normative—evaluative or prescriptive—judgements that are inherent to this discipline, and it highlights the importance of conceptual clarity. It then turns to the important task of providing reasons to justify our normative judgements, by explaining why reason giving is necessary, and examining what forms these reasons could take. In doing so it looks at the roles, and the limitations, of intuition, evidence, and established principles as sources of supporting reasons. The ideas of interests and rights are also introduced as possible tools of ethical reasoning. The section closes by offering a brief overview of some key features of a sound and well-reasoned bioethical argument.

1.5.1 THE LANGUAGE OF BIOETHICS: TALKING ABOUT RIGHT AND WRONG

Let us turn first to the language of bioethics and how we talk about what is at stake when we want to think, debate, and write about bioethics. As introduced at the start of this chapter, ethics—which includes bioethics—is concerned with making assessments about what is good and bad, right and wrong. These judgements are

---

[21] For further discussion see Edward Dove, 'Research Ethics Review' in Graeme Laurie et al. (eds.), *The Cambridge Handbook of Health Research Regulation* (CUP, 2021); Matthew Hunt and Beatrice Godard, 'Beyond Procedural Ethics: Foregrounding Questions of Justice in Global Health Research Ethics Training for Students' (2013) 8(6) Global Public Health 713.

often called for when there are difficult choices to be made. These might be choices between conflicting values or priorities, or when any outcome involves both risks and benefits. Health and medicine provide us with myriad examples of just these kinds of dilemmas. For example, providing one person with potentially lifesaving health information may breach someone else's confidentiality; or participants in a clinical trial might be exposed to non-trivial health risks as part of developing a vaccine that could benefit whole populations. In such circumstances, the best course of action may be one that still causes considerable harm or distress. When this is the case, the blunt language of good and bad may feel uncomfortable. We might instead think of these as cases in which the 'least bad' available option has been taken. In these circumstances we can still say, however, that the chosen course was the right one under the circumstances.

Sometimes the binary language of right and wrong is appropriate. However, we may want to introduce some further nuance to our ethical judgements and recommendations. One established, yet simplified, way of segmenting the ethical character of actions or states of affairs involves dividing them so that they are classified as being either forbidden, required, permissible, or supererogatory.[22] Most of these terms are familiar from everyday usage. One possible exception is 'supererogatory', which simply means going beyond what is required. We can also talk of actions (and other things such as choices or policies) as being justified, meaning that there are sufficiently strong, ethically relevant reasons to support taking them. Focusing more specifically on the moral character of the consequences of choices made, we can talk about actions, practices, and structures as being harmful or beneficial. Another set of terms relates to ideas of agency and accountability. For example, an action may be described as being blameworthy or praiseworthy, and a person may be identified as feeling regret or shame. The applicability of each of these concepts depends not only on the nature of what was done but also on the background of moral expectations, and on the role and responsibility of the person acting.

There is also a much wider range of terms that we may wish to use that capture our ethical assessments of a situation in yet more descriptively rich ways. For example, people, motives, and behaviours can be thought of as generous, disrespectful, or caring. And practices, processes, and institutions might be described as trustworthy, empowering, unjust, or oppressive. These represent just a tiny sample of possible moral descriptors and how they might be deployed. The connections between these evaluative terms and concepts, and those listed in the previous paragraphs, are complex and disputed. There is not the space to explore these complexities here. It is nevertheless useful to observe the variety of language we can use when engaging in bioethical reasoning and to reflect on what our choice of terminology might imply about the individual or societal impacts of the activity or situation under discussion, and the kinds of responses—again, individual or societal—that might be called for.

1.5.2 CONCEPTUAL CLARITY

Bioethics shares several features with its roots in philosophical scholarship. One of these is the importance it places on conceptual clarity—that is, in making explicit what we mean by the central concepts and terms on which our claims and arguments depend. In this section we will demonstrate why this clarity is so important by considering the use

---

[22] Roderick Chisholm, 'The Ethics of Requirement' (1964) 1(2) American Philosophical Quarterly 147.

of concepts that have in-built normative implications. However, the value of clarity is not limited to normative concepts such as those discussed here.

Bioethical claims and arguments are expressed not only in the kinds of overtly evaluative language such a 'right' and 'wrong' but also using a wide range of terms and concepts that incorporate value judgements in less explicit ways. These include, to give just a few examples, concepts such as fairness, autonomy, vulnerability, enhancement, dignity, commodification, and exploitation. We will return to explore many of these in Chapter 2. In reading this list of terms we can notice that some of these seem, almost by definition, to refer to something good or desirable—for example, we might include fairness amongst these. Other concepts, however, seem to refer to something bad, which should be remedied—such as distress. Yet others might be more ambiguous—for example, is enhancement always a good thing and is commodification always bad? Even where the value implied by a concept seems relatively clear—as with fairness—we might still not be sure what the person using this word thinks fairness looks like. We probably also want to hear more about *why* they think this kind of fairness is a good thing.

For the reasons just given, conceptual clarity is a key part of developing and expressing bioethical judgements. Two key questions to ask as part of achieving conceptual clarity are: what role is the concept playing in my current line of reasoning? And have I done enough to allow it to fulfil this role? In the current example, this could involve being clear what you mean by fairness in the current context, perhaps disambiguating it from competing interpretations of fairness and other related ideas such as equality, and explaining any evaluative or prescriptive weight you intend our use of 'fairness' to carry. It is rarely enough to allow the implicit normativity of a term do all the heavy-lifting of an ethical argument on its own. For example, if we were simply to say, 'commercial surrogacy is wrong because it is a form of exploitation', this alone is not yet a complete argument. Before we can justify a claim that commercial surrogacy is wrong on these specific grounds, we have to undertake the following steps:

- define exploitation (which itself may be subject to disagreement);
- argue and explain why exploitation under this definition is ethically problematic;
- show that commercial surrogacy is a form of exploitation in the way we have just defined this concept; and finally
- show that it is indeed this connection between the operative concept (exploitation) and commercial surrogacy, rather than some other reason, that explains (at least in part) why commercial surrogacy is ethically problematic.

As noted at the start of this section, the importance of conceptual clarity is not limited to use of concepts with normative implications. It is equally important that we are explicit and consistent about what we mean when we talk about, for example, 'the public', 'genetic engineering', 'health research', or 'identity'. This does not mean that we have to exhaustively define every term we use, but we do need to unpack those where the particular interpretation adopted makes a difference to the meaning, basis, and scope of our ethical claims, particularly where ambiguity or disagreements about interpretations are likely.

It is all very well identifying the appropriate language and concepts with which to express ethical judgements, but how do we go about making and defending these judgements? We start to address this question over the following sections, before returning in Chapter 2 to explore in greater depth the challenges and choices involved in identifying the who and what demands our attention when it comes to surveying the landscape and deciding what has ethical significance.

1.5.3 PROVIDING REASONS TO JUSTIFY ONE'S POSITION

Making a bioethical judgement, deciding whether something is right, wrong, or any of the subtle variants on these listed previously, requires us to provide reasons—relevant, plausible, and persuasive reasons—to justify our eventual judgement. It is natural in everyday language to talk about having 'an ethical belief' or a 'moral point of view'. However, as we saw earlier in this chapter, there are important differences between ethical judgements and mere matters of opinion. There are also important differences between ethical positions and more widespread and established norms like socially pervasive beliefs and widely adopted practices.

Two key features distinguish bioethical arguments from opinions and social conventions. First, when we disagree on bioethical matters, it makes sense to debate with or to try to persuade others who hold markedly different views from our own. This holds even if, in practice, reticence or politeness might mean that we do not feel comfortable arguing or persuading. The key point here, though, is that, even if it might feel uncomfortable, it would not be illogical or misplaced to do so. Indeed, the normativity at the heart of bioethical judgements—that they concern situations in which something of value is at stake and where something may need to be done to protect what is valuable—indicates exactly why persuasion makes sense. Moreover, in many areas of professional practice and scholarship, defending an ethical position by providing a supporting argument, is precisely what we are tasked with doing. When we talk of 'an argument' in bioethics, we are not referring to an ill-tempered quarrel. This expression simply means presenting and justifying one's considered position, while also countering alternative positions. This brings us to the second feature that distinguishes bioethical judgements from opinion and conventions: making an ethical judgement requires defending one's own position by providing reasons for it. It also involves reflecting upon and explaining why one does or does not support the, perhaps markedly different, reasons provided by others for their positions.

Bioethics is often characterised by dilemmas and hard choices. It may be extremely difficult to reach a judgement about what should be done when faced by a tragic dilemma—for example about when to cease life-sustaining care for a critically and minimally conscious patient. And our response to such a dilemma might differ from someone else's. This does not mean, however, that there are no better or worse ways of thinking about and discussing the ethical issues involved. The requirement to provide reasons in support of our ethical positions explains why we can talk of ethical arguments as being better or worse.[23] Their merits depend on the relevance, clarity, and consistency of the supporting reasons, their sensitivity to context and the detail and diversity of people's experience, and their ability to take into account and respond to challenges and alternative perspectives. In short, when we make an ethical judgement, we need to explain not only *what* should be done but also *why*.

The kinds of reasons involved in ethical discussion and deliberation always involve value judgements, even if they also frequently include descriptive and empirical (factual) claims. Providing robust ethical reasons requires identifying what kinds of valuable things are at stake in the given circumstances and characterising why we should be concerned about them. This means describing, for example, why the situation involves states of affairs, activities, attitudes, relationships, or outcomes

---

[23] James Rachels and Stuart Rachels, *The Elements of Moral Philosophy* (9th edn, McGraw Hill-Education 2022).

that are beneficial or harmful, virtuous or vicious, cause for celebration or dismay, or appropriate targets for praise or censure. How, though, do we go about working through what qualifies for any of these descriptions? Here we will make a start in addressing this question by looking at three candidates for potential ways of discerning 'what matters': our intuitions; observations of facts about the world; and popular and expert points of view. As we will see, while some of these, when handled with appropriate caution, can have useful roles to play, none of them simply offers an 'off-the-shelf' answer to what is morally valuable.

1.5.4 INTUITIONS AND REFLECTIVE EQUILIBRIUM

Even though ethical judgements are more than opinions or preferences, this does not mean that there is no place for emotions or intuitions in ethical thinking. Often, we recognise an ethical concern precisely because of our strong, intuitive reactions to it. Our initial feelings or emotional reactions can tell us that there might be an interesting or important moral issue at stake, and that we should explore this initial perspective further. However, intuitions—or what we might colloquially call 'our moral nose'—can also be problematic. Consider, for example, initial intuitions that might be racist, sexist, ableist, classist, xenophobic, or influenced by other biases and prejudices. Our intuitions might trigger our ethical or moral thinking, but they might also mislead us if we do not examine them further.

In order to achieve a considered ethical position, we need to practise the skills of critical thinking. Moral judgement is built on reasons, reasoning, and argumentation, and this requires subjecting our initial reactions to scrutiny from several angles. One way to test the usefulness and defensibility of our initial intuition in a certain case is to compare it with our reactions to other real or imagined circumstances that are similar in most respects while differing in some specific dimensions. For instance, to return to an earlier example, is my moral intuition about the detention of migrant children the same as my views about the detention of migrant adults, or about migrant children from a different part of the globe? If not, why not? More specifically, if my reactions differ, what seems to explain this difference: does this explanation hinge on a plausibly *morally relevant* distinction between the circumstances of these different categories of migrants? Or does it, perhaps, seem to rest on a trivial or arbitrary details, or reveal more about my own experiences and prejudices than about features inherent to the situation faced by migrant people living in detention. Intuitions that seem to hinge on arbitrary distinctions or personal preferences should, at very least, be treated with caution and subjected to further scrutiny.

Another way of testing the extent to which we can trust our intuitions—and a route by which we can subject them to further scrutiny—is to compare our reaction to a specific case with the broader principles by which we live and view the world. For example, how does my thinking about the treatment of child migrants live up to the principles of striving for a fair society and global order to which I profess to subscribe? Is there consistency between my specific judgement in this instance and my more established beliefs about what is right and good? And is there a way that I could achieve greater coherence between them?

Of course, it is possible that our more established beliefs and principles could themselves be askew. Perhaps we have adopted them without careful consideration, or maybe they are rather idealised and abstracted from the complex realities and diverse lived experiences. The details of particular cases, and of our own and others' reactions to these cases (provided we have checked that these reactions are not merely grounded in prejudice or arbitrary distinctions), can play a valuable role in bioethical reasoning precisely when they offer tools for checking and refining our broader, and potentially idealised, moral principles.

A key methodological approach in practical ethics, one that recognises the value of a two-way relationship between our value judgements about particular cases and more wider principles, is known as 'reflective equilibrium'.[24] This method seeks to arrive at well-reasoned and defensible assessments of practical ethical dilemmas and questions by moving systematically between consideration of case-specific details on one hand and broader theoretical lenses on the other, allowing each to inform and refine the other. For example, returning to our example, reflecting on our feelings about what is distressing and wrong about instances in which child and adult migrants have been detained, might prompt us to reconsider the decisive role that we had previously assigned to the idea of 'innocence' in determining when some kinds of deprivation of liberty are morally justified. We might instead come to think that the presence of various kinds of vulnerability are more meaningful and relevant considerations. A key aim of reflective equilibrium is to arrive at a picture of what ethical concerns and priorities are present and demand our attention in a given practical situation.

1.5.5 FACTS ABOUT THE WORLD

Let us turn now, then, to a second possible source of value claims on which to base our ethical arguments: empirical facts and observations. It is tempting to think that if we just knew enough of the appropriate kind of facts about the world, we could find out what is ethically required of us. Moral philosophers disagree about whether moral claims can be true, and can be proved to be true, in exactly the same way that scientific claims can be.[25] However, what is clear is that we cannot simply conduct empirical research to uncover the correct ethical position in the same way as we might settle debates about the causes of global heating by interrogating data about climate, industrial expansion, and concentrations of atmospheric greenhouse gases. Furthermore, just because a state of affairs is commonplace, well-established, or 'natural', does not mean that it is necessarily good or right. Consider, the following example:

> Country C is a low-resource country that has experienced consistently high levels of child mortality from malaria for centuries. Does this duration make these deaths right? Does it provide ethical justification for failures by better resourced nations to address their causes? The answer to these questions seems plainly to be no. It would be very odd to make these claims solely on the basis that the levels of child mortality have persisted for many generations. Similarly, if an effective and safe new vaccine is developed that could prevent many of these deaths, would it be morally wrong to use this vaccine just because it is the product of novel genetic engineering techniques, rather than naturally occurring? Again, the answer seems clearly to be no. The 'naturalness' of the intervention is irrelevant to the ethics of its use.

[24] John Arras, 'The Way We Reason Now: Reflective Equilibrium in Bioethics' in Bonnie Steinbock (ed.) *The Oxford Handbook of Bioethics* (OUP 2007); Norman Daniels, 'Wide Reflective Equilibrium and Theory Acceptance in Ethics' (1979) 76(5) The Journal of Philosophy 256.

[25] For further discussion see, Matthew Lutz and James Lenman, 'Moral Naturalism' (Stanford Encyclopedia of Philosophy 2018) available at <https://plato.stanford.edu/entries/naturalism-moral/> accessed 08 December 2022.

The misplaced assumption that what is natural is automatically good, and what is unnatural is bad, has been labelled the 'naturalistic fallacy'.[26] Indeed, a key underlying premise of this fallacy—that we can easily and cogently distinguish what is natural from what is unnatural—is itself contentious. Here we can consider, for example, the way that naturalness operates in one common topic of bioethical debate: the moral justifiability of so-called 'enhancement technologies', those that purport to boost user's cognitive, physical, or pro-social capabilities.[27] Before it is even possible to discuss whether such technologies are morally good or bad, we need to decide what constitutes enhancement. It is tempting to define enhancements in terms of interventions that raise users' capabilities beyond those that are 'natural' or 'normal'. However, this is far from an easy distinction to make. Not only is there a lack of consensus about what capacities or interventions are 'natural' and about where to draw the line between these and unnatural ones (do only those capacities bestowed by genetic inheritance count, or do they also include those attributable to parenting, nutrition, the social environment, or education and training?), but setting boundaries around what is considered normal or natural is itself ethically problematic. Labelling a people, and their capabilities and behaviours, as abnormal or unnatural can be discriminatory and stigmatising. Furthermore—recalling our earlier discussion about conceptual clarity—even if we were able to arrive at some kind of working conception of which interventions count as unnatural, we would still need to do further work to explain why their unnaturalness makes them morally impermissible.

1.5.6 POPULAR BELIEFS

Much as we cannot simply 'read off' what is morally right from the way the world happens to look and function, we cannot infer what is ethically right or wrong from conducting empirical observations to discern the prominence of a particular point of view in society, or among groups of 'experts'. Large numbers of people could, after all, have misplaced or questionable reasons for holding their views. And even if not obviously mistaken or problematic, these reasons might simply be different from those we ourselves find persuasive. Consider the following example:

> A respected research institution carries out a large study to gather the views of healthcare professionals who work in palliative care on a proposed change to the law to permit physician-assisted dying for terminally ill patients. The study draws on a large and representative sample of participants from this profession. The researchers find that the majority of participants are not supportive of such a legislative change. Does this mean, particularly given the medical expertise and professional experiences of the study participants, that changing the law would be unethical?

---

[26] George Edward Moore, *Principa Ethica* (CUP 1903); Nuffield Council on Bioethics, 'Ideas About Naturalness in Public and Political Debates About Science, Technology, and Medicine' (2015) available at <https://www.nuffieldbioethics.org/assets/pdfs/Naturalness-review-of-NCOB-reports.pdf> accessed 08 December 2022. For an example of a discussion of the concept of naturalness in the context of reproductive technologies, see Rosamund Scott, 'Women, Assisted Reproduction and the "Natural"' in Wendy Rogers et al. (eds.) *The Routledge Handbook of Feminist Bioethics* (Routledge 2022).

[27] For further discussion of enhancement, see Allen Buchanan, 'Human Nature and Enhancement' (2009) 23(3) Bioethics 141; Alberto Guibilini and Sagar Sanyal, 'The Ethics of Human Enhancement' (2015) 10(4) Philosophy Compass 233.

The findings from this study could be useful for many practical purposes. They might, for example, help legislators understand whether such a change in the law is likely to be well-received by those working in palliative care. However, the sheer fact that opposition to physician-assisted dying is widespread among the study's participants does not tell us whether or why it is actually morally justifiable. Knowing that particular ethical positions are prevalent among particular populations or professions, even when these groups are particularly close to the issue at hand, is no substitute for engagement with the underlying reasons.

To appreciate why this engagement is necessary, imagine that the researchers asked further follow-up questions of the same group of participants to learn their chief reasons for opposing physician-assisted dying. Suppose their findings reveal that one-quarter of participants explain that their primary reason is that they believe that hastening death is contrary to clinicians' professional duties; another quarter think that life is sacred and should never be intentionally taken; a further quarter are chiefly concerned that vulnerable patients will feel coerced into choosing assisted dying; while the final quarter do not trust the government to draft clear and workable legislation. This wide variety of explanations, each leading to what superficially looked like exactly the same ethical position on the defensibility of changing the law, indicates why it is necessary to identify and make plain our underlying reasons. It also indicates that not all possible reasons are equal. Some will strike us as being more compelling or well-founded than others. And some may not be ethical reasons at all, but rather practical ones—as in the reason given by the final quarter of participants. It may be necessary to seek more details, and to test how the various reasons stand up when we consider alternative perspectives or adjust the imagined circumstances, before we can assert with confidence that they provide sound justification.

1.5.7 EMPIRICAL BIOETHICS

None of what has been said so far means that empirical facts and findings have no place in bioethical reasoning. On the contrary, they can play a number of important roles. At the most basic level, we need to know that our inquiries address genuine ethical concerns, and whether debates that look as if they are about ethical matters are actually disagreements about matters of underlying fact. We can recall here the disagreement between Mae and Sasha introduced earlier in this chapter. Sasha's belief that legal protection of healthcare professionals' conscience-based exemptions from participating in abortion care is essential to the recruitment of sufficient numbers of dedicated and well-trained staff—itself an ethical priority—is her reason for supporting such exemptions. Therefore, finding out whether a lack of legal protection would indeed be a deterrent to recruitment is key to the relevance and persuasiveness of Sasha's position and to the clarity of her debate with Mae. Excessively speculative bioethical debates may be unproductive and detract attention from more pressing ethical concerns. An area in which speculative bioethics can be particularly problematic is in debates about emerging technologies. When debates are premised on unrealistic or premature expectations about the promises or threats of these technologies they may contribute to unwarranted hyperbole and hope, or mistrust of innovation.[28]

[28] For further discussion of speculative ethics see Eric Racine et al., 'The Value and Pitfalls of Speculation About Science and Technology in Bioethics: The Case of Cognitive Enhancement' (2014) 17(3) Medicine, Health Care and Philosophy 325.

Another illustration of the potential value of empirical findings is provided by the previous example of attitudes to physician-assisted dying. Engaging carefully with insights into palliative care professionals' reasons for opposing changes to the law could, for example, open our eyes to perspectives that we had not previously considered, or alert us to the ways that healthcare professionals' own well-being could be impacted by end-of-life care and decision-making.

A key reason to attend to empirical findings is that robust ethical analysis cannot proceed from purely abstract or theoretical foundations. It needs to be informed by, and responsive to, the real world if it is to be appropriately nuanced, relevant, and applicable. In recognition of this, there has been a move towards greater integration of the methods from the social sciences, including psychology, sociology, and anthropology, and greater use of empirical data in bioethics. Approaches that make marked use of these methods, and the resultant data, can be thought of as examples of 'empirical bioethics'.[29] However, *any* bioethical analysis, not only that falling under this label, will benefit from reflecting upon the lived realities of those implicated by the topic at hand. Empirical observations and personal testimonies can enrich our applied ethical arguments, helping to make them sensitive to the particularities of how people experience the world, where their priorities lie, and what their encounters with institutions and social structures are like. The value of these insights comes vividly to life when we think about the key importance of, for example, reflecting patients' experiences of care when assessing what makes for good healthcare services. Observation also brings into sharp focus the fact that 'patients' experiences'—or those of 'citizens', 'research participants', or 'the public'—are not homogeneous, thus highlighting the importance of listening and responding to insights from people with diverse lives, different experiences of embodiment, and intersectional identities.[30] We return to explore themes of embodiment and intersectionality in Chapter 2.

1.5.8 PRINCIPLES AND PRINCIPLISM

Thus far we have emphasised the necessity of justifying our bioethical judgements by providing reasons to support them. This involves identifying what valuable things are at stake and how these things might best be protected or enabled. We have looked at three possible routes to identifying where value lies—intuitions, facts, and widespread attitudes—and noted that these can often make useful contributions but must be approached with care and in a critical spirit. Being critical in this way, and resisting easy assumptions, are undeniably challenging intellectual and practical tasks. It is reasonable to wonder, therefore, whether there are any short-cuts or 'off-the-peg' frameworks that could help us get more swiftly to the heart of what is at stake.

One famous example of just such a device is the set of four priorities known collectively as the 'principles of biomedical ethics'.[31] The application of these principles as the chief means of bioethical decision-making, an approach known as 'principlism', was originally

[29] Pascal Borry, Paul Schotsmans, and Kris Dierickx, 'What is the Role of Empirical Research in Bioethical Reflection and Decision-Making? An Ethical Analysis' (2004) 7(1) Medicine, Health Care and Philosophy 41; Jonathan Ives, Michael Dunn, and Alan Cribb, *Empirical Bioethics: Theoretical and Practical Perspectives* (CUP 2016).

[30] Stacy Carter and Vikki Entwistle, 'Feminist Bioethics and Empirical Research' in Wendy Rogers et al. (eds.), *The Routledge Handbook of Feminist Bioethics* (Routledge, 2022).

[31] Tom Beauchamp and James Childress, *Principles of Biomedical Ethics* (8th edn, OUP 2019).

conceived in North America in the mid-twentieth century to provide a framework for guiding ethical medical research. The four principles of principlism are:

- Autonomy: this points to the importance of respecting self-determination.
- Beneficence: this requires promoting the well-being of others.
- Non-maleficence: this requires refraining from causing harm.
- Justice: at its simplest, this means securing equitable distribution of benefits.[32]

Proponents of principlism maintain that these four principles have the strengths of being universally endorsed, capturing core priority concerns, and providing simplified rules of thumb, which are especially useful for guiding the activities of busy healthcare professionals and medical researchers. Principlism remains influential in many practical contexts. For example, it is sometimes cited in research ethics guidance or taught as part of medical curricula. And this set of four principles does capture relevant concerns in many situations. However, whether principlism actually exhibits the strengths and simplicity claimed for it remains a matter of vigorous debate.[33] Several key questions remain largely unresolved. These include, what should be done when following one principle brings one into conflicts with another of the four? For example, when someone volunteers to participate in a research study that they know carries a high risk of significant harm to their health, should respect for their choice or the responsibility to protect them from harm take precedence? Furthermore, the meanings of each principle are open to multiple, competing interpretations, and principlism does not obviously get around the challenging task of deciding which of these to adopt. We will explore the divergent ways in which well-being, autonomy, and justice can be interpreted, each interpretation carrying different implications for what the principle in question would require of us, in the next chapter. The four principles have also been critiqued for being culturally imperialist, giving priority to values that are specific to and particularly valorised in Anglo-American contexts.

Most fundamentally, perhaps, there is no obvious reason why our ethical analyses should be limited to the application of these four, and only these four, principles. Consider the following example:

For some periods during the Covid-19 pandemic, people living in or visiting the United Kingdom were required to inform the National Health Service when they tested positive for the virus, via an app, online service, or telephone number. Those testing positive, and those they lived with, were also required to self-isolate and to notify close contacts. These measures were intended to serve public health goals in a number of ways, including facilitating contact tracing, tracking rates of infection in the population, and targeting health advice to reduce the spread of the virus. Depending on the laws and guidance in place at different points, this process involved at the very least some inconvenience for members of the population, with potentially more serious burdens, including restricted freedom of movement, harms to mental and physical health from isolation, lost earnings, missed education, and intrusions associated with contact tracing and official checks on adherence with isolation rules. Suppose we are asked whether imposing these kinds of burdens was ethically justified. Which values and concerns should we attend to in attempting to answer this question appropriately? What would we want to take into account and weigh up?

---

[32] We discuss the concepts of autonomy, well-being, and justice in greater detail in Chapter 2.

[33] Richard Huxtable, 'For and Against the Four Principles of Biomedical Ethics' (2013) 8 Clinical Ethics 39; Tuija Takala, 'What is Wrong with Global Bioethics? On the Limitations of the Four Principles Approach' (2001) 10 Cambridge Quarterly of Healthcare Ethics 72.

It is not obvious that the four principles of principlism provide the most suitable set of tools with which to address this question. Rather than adhering strictly to this limited framework, we might think that it is equally—or more—relevant to ask:

- What would solidarity require of us?
- How is privacy affected?
- Who is at risk of being stigmatised by adhering to these rules?
- Is our shared interest in protecting population health well-served?
- Are there risks associated with normalising state surveillance of populations?
- What measures would best preserve trust in public institutions?

Earning trust, protecting privacy, averting stigma, promoting public interests, managing relationships of power, and exercising solidarity are also ethical principles, no less so than the four proposed by principlism. And they themselves do not exhaust of the gallery of further ethical considerations that might demand our attention in these, or any other, circumstances.

As this example illustrates, treating the four principles as the only relevant ethical concerns in all circumstances, or those that deserve highest priority consideration, can seem both arbitrary and limiting. Doing bioethics is a reflective and critical undertaking. It should not, therefore, involve simply running through a standardised checklist, whether this is the four principles or any other default set. Instead, we need to make sure we identify what specific principles, concerns, and values are at stake in the circumstances at hand. This may seem like a daunting task for busy students and professionals who are not professional bioethicists. One pragmatic step we can take to make it more approachable is to examine, with a critical eye, what considerations existing debates, guidance, or policies have judged important and assess which of these, if any, we think are relevant and why. A further complementary approach is to consider whose *interests* are affected, for better or worse, by the given situation, how much weight ought to be given to these interests, and if they warrant attention, how might they best be protected. What, though, is meant by 'interests' in this context?

1.5.9 INTERESTS AND RIGHTS

The term 'interests' is commonly used in bioethical discussions, in a way that is perhaps unfamiliar. Interests here do not refer to hobbies or objects of study. In ethics, to say someone has an interest in something—a situation, an outcome, or a relationship, for example—is to say they have something at stake, something to lose or gain, depending on how that thing goes.[34] We benefit to the extent our interests are met, and harmed when they are not. As such, interests identify specific aspects or components of well-being.[35] For example, we may be said to have interests in remaining healthy, taking part in a clinical trial, spending time with those we love, having sufficient food and shelter, living in accordance with our plans and values, or experiencing good weather on our holiday. As this suggests, interests can be strong or weak, ephemeral or life-long, critical or trivial. More specific interests can serve more general, underlying ones. For example, someone's interest in being included in a clinical trial of a new drug could promote their

---

[34] See for example Richard Dworkin, *Life's Dominion: An Argument About Abortion, Euthanasia, and Individual Freedom* (Vintage 2011); John Feinberg, *Harm to Others: The Moral Limits of the Criminal Law Vol. 1* (OUP 1984).

[35] The concept of well-being is examined in more detail in Chapter 2.

more fundamental interest in being healthy. Our most basic or vital interests are those on which our survival depends. These might also be described as 'needs'.

As well as thinking of individuals as having interests, we can also think of groups, which have attributes or causes in common, as having shared group interests. For example, we might talk about families of children living with a rare genetic disease as having a shared interest in promoting research into the condition. At a wider scale yet, we can also talk about 'the public interest'. For example, a healthcare professional may justify breaching patient confidentiality where this is the only way to serve the public interest in averting the risk of the spread of a serious infectious disease and where this breach, in turn, does not significantly threaten a further public interest, that in being able to trust that healthcare professionals will generally respect confidentiality.[36]

One *legal* context in which interests are prominently discussed is when a patient lacks the capacity to make or communicate their own wishes about their care. In these circumstances, decisions can be made by others in line with their 'best interests'.[37] Interests, in this legal context, also refers to those things in which the patient has a stake, those that would make their life go better, and thus identifying them involves ethical deliberation. However, 'best interests' cases represent a relatively narrow application of the idea of interests. We all have interests throughout our lives, not only when decisions must be made about our care while we lack capacity.

Beyond attention to 'best interests', it may be more common in legal contexts to use the language of rights, rather than interests, when some aspect of well-being or liberty is at stake, for example the 'right to privacy', or the 'right to reproductive autonomy'. The relationship between rights and interests is a matter of debate. However, on many views, a plausible claim to have a right will be predicated on the existence of a corresponding interest or set of interests.[38] It only makes sense, for example, to talk of an ethical right to reproductive autonomy if we can point to the ways in which being constrained and coerced in our reproductive choices represent a threat to our interests in deciding the shape of our own families, in what happens to our bodies, and in living according to our values and chosen projects.[39] Simply labelling something an ethical right neither places it beyond question nor removes the need to provide justifying reasons. And just because something is plausibly an ethical right does not mean that it will automatically be recognised in law or protected by a legal instrument such as European Convention on Human Rights.

The phase 'human right' is itself ambiguous, frequently being used to refer both to broad normative claims about which freedoms and protections people are, morally, entitled to, *and* the specific provisions of human rights law. So, when referring to rights, it is important to be clear whether one is talking about ethical or legal entitlements, or both. Unless we are specifically referring to specific protections under human rights law, talking about interests rather than rights can often be more straightforward and illuminating. It allows us to unpack the harms and benefits at stake rather than just wielding talk

---

[36] See, for example, BMA, 'BMA Guidance: Confidentiality and Health Records Toolkit' (2021) available at <https://www.bma.org.uk/advice-and-support/ethics/confidentiality-and-health-records/confidentiality-and-health-records-toolkit> accessed 08 December 2022. For a discussion of the role of public interest in the context of health research, see for example, Angela Ballantyne and G. Owen Schaefer, 'Public Interest in Health Data Research: Laying Out the Conceptual Groundwork' (2020) 46(9) Journal of Medical Ethics 610.

[37] The topic of best interests is discussed in detail in Chapters 9 and 10.

[38] See, for example, Joseph Raz, *The Morality of Freedom* (Clarendon Press 1986).

[39] Emily Jackson, *Regulating Reproduction: Law, Technology and Autonomy* (Bloomsbury Publishing, 2001).

of rights as a trump card, or getting stuck invoking a set of apparently conflicting rights, without the language to discuss how they might be weighed or reconciled. Debates about disclosures of an individual's genetic test results to their family members, for example, are often framed in terms of conflicts between the various parties' respective rights: rights to confidentiality, to know, and to not know.[40] To have any hope of resolving conflicts between these rights we need to explore the nature and strength of the interests involved.

1.5.10 LIMITS OF RATIONALITY AND IMPARTIALITY

The preceding sections have reviewed the kinds of terminology we use when doing bio-ethics and some of the key features of well-grounded, persuasive bioethical argumenta-tion. The risks of relying on intuition, social norms, and widespread opinions have been noted. Meanwhile, the importance of critically examining our intuitions and initial reac-tions, attending to how the world works, and recognising the diversity of people's lived experiences has been emphasised, as has the importance of testing the consistency of our reasoning across a range of scenarios and assessing its strengths relative to alternative perspectives. The objective is to arrive at ethical judgements that would, as far as possible, apply equally to all relevantly similar cases, and to identify and rectify instances when our judgements depend on arbitrary distinctions or unwarranted assumptions. However, despite the emphasis on reason-giving as part of robust ethical analysis, we should always remember that none of us is perfectly rational, and we all have limited experiences, and our understandings of the world are filtered through the lenses of our particular social and embodied position. Our judgements are also subject to bias and prejudice. In doing bioethics we must be ready to listen to others, develop our thinking, and change our minds. Furthermore, we should acknowledge that even if ethical positions are more than mere opinions or social conventions, our assumptions and methods of reasoning are nev-ertheless shaped by who we are, our position our communities, and the social contexts we inhabit.

1.6 CONCLUSION

In this chapter we have introduced the discipline of bioethics, its aims, scope, and meth-ods. The discussion has been framed around three key questions: What is ethics? What is bioethics? And, how does one do bioethics? The chapter opened, however, by addressing the question of how law and ethics are related in the contexts of health and medicine and in the combined discipline of 'health law and ethics' with which this textbook is concerned. We then took a step back to look at the distinguishing features of ethics itself, the field in which the applied discipline of bioethics is located. We outlined how ethical questions can be distinguished from questions about matters of fact, personal preferences, and pre-vailing community norms, and explained why these distinctions are important. The core idea that ethics is concerned with normative—evaluative and prescriptive—questions was introduced. We then turned to look at the discipline of bioethics itself: introducing the kinds of questions and practical contexts with which it is concerned; the language in which these questions are couched; and the sub-disciplines—such as research and public health ethics—that have developed within it.

---

[40] See, for example, discussions in Ruth Chadwick, Mairi Levitt, and Darren Shickle, *The Right to Know and the Right Not to Know: Genetic Privacy and Responsibility* (2nd edn, CUP 2014).

This chapter is the first of two in this textbook whose aim is to begin to equip readers with the tools to actually do bioethics: to engage in critical analysis and reasoned argumentation in order to defend robust and plausible ethical positions on matters relating to health and medicine. This chapter has emphasised the crucial importance of reason-giving and conceptual clarity in these endeavours. It has interrogated some of the places we might initially be tempted to look for reasons to support our ethical arguments, including: observable facts about the world; our own intuitions; others' opinions; and prescribed checklists of principles. We have seen that, while each of these could provide useful starting points and material for critical reflection, it is rarely possible to draw inferences from these elements taken in isolation to defensible ethical conclusions. We have suggested that two illuminating and useful approaches to locating what of value is at stake in ethical dilemmas—and thus considering and explaining our responses to such dilemmas—can be to ask which specific principles might be engaged and whose interests are affected and in what ways.

The discussion up to this point has laid the foundations for identifying and describing the interests of those affected by ethical dilemmas. More detailed discussions of how we can start to think about *whose* interests demand our attention, and how to work out *what* these interests might be, follows in Chapter 2. In the coming chapter we will explore key ethical concepts such as well-being, autonomy, and justice. We will look at the role of moral theories in applied bioethical thinking. And we will highlight the central importance of doing bioethics in a way that prioritises addressing injustices and sources of oppression.

FURTHER READING

1. Stephen Darwall, *Philosophical Ethics* (Westview Press 1998).

2. Richard Edmund Ashcroft et al. (eds.), *Principles of Health Care Ethics* (2nd edn, Wiley 2007).

3. Helga Kuhse and Peter Singer (eds.), *A Companion to Bioethics* (2nd edn, Wiley 2009).

4. Udo Schüklenk and Peter Singer (eds.), *Bioethics: An Anthology* (4th edn, Wiley-Blackwell 2021).

5. Wendy Rogers et al. (eds.), *The Routledge Handbook of Feminist Bioethics* (Routledge 2022).

6. Bonnie Steinbock (ed.), *The Oxford Handbook of Bioethics* (OUP 2007).

7. Simon Blackburn (ed.), *Being Good: A Short Introduction to Ethics* (OUP 2002).

2

CRITICAL FRAMEWORKS
IN BIOETHICS

2.1 INTRODUCTION

In Chapter 1 we looked at the central importance to good bioethical reasoning of supplying well-grounded reasons for the moral judgements we make. We considered the potentially useful roles of intuition, empirical observations, and widespread attitudes as possible starting points for identifying these reasons, while highlighting why their usefulness might be limited and when invoking them might be problematic. We also discussed how identifying the principles and interests at stake in a particular situation can be a key step in explaining the reasons behind our ethical judgements. And we briefly introduced the idea that high-level moral theories and principles about what is right and wrong can provide counterpoints for reflecting on and refining our initial reactions to specific circumstances. In this chapter we pick up the threads of each these proposals. Here, we will dig a little deeper into the theories and critical frameworks that are widely used to characterise the concerns, interests, and principles at stake in ethical challenges arising in medicine and health-related contexts and that we can use to justify our responses to these challenges.

We start this chapter by asking two broad questions: What matters? And who matters? The first of these questions could, admittedly, be dauntingly broad, so here we focus specifically on key concepts that are commonly used to capture what is valuable in the lives of people affected by the kinds of dilemmas with which bioethics is concerned. The second question—who matters?—looks at how we identify *whose* needs and interests must be taken into account in any ethical analysis and indeed, who is capable of having interests at all. Thereafter, we turn to examine a suite of dominant high-level moral theories—that is, theories about what features of a situation determine whether it should be seen as morally right or wrong. We look at the claims of three different theories, before noting their limitations and suggesting when theories of this kind are useful to the practical task of doing applied bioethics and when they are not. The final section of the chapter addresses concerns with justice and inequalities and the central role that these play in any bioethical analysis that purports to respond to diverse lived experiences and to many of the most pressing challenges in health and health care. This section highlights the way that political philosophy is just as much part of the critical tools of bioethics as moral philosophy.

Bioethics is, as we noted in the previous chapter, an inherently critical discipline. In doing bioethics we are required to challenge easy assumptions and to interrogate the relevance and persuasiveness of reasons we, and other people, give for our ethical positions. The range of responses to the four questions surveyed in this chapter—What matters? Who matters? What defines right and wrong? And what does justice demand of us?—provide a range of frameworks that can be used in this critical endeavour. As we progress it will become apparent that multiple, and sometimes competing, responses have been offered to these four questions. This chapter does not prescribe which of these responses is correct. It is not possible to do this. In many cases, debates about their relative merits remain unresolved. The aim here, then, is to outline the reasons that have been offered for endorsing particular conceptions of value, moral status, and right and wrong, while also highlighting some of their attendant limitations. As scholars and practitioners engaged in the practical work of doing bioethics, the unresolved nature of these debates and the sense that there is no 'one right answer' can be frustrating. However, recognising the different perspectives from which it is possible to approach ethical questions helps to strengthen our own arguments—both by offering us a range of lenses through which to consider dilemmas, and by showing us what we need to do to sharpen and defend our reasons for the eventual position we take. It also teaches us humility, in recognising that even our most firmly held ethical conclusions may only ever be provisional in anticipation of fresh challenges and insights.

2.2 WHAT MATTERS?

An essential part of deciding what is the right thing to do involves identifying what kinds of important concerns are at stake in the circumstances in question. In order to do this, we need to be able to identify what is valuable and worthy of protection or promotion, and what kinds of harms and wrongs could occur and should be avoided. We should also be able to explain *why* any of these things matter and *how* they are relevant to the given situation. This section provides an introduction to some of the answers that have been offered in response to these kinds of questions. More specifically, it looks at what matters to us in our human lives. Here we will look at seven aspects of people's lives and experiences that, it is commonly suggested, tend to make things go significantly better or worse for them, and thus warrant our ethical attention. These are:

- well-being;
- health;
- autonomy;
- dignity;
- embodied experiences;
- vulnerability;
- relationships.

2.2.1 WELL-BEING

A key facet of 'what matters', ethically speaking, in any situation is how it affects the well-being of the people involved. In Chapter 1 we encountered the idea of 'interests' and the importance, when attempting to make moral judgements, of looking at how people's interests are, or would be, impacted. What is in someone's interests is usually understood to align with what would protect or promote their well-being.[1] But what does well-being entail? This may seem like an odd question. Surely, we all know what 'well-being' means? However, the following example illustrates how challenging it is to decide what actually contributes to or constitutes this valued state.

---

[1] Joel Feinberg, *Harm to Others: The Moral Limits of the Criminal Law Vol. 1* (OUP 1984).

Pablo is seriously ill with a movement disorder. He suffers from tremors and stiffness in his joints, which cause him pain and present difficulties for his mobility and dexterity. His care team must decide whether to try a new kind of neurological treatment using Deep Brain Stimulation (DBS). This treatment could alleviate Pablo's physical symptoms better than his existing drug regime, but it carries a risk of side-effects including marked cognitive, behavioural, and mood changes. These in turn could affect Pablo's priorities, decision-making abilities, and personal relationships.[2]

When it comes to assessing whether the proposed treatment would improve Pablo's well-being, there is a need to consider which of the following should be taken into account:

- minimising Pablo's pain;
- prolonging his life;
- improving his mood and emotions;
- improving his mobility;
- enabling Pablo to live independently;
- boosting his cognitive capacities;
- supporting his relationships with his family and friends; or
- respecting Pablo's choices.

This list is not intended to be exhaustive. As bioethicists, we also need to consider not only which of these factors are relevant to Pablo's well-being but also which apply in the given circumstances, and what weight should be afforded to each of those that does apply.

An extremely minimalist conception of what is good or bad for us might equate what is good for us simply with being alive, while taking death to be the greatest possible harm.[3] However, this narrow pair of options does not allow for the possibility that our lives can go better or worse, and that what matters to us is not simply being alive, but the *quality* of our lives. For example, imagine that Pablo's doctors expect DBS will have little impact on his life-expectancy, but result in marked impacts on several other factors in the list. It seems unlikely that we, or Pablo, would dismiss these other factors as irrelevant to the question of whether he would want to pursue this treatment and whether it would be best for him to do so.

In ethical discussions we can capture the idea of 'what would be best' for Pablo using the related (though not totally synonymous) concepts of well-being, quality of life, and flourishing. In some contexts, we might also encounter the term 'welfare' used in this way. Working out what well-being looks like, or what would make for a high quality of life, or a fulfilling existence, requires that we have some way of thinking about which opportunities, experiences, and activities really matter to us for their own sake, and what kinds of things would tend to make an individual's life better or worse. Various attempts

---

[2] For further discussion of ethical concerns about DBS, see Jonathan Pugh, 'Clarifying the Normative Significance of "Personality Changes" Following Deep Brain Stimulation' (2020) 26(3) Science and Engineering Ethics 1655.

[3] Jonathan Glover, *Causing Death and Saving Lives: The Moral Problems of Abortion, Infanticide, Suicide, Euthanasia, Capital Punishment, War and Other Life-or-Death Choices* (Penguin UK 1990).

have been made to answer these high-level questions.[4] We will briefly review in turn the following three prominent accounts:

- Hedonism, which takes well-being to be synonymous with happiness or pleasure, and the absence of suffering and pain.
- The idea that well-being lies in the satisfaction of one's individual preferences.
- The position that holds that there is an objective list of the kinds of experiences and pursuits that invariably contribute to human well-being.

As an interpretation of what well-being consists in, hedonism has intuitive appeal. What could be more important than being happy? And prioritising happiness, rather than specific causes of happiness, makes space for respecting the value of diverse ways of living, as what makes different people happy will vary. However, hedonism also attracts critique.[5] We might question whether it is really true that we only value happiness and value it for its own sake. Many pursuits that people value, such as challenging creative projects, are onerous or even painful. Imagine that DBS makes Pablo experience feelings of euphoria but also impairs his concentration and memory, making it harder for him to pursue his beloved side-project as a songwriter. Would we necessarily agree that the heightened euphoria improves his well-being? Would Pablo? We also might worry that hedonism positions the relationship between happiness and value the wrong way round, implying that an experience like songwriting is valuable only because and when it makes us happy, rather than happiness being the response to the inherent value of the creative process.

A second suggestion that attempts to avoid some of these objections is that well-being consists in the fulfilment of one's preferences or desires.[6] Unlike hedonism, this makes space for recognising the contribution of valued pursuits that are not necessarily accompanied by happiness. It also reflects widespread assumptions about the importance of a fulfilling life of being able to follow one's desires and choices. However, this interpretation also faces challenges. These include doubts that all preferences contribute equally to well-being, and difficulties in distinguishing those that do from those that do not. After all, most of us have at least some self- or other-harming or ill-considered preferences. And our short-term desires may fail to serve our longer-term goals. For example, we might question whether Pablo's well-being has necessarily been enhanced if, once his mobility and dexterity problems are relieved, he is able once again to indulge his passion for online gambling, a hobby which he then pursues at considerable financial expense and at the cost of time spent with family and friends.

A third conception moves away from a focus on the individual's subjective moods and desires, suggesting that well-being consists in particular experiences and pursuits that are inherently valuable. Conceptions such as this are often referred to as 'objective list'

---

[4] Dan Brock, 'Quality of Life Measured in Health Care and Medical Ethics' in Martha Nussbaum and Amartya Sen (eds.) *The Quality of Life* (Clarendon Press, 1993) 95–133; Roger Crisp, 'Well-Being' (The Stanford Encyclopedia of Philosophy Archive, 06 November 2001) available at <https://plato.stanford.edu/archives/win2021/entries/well-being/> accessed 19 December 2022; Guy Fletcher, *The Philosophy of Well-Being: An Introduction* (Routledge 2016).

[5] One widely discussed challenge to the idea that we value happiness for its own sake may be found in Nozick's 'experience machine' thought experiment in Robert Nozick, *Anarchy, State, and Utopia* (Basil Blackwell, 1974); see also Roger Crisp, 'Hedonism Reconsidered' (2006) 73(3) Philosophy and Phenomenological Research 619.

[6] Chris Heathwood, 'Desire-Fulfillment Theory' in Guy Fletcher (ed.) *The Routledge Handbook of the Philosophy of Well-Being* (Routledge 2016).

accounts.[7] The proposed contents of such lists vary from version to version. Some versions, such as 'capabilities approaches', focus on the most basic conditions for essential human existence. These include, for example, the capacities to enjoy good health and preserve one's physical integrity and self-respect, as well as opportunities for play and to pursue personal relationships.[8] Other versions might place particular emphasis on, for example, being able to exercise one's autonomy, engage in intellectual projects, or being creative. A key challenge faced by any objective list account, however, is justifying the chosen items on the list, particularly when these extend beyond the basic capabilities needed for survival. We may also question whether any criteria beyond these basics are really universal and objective, or whether they instead simply reflect the particular preferences and social contexts of those who espouse them.[9]

In practice we may not need to make an all-or-nothing choice between these three conceptions of well-being. It may be possible to combine elements and strengths of each.[10] However, in doing so it is important that we remain alert to the possible limitations of the various approaches and to possible tensions between them. It is also worth noting that certain conceptions provide the (more, or less, explicit) foundations for other ethical positions. For example, as we shall see later in this chapter, the idea that happiness is what matters most underpins the ethical theory of right and wrong known as utilitarianism.

2.2.2 HEALTH

It is unsurprising that the impact on people's health is a key facet of the features we need to attend to in ethical decision-making, particularly in bioethics. Illness is often a key factor in impaired well-being and quality of life. However, when we think about the relationship between health and well-being, we need not only to examine the nature of this relationship but also to be clear what we mean when we talk about 'health'. Again, this may seem like a surprising problem to introduce about a term we use every day without difficulty. However, defining 'health' is not necessarily simple and this is reflected in the differences in how various thinkers and disciplines have delineated what counts as health. It is difficult to label and distinguish between approaches in a systematic manner, but distinctions are often drawn between the following four approaches:

- medical;
- holistic;
- social;
- planetary.

We will briefly examine each in turn.

Medical models define health as the absence of disease and the possession of a high level of typical functioning. They often attract criticism for neglecting to pay sufficient attention to influences external to our own bodies that contribute to ill health and our experiences of illness—influences such as social and environmental factors.[11] This model

[7] Guy Fletcher, 'Objective List Theories' in Guy Fletcher (ed.) *The Routledge Handbook of the Philosophy of Well-Being* (Routledge 2016).
[8] Marta Nussbaum, 'Capabilities as Fundamental Entitlements: Sen and Social Justice' (2003) 9(2–3) Feminist Economics 33.
[9] Gwen Bradford, 'Problems for Perfectionism' (2016) 29(3) Utilitas 344.
[10] Thomas Hurka, 'On "Hybrid" Theories of Personal Good' (2019) 31(4) Utilitas 450; Derek Parfit, *Reasons and Persons* (OUP, 1984).
[11] Michael Marmot and Richard Wilkinson (eds.), *Social Determinants of Health* (OUP 2005).

also relies on the idea that there are objective standards of normality or typical function-ing against which ill health can be defined, and apparent presumptions that normality corresponds to what is best or good for us. As we saw in the discussion of the naturalistic fallacy in the previous chapter, these presumptions are problematic. We will return to some of these themes again shortly.

The holistic model of health adopted by the World Health Organization (WHO) defines health as 'a state of complete physical, mental and social well-being and not merely the absence of disease or infirmity'.[12] Models such as this represent attempts to move away from purely biomedical approaches. They also tend to make explicit the importance of mental as well as physical health. These kinds of models are influential, though are some-times criticised for being unhelpfully vague.[13]

Social models of health, meanwhile, emphasise a diverse range of influences, includ-ing environmental, societal, cultural, and political factors, which affect our physical and mental health. These models better reflect current understandings of the complex interactions between health, experiences of health, and structural features of our lived environments, and they are increasingly influential in bioethics and policymaking.[14] For example, social models of disability direct us to notice the extent to which disability is at least as, if not more, attributable to the built environment and to social structures and attitudes, than it is to differently functioning bodies.[15] Identifying what are often (more concisely) referred to as the 'social determinants of health' is especially important when it comes to addressing public health concerns, recognising the roots of health inequalities, and identifying institutions and structures beyond the clinic that are key to supporting health.[16] In particular, attending to the ways in which social determinants of health are unequally distributed across society, and the ways they may intersect with and compound other sources of oppression, is key to ensuring effective and ethical responses to health and healthcare challenges.

Planetary, ecosystem-based, or One Health models of health meanwhile, emphasise the inevitable interdependencies between human, non-human animal, and environmen-tal health, in ways that have often been integral to many Indigenous and non-Western perspectives, but have only recently been taken up by Eurocentric perspectives.[17] The importance of recognising the connections between the environment, humans and non-human animals is brought into particular focus by several contemporary global challenges, including zoonotic diseases (infectious diseases that move from animals to human populations) such as Covid-19, and antimicrobial resistance.

As discussed, one critique of so-called objective list accounts of well-being is that they might not actually be as universal and objective as they claim. These list-based accounts also risk being exclusionary to the extent that they emphasise the importance of some activities, while ignoring those valued by minoritised or marginalised groups. This is

[12] WHO, 'Constitution of the World Health Organization' (1948) p 1, available at <https://apps.who.int/gb/bd/PDF/bd47/EN/constitution-en.pdf?ua=1> accessed 12 December 2022.

[13] Rodolfo Saracci, 'The World Health Organisation Needs to Reconsider its Definition of Health' (1997) 314(7091) BMJ 1409.

[14] Marmot and Wilkinson (n 11).

[15] Colin Barnes, 'Understanding the Social Model of Disability: Past, Present and Future' in Nick Watson, Alan Roulstone, and Carol Thomas (eds.) Routledge Handbook of Disability Studies (2nd edn Routledge 2019) pp 14–31.

[16] Michael Marmot, 'Social Determinants of Health Inequalities' (2005) 365(9464) The Lancet 1099.

[17] Ronald Atlas, 'One Health: Its Origins and Future' (2013) 365 Current Topics in Microbiology and Immunology 1; John Mackenzie et al., One Health: The Human-Animal-Environment Interfaces in Emerging Infection Diseases (Springer 2013).

relevant to the present discussion of different conceptions of health, as some lists may exhibit ableist preconceptions (those that discriminate against people perceived to have disabilities and presume the superiority of more typical abilities) by affording disproportionate prominence to particular kinds of physical, social, or intellectual activities or to having children—pursuits that may not be valuable or accessible to all.[18]

A related concern, borne out by empirical research, is that non-disabled and neurotypical people can over-estimate the negative impacts on well-being and quality of life of living with a disability, mistakenly imagining the quality of life of people living with a disability to be much lower than it actually is. This is sometimes referred to as the 'disability paradox'.[19] The serious consequences of the underlying misconception may be evident in healthcare rationing policies that use unsuitable proxies for quality of life as grounds for allocating scarce healthcare resources. For example, guidelines released in the UK in the early months of the Covid-19 pandemic made a person's dependency on others for assistance with everyday activities a criterion for lower priority in allocation of critical care resources.[20] Policies such as those just mentioned are discriminatory and unjustifiably conflate particular kinds of support needs with impaired health and quality of life. The risks of serious injustices of this kind illustrate why it is so important that we critically interrogate the relationship between health and well-being.

It is clear that people can lead full and fulfilling lives while living with chronic disease or disability. And enjoying a high quality of life seems likely to consist in more than simply being healthy. Given this, it seems that health is important, but perhaps neither necessary nor sufficient for well-being. This suggests that it may make sense to view health as playing an instrumental role in a good life, albeit an important one. That is, it is ethically significant insofar as it enables the enjoyment of other valuable experiences and activities, rather than because it is a valuable goal in its own right. From a different perspective, however, it is interesting to note that the WHO's holistic definition inverts this relationship, presenting well-being as contributing to health, rather than the other way round. As the preceding paragraphs indicate, while the close connection between health and well-being seems intuitive, the precise nature and direction of the relationship between the two is more complex.[21]

2.2.3 AUTONOMY

The idea that it matters a great deal, perhaps above all else, that our desires and choices are respected and that we are in a position to act on them, is strikingly prominent in contemporary Anglo-American bioethical thinking.[22] These ideas are captured under the concept of 'autonomy'. Before exploring in greater depth what is required in order to be autonomous, it is worth asking why autonomy is widely seen as such an important aspect of 'what matters', rather than assuming that this is self-evident.

One answer is that, determining the course of one's life in line with one's own goals, and being true to one's own identity and values, are widely considered to be extremely

[18] Disability ethics is discussed further later in this chapter.
[19] Gary Albrecht and Patrick Devlieger, 'The Disability Paradox: High Quality of Life Against All Odds' (1999) 48(8) Social Science & Medicine 977.
[20] Jackie Leach Scully, 'Disability, Disablism, and COVID-19 Pandemic Triage' (2020) 17(4) Journal of Bioethical Inquiry 601.
[21] For further discussion of one influential perspective on the relationship between health and well-being, see Norman Daniels, *Just Health: Meeting Health Needs Fairly* (CUP 2007).
[22] Tom Beauchamp and James Childress, *Principles of Biomedical Ethics* (8th edn OUP 2019).

valuable.[23] Autonomy is also closely associated with related valued attributes such as freedom and authenticity. However, independence and self-determination are not universally valorised. Some ethical perspectives may give greater priority to other things such as interpersonal responsibilities, or collective well-being.[24] And even if we do recognise the value of autonomy, we can still ask (as we did with health) whether it is valuable for its own sake, or whether autonomy is principally valuable in an instrumental sense. That is, does it matter because self-determination is inherently important whatever we end up using it for and whatever the consequences of doing so, or is supporting people's autonomy simply the most effective, if imperfect, means of making space for them to identify and pursue other goals that contribute to their well-being?

The question of whether autonomy is of intrinsic or instrumental value is not just an abstract philosophical puzzle. Its practical relevance comes to life, for example, when we are called to consider the ethics of permitting apparently self-harming choices made by autonomous individuals in healthcare contexts, such as refusals of life-saving blood-transfusions.[25] In these cases, we may have to ask which is more important: respecting someone's choice or saving their life? And as with many concepts that comprise staple tools of bioethics, there are several different and contested interpretations of autonomy.[26] As we will now explore, what kind of—and how much—value we invest in autonomy will depend on which interpretation we adopt.

The first thing to note is that the term 'autonomous' can be applied across a number of different dimensions. We can, for example, refer to a choice, an action, a course of conduct, a way of living, a person, or a life, as being autonomous. These different dimensions of autonomy do not necessarily go hand-in-hand. For example, a person with the capacity to be autonomous in most areas of their life may sometimes act in non-autonomous ways, perhaps due to external coercion or impulse. Or someone with dementia, whose cognitive impairment makes it hard for them sustain long-term goals and engage in complex deliberations, may be well able to understand and choose if they want to be visited by particular family members. These kinds of disjunction are significant when it comes to making practical ethical judgements, because factors that enable autonomy in one dimension could undermine it in another. Respecting someone's refusal of treatment for a progressive illness (that is, respecting their autonomous choice) could, in time, threaten their capacities to make decisions or act on their desires (thereby, threatening their future as an autonomous person), for example. Identifying which dimension of autonomy one is concerned with in a particular instance is key to working out how strong an interest is at stake and how one might go about supporting this interest.

In healthcare contexts—and indeed in health and medical law—it is often implied that autonomy it is synonymous with 'valid consent'. Valid consent must be voluntary, informed, and given by a person (a patient or research participant, for example) with

---

[23] John Christman, 'Autonomy in Moral and Political Philosophy' (The Stanford Encyclopedia of Philosophy, 2020) available at <https://plato.stanford.edu/archives/fall2020/entries/autonomy-moral/> accessed 12 December 2022; Ronald Dworkin, *Life's Dominion: An Argument About Abortion, Euthanasia, and Individual Freedom* (Vintage 2011).

[24] See, for example, Henk ten Have, 'Global Bioethics and Communitarianism' (2011) 32(5) Theoretical Medicine and Bioethics 315.

[25] These kinds of cases are discussed in Chapter 8.

[26] For further discussions see, John Christman, 'Constructing the Inner Citadel: Recent Work on the Concept of Autonomy' (1988) 99(1) Ethics 109.

capacity to make a reasoned decision on the specific matter at hand.[27] In an ideal world, consent procedures would indeed support and enable patients' and participants' autonomy by allowing them to weigh up their options and decide what course of action would best express and support their values and objectives. However, the relationship between autonomy and consent is actually less direct and more nuanced than this might suggest. Informed consent—to submit to treatment or to take part in a clinical trial, for example— might not always be sufficient to promote the individual's wider interests in leading a life informed by what they value.[28] Isolated choices, even informed ones, may fail to reflect the goals of such a life. This is particularly so when consent procedures are conducted when a person is ill, dealing with an unfamiliar healthcare environment, or when their options are limited to assenting to or refusing a predetermined course of action, such as the sole treatment option proposed by their doctor.[29]

Consider the earlier example of Pablo. Let us imagine that Pablo understands the risks of embarking on DBS therapy and agrees to undergo the surgery and subsequent regime of neurostimulation this involves. His choice, however, is made following advice from his healthcare team that all other therapeutic options for his serious and debilitating movement disorder have been exhausted. And this treatment carries the risks of cognitive impairment and personality changes that may change his life in many profound ways. In this case, we can see how Pablo's consent may meet the criteria for validity, while also recognising that his choice may fall some way short of truly expressing his identity or enabling his continued authorship of his life in line with his values. It may be too strong to claim that Pablo's decision is categorically non-autonomous in this case. But we might still have grounds to question whether it attains the most valuable aspects of autonomy, or whether his autonomy could have been better supported.

A second question we need to consider if we want to invoke autonomy as a relevant consideration in bioethical reasoning is how we would distinguish autonomous from non-autonomous choices, activities, or lives. As the previous paragraphs indicate, according to some minimal conceptions, autonomy may be seen as consisting in little more than merely 'getting to choose'. However, as we have noted, this seems to fall short of capturing the full spirit of the kind of self-determination that justifies ethical attention and protection. There are, it will come as little surprise to hear, different views about what else is required for a richer and more ethically significant form of autonomy.[30] Some accounts, for example, focus on the presence or absence of contextual features, such as the availability of meaningful options to choose from, or freedom from constraint or coercion by others.[31] However, freedom from constraint may fail to capture all of what seems to be important, as we will return to discuss shortly.[32] An emphasis on available choices may encourage simplistic assumptions that living within particular social constraints automatically undermines autonomy. For example, simply because a woman entering into a commercial reproductive arrangement as a surrogate lives in a low-resource country with limited opportunities for well-paid employment may not be sufficient grounds for

---

[27] Alasdair Maclean, *Autonomy, Informed Consent and Medical Law: A Relational Challenge* (CUP 2009).

[28] Onora O'Neill, *Autonomy and Trust in Bioethics* (CUP 2002).

[29] The issue of consent is examined in more detail in relation to adults in Chapter 8 and in relation to children and young people in Chapter 9.

[30] Christman (2020) (n 26); Lisa Dive and Ainsley Newson, 'Reconceptualizing Autonomy for Bioethics' (2018) 28(2) Kennedy Institute of Ethics Journal 171.

[31] Joseph Raz, *The Morality of Freedom* (Clarendon Press 1986).

[32] For discussion of the distinction between 'freedom from' and 'freedom to' see Isaiah Berlin, 'Two Concepts of Liberty' in Isaiah Berlin (ed.) *Four Essays on Liberty* (OUP 1969).

assuming that she is necessarily non-autonomous. It is possible that her entering into this arrangement is a considered response to her economic realities and personal priorities. Of course, this does not mean that the underlying structural inequalities in this example raise no further ethical concerns on other grounds—autonomy is not the only ethical dimension in cases like this.[33]

Rather than focusing solely on absence of constraint, many thinkers have suggested that a rounded conception of autonomy needs to include an account of the kinds of the critical and reflective processes that underpin an agent's choices and conduct. These might include thoughtful weighing of options; critical reflection on how one's different motives fit together; or endorsement, rather than mere adoption, of a chosen course of action, for example.[34] Yet other accounts suggest that being autonomous rests on developing and exercising particular kinds of skills: not only those for reflecting and choosing but also for self-understanding and self-respect.[35] What these various accounts share is the broad idea that being autonomous involves living in accordance with values and aims that one has considered, with which one identifies, and which coexist as part of a meaningful life. These kinds of conceptions reflect a richer conception of autonomy than the mere exercise of choice and go some way to explain the value of autonomy. However, in defining autonomy we must take care not to set such a high threshold—demanding deep psychological insight and intellectual engagement, for example—that it is unattainable by most people.

One school of thought that has developed in reaction to what it sees as unrealistic criteria for being autonomous is *relational autonomy*. Relational approaches have their roots in feminist thinking. They suggest that there is something both factually implausible and morally wanting and about the supposed ideal of an isolated individual exercising rational deliberation in the absence of external influences—these are individualistic features shared by many conceptions of autonomy.[36] In contrast, relational approaches point out that our values and motives are informed by our personal relationships, and that we inevitably develop and exercise our abilities to weigh and direct our actions through our relationships. They also note that autonomous decisions are not always self-regarding but are often quite properly shaped and constrained by our concern for and responsibilities towards others. For these reasons, relational approaches reject individualist and rationalist accounts of autonomy that require our choices to be independent of the influence of others. Instead, they emphasise our inherent interdependence and the importance of collaboration to achieve our goals. Relational interpretations can provide important tools for interrogating many topics in contemporary bioethics, including how to approach the intersecting interests of family members regarding their shared genomic data and collaborative decision-making in health care.

---

[33] See, for example, Ganguli-Mitra A. 'Exploitation through the lens of structural injustice: Revisiting global commercial surrogacy' in Monique Deveaux and Vida Panitch (eds.) *Exploitation: From Practice to Theory* (Rowman & Littlefield 2014).

[34] See, for example, Harry Frankfurt, 'Freedom of the Will and the Concept of a Person' in Harry Frankfurt (ed.) *The Importance of What We Care About* (CUP, 1987); for further discussion see Christman (2020) (n 26).

[35] See for example Diana Tietjens Meyers, *Being Yourself: Essays on Identity, Action and Social Life (Feminist Constructions)* (Rowman & Littlefield Publishers 2004); Carolyn McLeod and Susan Sherwin, 'Relational Autonomy, Self-Trust, and Health Care for Patients Who are Oppressed' in Catriona Mackenzie and Natalie Stoljar (eds.) *Relational Autonomy: Feminist Perspectives on Autonomy, Agency, and the Social Self* (OUP 2000).

[36] For further discussion, see generally, Mackenzie and Stoljar (n 35).

The preceding discussion highlights a close connection between the concept of auton-omy and the medical and legal concepts of capacity and competence. A person's mental (or cognitive) capacity is assessed with respect to their ability to understand and make use of information to reach a particular decision. This is instrumental in determining whether they are legally competent to decide or act in that context.[37] A nuanced under-standing of what autonomy entails, the nature of its value and its relational aspects, pro-vides a useful set of critical tools when it comes to reflecting on whether existing tests for capacity protect what matters and what the proper role of family, carers, and healthcare professionals should be in supporting capacity.

Respect for autonomy is often contrasted with paternalism.[38] Paternalism refers to one party, particularly a party with greater power, making decisions on behalf of someone else on the basis of what they, rather than the person themselves, thinks is in the other's interests. For example, an obstetrician's decision not to offer a woman the choice of deliv-ery by Caesarean section, or a government policy to raise the minimum price of alcohol to reduce problem drinking, might attract accusations of paternalism. Paternalism is often not only seen as antithetical to respect for autonomy but, given the value ascribed to autonomy in contemporary bioethics, also viewed as inherently wrong. However, this may be too simplistic. In some cases, actions potentially labelled as paternalistic—for example intervening to prevent someone agreeing to undergo a risky and unlicensed therapy—might not only be defensible but perhaps also protect their longer-term capacity for living autonomously.

When unpacking cases such as the preceding example, a distinction between strong and weak forms of paternalism can be useful.[39] Strong paternalism involves overriding someone's free, informed choice. Meanwhile weak paternalism is generally understood to involve overriding non-voluntary or ill-informed choices, or redirecting the individual to a course of action that would better fulfil their known wishes; the example of inter-vening to stop someone undergoing experimental therapy could fall into this category. The distinction between strong and weak forms of paternalism may not always be clear in practice. However, interventions meeting the weaker definition may be seen as more ethically defensible from a perspective where autonomy matters. From a slightly differ-ent perspective, we can also question whether all interventions by other people in our decision-making should invariably be labelled as paternalistic. The preceding discussion of relational autonomy highlights that the exercise of autonomy need not preclude—and might actually require—the involvement and support of others, particularly others who know us well and share our lives, or have particular expertise in, for example, the medi-cal procedures under consideration. The broader lesson here is that it is often important to distinguish between cases in which other people are simply involved in someone's decision-making, and cases when this involvement is ethically problematic.

2.2.4 DIGNITY

A concept often associated with the idea of autonomy is that of dignity—although, as we shall see shortly, this connection is contested. References to dignity are ubiquitous in human rights instruments and other international legal instruments, where the concept is called upon to do a lot of moral work denoting broad conceptions of doing well by others

---

[37] The topics of capacity and competence are discussed further in Chapter 10.
[38] Robert Young, 'Autonomy and Paternalism' (1982) 8 Canadian Journal of Philosophy 47.
[39] ibid.

and a close, if somewhat vague, connection between dignity and well-being or human flourishing.[40] It is also invoked in more pointed ways in connection with protection from particular kinds of suffering caused by torture, infringements of privacy or bodily integrity, and deprivations of liberty. Beyond the context of human rights law, the capabilities approach, mentioned earlier in this chapter, is sometimes described as characterising the essential conditions for a minimally dignified human life.[41] In healthcare settings, patient dignity is associated with respectful, attentive, person-centred care. Other notable uses of the term include close associations between dignity and self-determination; dignity as the basis for prohibitions on treating other people as having merely instrumental value; and respect for dignity requiring non-interference with inviolable, sacred, or God-given aspects of human existence or the natural world.[42]

These various disputed and potentially incommensurable interpretations mean it is far from clear to what extent dignity should be counted among 'what matters' in ethical debate and evoked as a reason for taking a moral position. For example, consider ethical questions about the prospect of using human genome editing to prevent serious hereditary disease by removing the genes responsible of these diseases from pre-implantation human embryos. If dignity is understood as inextricably linked to respect for self-determination, then such uses of genome editing could be seen as promoting dignity by supporting parental autonomy and the health of their future children. In contrast, if dignity is a quality that demands to be met with humility and respect for God-given qualities and the shared heritage of humankind, then changes to the human genome achieved through technological interventions could be seen as violating dignity. As this indicates, when engaging in bioethical reasoning, the term 'dignity' should only be used with appropriate caution, making it clear which of the many conflicting interpretations is being adopted.

2.2.5 EMBODIED EXPERIENCE

Given that bioethics is concerned with moral questions raised by human health, it is perhaps surprising that the discipline has historically paid little attention to the fact that we are inescapably material, embodied beings. In recent years, there have been calls to pay more attention to the significance of the body in identifying and characterising how our lives progress and what matters to us.[43] In discussions of autonomy, well-being, and even our status as beings worthy of moral attention, it is often assumed that this depends primarily on our mental health, cognitive capacities, and rational choices. However, we are not just *thinking* beings, but also embodied, material, mortal ones. Our encounters with, and experiences of, the world are mediated by our bodies.[44] Moreover, the specific and diverse characteristics of our bodies, for example, our size, reproductive status,

[40] See, for example, the Universal Declaration of Human Rights (United Nations General Assembly, 1948) and the Universal Declaration on Bioethics and Human Rights (UNESCO 2005).

[41] Paul Formosa and Catriona Mackenzie, 'Nussbaum, Kant, and the Capabilities Approach to Dignity' (2014) 17(5) Ethical Theory and Moral Practice 875.

[42] For further discussion, see Richard Ashcroft, 'Making Sense of Dignity' (2005) 31(11) Journal of Medical Ethics 679; Deryck Beyleyeld and Roger Brownsword, *Human Dignity in Bioethics and Biolaw* (OUP 2001).

[43] Jackie Leach Scully, 'Moral Bodies: Epistemologies of Embodiment' in Hilde Lindemann, Marian Verkerk, and Margaret Urban Walker (eds.), *Naturalised Bioethics: Toward Responsible Knowing and Practice* (CUP 2008).

[44] Shaun Gallagher, *How the Body Shapes the Mind* (Clarendon Press 2006).

dexterity, mobility, skin colour, sensory functions, neurodiversity, and health can enable or obstruct our abilities to navigate and thrive in our social and built environments.[45] The kinds of bodily characteristics listed here can shape others' ideas of what we are like, and how they treat us. Later in this chapter we will look at the ways that these responses can manifest ableism and racism, for example, and the specific injustices these can lead to in the contexts of health and medicine.

Our embodiment is at the heart of our relationships with other people. All of us at various points in our lives will be responsible for, and dependent upon, others because of our respective bodily needs and vulnerabilities. We give birth to, and are born from, other bodies. We may experience connections and mutual interests with others grounded in shared features of our embodiment, such as susceptibility to the same disease or biological relatedness. If we neglect to take account of the embodied aspects of our lives and experiences, then we may lack a nuanced appreciation of key of what matters to us, our needs, and where our interests lie.

2.2.6 VULNERABILITY

An important feature of our embodied lives is that all of us are vulnerable to injury, ill-health, physical and psychological trauma, and death. It is an inescapable feature of the human condition and provides the basis for our mutual dependency as human beings.[46] However, it is also the case that some of us, under some conditions, might be more vulnerable than others, such as children for example, and therefore are worthy of additional moral concern and protection. It is an important normative concept, not merely a descriptive term, in that it suggests that situations or states should be of moral concern, or require moral attention. The concept of vulnerability has a long history in bioethics, as well as in health and medical law, featuring prominently in guidelines and protection mechanisms in research ethics, for example. In early clinical research guidelines, it was common to find entire groups labelled as vulnerable, including children, prisoners of war, and pregnant women. There are historical reasons why this came to be, chief among which is the fact that several research ethics guidelines were developed in response to atrocities and abuses in research. Therefore, those devising such guidelines were particularly attuned to protecting those considered vulnerable.

In health and medical law, vulnerable persons are often those considered unable to exercise their autonomy and therefore unable to look after their own interests. In other words, autonomous and vulnerable are presented as oppositional terms, primarily focused on capacity to consent. This approach has been criticised on various fronts. Associating vulnerability with autonomy suggests that vulnerable persons are never able to exercise their autonomy. This might be true in some cases, such as those involving very young children for example. However, other groups, such as pregnant women, are perfectly capable of exercising their autonomy, and therefore the label is misleading. This results in what is often known as protectionism, which involves unreasonably restricting people's self-determination in the name of protection. Additionally, labelling individuals and groups as vulnerable presents us with the problem that any such label might either be too wide, potentially encompassing those who might perfectly be capable of looking after their own

---

[45] For further discussion, see Stacy Alaimo and Susan Hekman, *Material Feminisms* (Indiana University Press 2008).

[46] Martha Albertson Fineman, 'The Vulnerable Subject: Anchoring Equality in the Human Condition' (2008) 20(1) Yale Journal of Law and Feminism 1.

interests, or too narrow in that any list will fail to capture some forms of vulnerability.[47] In recent years, feminist scholars have presented a more nuanced taxonomy of vulnerability, involving one that captures universal and specific types of vulnerabilities (e.g. The fact that we all have bodies susceptible to illness and injury versus suffering from chronic illness) and inherent and situational vulnerability (e.g. being in a permanent vegetative state versus working in a conflict zone). This is in addition to bringing attention to the ways in which individuals can be made vulnerable in certain situation, even by measures that are meant to protect them (this is referred to as pathological vulnerability). An important feature of such approaches is that not only do they not assume a lack of capacity, they also encourage us to consider addressing vulnerability in a manner that enhances autonomy.[48]

2.2.7 RELATIONSHIPS

The preceding sections offer illustrations of the limitations and pitfalls of installing an overly individualistic worldview at the heart of bioethical thinking. Relational approaches—not only to autonomy but also to subjects including reproductive decision-making, public heath, and recognition of moral status (as discussed later in this chapter)—are increasingly influential in bioethics.[49] These reflect a recognition, perhaps long overdue, that much of the value and meaning in our lives is be derived not solely from our own happiness or fulfilment of our individual preferences, but also from our relationships with others, our membership of families and communities, and the roles we play in each other's lives. Some of these roles may be ones of dependency, but they are no less valuable and life-enhancing for that.

If we adopt an excessively individualistic outlook, then valuable relational aspects of our lives may be overlooked. In many cases our well-being and fulfilment rests not only on how our own lives go but also on the well-being of the people we care about and the groups we belong to. Our well-being also depends on the extent to which we feel that we are valued and equal members of our communities and are able to participate on an equal, respected footing with others in economic, civic, and political life. Empirical research on social and health inequalities has highlighted that our health and well-being suffer not only in relation to absolute levels of deprivation but also to a considerable degree in relation to levels of deprivation relative to other people living in our communities.[50] So, good lives and well-being depend not only on access to opportunities and resources but also on the extent to which such lives are free from oppression, domination, and exploitation. For these reasons, justice—as manifest both in the distribution of resources and opportunities, and in equitable access to mechanisms of power, representation, and decision-making—must be recognised as an important aspect of human flourishing. Later in this chapter we will turn to examine the crucial part that justice plays in the ethical landscape.

The overview of the different aspects of what matters to us, what constitutes our well-being, and where our interests lie offered in this chapter has not been exhaustive. Given

---

[47] Carol Levine et al., 'The Limitations of "Vulnerability" as a Protection for Human Research Participants' (2004) 4(3) American Journal of Bioethics 44.

[48] Catriona Mackenzie, Wendy Rogers, and Susan Dodds, 'Introduction: What is Vulnerability and Why Does it Matter for Moral Theory' in Catriona Mackenzie, Wendy Rogers, and Susan Dodds (eds.), *Vulnerability: New Essays in Ethics and Feminist Philosophy* (OUP 2014).

[49] Bruce Jennings, 'Reconceptualizing Autonomy: A Relational Turn in Bioethics' (2016) 46(3) Hastings Center Report 11.

[50] Kate Pickett and Richard Wilkinson, 'Income Inequality and Health: A Causal Review' (2015) 128 Social Science & Medicine 316.

more space we could have also discussed the extent to which privacy,[51] identity develop-ment,[52] and trust,[53] among myriad other features, may also ground important interests and are also subject to contested interpretations. The preceding discussions cannot tell us definitively which particular conceptions of a well-being to adopt, what matters most to a good life, or which priorities are most salient in any particular circumstance. Instead, the ideas introduced here are intended to assist in developing the language and conceptual tools that we can bring to articulating the various capacities, experiences and activities that matter when addressing practical ethical questions and dilemmas. In order to work out what is the morally right thing to do in practical contexts, we need to find ways of articulating and comparing what would best support the well-being interests of the par-ties affected, and how avoidable harms can be averted or minimised. However, before we can properly assess which values and interests to take into account, we need to be able identify *whose* interests we are required to focus upon. This is the question examined in the following section.

2.3 WHO MATTERS?

Part of the work that needs to be done when addressing practical ethical questions involves making judgements about the scope of relevant impacts, specifically—who is affected in ways that we need to care about? So, for example, when thinking about the ethical justifi-ability of including pregnant women in clinical research, we might need to think about the potential consequences not only for participating women, but also for their families and future children, as well as for all those who might benefit from the research findings in the future. However, prior to making these kinds of judgements, we need to consider an underlying conceptual question: what distinguishes those *beings* who count as potential candidates for consideration in any ethical judgements from those who do not?

At first instance, this may seem like an odd question. We might assume we simply need to think about all the people potentially affected. However, it may not be self-evident who this includes. In the example just given there may, for instance, be disagreement about whether the foetuses of pregnant women participating in health research should be taken into account. Moreover, it is not clear that all individuals are, or have been, afforded equal status when it comes to taking account of, let alone protecting, their interests and well-being. The colour of people's skin, their gender, and their disabilities have all been used as grounds to deny that they are worthy of moral consideration. This is evident to varying degrees when, for example:

- populations in the Global South are treated merely as useful resources for clinical trials, with little or no attention paid to the need to involve them in decision-making about such trials, or post-trial access to treatment;
- young people with learning disabilities are sterilised against their wishes;
- elderly people's health is accorded lower priority in a public health crisis; or
- pregnant women's needs are respected only insofar as these coincide with the birth of a healthy infant.

---

[51] See, for example, Graeme Laurie, *Genetic Privacy: A Challenge to Medico-Legal Norms* (CUP 2002).
[52] See, for example, Emily Postan, *Embodied Narratives: Protecting Identity Interests Through Ethical Governance of Bioinformation* (CUP 2022).
[53] See, for example, Onora O'Neill (n 28).

In the language of bioethics, and ethics more widely, we can say that these are instances of people being treated as if they are 'not persons' or, at the very least, instances in which they are denied the care and respect due to 'persons'.

2.3.1 PERSONHOOD AND MORAL STATUS

The term 'person', when used in bioethics, does not just mean the singular of 'people'. It is often used in a more technical sense with prescriptive and value-laden implications. First, it carries implications for how beings classed as persons ought to be treated and, on some views, how persons ought to behave. And second, being a person is understood to depend on possession of particular qualities that justify these prescriptions.

Ethical personhood demarcates the category of beings (paradigmatically, but not necessarily, human ones) who warrant a particular kind of moral attention and concern in their own right, as members of our shared moral community.[54] Beings who warrant this kind of moral consideration are also referred to as having 'moral status'. Moral status differs from instrumental moral value. The latter refers to the quality of being valuable or useful *for* someone else, and in order to fulfil some further purpose. A transplant organ, for example, has instrumental value. It would be wrong to needlessly destroy this organ. However, this would be because it would show a lack of respect to donors and cause harm to potential recipients, not because the organ itself is wronged. In contrast, we care or should care about beings with moral status for their own sakes. Someone with moral status is recognised as having interests, the fulfilment of which matters to them and should also matter to others. Personhood is also seen as intrinsically linked to capacities for moral agency. This said, our focus here is chiefly on how it intersects with moral status. Persons, by definition, have moral status.

It is worth noting at this point that although *legal* personhood and *ethical* personhood are both normative concepts—in that they tell each of us that those holding these types of status have particular entitlements and responsibilities—and there will be overlap between the membership of the categories of legal and ethical personhood, these two kinds of status are not synonymous. Someone may possess one while lacking the other. For example, a corporation may have legal personhood, but is not a person in the ethical sense. Meanwhile an eight-year-old child may be a person in the ethical, but not the legal, sense.

2.3.2 QUALITIES DEFINING PERSONHOOD

There is much heated and unresolved debate, however, about who or what counts as a person in the ethical sense. These disputes often focus on the moral status of human embryos and foetuses, non-human animals such as great apes and octopuses, brain organoids, and future highly sophisticated artificial intelligence (AI) systems.[55] These entities provide the paradigmatic examples of hard cases and grey areas in bioethical debate about moral status and personhood. However, we must not lose sight of the fact that many of the practical circumstances in which individuals are seriously harmed by the denial of their personhood are not these types of hard cases. Instead, they occur in circumstances where, under any reasonable criteria, an individual's personhood should not be in dispute, but

---

[54] Lisa Bortolotti, 'Disputes Over Moral Status: Philosophy and Science in the Future of Bioethics' (2007) 15(2) Health Care Analysis 153.
[55] ibid.

they are nevertheless denied respect. Nevertheless, debates about hard cases remain fraught because there is disagreement about the qualities on which personhood depends and there are real ethical and practical consequences of something falling outside this category. Some examples of the qualities that have been proposed are:

- possession of the kinds of cognitive abilities that allow someone to be aware of themselves as subjects of their own life and experiences, invested in their future, and capable of making autonomous decisions;[56]
- prior or probable future or possession of these kinds of abilities and experiences;[57]
- sentience, in particular the ability to feel pain; or[58]
- membership of the human species.[59]

Some of these criteria entail troubling exclusions. For example, a requirement for sophisticated cognitive capacities rules out infants and people in minimally conscious states. Approaches that limit moral status to all and only human beings have attracted charges of arbitrary speciesism. Meanwhile, other options, such as sentience, may seem too inclusive and therefore unreasonably ethically demanding. Imagine if we were obliged not only to avoid causing undue suffering to all sentient non-human animals and reject their use as sources of food or clothing but also to treat them as full members of our moral communities. This is a vivid reminder that recognition of personhood and moral status has real ethical and practical consequences for how we live our lives. The examples of hard cases cited in the previous paragraph indicate the challenges of locating a single quality to demarcate the boundaries of personhood or moral status that satisfies our intuitions about who deserves moral attention and widespread ethical norms. Due to these challenges, it is sometimes suggested that personhood and moral status depend on a mixture of qualities, not all of which need be present in every case, or that moral status is not an all-or-nothing property, but exists on a sliding scale.

Notably, each of the potential criteria for moral status just listed appeals to intrinsic qualities of individuals viewed on their own. Some feminist thinkers take a different route, arguing that being a member of a moral community is inescapably about interpersonal relationships. According to such views, personhood is sustained by relationships of care and recognition.[60] So, for example, the personhood of a loved child or old friend is not diminished simply because they lack capacities for reasoning or self-awareness due to age or cognitive impairment. They are persons, deserving of moral attention and respect, precisely because their interests, needs, and unique qualities are recognised by those close to them, and because they respond to and thrive within these relationships. Whichever qualities, relationships, or set of mixed features we recognise as defining personhood, one thing is non-negotiable: these features must be relevant to what it means to have moral status. That is, these qualities must themselves explain *why* someone has interests that warrant our moral attention and explain why we should be concerned for them for their own sake. For example, it might be argued that capacities for self-awareness and self-concern underpin personhood because they explain why abusing, instrumentalising, or otherwise constraining the freedoms of someone with these qualities causes fear, pain,

---

[56] Michael Tooley, 'Abortion and Infanticide' (1972) 2(1) Philosophy and Public Affairs 37.
[57] Don Marquis, 'Why Abortion is Immoral' (1989) 86(4) The Journal of Philosophy 183.
[58] Tom Regan, *The Case for Animal Rights* (University of California Press, 2004).
[59] Stanley Benn, 'Egalitarianism and Equal Consideration of Interests' in J. Roland Pennock and John Chapmans (eds.) *Nomos IX: Equality* (Atherton Press 1967) pp 61–78.
[60] Eva Kittay, 'At the Margins of Moral Personhood' (2008) 5(2) Journal of Bioethical Inquiry 137.

and other kinds of harm, and thus would be ethically wrong. The defining qualities we settle upon cannot simply reflect our arbitrary preferences or fears of exclusivity.

2.3.3 BEYOND THE INDIVIDUAL

While the focus of bioethics is often on the individual, the reality is that we do not live as isolated beings in the world. We are formed and continually influenced by the relationships we have with family, friends, and the many actors around us that shape our lives in important and sometimes invisible ways. Our interests are related to those of others around us, and vice versa. We are also enabled and constrained by our position within social structures and our identities within these. Each of us is placed at particular intersections of power, oppression and privilege, which affects how much we are able to flourish, live freely, and exercise our interests. Our moral radar neglects systematic forms of domination or oppression when we tend to focus on the individual, without attention to the historical, social, and structural aspects of the lives of individuals. We return to such considerations in more detail when we examine the concept of justice later in this chapter.

Individual persons are not the only entities that can be thought of as having interests and as being the proper objects of our moral concern. Communities and groups can also be respected or wronged, benefited or harmed by what happens to them and how they are treated. In many cases, the ethical significance of these impacts can only be properly appreciated when we understand these as impacts on the group as a whole and not just as an aggregation of impacts on individual members of the group. These kinds of group interests have been brought into sharp focus by the increased prevalence of genomic research and medicine, due to the inherently shared nature of genetic information.[61] For example, we may appreciate how a family, including its integral relationships, bonds of care, trust, interdependence, and shared history could benefit from the eventual identification of a rare genetic disorder that has affected successive generations. We may also understand how the identity and self-esteem of an entire ethnic group might suffer from unethical and poorly conducted research that purports to identify high prevalence of a particular genetic marker within the group that is also closely associated, for example, with psychiatric illness or propensity to violence.[62] Group interests are not, however, limited to the realm of genomics. For example, group interests can also arise from shared histories, geographies, and politics. While a focus on health and medicine means that our focus tends inevitably to fall on people and groups of people, planetary and other wider perspectives may give us cause to interrogate whether entities such as ecosystems, or cultural and linguistic heritage have inherent moral value.

This and the preceding section have examined the questions of 'what matters?' and 'who matters?' These are questions about what makes someone an appropriate subject of ethical attention, and what kinds of valuable moral things our attention should then focus upon. The answers to these questions provide some of the basic conceptual building blocks of ethical reasoning—although, as we have seen, many of these concepts are interpreted in diverse and contested ways. Having gained a sense of what kinds of things are valuable, the next step is to understand how to approach questions about what is the right thing to do. The following section explores the key theoretical tools that we can use in engaging in this kind of practical analysis and in arriving at answers that are supported by explicit and persuasive reasons.

[61] Heather Widdows, *The Connected Self: The Ethics and Governance of the Genetic Individual* (CUP 2013).
[62] For discussion of one such example see, Nanibaa Garrison, 'Genomic Justice for Native Americans: Impact of the Havasupai Case on Genetic Research' (2013) 38(2) Science, Technology and Human Values 201.

2.4 USING MORAL THEORIES IN BIOETHICS

We turn now to quite a different set of considerations that will allow us to further equip our toolkit for making and defending reasoned, well-justified ethical arguments. Here we examine three of the most prominent schools of thought in moral philosophy about what features of any situation make it right or wrong. These schools of thought are:

- consequentialism;
- rules-based (sometimes known as 'deontological') theories;
- virtue ethics.

These three schools (which in actuality contain a multitude of variants and disagreements) are commonly referred to when people talk about normative moral theories. 'Moral theory' here refers to a set of long-standing, somewhat abstracted and idealised interpretations of which factors actually determine whether something (an action, practice, or state of affairs) is morally right or wrong. Different theories hold that different aspects of the practical landscape—consequences on the horizon, the signposts to rules, the subterranean motives, or the pattern of benefits and harms distributed across the scene—are most salient to moral judgement. Each theory directs us to look towards their favoured aspect to decide what would be the right thing to do. To illustrate what this means in practice, we can consider the following example:

> Layla has been on dialysis and awaiting a suitable donor kidney for 18 of the 36 years she has been alive. Her health is fast deteriorating and the need for donor kidneys far exceeds availability in her country. Layla's doctors have told her that she may not live long enough to receive an organ donation. Her family and friends have gathered sufficient crowd-sourced funds for Layla to pay to undergo private transplant surgery in another country where kidneys are available from healthy live donors who receive payment for their organs. If Layla undergoes a transplant with a kidney that she has paid for, she is likely to make a full recovery.

What would be the morally right thing for Layla to do: stay—at risk to her life, or travel for surgery? We can perhaps imagine ourselves, and our friends and colleagues, coming up with different answers to this question. One of the reasons these answers might differ is that we each identify different aspects of Layla's situation as being relevant to our judgements about what is morally good or bad about the options available to her. For example:

- Some might think that what really matters are the *outcomes* of the different available options. They recognise that the purchase of a donor organ is not without some risk to the donor and to Layla, but believe that the magnitude of the benefit to Layla, and to those who love her, of travelling for this surgery outweighs these risks.

- Meanwhile, someone else could believe that the most important thing is to abide by any established *rules* that prohibit or require particular conduct. Perhaps they think that it is always wrong to conduct risky surgery on a healthy individual who will not benefit from it, or they might think that body parts should never be bought or sold irrespective of the possible benefits of doing so in some circumstances.

- Others might place greatest weight on the nature of the *attitudes and motives* of those involved. They might judge that, while unpaid, altruistic organ donation exemplifies admirable generosity, mutual concern, and empathy, a trade in paid-for organs perpetuates troubling commodifying and instrumentalising attitudes towards both organs and people.

Each of these three different ways of looking at the ethical dilemma facing Layla broadly reflects approaches characteristic to one of the three prominent moral theories listed previously. In this section, we will suggest that in order to undertake bioethical analysis and argumentation, it may be neither necessary nor realistic to adopt, defend, and apply one theoretical approach to the exclusion of all others. Rather, we suggest that these theories provide a suite of valuable critical lenses through which to assess ethical problems and develop one's response. To get a fuller sense of these useful lenses, we will now look a little more closely at the claims, merits, and weaknesses of each of the three positions.

2.4.1 CONSEQUENCES

Consequentialism is the label given to the family of moral theories that holds that an action or practice is morally right when, and only when, it delivers the best overall outcomes of the available options. According to consequentialist thinking, morally right actions are those in which the aggregate good consequences outweigh the bad ones.[63] The motives from or means by which these consequences are achieved are only relevant to ethical assessment insofar as they affect the outcomes.

This broad definition leaves room for different interpretations as to what counts as a good or a bad consequence and there are, accordingly, several different versions of consequentialism. One of the best-known versions is utilitarianism. Utilitarianism holds that a right action is one that results in a greater total balance of happiness and pleasure over pain, while wrong actions are those resulting in net aggregate suffering.[64] As we have seen earlier in this chapter, we can question whether pursuit of happiness is really the only or most valuable goal in life. If we have doubts about the truth of hedonism, we should also be doubtful about the validity of utilitarian thinking. Nevertheless, it is possible to adopt different kinds of consequentialist approaches that take a wider and more heterogeneous view of what kinds of things can count as good or bad consequences. In the earlier sections of this chapter, we explored a range of ways of interpreting what would harm or enhance people's well-being and identifying 'what matters' to them and where their interests lie. In principle, any of these could be used to populate the list of harms and benefits that are entered into the consequentialist calculation.

Consequentialist thinking is highly influential in many areas of healthcare decision-making. For example:

- it lies at the heart of triage arrangements in emergency care, where the aim is to target limited resources at those patients thought most likely to benefit, and to benefit to the greatest degree, from the intervention, thus maximising the overall good achievable;[65] and

- when ethical assessments of, for example, introducing a new therapy or conducting health research, is framed in terms of the ratio of the expected resultant benefits to risks.

---

[63] Samuel Scheffler, 'Introduction' in Samuel Scheffler (ed.), *Consequentialism and its Critics* (OUP 1988).
[64] John Jamieson Smart and Bernard Williams, *Utilitarianism: For & Against* (CUP 1973).
[65] See, for example, Julian Savulescu, Ingmar Persson, and Dominic Wilkinson, 'Utilitarianism and the Pandemic' (2020) 34(6) Bioethics 620.

We will return shortly to reviewing some of the reasons why consequentialist thinking—and the positions of the other theories considered here—might be viewed as incomplete or problematic.

2.4.2 RULES

Another prominent family of theories is illustrated by the second of the imagined responses to Layla's decision. It locates the rightness or wrongness of an action or set of circumstances in the extent to which it complies with pre-existing rules about permissible, prohibited, or obligatory conduct.[66] This family of theories is often referred to as 'deontological', its etymology signalling the emphasis on following duties. There is no single set of rules shared by all deontological approaches. Different approaches vary in both the precise rules they prescribe and the source of these rules. For example, some derive binding ethical rules from the teachings of particular faiths, while others suggest that we can identify rules from considering what standards are needed to sustain harmonious social existence, or that ethical rules can be discerned through impartial, rational deliberation.

Examples of the kinds of ethical rules that are most widely evoked in healthcare contexts include:

- the requirement always to protect the safety of human participants in clinical research and to refrain from treating them merely as instrumental means to the contribution of research to scientific knowledge;[67] and

- obligations to respect patient confidentiality in the absence of strong overriding reasons.[68]

2.4.3 VIRTUE

The third example of a possible response to Layla's situation reflects an approach known as virtue theory. This treats the motives, attitudes, and character of people involved as the appropriate locus of moral judgements.[69] Good people and good actions are those that exemplify virtuous characteristics. Departing somewhat from everyday usage, in which virtue is commonly associated with abstinence or piety, virtue here refers more broadly to character traits that are appropriate objects of admiration, that contribute to good lives for those who have them and, just as importantly, contribute to the flourishing of those whose lives are affected by others' attitudes and conduct. Common examples of virtues include kindness, honesty, courage, and practical wisdom. However, once again, different virtue-led approaches come in different forms and may differ on what counts as a virtue or a vice.

---

[66] Joseph Boyle, 'Exceptionless Rule Approaches' in Helga Khuse and Peter Singer (eds.) *A Companion to Bioethics* (2nd edn, Wiley Blackwell 2012).

[67] Research ethics are discussed further in Chapter 6.

[68] Confidentiality is discussed further in Chapter 11.

[69] Justin Oakley, 'Virtue Ethics and Bioethics' in Daniel Russel (ed.) *The Cambridge Companion to Virtue Ethics* (CUP 2013) 197–220; Roger Crisp and Michael Slote (eds.), *Virtue Ethics: Oxford Readings in Philosophy* (OUP 1997).

Although the term 'virtue' is rarely explicitly used in relation to ethical conduct in health care, it is not uncommon for claims to be made about the importance of health-care professionals or policymakers exhibiting particular virtuous character traits. For example:

- In recent years there have been public debates in the UK, often precipitated by findings of institutional failings in regional health authorities, about the value of compassion in patient care, and the need for candour when mistakes have been made.[70]
- The importance of the trustworthiness of public institutions and large projects funded or overseen by these institutions—such as the roll-out of population-wide Covid-19 vaccination programmes, or the introduction of population-wide projects for sharing and linking patient data—is also widely emphasised.[71]

As these examples indicate, virtues can be seen as desirable attributes of institutions and groups as well as of individuals.

The 'ethics of care' or 'care ethics' approach can be seen as a sub-set of contemporary virtue theory that has particular salience in healthcare contexts.[72] This approach holds that the character of our personal relationships with and attitudes to other people are at the heart of doing the right thing and that good actions are those that are characterised by attitudes of care and benevolence. Care ethics particularly emphasises the importance of being appropriately attentive and responsive to other people's interests, and observes that this importance arises from the fact that we are dependent on one another as result of our inevitable human needs and vulnerabilities.

2.4.4 USING MORAL THEORIES AS CRITICAL LENSES

It is important to appreciate the nature of work each of these moral theories is seeking to do and what this means for their role and utility in bioethics, a discipline that is foremost an applied one. These theories do not chiefly aim to tell us precisely what ought to be done in responding to particular practical situations like Layla's. They are more ambitious in their aims and intended scope. Each purports to define what actually makes something morally right or wrong, and does so in all and any circumstances. As such, the claims of each theory are largely incommensurable and do not lend themselves to being easily mixed and matched. Each could deliver contradictory advice on what should be done in practical dilemmas, and provide different reasons for this advice.

Having said this, it is important not to overstate the distance between all aspects of these theories. For example, while consequentialist approaches place all the emphasis on outcomes, almost any ethical theory—whether concerned with rules or virtues—is likely to take outcomes into account in some way, when assessing inequities in distribution or desirable traits, for example. Similarly, approaches that appeal to binding moral rules

---

[70] See, for example, Oliver Quick, 'Duties of Candour in Healthcare: The Truth, the Whole Truth, and Nothing but the Truth?' (2022) 30(2) Medical Law Review 324; Robert Francis, 'Report of the Mid Staffordshire NHS Foundation Trust Public Inquiry – Executive Summary' (Stationary Office 2013).

[71] See, for example, Felix Gille, Sarah Smith, and Nicholas Mays, 'Towards a Broader Conceptualisation of "Public Trust" in the Health Care System' (2017) 15(1) Social Theory & Health 23.

[72] Rita Manning, 'A Care Approach' in Helga Kuhse and Peter Singer (eds.), *A Companion to Bioethics* (2nd edn, Wiley Blackwell 2012); see also Tove Pettersen, *Comprehending Care: The Problems and Possibilities in the Ethics of Care* (Rowman & Littlefield, 2008).

may well derive these rules from broadly consequentialist calculations, or with the aim of formalising expectations of virtuous behaviour. These commonalities notwithstanding, when it comes to pursuing the practical aims of bioethics, it is generally not possible, for the reasons just given, to employ all of these theoretical approaches fulsomely and simultaneously without running into difficulties. It is tempting to ask, therefore, which of these theories is the 'best' and which one we, therefore, ought to take up and apply across all our bioethical analyses and debates.

Unfortunately, this is not the simple or appealing solution it might seem. For a start, idealised moral theories may be too abstract and inflexible to apply under the pressures of ethical decision-making especially, for example, in acute clinical cases or in the midst of global health emergencies. More fundamentally, there is the problem of deciding which theory is 'best'. Debates about this remain live and unresolved in the field of ethics itself. While each theory highlights potentially relevant considerations, each is also vulnerable to ready critique. For example, although utilitarian thinking might look appealingly intuitive, we might query whether maximising pleasure is really all we care about. We might also feel uncomfortable about agreeing that a net balance of overall happiness achieved at the expense of terrible suffering to some people is morally good. Rule-based theories seem to offer practical clarity, but are vulnerable to disputes about the proper source of authoritative moral rules, and about what should be done when rules conflict rule, or when following them would lead to serious harm. Virtue theory reminds us that motives and attitudes matter, a feature missing from other theories, but we may question whether thinking in terms of virtuous character traits is a practical way to work out what would be the right thing to do in particular dilemmas, or doubt the possibility of universal definition of a good character or flourishing life. Furthermore, each of these theories is drawn from the relatively narrow scope of Western traditions of analytic moral philosophy, and each risks incorporating omissions and biases arising from its origins.

Proponents of each of these theories, unsurprisingly, offer responses to the kinds of critiques just sketched. Nevertheless, fundamental disagreements and criticisms persist, and each headline 'theory family' includes multiple different versions that differ on key points. It is simply not possible to resolve these disputes while engaged in practically focused bioethical decision-making. It is usually, therefore, neither desirable nor realistic to attempt to endorse and apply any one theoretical approach to the exclusion of all others when doing applied ethics of the kind required by critical bioethical thinking.

Why introduce these theories at all then? We have already encountered one kind of answer to this question in Chapter 1. Moral theories can, along with other broad principles, provide a critical counterpoint to our initial intuitions and reactions to particular ethical cases and dilemmas, allowing us to practise reflective equilibrium in order to arrive at a considered response to the situation. A second answer is that each theory can provide us with a different and potentially useful lens through which to view ethical problems, compare perspectives and options, and decide which considerations are most relevant and urgent in the circumstances.[73] For example, in the case of Layla we might decide that the likely positive outcomes for her health carry a great deal of weight but should only prevail if other concerns can be addressed. For example, we might also judge that it also matters that the healthcare system in the destination country treats donors with respect, meets their health needs, and compensates them fairly, while the state offers meaningful alternative sources of income for those choosing not to donate. This assessment of the

---

[73] Susan Sherman, 'Foundations, frameworks, lenses: The role of theories in bioethics' (1999) 13(3–4) Bioethics 198.

dilemma places considerable emphasis on maximising well-being, but not at the expense of perpetuating instrumentalising attitudes towards donors, or supporting a system that constrains donors' options in ways that render them vulnerable.

Doing practically focused bioethics is never just a matter of taking a single theory down from the shelf and applying it like a cookie-cutter to the practical situation at hand.[74] Nor should it involve running through a shopping list in an attempt to detail what every permutation of each theory family would prescribe in the circumstances. Even if it were possible to populate such a lengthy list, this would not get one any closer to a workable ethical judgement or a consistent set of reasons for this judgement. Moreover, the three canonical moral theories discussed here are not the only possible sources of perspectives we may bring to addressing moral questions and dilemmas. A further set of considerations arise when we look through lenses informed by concerns about justice.

Justice can, of course, be understood as referring to the institutions and operation of the law. However, in ethics, talk of justice is associated with the just or fair distribution of opportunities and outcomes, processes, and the ways in which we treat each other. Considerations of justice, while rooted in political philosophy, are closely tied to questions of morality. If we say something is just, we mean that it is also the right state of affairs, or that it is a state that we should strive to achieve. Giving someone their due is 'the right thing to do', or that organising society, its benefits, and burdens in a fair manner is a good aim, ethically speaking. This in turn implies that someone else has the responsibility to provide what is due, or that society—as a collective—has the responsibility to ensure that people get what is owed to them as a matter of justice, a responsibility usually disbursed through its institutions. Regarding Layla's decision about whether to travel abroad to receive a paid-for transplant organ, focusing on questions of justice might lead us to ask the following questions:

- What is a fair allocation of organs within a health system?
- Is it fair that some patients might have access to life-saving treatments outside of their countries when others do not?
- Is receiving an organ in exchange for payment a form of unfair transaction? Are there terms of exchange that might make the arrangement fairer?
- If the potential 'donors' are in fact selling their organs, due to their socio-economic disadvantage, does this make the arrangement (particularly) unjust?

In the following section we will turn to look at various conceptions of justice and injustice in greater detail, as well as considering the ways that inequalities manifest in health and medical contexts and the kinds of bioethical concerns that come into focus when viewed through the lenses of justice and critical theory.

2.5 JUSTICE AND INEQUALITY

2.5.1 STANDARD APPROACHES TO JUSTICE IN BIOETHICS

While we have stated the ways in which moral philosophy and its tools are important to bioethical questions, another discipline -political philosophy- has had, and is gaining further importance in bioethical thinking and deliberation. Political philosophy can, in

---

[74] For further discussion of the role of theory in bioethics, see James Rachels, 'Ethical Theory and Bioethics' in Helga Khuse and Peter Singer (eds.), *A Companion to Bioethics* (2nd edn, Wiley Blackwell 2012).

the first instance, be described by the questions: 'Who gets what?' and 'Says who?'[75] in society. The first question is about the distribution of resources, entitlements, and burdens within a society. The second question is about who has the (political) power to make decisions about the first question. These are of course not the only questions that are morally relevant in this area. Just like moral philosophy, political philosophy is often a source of critical lenses in bioethics. The most relevant aspects of political philosophy to bioethics are the considerations of justice. Take, for example, the following questions:

- If there is a waiting list for a life-saving surgery, what is a fair way of establishing priority?
- What kind of health care should undocumented migrants receive in a country that has not yet recognised their status?
- Is it right to undertake biomedical research in low-income contexts and sell the products of that research to high-income markets?
- Is international commercial surrogacy unfairly exploitative?
- If the tools of genetic enhancement are perfected, does it matter if only a small number of privileged individuals have access to it?
- Should health care be distributed according to need, priority, or ability to pay?
- How should we address socially mediated health inequalities?

Each of these questions might require engaging with the concepts of fairness and justice. There are several ways of thinking about justice, and different approaches highlight different interests or values at stake. Approaches might differ also on what counts as equality, or what we might need to compare when we think about what is owed to others in terms of equality or fairness. Political philosophers will disagree on the answers, as well as their justifications, just as moral philosophers might. Some approaches to justice might argue that a fair state of affairs (and by extension, a morally correct one) is achieved by using fair procedures, regardless of the substantive outcomes of those procedures. Other approaches might emphasise the principle that, in trying to achieve a fair society, no one should be considered more important than anyone else. Several approaches to justice propose a specific understanding of equality as the aim of justice, for example, one where access to the basic goods and opportunities of society are not based on one's ability to pay, or one's hereditary advantages.

Consider the following questions around access to basic health care as exemplifying different approaches to justice in health. In society, how should access to health care be distributed:

- According to one's ability to pay for them?
- According to need, that is, those who need it the most have priority?
- Equally, regardless of need or ability to pay?
- Sufficiently, so that everyone's basic needs are covered first?
- So that those who are most disadvantaged in society have priority?

Different (aspects of) healthcare systems are based on one or a combination of these considerations. For example, a universal healthcare system is not dependent on anyone's ability to pay for care; or by way of alternative, health care might be organised so that everyone has access to a certain level of basic care, free of charge, but might be able to access non-emergency care upon payment.

---

[75] Jonathan Wolff, *An Introduction to Political Philosophy* (OUP 2006).

Many of the well-established frameworks of justice that are encountered in bioethical scholarship engage with the following question: what would an ideal just society or a just state of affairs look like, and what steps do we need to take to aim for that state? Such approaches have been criticised for failing to engage with the world as it is now, and for failing to incorporate historical existing inequalities and oppressions in thinking about the issue. A different set of approaches begins by considering not what justice might look like to achieve an ideal state of affairs, but rather how to address existing social and health inequalities. We consider some of these approaches in the following sections.

A second area of criticism arises from the justice-related questions we have historically considered in bioethics. Traditionally, we have tended to think of concerns of justice as amounting to considerable emphasis on fair resource allocation. For example, we can ask: how do we fairly distribute scarce health resources? In a fair system, how should we place people on the waiting list for an organ? Who should get the vaccine first? As exemplified in Layla's case, such questions have a far broader reach.

Our moral gaze remains incomplete when we assume that justice and its requirements will affect all people equally. Society (and the world) as we find it are characterised by various forms of historical and current oppressions, as well as socially, politically, and commercially mediated determinants of health. While it might appear strange to begin by focusing on inequalities and injustices instead of directly aiming for justice, this exercise allows us to see the ways in which inequality or suffering are not merely unfortunate, but also unjust, and how these are strongly embedded in our social structures and processes. Indeed, some critical philosophical lenses and approaches have been gaining prominence; they stress the need to centre social inequalities in our moral and political concerns about health.

2.5.2 FEMINIST APPROACHES

At the core of feminist approaches to philosophy and bioethics is a quest for social justice and, as such, an intrinsically political movement aiming for equality. Some feminist approaches focus on the radical aspects of the movement, others are pragmatic or intersectional. Feminist bioethics emerged as a critique of mainstream bioethics, invigorated by women's health movements, and focused on issues that were often neglected by more traditional approaches in bioethics. These include access to reproductive and sexual health for women, questions of justice for women in the family and the public sphere, and the involvement of women in research. Feminist approaches also criticise tendencies towards philosophical abstraction[76] and the use of broad principles in relation to the moral and justice-based issues arising from the realities of those who are less powerful and visible in society.

Such approaches have been particularly successful in making power visible within and beyond the medical establishment. Feminist concerns in bioethics might include:

- Considering the ways in which the male-dominated field of medicine has systematically failed women, non-binary, and other marginalised genders and bodies.
- Highlighting how reproductive issues in medicine are problematically addressed through heteronormative and cis-gendered lenses.

---

[76] Herjeet Marway and Heather Widdows, *Philosophical Feminist Bioethics: Past, Present, and Future* (2015) 24(2) Cambridge Quarterly of Healthcare Ethics 165; Camisha Russell, 'Questions of Race in Bioethics: Deceit, Disregard, Disparity, and the Work of Decentering' (2016) 11(1) Philosophy Compass 43.

- Addressing access to abortion as a matter of health care and reproductive justice.
- Advocating for the inclusion of pregnant women in research so that their interests are represented in such research.
- How global beauty norms add to specific forms of injustices across genders.

Feminist approaches do not only attend to matters related to reproduction and to women's interests. They also have made crucial contributions to conceptual and theoretical discussions, for example on autonomy, vulnerability, embodiment, and justice, as we have discussed previously in this chapter.

2.5.3 BIOETHICS AND DISABILITY

A critique of a bioethics, which abstracts and generalises the lived experiences of those with standard bodies and a certain amount of privilege, is also prominent in bioethical lenses informed by disability theory and approaches. Feminist disability scholars have long engaged with the ethical considerations arising from living in a 'non-standard' body, using this to critique approaches to health, impairment, and normality entrenched in mainstream bioethics.[77] They have engaged with political and justice concerns arising from ableist approaches and practices in the field. Disability studies and bioethics might:

- Engage with the expertise that people with disability bring to navigating health, health technologies, and the built environment.
- Highlight the ways our understandings and approaches to health might adversely affect those with disabilities, or conversely enable those who live with non-standard bodies in the world.
- Consider the lived experiences of impairment and what that might mean for the ethics of relationships, moral obligations, or the requirements of justice.
- Engage with the ways in which our built environments, social and health policies, structures, and processes might make those with disability particularly vulnerable to harm, injury, ill-health, or discrimination.

2.5.4 BIOETHICS AND RACE

A similarly critical approach and one that also been problematically ignored by mainstream bioethics arises in relation to race. The history of global health, public health, and biomedical research is rife with conceptions, processes, and institutions that build on oppressive, exploitative, and marginalising ideology and practices, including racism and racist oppression. While bioethics in part arose as a response to abuses of vulnerable and historically oppressed groups, racism has rarely been a focus in the context of a systematic approach to theorising and development of the field. Bioethics has also neglected its own participation in global and local white privilege, coloniality, and racial injustice. Recent scholarship based on critical race theory, intersectionality, anti-racist and anti-colonial thought and practice is gaining much-needed attention in the field.

---

[77] Jackie Leach Scully, *Disability Bioethics: Moral Bodies, Moral Difference* (Rowman and Littlefield 2008).

A bioethics that is informed by race and racism might engage with concerns such as:

- Racial disparities in health outcomes, including for, example, the existing higher level of maternal mortality for Black women in comparison to their white counterparts, or access to reproductive care.
- Historical and ongoing oppression of Black and minority populations within the medical and biomedical research establishments, as well as the lack of representation of non-white bodies in such disciplines.
- The ways in which historical understandings of the liberal individual, their interests, entitlements, and rights have systematically depended on the exclusion of others.
- How health technologies and algorithms systematically reproduce structural and other forms of racism.

2.5.5 INTERSECTIONALITY

An important concept from critical race theory is that of intersectionality.[78] This concept comes from the idea that every individual, depending on their social and political identities, is situated at an intersection between several sources of oppression, for example, gender and race. Intersectionality is a significant concept at the heart of Black feminist scholarship. The motivation behind such scholarship and activism arose from the realisation that emancipatory and justice-based movements, while focusing on one form of oppression, were failing those experiencing several forms of injustices. In this particular case, Black women's race-based oppression was ignored by white feminist movements, and civil rights movements were often dominated by men who failed to engage with gendered oppression. Intersectionality, a term coined by Black feminist scholar Kimberlé Crenshaw in the late 1908s, gives us an important tool in engaging with the ways in which individuals may experience many forms of oppression (class, gender, race, disability, caste, religion, nationality), which give rise to new forms of injustices, and leads to specific forms of social, political, and health-based inequalities. Failing to engage with oppression and privilege at these intersections leaves us ill-informed with respect to some of the most egregious harms and injustices.

2.5.6 STRUCTURAL AND EPISTEMIC INJUSTICE

Understanding the ways in which sexism, racism, ableism, oppression, and power operate in and beyond health means that there is a need to address inequalities and injustices beyond interpersonal relationships and interactions. The fact that many social and health inequalities arise and are sustained in social patterns means that in thinking about justice, we need to focus further on the structures and processes of society. Moving away from the use of abstraction (as explored earlier in the chapter), especially with the tools offered by feminist and other critical approaches, allows us to see how power and oppression are socially and institutionally mediated and do not necessarily arise from specific morally problematic actions or policies. An approach based on structural injustice, for example, allows us to see how our societies have often been organised in a way that considers some lives as less valuable than others and leads to systematic patterns of

---

[78] Kimberlé Crenshaw, 'Demarginalizing the Intersection of Race and Sex: A Black Feminist Critique of Antidiscrimination Doctrine, Feminist Theory and Antiracist Politics' (1989) 8(1) University of Chicago Legal Forum 139.

disadvantage.[79] Oppression and power, unlike social resources and burdens that are distributed, are structural, existing in everyday social processes and institutions, and do not solely arise from morally problematic behaviour.[80]

A specific kind of structural injustice arises in the context of knowledge and is referred to as epistemic injustice.[81] Although a recently coined philosophical term, the concept of epistemic injustice originally arises from the scholarship and activism of Black feminists. This particular form of injustice arises from the ways in which we are socialised to accept and understand certain forms of knowledge, authority, or testimony over others. The fact that women's pain is systematically disregarded in the medical encounter is a form of testimonial injustice that arises from how we all (and therefore healthcare professionals too) are socialised into viewing women's expression of pain and the importance it should be given. Other examples include the manner in which Black and marginalised women's suffering is often viewed with additional contempt, suspicion, and surveillance;[82] or the ways in which people with disability are systematically excluded from decision-making that pertains to their care.[83] In other words, our socially mediated understanding of individuals, their bodies, and how they live in the world also result in further silencing and discrimination.

2.6 CONCLUSION

In this chapter, we have explored various concepts, ideas, frameworks and values that lie at the core of doing bioethics. One way to approach bioethical problems, we suggest is to ask: who matters and what matters? The first of these two questions directs us to think about whose interests are at stake in a particular context and whose interests we need to attend to for their own sake. To this end we have explored the concepts of moral status and personhood. The second of these questions requires us to evaluate situations and decisions in terms of how they might give rise to benefits and harms. To equip us to make these kinds of assessments we have looked at the different ways in which well-being may be conceptualised, alongside as core concepts in bioethics such as health, autonomy, embodiment, and vulnerability.

A second aim of this chapter has been to survey how existing schools of Western moral philosophy have defined some of these core questions and ideas, and the characteristic ways in which they approach ethical problems, as well as the advantages and limitations of such approaches. We have suggested that such theories act best as critical lenses, allowing us to highlight important aspects of moral problems. Finally, we have explored the relevance of Western, liberal political philosophy and theories of justice in bioethical scholarship, as well as some critical approaches which problematise the dominant scholarship, from the perspectives of those who are systematically marginalised by the inherent ableism, sexism, and racism of well-established approaches to justice in bioethics. This chapter then presents a range of critical ideas, framings, and approaches in bioethics that students and researchers will generally encounter, as well as those that are shaping the bioethics discourse going forward.

---

[79] Madison Powers and Ruth Faden, *Structural Injustice: Power, Advantage and Human Rights* (OUP 2019).

[80] Iris Young, *Justice and the Politics of Difference* (Princeton University Press 1990).

[81] Miranda Fricker, *Epistemic Injustice: Power and the Ethics of Knowing* (OUP 2007).

[82] Yolanda Yvette Wilson, 'Bioethics, Race and Contempt' (2021) 18 Bioethical Inquiry 13–22.

[83] Jackie Leach Scully (n 77).

FURTHER READING

1. Alastair Campbell, *The Body in Bioethics* (Routledge-Cavendish 2009).

2. John Christman (ed.), *The Inner Citadel: Essays on Individual Autonomy* (OUP 1990).

3. Norman Daniels, *Just Health: Meeting Health Needs Fairly* (CUP 2007).

4. Helga Kuhse and Peter Singer (eds.), *A Companion to Bioethics* (2nd edn, Blackwell Publishing 2009).

5. Patricia Hill Collins and Sirma Bilge, *Intersectionality* (Polity Press 2016).

6. Michael Marmot and Richard Wilkinson (eds.), *Social Determinants of Health* (OUP 2005).

7. Martha Nussbaum and Amartya Sen (eds.), *The Quality of Life* (Clarendon Press 1993).

8. Miranda Fricker, *Epistemic Injustice: Power and the Ethics of Knowing* (OUP 2007).

9. Onora O'Neill, *Autonomy and Trust in Bioethics* (CUP 2002).

10. Madison Powers and Ruth Faden, *Structural Injustice: Power, Advantage and Human Rights* (OUP 2019).

11. Wendy Rogers et al. (eds.), *The Routledge Handbook of Feminist Bioethics* (Routledge 2022).

12. Jackie Leach Scully, *Disability Bioethics: Moral Bodies, Moral Difference* (Rowman and Littlefield 2008).

13. Iris Young, *Justice and the Politics of Difference* (Princeton University Press 1990).

3

THE GOVERNANCE OF THE HEALTH SYSTEM

3.1 INTRODUCTION

This chapter examines the governance of the health system in the UK. In the UK, there are four health services which are often referred to collectively as the 'National Health Service' (NHS). We use the term 'governance' in this context because it describes the way in which health systems cope with everyday challenges, new policies and problems, and the way in which decisions are made and implemented about the management and delivery of health care and related services.[1] In this context, governance also means taking account of political leaders who make and are accountable for health policy and services to legislatures, soft and hard law and regulation, institutional arrangements for the delivery of health services, and the role of key stakeholders from within the system such as patients and healthcare professionals (HCPs). Key aspects of health governance include accountability, transparency, participation of key stakeholders, integrity, and policy capacity.[2]

When things go wrong in the governance of health systems, it usually means that one of these aspects is not working well—or it is not working in the right way and as such may contribute to health inequities and poor health outcomes for patients,[3] as well as dissatisfaction on the part of the health workforce.[4] Law and regulation, at times underpinned by ethical considerations, are tools that are used by political leaders in seeking to reform aspects of health governance that do not work well. In this chapter, we first proceed with providing a general overview of the UK health system, which includes examining how health policy is made and how health decision-makers are held to account, what public bodies are involved in the health system, and how the health system is financed. Thereafter, we consider current constitutional arrangements in the UK which have resulted in the devolved administrations of Northern Ireland (NI), Scotland, and Wales now being responsible for health care and public health. We consider the nature and remit of this devolved health competence, its advantages and disadvantages, as well as the newly established internal market in the UK and its impact on health policy in the devolved administrations. We then turn to examine in more detail each of

---

[1] Scott Greer, Matthias Wiesmar, and Josep Figueras (eds), *Strengthening Health System Governance: Better Policies, Stronger Performance* (Open University Press 2016) 4–5.

[2] ibid.

[3] ibid 3; see also Ole Petter Ottersen et al., 'The Political Origins of Health Inequity: Prospects for Change' (2014) 383(9917) Lancet 630.

[4] See e.g. Peter Walker, 'Endemic Low Pay Threatens Future of NHS, Says Union Boss', *The Guardian* (17 October 2022); Benjamin Cooper, 'Two-thirds of Junior Doctors Considering Leaving NHS as Industrial Action Looms' *Evening Standard* (27 December 2022).

the healthcare services in England, NI, Scotland, and Wales, focusing on their values, organisational structure, specific health initiatives, and their approach to patient safety and quality improvement.

3.2 THE UK HEALTH SYSTEM

3.2.1 GENERAL OVERVIEW

The NHS was founded in 1948 as a publicly funded health service.[5] Access is determined on the basis of clinical need and not an individual's ability to pay,[6] and is available to all persons ordinarily resident in the UK.[7] It is now the largest such health service in the world and it also 'leads the world in terms of equity of access and ensuring people do not suffer financial hardship when they are ill'.[8] It also performs well in terms of managing a range of chronic conditions, like diabetes. However, it is comparatively under-resourced in terms of its overall funding, 'has markedly fewer doctors and nurses, and among the lowest number of hospital beds' and healthcare technologies among OECD countries (an organisation representing the 38 wealthiest countries in the world).[9] For NHS England, its budget for 2023/24 is £160.4 billion in cash terms, which has risen from £115.5 billion in 2013/14.[10] The NHS is also the fifth-largest employer in the world, with 1.7 million employees across the UK's four jurisdictions.[11] This is quite apart from the role played by general practitioners (GPs) and dentists, who are self-employed, but nevertheless contribute to the health service as well. In the 2000s, it was estimated that NHS activity amounted to seeing 1 million people every 36 hours, but this grew to 1.5 million people prior to the Covid-19 outbreak in 2020.[12]

All the UK's four health services are publicly funded and are often collectively referred to as the NHS. Scotland's NHS was established at the same time as the English and Wales NHS in 1948, although the Welsh NHS became separate from the English NHS in 1969. In NI, its publicly funded health service is known as Health and Social Care (HSC). The naming of the health service in this way in NI reflects the fact that health and social care

---

[5] Geoffrey Rivett, *The History of the NHS*, The Nuffield Trust, available at <https://www.nuffieldtrust.org.uk/health-and-social-care-explained/the-history-of-the-nhs> accessed 12 January 2023.

[6] See e.g. The NHS Constitution for England, updated 1 January 2021, Principle 2, available at <https://www.gov.uk/government/publications/the-nhs-constitution-for-england/the-nhs-constitution-for-england> accessed 12 January 2023.

[7] For exceptions to the principle of the NHS being free at point of access, see Department of Health and Social Care, 'NHS Visitor and Migrant Cost Recovery Programme', updated 8 October 2020, available at <https://www.gov.uk/government/collections/nhs-visitor-and-migrant-cost-recovery-programme> accessed 12 January 2023.

[8] Tim Gardner and Elaine Kelly, 'The NHS at 70: How Good is the NHS?' The Health Foundation, March 2018.

[9] ibid. See also Organisation for Economic Cooperation and Development, OECD Health Statistics 2022, available at <https://www.oecd.org/els/health-systems/health-data.htm> accessed 12 January 2023.

[10] Siva Anandaciva, 'The Autumn Budget 2022: What Has Been Announced and What Does it Mean for Health and Care Spending?' The King's Fund, 21 November 2022, available at <https://www.kingsfund.org.uk/blog/2022/11/autumn-budget-2022-announced-what-does-it-mean-health-and-care-spending> accessed 12 January 2023.

[11] BBC News, 'Which is the World's Biggest Employer?' 20 March 2012, available at <https://www.bbc.co.uk/news/magazine-17429786> accessed 12 January 2023.

[12] The King's Fund, 'Activity in the NHS', 23 October 2020, available at <https://www.kingsfund.org.uk/projects/nhs-in-a-nutshell/NHS-activity> accessed 12 January 2023.

have been formally merged since the 1970s.[13] Similarities between the four UK health systems include a high degree of service integration, low costs, effective gatekeeping, and planning (by international standards). They also share similar disadvantages, such as vulnerability to underfunding, a propensity towards centralisation, and regular rounds of organisational reform.[14] Where there has been clear convergence between the devolved administrations of NI, Scotland, and Wales is in relation to models of healthcare services and the financing of their health systems: they all share a 'basic integrated structure with territorial organisations that organise and provide integrated health services in their area.'[15] The divide between purchasers of care and providers of care that has been the core of NHS England since the late 1980s does not apply in Scotland and Wales. Both devolved administrations have large health boards that are the focus of policy and planning, with accountability resting with the boards, which in turn are responsible to their respective Ministers for Health. While NI technically preserves the purchaser-provide divide, its centralised commissioning process, which essentially functions like an arm of the NI Department of Health, means its 'divide' in this regard has been described as 'largely a distinction without a difference'.[16]

3.2.2 HEALTH POLICYMAKING

In the UK, the administrative and now constitutional devolution of health care has resulted in a significant level of delegation of decision-making and responsibility to a range of bodies and parts of the health system. In NHS England, for example, implementation of policy that has been arrived at by 'the centre' is unusually complex, involving a plethora of bodies, including local authorities, NHS (Foundation) Trusts and Integrated Care Systems (ICSs), and general practitioner (GP) practices. This is also reflected in each of the other jurisdictions, with each taking their own separate approach to health policy and delivery.[17] At the apex, the Secretary of State for Health and Social Care has specific duties and obligations in relation to the NHS, including having overall responsibility for financing delivery and performance in relation to the provision of healthcare services.[18] They report and are accountable to the UK Parliament, and there are specific committees which scrutinise various aspects of health policy, administration, and regulation in England. They include:

- the Health and Social Care Committee, which examines expenditure, administration, and policy-making;[19]

- the Public Accounts Committee, which reviews whether the NHS is run economically, efficiently, and effectively;[20] and

---

[13] Kelly Shuttleworth and Elspeth Nicholson, 'Devolution and the NHS', Institute for Government, 18 August 2020, available at <https://www.instituteforgovernment.org.uk/explainer/devolution-and-nhs> accessed January 2023.

[14] Scott Greer, 'Devolution and Health in the UK: Policy and Its Lessons Since 1998' (2016) 118(1) British Medical Bulletin 16; Srinivasa Katikreddi et al., 'Devolution of Power, Revolution in Public Health' (2017) 39(2) Journal of Public Health 241.

[15] ibid.

[16] ibid., 19, but see the discussion re the planned reforms to the NI health service later in this chapter.

[17] Expert Report to the Infected Blood Inquiry: Public Health and Administration, August 2022, 17–18 ('Expert Report: Public Health and Administration').

[18] See e.g. Health and Care Act 2022 (HCA 2022), Part 1, ss 40–47 and Part 3.

[19] UK Parliament, Health and Social Care Committee, available at <https://committees.parliament.uk/committee/81/health-and-social-care-committee/> accessed 12 January 2023.

[20] UK Parliament, Public Accounts Committee, available at <https://committees.parliament.uk/committee/127/public-accounts-committee/> accessed 12 January 2023.

- the Public Administration and Constitutional Affairs Committee,[21] which analyses the reports of the Parliamentary and Health Service Ombudsman which operates as an independent complaint handling service for complaints that have not been resolved by the NHS and UK government departments.[22]

This type of parliamentary scrutiny of health policy and administration is also mirrored in the devolved administrations of NI, Scotland, and Wales.[23]

The Department of Health and Social Care (DHSC) sits at the heart of health policy-making in England, although this has lessened since the creation of NHS England in 2012. Most of its annual budget is devolved to NHS England. On behalf of the Secretary of State for Health and Social Care, it is the only body with oversight of the whole English health system and acts as a 'system steward' to ensure that the system's various components coordinate to deliver on policy priorities,[24] including NHS England's Long Term Plan.[25] The DHSC also creates and updates the policy and legislative frameworks within which the health system operates, which is a departmental role that is mirrored in the UK's other jurisdictions. In Scotland, for example, it is known as the Health and Social Care Directorate; in Wales as the Welsh Health Department; and in NI, it is the Department of Health. Devolved administrations are much more directly involved in the management of their health services, with stronger ministerial oversight.[26] Policy development often involves a series of stages including the following: 'outlining the *rationale* behind the policy; defining the *objectives*; conducting an *appraisal* of policy options, *monitoring* and then *evaluating* the impact; and capturing that as *feedback* to inform future policies.'[27] Major decisions about which policies to pursue and when, or any that have novel spending implications, are usually made by ministers. Others might be delegated to senior civil servants, with executive agencies also delegated authority to act in certain policy areas.

Throughout the policymaking process, officials, and ministers draw on a range of expertise. Some of this is internal: the Chief Medical Officer plays a central role with respect to health policy, especially in supporting Ministerial decision making, and is in turn supported by deputies and a team of civil servants. In England, for example, much of it comes from outside the DHSC, which used to have a range of medical advisors that functioned in a parallel hierarchy to civil servants. It is now more common to

---

[21] UK Parliament, Public Administration and Constitutional Affairs Committee, available at <https://committees.parliament.uk/committee/327/public-administration-and-constitutional-affairs-committee/> accessed 12 January 2023.

[22] Parliamentary and Health Service Ombudsman, 'Who We Are', available at <https://www.ombudsman.org.uk/about-us/who-we-are> accessed 12 January 2023.

[23] See e.g. Northern Ireland Assembly, Committee for Health available at <http://www.niassembly.gov.uk/assembly-business/committees/2017-2022/health/> accessed 12 January 2023; Scottish Parliament, Health, Social Care and Sport Committee, available at <https://www.parliament.scot/chamber-and-committees/committees/current-and-previous-committees/session-6-health-social-care-and-sport-committee> accessed 12 January 2023; Welsh Parliament (Senedd Cymru), Health and Social Care Committee, available at <https://senedd.wales/committees/health-and-social-care-committee/> accessed 12 January 2023.

[24] Department of Health and Social Care, 'Guide to the Healthcare System in England', 3 May 2013, available at <https://www.gov.uk/government/publications/guide-to-the-healthcare-system-in-england> accessed 12 January 2023.

[25] NHS England, 'The NHS Long Term Plan', updated 21 August 2019, available at <https://www.longtermplan.nhs.uk/> accessed 12 January 2023.

[26] Expert Report: Public Health and Administration (n 17) 17.

[27] ibid., drawing on HM Treasury, Green Book, updated 18 November 2022, available at <https://www.gov.uk/government/publications/the-green-book-appraisal-and-evaluation-in-central-governent/the-green-book-2020> accessed 12 January 2023.

find such experts embedded in a range of arm's-length bodies (see 3.2.3) that support the Department and the work it does, including the Care Quality Commission (CQC), the National Institute for Health and Care Excellence (NICE), and the Medicines and Healthcare products Regulatory Agency (MHRA).[28] In addition, the Department also convenes a range of expert advisory committees which often bring greater specialist expertise to particular areas. They feed their advice back to the Chief Medical Officer, who then liaises with key policy officials and those in political leadership.[29]

Overall, though, there has been a gradual shift away from a centralised to a more local-ised approach, as well as towards delegating health policymaking and this has also been mirrored in institutional arrangements in the NHS. This delegation reflects the 'sheer complexity of the health system', which is seen as limiting the effectiveness of a central-ised approach to managing and improving health care.[30] This has been made even more complicated by the political preference towards regular organisational reform of the NHS, and a tendency towards the creation of 'silos' of policymakers and the use of experts in specific areas. There are examples of more centralised collaboration and cooperation in health policymaking, of which the management of the initial stages of the Covid-19 pandemic during the period 2020–21 is a clear example. However, over time the manage-ment of the pandemic has led to a more independent approach on the part of the devolved administrations in line with local political preferences and population needs.[31]

3.2.3 PUBLIC BODIES

There are a range of public bodies that play an important role in providing advice and undertaking specialist tasks or services in support of the health and care system in the UK. They are commonly referred to as the 'Arm's-Length Bodies' (ALB), a general term that is used to describe public bodies which have been established with a degree of auton-omy from the UK Secretary of State for Health, as well as Ministers for Health in the devolved administrations.[32] Reference will be made to specific ALBs in this and other chapters in the book, examples of which include the following:

- NHS England;
- CQC;
- NICE;
- Health Research Authority (HRA);

---

[28] DHSC, 'DHSC's Agencies and Partner Organisations', updated 6 October 2022, available at <https://www.gov.uk/government/publications/how-to-contact-department-of-health-arms-length-bodies/department-of-healths-agencies-and-partner-organisations> accessed 12 January 2023.

[29] Expert Report: Public Health and Administration (n 17) 18.

[30] Christopher Ham, *Governance of the Health and Care System in England: Creating the Conditions for Success*, NHS Confederation, February 2022, available at <https://www.nhsconfed.org/publications/governing-health-and-care-system-england> accessed 12 January 2023.

[31] Anne-Maree Farrell and Rhiannon Frowde, 'Scottish Covid-19 Inquiry: The Provision of Health and Social Care Services', Final Report, 1 March 2022, 15, available at <https://www.covid19inquiry.scot/introductory-academic-research> accessed 12 January 2023.

[32] There are three types of Arm's-Length Bodies: executive agencies, non-departmental public bod-ies and non-ministerial departments. See UK Government, Cabinet Office, 'Public Bodies', last updated 27 September 2022, available at <https://www.gov.uk/guidance/public-bodies-reform#arms-length-bodies> accessed 12 January 2023. Note that in Scotland, the preference is to refer to ALBs as 'public bodies', see Scottish Government, 'Public Bodies', available at <https://www.gov.scot/policies/public-bodies/> accessed 12 January 2023.

- NHS Blood and Transplant (NHSBT);

- MHRA;

- NHS Resolution;

- Human Fertilisation and Embryology Authority (HFEA);

- Human Tissue Authority (HTA).[33]

Specifically, under the Health and Care Act 2022 (HCA 2022), provision has now been made to enable a change or transfer of functions involving ALBs known as Non-Departmental Public Bodies (NDPBs). This is to enable more flexibility to adapt to changing or emerging priorities. However, there are certain NDPBs that will not be included in this legislative reform, such as the CQC and NICE, as well as the Health Service Safety Investigation Body (HSSIB) which is discussed later in this chapter.[34]

There are also ALBs that focus specifically on public health prevention and protection. As a result of several rounds of reform of public health policy, these bodies have been re-organised and even given new titles in recent years. In England, Public Health England (PHE) was created in 2013 to provide national oversight and leadership on public health protection issues. It was a relatively small, centralised agency, with most public health staff and public funds being transferred to local governments. In the wake of the Covid-19 pandemic and ongoing concerns on the part of the UK Government about its work, PHE has now been disbanded and replaced by two separate public health bodies. The first is the UK Public Health Security Agency, which operates as an executive agency sponsored by the DHSC. It is responsible for public health protection activities in relation to the impact of infectious diseases, chemical, biological, radiological and nuclear incidents, and other health threats.[35] The second is the Office for Health Improvement and Disparities (OHID), which is part of the DHSC, and is focused on public health promotion, as well as activities relating to addressing health disparities in England.[36]

In the devolved administrations, there are also separate public bodies for managing public health and protection activities.[37] In Scotland, for example, Public Health Scotland was established in April 2020, which consolidated several health functions into a single body. It is responsible for the public health domains of health protection and healthcare improvement and for providing services in respect of public health related research, development, training, and education. It also has a duty to promote the improvement of the physical and mental health of the people of Scotland, as well as addressing persistent inequalities in health outcomes.[38] Such bodies focus on health inequalities as part of their public health activities. This is particularly so in light of the fact that available evidence

---

[33] Department of Health and Social Care, 'DHSC's Agencies and Partner Organisations', updated 6 October 2022, available at <https://www.gov.uk/government/publications/how-to-contact-department-of-health-arms-length-bodies/department-of-healths-agencies-and-partner-organisations> accessed 12 January 2023.

[34] See HCA 2022 (n 18), Explanatory Notes, paras 130–136.

[35] UK Health Security Agency, 'What We Do', available at <www.gov.uk/government/organisations/uk-health-security-agency> accessed 12 January 2023.

[36] Office for Health Improvement and Disparities, 'What We Do', available at <www.gov.uk/government/organisations/office-for-health-improvement-and-disparities> accessed 12 January 2023.

[37] In Northern Ireland, see Public Health Agency, 'About Us', available at <https://www.publichealth.hscni.net/about-us> accessed 12 January 2023; in Wales, Public Health Wales, 'About Public Health Wales', available at <https://phw.nhs.wales/about-us/> accessed 12 January 2023.

[38] Public Health Scotland, 'Our Areas of Work' available at <www.publichealthscotland.scot/our-areas-of-work/> accessed 12 January 2023.

points to such inequalities widening and worsening within and across the UK's four jurisdictions.[39] In England, for example, life expectancy has stalled since 2010; this has not happened since at least 1900.[40] The amount of time people spend in poor health has also increased over the past ten years, with evidence of significant decreases in male and female life expectancy in the most deprived areas. In recognition of such developments, NHS England set out the key actions it planned to take to strengthen its contribution to addressing health inequalities in its Long Term Plan, published in 2019.[41] In 2021, the National Healthcare Inequalities Improvement Programme was also established to facilitate 'equitable access, excellent experience and optimal outcomes' for patients in NHS England, as well as creating a 'positive improvement culture' using data to 'reduce and prevent healthcare inequalities.'[42]

In 2022, the UK Government also published its White Paper on Levelling Up, which has an ambitious target of improving health life expectancy by five years by the year 2035, while narrowing the gap between the experience of the richest and poorest people.[43] Recent research published by the Health Foundation, however, has argued that on the basis of current evidence in relation to worsening health inequalities it would take 192 years to reach this government target. Instead, what was needed was a 'whole-of-government' approach, as well as a focus on the social determinants of health, in order to establish the baseline conditions for improving health.[44] This requires leadership on the part of not only UK public bodies responsible for public health promotion and protection but also political leaders.[45] For a detailed analysis of this and other issues in public health, see Chapter 7. Having provided an overview of key elements of the health system, we now turn to consider recent developments in relation to political devolution and its impact on the design and delivery of health care and related services in the UK.

3.3 DEVOLUTION AND HEALTH

When we speak of devolution and health, it is important to distinguish between the following: (i) *political devolution*, which involves the transfer of responsibility for health care to locally elected politicians in devolved administrations; (ii) *administrative devolution*, which involves the separate administration of health care, public health regimes, and policymaking within the UK's four jurisdictions, overseen by the same elected government based at Westminster; and (iii) *delegation*, which involves centralised policymaking

---

[39] In relation to the devolved administrations, see Adam Lang, 'Ambition and Long-Term Thinking Needed to Tackle Scotland's Health Inequalities', The Health Foundation, 15 December 2022; Northern Ireland Health Inequalities Annual Report 2022; Welsh NHS Confederation, Mind the Gap: What's Stopping Change? The Cost-of-Living Crisis and the Rise in Inequalities in Wales, July 2022.

[40] Michael Marmot et al., *Health Equity in England: The Marmot Review 10 Years On* (Health Foundation 2020).

[41] NHS England, 'The NHS Long Term Plan' (n 25).

[42] NHS England, 'National Healthcare Inequalities Improvement Programme', available at <https://www.england.nhs.uk/about/equality/equality-hub/national-healthcare-inequalities-improvement-programme/> accessed 12 January 2023.

[43] Department for Levelling Up, Housing and Communities, 'Levelling up the United Kingdom' February 2022, available at <https://www.gov.uk/government/publications/levelling-up-the-united-kingdom> accessed 12 January 2023.

[44] Emilie L'Hôte et al., *A Matter of Life and Death: Explaining the Wider Determinants of Health in the UK* (Health Foundation 2022).

[45] Jacqui Wise, 'Life Expectancy: Parts of England and Wales See Shocking Fall' (2022) 377 Lancet o1056.

at the UK Government level, with responsibility for policy implementation taking place at the devolved level. Administrative devolution is longstanding in the UK, whereas political devolution is a relatively new phenomenon.[46] Nevertheless, a brief historical overview is required of both administrative and political devolution arrangements if we are to understand current developments with respect to devolved health competence in the UK.

3.3.1 HISTORICAL OVERVIEW

From 1919 onwards, England and Wales were under the control and direction of the UK Secretary of State for Health. In contrast, Scottish health care remained under the control of the Secretary of State for Scotland. It therefore retained administrative devolution, which was separate from England and Wales, albeit with more central oversight. In 1921, responsibility for health care in NI was devolved to a new NI Parliament and government and civil service. When the NHS was founded in 1948, these arrangements remained in place with political devolution in NI, administrative devolution in Scotland, and no devolution in Wales.[47] Therefore, any claim to there being a truly national health service was not in fact the case in practice. Instead, there were three separate health services: England and Wales, Scotland, and NI. All were founded on similar principles (e.g. free at point of access based on need, not ability to pay), but they were formally established under separate pieces of legislation. In 1969, responsibility for health care in Wales was transferred to the Secretary of State for Wales. However, key policy regarding the design and provision of healthcare services continued to be made on an 'England and Wales' basis. From this point on, there was administrative devolution in Scotland, delegation of executive responsibilities in Wales, and political devolution in NI. This would change in the early 1970s with the imposition of direct rule by the UK Government following the eruption of violent sectarian conflict in NI.[48]

During the 1970s, further reorganisation of the healthcare services took place, with a regional-area and district health authority structure being established in England and Wales; the creation of 15 health boards in Scotland, with new local health councils, and the creation of an integrated structure for health and social care in NI. For the next 25 years, the three health services were 'administratively separate, albeit overseen by the same government based at Westminster. The Secretaries of State for Scotland, Wales, and NI were not answerable to the UK Secretary of State for Health' based at Westminster for their decisions in relation to health matters and a 'considerable degree of autonomy' was exercised by key decision-makers in both NI and Scotland.[49]

3.3.2 POLITICAL DEVOLUTION AND HEALTH COMPETENCE

In 1999, the next major development took place following referendums in NI, Scotland, and Wales, which led to the establishment of new devolved institutions. More recently, there have been calls for more political devolution from Westminster to the English regions. For example, some healthcare responsibilities have now been devolved to the Greater Manchester Combined Authority, which now controls the region's £6bn health and social care budget, as well as Cornwall as part of their 'devolution deals' with the UK Government.[50] Devolving further healthcare functions to

---

[46] Expert Report: Public Health and Administration (n 17) 31.   [47] ibid., 31–32.   [48] ibid., 32.
[49] ibid.   [50] Shuttleworth and Nicholson (n 13).

combined local authorities through negotiation with the UK Government continues to remain an option provided for under legislation.[51]

As a result of these recent shifts in political devolution arrangements, many health matters now come within the remit of the devolved administrations of NI, Scotland, and Wales. However, there are still some health matters that remain 'reserved' to Westminster. These include the regulation of healthcare professionals (HCPs), product safety and labelling, employment rights, and duties. Note that medicines and medical supplies and the standards for and testing of biological substances are not devolved in Scotland and Wales. In contrast, medicines and medical supplies are fully devolved in NI; however, legislation on matters relating to standards for, and testing of, biological substances still require the consent of the Secretary of State for Northern Ireland.[52]

Prior to the most recent shift towards political devolution, much of health policy was developed at Westminster and was then sought to be replicated across the UK, without much change to take account of local considerations. This has now changed, with the option of a more tailored approach enacted by locally elected politicians who may be more attuned to local needs. They are also likely to be much more locally accountable and subject to scrutiny by local media, as well as more able to listen to and respond to the concerns of patients and their families regarding access to, as well as delivery of, quality and safety in health care. Increased devolution has made coordination across the UK more challenging.[53] With different political parties in power in each of the UK's four administrations, it is inevitable that their health policies will move in different directions. Each devolved administration will have its own unique set of interests and concerns. Finding suitable mechanisms for managing such differences has proved problematic, as has been recently highlighted during the Covid-19 pandemic.[54]

3.3.3 FUNDING

Funding for the UK's four health systems is organised on the basis of an annual block grant to the devolved administrations, which consists of a baseline allocation, plus an annual increment. Each year the baseline consists of the total block grant from the previous year. What is known as the Barnett Formula determines the increment and reflects the change in spending in England, the extent to which the relevant English departmental programme is comparable with the services carried out by the devolved administration, and the proportion of the population in each devolved administration in relation to the appropriate one used for the UK Government's programmes.[55] Around 83% of total health spending in the UK is publicly funded. The remainder comes from direct payments for dental care, ophthalmic services, and private treatment in independent or NHS facilities.

---

[51] See Cities and Local Government Devolution Act 2016.
[52] Expert Report: Public Health and Administration (n 17) 32.   [53] ibid., 33–34.
[54] Akash Paun et al., 'Coronavirus and Devolution', Institute for Government, 1 July 2020, available at <https://www.instituteforgovernment.org.uk/explainers/coronavirus-and-devolution> accessed 12 January 2023.
[55] In 2019–20, for example, the application of the formula resulted in an allocation of £32bn to Scotland, £16bn to Wales and £12bn to Northern Ireland, before adjustments to account for tax devolution. See Institute for Government, 'The Barnett Formula', 5 November 2020, available at <https://www.instituteforgovernment.org.uk/explainers/barnett-formula> accessed 12 January 2023; Matthew Keep, The Barnett Formula and Fiscal Devolution, House of Commons Library, 11 July 2022, available at <https://commonslibrary.parliament.uk/research-briefings/cbp-7386/> accessed 12 January 2023.

This funding approach for the UK's health services, which makes use of the Barnett formula, has been subject to ongoing criticism. It was a formula that was created prior to recent political devolution arrangements which has resulted in increased health competence powers being granted to the devolved administrations. It has been suggested that it fails to properly consider socio-economic, demographic, geographic, and institutional variations across the UK. In England, for example, there is a divide between purchasers of care and providers of health care. This purchaser-provider divide does not exist in the devolved administrations of Scotland and Wales, and only formally so in NI.[56] What constitutes 'England-only' expenditure is pivotal but difficult to define, and fundamentally affects the freedom of choice available to devolved administrations in terms of how best to deliver health care in line with the needs of their respective populations.

3.3.4 THE INTERNAL MARKET

Of particular interest in the area of devolution and health is the development of an internal market structure post Brexit.[57] Pursuant to the UK Internal Market Act 2020, two key principles now guide access to the UK's internal market: mutual recognition and non-discrimination.[58] Mutual recognition for goods involves the principle that goods which have been produced in, or imported into, one part of the UK (originating part), and can be sold there without contravening any relevant requirements that would apply to their sale, should be able to be sold in any other part of the UK, free from any relevant requirements that would otherwise apply to the sale.[59] Non-discrimination for goods involves the principle that the sale of goods in one part of the UK (originating part) should not be affected by relevant requirements that directly or indirectly discriminate against goods (incoming goods) that have a relevant connection with another part of the UK (destination part).[60] Designed to 'prevent potentially harmful trade barriers', these principles apply not only to goods but also to services (Part 2) and professional qualifications (Part 3) under the Act.[61] In the area of health care services, the Act provides for exclusion of the two key market access principles in relation to healthcare services provided in hospitals, other healthcare facilities or at other places, xenotransplantation, human genetics, human fertilisation, embryology, and services in connection with surrogacy.[62] This is in addition to the exclusion of social services which may intersect with matters of health, or the social determinants of health, including social housing, childcare, adult social care, and support of families and persons permanently or temporarily in need.[63]

---

[56] Greer (n 14) 19.

[57] The term 'Brexit' is used to refer to the UK's withdrawal from the European Union, which took place on 31 January 2020. There was a transition period where the UK and the EU continued to negotiate over trade matters, which culminated in the EU-UK Trade and Cooperation Agreement which was signed on 30 December 2020. The Cooperation Agreement subsequently underwent further legal revision, being finalised in April 2021. For further details, see UK Government, Foreign, Commonwealth & Development Office, 'UK/EU and EAEC: Trade and Cooperation Agreement [TS No.8/2021]', last updated 8 June 2021, available at <https://www.gov.uk/government/publications/ukeu-and-eaec-trade-and-cooperation-agreement-ts-no82021> accessed 12 January 2023.

[58] Internal Market Act 2020, Part 1, ss 2–4 (mutual recognition) and ss 5–9 (non-discrimination).

[59] ibid., s 2(1).   [60] ibid., s 5(1) and (2).

[61] UK Government, Department for Business, Energy and Industrial Strategy, 'An Introduction to the UK Internal Market Act', updated 16 February 2022, available at <https://www.gov.uk/government/publications/complying-with-the-uk-internal-market-act-2020/an-introduction-to-the-uk-internal-market-act> accessed 12 January 2023.

[62] See UK Internal Market Act 2020, Sch 2, Parts 1 and 2.   [63] ibid.

Although it is early days in terms of implementing the Act, concerns have already been expressed about the levels of uncertainty that continue to exist about how the internal market will now operate in the context of devolved health competence. In the area of health care, particular concerns have been raised in relation to the range and type of pharmaceuticals and medical devices that will continue to be made available for patients, as well as how supply chains will operate in the internal market with respect to the supply of such goods.[64] This is made more complex in the case of NI. The border between NI and Ireland now represents the only land border between the UK and the European Union (EU). As part of Brexit, the UK Government and the EU reached agreement on how to deal with customs and related matters in the context of managing this border, which is set out in what is known as the Northern Ireland Protocol.[65] In order to avoid a potentially 'hard' border created by Brexit, the Protocol requires that goods produced or sold in NI should 'align with certain EU rules and regulations in order to allow goods to move freely across the island of Ireland'. In addition, the UK Government has agreed that it will be responsible for 'ensuring that checks take place on goods entering Northern Ireland from Great Britain to ensure they are compliant, creating barriers to intra-UK trade.'[66] This has the potential to impact the supply of healthcare goods, such as medicines and medical supplies, to NI.[67] In a post-Brexit world, there has been much ongoing debate about the merits or otherwise of the Protocol, with the UK Government arguing that it creates unacceptable barriers to trade within the UK internal market. In March 2023, the Windsor Framework was adopted, a UK–EU political agreement which amends the provisions of the original NI Protocol.[68] Once implemented, it aims to deliver a form of dual regulation which will facilitate NI's place in the UK's internal market, while also complying with relevant laws relating to the EU's Single Market, to which NI has 'unique access'.[69] In particular, 'all medicines placed on the market in NI will now be regulated by the UK regulator, the Medicines and Healthcare Products Regulatory Agency, rather than the EU's regulator, with all UK-approved medicines available for sale there'.[70]

Of particular concern to devolved administrations, such as Scotland and Wales, is whether these new internal market laws will result in market access principles overriding their existing competence with regards to policymaking and laws in the areas of healthcare services and public health. From their perspective, it represents an 'unwarranted

[64] See e.g. Jean McHale et al., 'Health Law and Policy, Devolution and Brexit' (2020) 55(9) Regional Studies 1561; Mark Dayan et al., *Going it Alone: Health and Brexit in the UK* (Nuffield Trust 2021) available at <https://www.nuffieldtrust.org.uk/research/going-it-alone-health-and-brexit-in-the-uk> accessed 12 January 2023.

[65] UK Government, Cabinet Office, Northern Ireland Protocol, last updated 5 January 2021, available at <https://www.gov.uk/government/publications/the-northern-ireland-protocol> accessed 12 January 2023.

[66] Maddy T Jack, 'Devolution: UK Internal Market', Institute for Government, 24 July 2020, available at <https://www.instituteforgovernment.org.uk/article/explainer/devolution-uk-internal-market> accessed 12 January 2023.

[67] See Dayan et al. (n 64); BBC News, 'NI Protocol: Medicine Supply Still Faces "Significant Issue"' 16 November 2022.

[68] UK Government, The Windsor Framework: A New Way Forward, updated 24 March 2023, available at <https://www.gov.uk/government/publications/the-windsor-framework> accessed 30 March 2023.

[69] European Commission, Protocol on Ireland and Northern Ireland, 24 March 2023, available at <https://commission.europa.eu/strategy-and-policy/relations-non-eu-countries/relations-united-kingdom/eu-uk-withdrawal-agreement/protocol-ireland-and-northern-ireland_en> accessed 30 March 2023.

[70] UK Parliament, House of Commons Library, Northern Ireland Protocol: The Windsor Framework, 21 March 2023, available at <https://commonslibrary.parliament.uk/research-briefings/cbp-9736/> accessed 30 March 2023.

attack on devolution' and the right of devolved legislatures to makes laws without inter-ference in areas of devolved competence.[71] With support from Scotland, Wales launched a constitutional challenge against the UK Government in relation to such laws.[72] Although the challenge was ultimately unsuccessful in the Supreme Court,[73] it points to ongoing tensions that exist between the UK Government and the devolved administrations over the control of policymaking and laws within areas of devolved competence, such as health care and public health, in a post-Brexit world.[74] It remains to be seen whether the recently established independent body, known as the Office for the Internal Market (OIM), will assist or frustrate relations between the UK Government and the devolved administra-tions over internal market regulatory initiatives going forward.[75] More generally, a range of concerns persist in relation to the medium to longer term impact of Brexit on health care in the UK. This was evidenced in a recently published report pointing to ongoing problems with regards to health and social care workforce and planning, given the dif-ficulties in recruiting and registering EU staff, as well as persistent medicines shortages, which it was suggested were likely to be associated with new trade barriers.[76] In the fol-lowing sections of the chapter, we examine each of the UK's health systems in more detail, focusing on values, organisational structure, specific health initiatives, and their respec-tive approaches to patient safety and quality improvement.

3.4 ENGLAND

The English NHS is a very large, complex organisation which is required to manage the healthcare needs of the English population, which currently stands at just under 57 million people, representing 84% of the UK's total population.[77] Funding for the NHS in England comes from the DHSC budget. In 2022/23, the DHSC's budget stood at £180.2 billion, with £152.6 billion in funding earmarked for NHS England for spend-ing on healthcare services.[78] The source of this funding is derived mainly from general taxation, which is supplemented by national insurance contributions. This is in addition

---

[71] See Welsh Government, Mick Antoniw MS, Counsel General and Minister for the Constitution, Written Statement: Legal challenge to the UK Internal Market Act 2020, 18 August 2022, available at <https://www.gov.wales/written-statement-legal-challenge-uk-internal-market-act-2020-0> accessed 12 January 2023.

[72] ibid.

[73] In *R (on the application of the Counsel General for Wales) (Appellant)* v *Secretary of State for Business, Energy and Industrial Strategy) (Respondent)* UKSC 2022/0055, the Supreme Court refused permission to appeal because the application did not raise an arguable point of law.

[74] See e.g. Scottish Government, 'After Brexit: The UK Internal Market Act and Devolution', 8 March 2021, available at <https://www.gov.scot/publications/brexit-uk-internal-market-act-devolution/pages/5/> accessed 12 January 2023. See generally Graeme Atkins and Grant Dalton, 'Devolved Public Services: The NHS, Schools, and Social Care in the Four Nations' Institute for Government, 20 April 2021, available at <https://www.instituteforgovernment.org.uk/publications/devolved-public-services> accessed 12 January 2023.

[75] UK Government, Department for Business, Energy & Industrial Strategy, 'Introduction to the UK Internal Market Act 2020', available at <https://www.gov.uk/government/publications/complying-with-the-uk-internal-market-act-2020/an-introduction-to-the-uk-internal-market-act> accessed 12 January 2023.

[76] Martha McCarey et al., *Health and Brexit: Six Years On* (Nuffield Trust 2022).

[77] UK Population Data, Population of England 2022, available at <https://populationdata.org.uk/population-of-england/> accessed 12 January 2023.

[78] The King's Fund, 'The NHS Budget and How It Has Changed', 8 December 2022, available at <https://www.kingsfund.org.uk/projects/nhs-in-a-nutshell/nhs-budget> accessed 23 January 2023.

to patient charges, which refers to charges for prescriptions and dental treatment, which were first introduced in the mid-twentieth century. Income from these types of patient charges represents just over 1% of the total DHSC budget. The level of funding provided to NHS England each year is determined by the UK Government as part of a spending review process, which considers what income the NHS is likely to generate and the extent to which further funds will be needed from general taxation to deliver healthcare services to the population of England. Apart from the provision of central funds, individual NHS organisations, such as hospital trusts, can generate their own income through parking charges, land sales, and treating private patients, for example.[79]

3.4.1 STRUCTURE AND ORGANISATION

The English NHS was established in 1948. Prior to the closing decades of the twentieth century, the medical profession enjoyed a high degree of autonomy in decision-making regarding clinical and managerial matters, which had been facilitated by the desire on the part of the state to have the support and participation of the medical profession in the work of the NHS. This was described as a situation of 'mutual dependency' between the state and the profession to encourage them to be part of a publicly funded health service.[80] From the 1980s onwards, however, this began to change, with a rise in managerialism under the then Thatcher Government, as well as a commitment to developing competition and fostering market incentives. In the early 1990s, this led to the introduction of an internal market in the NHS, which involved a purchaser-provider split, where health authorities were required to 'purchase' healthcare services from NHS Trusts.[81]

From this period onwards, the NHS also underwent successive waves of restructuring. At times this involved a shift towards centralisation, whereas at other times it led to a swing back towards decentralisation. There is a range of national and local bodies both internal and external to the NHS that contribute to both the provision and oversight of its delivery of healthcare services. There are integrated care systems (ICSs) which plan and commission care for local populations within given geographical areas, as well as primary care organisations, which are independent contractors offering NHS health care services such as GP practices, dental practices, and opticians. Within the NHS itself, there are organisational and legal entities known as NHS Trusts, which deal with both general and specialist healthcare activities within a given geographical area. They are also allowed to offer private health care or extra amenities to NHS patients for a fee. They can also borrow money within agreed limits, but they must be spent in line with Trusts' statutory powers, which translates into not making a profit as a result of such spending. Different types of NHS Trusts include the following:

- acute (hospital) trusts, which provide hospital-based NHS services;
- mental health trusts, which offer mental health and social care services;

---

[79] The King's Fund, 'How the NHS Is Funded', 1 March 2021, available at <https://www.kingsfund.org.uk/projects/nhs-in-a-nutshell/how-nhs-funded> accessed 23 January 2023.

[80] Rudolf Klein, 'The State and the Profession: The Politics of the Double Bed' (199) 301 British Medical Journal 700; Michael Moran, *Governing the Health Care System: A Comparative Study of the United Kingdom, the United States and Germany* (Manchester University Press 1999).

[81] For an historical overview of such developments, see David Hughes and Peter Vincent Jones, 'Schisms in the Church: National Health Service Systems and Institutional Divergence in England and Wales' (2008) 49(4) Journal of Health and Social Behavior 400.

- community trusts, which provide healthcare services such as district nursing, physiotherapy, as well as speech and language therapy; and

- ambulance trusts, which provide transportation services emergency and non-emergency care within the NHS.

Another type of NHS Trust is known as a Foundation Trust, which is described in enabling legislation as a 'public benefit corporation'.[82] Foundation Trusts have been designed to have much more financial and organisational freedom, so as to allow them to offer more tailored services to patients using their services in their area. While much has been promised with respect to achieving Foundation Trust status, it has proved to be somewhat different in practice. In recent years, they have been subject to increasing centralised control, particularly in relation to financial matters and how they deliver healthcare services. As a result, Foundation Trusts have been described as inhabiting 'a precarious halfway house between the public and private sectors: independent corporations on paper yet entirely dependent on the state in reality—for funding, capital investment and bailouts when things went wrong.'[83] Although the UK Government had anticipated that all NHS Trusts would eventually become NHS Foundation Trusts, this has not in fact happened. As things stand, at least a third of all Trusts do not have foundation status and this is likely to remain the case. In the circumstances, the HCA 2022 has repealed earlier legislative provisions which provided for the abolition of NHS Trusts.[84] The 2022 Act now permits the continuation of legislative provisions applicable to such Trusts, including the power to establish new Trusts. The DHSC views this legislative flexibility as important, as it considers that applications are likely to be made from integrated care boards to the Secretary of State for Health and Social Care (SSHSC) to establish new NHS Trusts in the future.[85]

The latest organisational reform of the NHS in England took place in 2022.[86] It brought together a number of bodies, such as the NHS Commissioning Board, Monitor, the NHS Trust Development Authority, and NHS Improvement into a single body called NHS England.[87] The rationale for this structural reform was to 'provide national leadership which speaks with one voice to providers, commissioners and local health systems; to remove potential duplication; and to use collective resources more efficiently and effectively to support local health systems and ultimately make effective use of public money.'[88] New powers were also given to the SSHSC to intervene in local service provision, but it is limited to complex and substantial changes to services, although concerns have been expressed at the potential for high-level ministerial involvement in local service changes and to delay decisions about any such changes.[89] The SSHSC also now has the power to direct NHS England to take action beyond the objective set out in the NHS Mandate, which is the annual list of priorities that the DHSC issues to NHS England and for which NHS England is accountable.[90] Again, concerns have been expressed as to how this might

[82] National Health Service Act 2006, Sch 7.
[83] Ben Collins, 'The Foundation Trust Model: Death by A Thousand Cuts' The King's Fund, 15 February 2016, available at <https://www.kingsfund.org.uk/blog/2016/02/foundation-trust-model> accessed 12 January 2023.
[84] See Health and Social Care Act 2012, Part 4, s 179.
[85] HCA 2022, Explanatory Notes, paras 69 and 70.   [86] HCA 2022, Part 1, ss 18–32.
[87] ibid., ss 33–39.   [88] HCA 2022, Explanatory Notes, paras 11 and 12.
[89] See The King's Fund, 'Integrated Care Systems: How Will They Work Under the Health and Care Act?' 23 May 2022, available at <https://www.kingsfund.org.uk/audio-video/integrated-care-systems-health-and-care-act> accessed 12 January 2023.
[90] As to the legislative requirements for the NHS Mandate, see NHS Act 2006, s 13A. More generally, see UK Government, NHS Mandate 2022/23, last updated 30 June 2022, available at <https://www.gov.uk/government/publications/nhs-mandate-2022-to-2023> accessed 12 January 2023.

work in practice, including the potential for interfering with the operational and clinical independence of NHS England.[91] In addition, further powers have also now been given to the SSHSC to require that NHS England take on public health functions. This offers the potential to facilitate better liaison between NHS England and public health and social care bodies in order to 'support integration and tackle broader priorities such as health inequalities'.[92]

The key organisational reform has been the creation of ICSs, which are designed to promote further integration of health and social care in England.[93] On 1 July 2022, NHS England formally established 42 statutory integrated care boards (ICBs)[94] as part of creating ICSs. Each ICS now has an ICB, which is a statutory NHS organisation responsible for developing a plan in collaboration with NHS (Foundation) Trusts and other system partners for meeting the health needs of the population, managing the NHS budget, and arranging for the provision of health services in its defined area. This means that what were previously known as Clinical Commissioning Groups (CCGs), which had responsibility for many of the aforementioned tasks, were closed down on 1 July 2022, when ICBs were established on a statutory basis.[95]

ICSs are partnerships that bring providers and commissioners of NHS services across a geographical area together with local authorities and other local partners to collectively plan health and care services to meet the needs of their local population. Each ICS is now made up of an ICB and an integrated care partnership (ICP). ICBs are responsible for commissioning and oversight of most NHS services and will be accountable to NHS England for NHS spending and performance. ICPs will bring together a wider range of partners, not just the NHS, to develop a plan to address the broader health, public health, and social care needs of the population for which they are responsible within a given area. ICSs can also choose to work alongside local authorities and other partners to address the wider determinants of health. Much of the work undertaken by ICPs to integrate care and improve population health will be driven by organisations collaborating in a flexible way over smaller geographies within ICSs, referred to as 'places'. They will work through teams delivering services working together on even smaller footprints, usually referred to as 'neighbourhoods'.[96] For an overview of how ICSs will operate, see **Figure 3.1**.

---

[91] The King's Fund (n 87).

[92] HCA 2022, Explanatory Notes, para 55.

[93] The HCA 2022 gives effect to the NHS's recommendations for legislative reform set out in the NHS Long Term Plan and the DHSC White Paper: Integration and Innovation: Working Together to Improve Health and Social Care for All, 2021, available at <https://www.gov.uk/government/publications/working-together-to-improve-health-and-social-care-for-all/integration-and-innovation-working-together-to-improve-health-and-social-care-for-all-html-version> accessed 12 January 2023.

[94] See HCA 2022, Part 1 ss 18–32. Pursuant to the Integrated Care Boards (Establishment) Order 2022, under s 14Z25 of the NHS Act 2006 (as inserted by the HCA 2022), NHS England established the 42 ICBs with effect from 1 July 2022. The Order specifies the name and area of each ICB, which are also included in each board's constitution, and gives legal effect to the constitutions, see NHS England, 'Integrated Care in Your Area', available at <https://www.england.nhs.uk/integratedcare/integrated-care-in-your-area/> accessed 12 January 2023.

[95] ibid.

[96] See 'Integrated care systems: how will they work under the Health and Care Act?' on The King's Fund website. Available at <www.kingsfund.org.uk/audio-video/integrated-care-systems-health-and-care-act> accessed 26 January 2023.

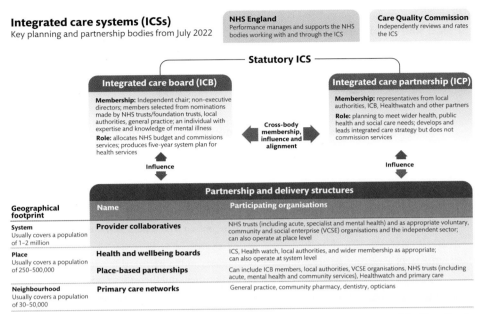

Figure 3.1 Integrated Care Systems in England[97]

3.4.2 THE NHS CONSTITUTION

The NHS Constitution for England sets out rights for patients, public, and staff, outlining NHS commitments to patients and staff, and the responsibilities that the public, patients, and staff owe to one another to ensure that the NHS operates fairly and effectively. All NHS bodies and private and third sector providers supplying NHS services are required by law to take account of the constitution in their decisions and actions.[98] In line with principle 7 of the Constitution, the DHSC publishes an accountability statement which explains how decision-making works in the NHS, which is set out in the Guide to the Healthcare System in England, which is updated annually.[99] The complaints guidance explains how patients can give feedback or make a complaint about NHS care or treatment. It includes information on the NHS complaints arrangements, and what patients can expect when they make a complaint and how it should be read in conjunction with the NHS Constitution.[100] The DHSC has also produced further detailed guidance on how the values and principles in the NHS Constitution work in practice. It is set out in the NHS Constitution Handbook and covers the values and the principles that guide the NHS; it

---

[97] ibid.

[98] NHS Constitution for England, last updated on 1 January 2021, available at <https://www.gov.uk/government/publications/the-nhs-constitution-for-england> accessed 12 January 2023.

[99] DHSC, 'Guide to the Healthcare System in England', available at <https://www.gov.uk/government/publications/guide-to-the-healthcare-system-in-england> accessed 12 January 2023.

[100] Note that NHS England handles complaints in line with the Local Authority Social Services and NHS Complaints Regulations 2009. For an overview, see NHS England Complaints Policy, last updated 16 November 2021, available at <https://www.england.nhs.uk/publication/nhs-england-complaints-policy/> accessed 12 January 2023.

also provides explanations of the rights and pledges in the NHS Constitution; identifies the legal sources of patient and staff rights; and sets out the roles the public, patients, carers, families, and the NHS play in protecting and developing the NHS.[101] The NHS Constitution is required to be renewed every ten years. In the Constitution, there are seven key principles that guide NHS England, which are set out in the following section.

NHS Constitution for England: Seven Key Principles

1. The NHS provides a comprehensive service, available to all irrespective of gender, race, disability, age, sexual orientation, religion, or belief.

2. Access to NHS services is based on clinical need, not an individual's ability to pay.

3. The NHS aspires to the highest standards of excellence and professionalism.

4. NHS services must reflect the needs and preferences of patients, their families, and their carers.

5. The NHS works across organisational boundaries and in partnership with other organisations in the interest of patients, local communities, and the wider population.

6. The NHS is committed to providing best value for taxpayers' money and the most effective, fair, and sustainable use of finite resources.

7. The NHS is accountable to the public, communities, and patients that it serves.

There are also six values that all NHS staff are expected to demonstrate: (i) working together for patients; (ii) respect and dignity; (iii) commitment to quality of care; (iv) compassion; (v) improving lives; and (vi) everyone counts. The Constitution sets out legal rights for patients and what they can do if they do not receive access to such rights. The sources of the identified rights are a mix of common law (law of negligence, administrative law, and case law), Acts of Parliament, and Regulations, although the extent to which these rights are legally enforceable is not clear. The Constitution also contains pledges that the NHS is committed to achieving, but they are not legally binding or enforceable. The pledges are set out on a thematic basis. Particular rights are linked with each identified theme, which include access to health services, quality of care and environment, nationally approved treatments, drugs and programmes, respect, consent and confidentiality, informed choice, involvement in one's health care and in the NHS, and complaints and redress.

By way of example, the theme of complaints and redress, the latter of which is examined in more detail in Chapter 12, makes clear individuals have the right to have any complaint made about NHS services dealt with efficiently and to have it properly investigated and to know the outcome of any investigation into a complaint. There is also a right to bring a judicial review if a person considers that they have been directly affected by an unlawful act or decision of an NHS body. Finally, a person has the right to compensation where they have been harmed by negligent treatment. As part of the commitment to redress where appropriate, it also commits the NHS to treating individuals with courtesy and to ensuring that they receive appropriate support throughout the handling of a complaint. Where individuals do make a complaint, a pledge is made that this will not adversely affect their future medical

---

[101] DHSC, Handbook to the NHS Constitution for England, last updated 27 January 2022, available at <https://www.gov.uk/government/publications/supplements-to-the-nhs-constitution-for-england> accessed 12 January 2023.

treatment. Additional pledges make up what would be understood as a redress package includes the following: when mistakes happen, they will be acknowledged; apologies and explanations should be provided as to what went wrong; and things should be put right quickly and effectively. In addition, NHS organisations should learn lessons from complaints and claims, and use such lesson-learning to improve NHS services.

The Constitution also makes clear that patient rights are accompanied by responsibilities as well. It is a matter which has been subject of academic commentary, where it has been argued that while it is important to show due respect for patient autonomy in the context of rights talk, account should also be taken of moral (if not legal) responsibilities that should accompany respect for patient rights.[102] On this issue, the Constitution broadly states that 'the NHS belongs to all of us. There are things that we can all do for ourselves and for one another to help it work effectively, and to ensure resources are used responsibly.'[103] This includes treating NHS staff and other patients with respect; recognising that causing a nuisance or disturbance on NHS premises could result in prosecution; providing accurate information about one's health, condition, and status; and attending appointments or cancelling within a reasonable period of time. Patients should follow the agreed course of treatment, and talk to their treating clinician if this is proving difficult to do. They should also offer feedback, whether positive or negative, about the treatment and care they have received, including any adverse reactions experienced. Finally, it is emphasised that patients should participate in important public health programmes, such as vaccination, and advise family and friends regarding their views on organ donation.[104] Recently, academic commentators have argued that it is time to revisit the values and rights espoused in the NHS Constitution to offer a more relational approach 'within which the rights and responsibilities of NHS stakeholders (patients, the public, and members of NHS staff) are experienced and enacted, and the values that inform them.' This would lead to greater emphasis being place on solidarity and care in order to address concerns about growing health inequalities which have only been exacerbated as a result of the Covid-19 pandemic.[105] It remains to be seen whether such arguments will find traction in future iterations of the Constitution.

3.4.3 PATIENT SAFETY AND QUALITY IMPROVEMENT

The promotion of patient safety and quality improvement have long been priorities within the NHS in England, with the publication of successive strategic plans over the decades designed to enhance patient safety culture, improve systems learning from patient safety incidents, and to minimise the occurrence of such incidents.[106] This is in addition to establishing mechanisms for inspections and regulation of quality improvement in the delivery of healthcare services involving both the NHS and the independent (private)

---

[102] For academic commentary on the relationship between patient rights and responsibilities, see Heather Draper and Tom Sorell, 'Patients' Responsibilities in Medical Ethics' (2002) 16(4) Bioethics 335; Margaret Brazier, 'Do No Harm: Do Patients Have Responsibilities Too?' (2006) 65(2) Cambridge Law Journal 397.

[103] NHS Constitution for England (n 96).   [104] ibid.

[105] Caroline A.B. Redhead et al., 'Relationships, Rights and Responsibilities: (Re)viewing The NHS Constitution for the Post-Pandemic "New Normal"' Medical Law Review, published 25 August 2022, <https://doi.org/10.1093/medlaw/fwac028>.

[106] For an historical overview, see UK Department of Health, *An Organisation with a Memory: Report of an Expert Group on Learning from Adverse Events in the NHS* (TSO 2000). With regard to medical errors, see Alan Merry and Warren Brookbanks, *Merry and McCall Smith's Errors, Medicine and the Law* (2nd edn, CUP 2017).

sector. In recent decades, policy and regulatory developments in relation to patient safety and quality improvement have been driven in part by an upsurge in healthcare scandals in England, with successive reports highlighting episodes of substandard health care being provided to patients, resulting in injury and/or death.[107] For example, recommendations from one such inquiry (otherwise known as the Francis or Mid-Staffs Inquiry) led to legal reform involving the reorganisation of regulation of health and social care in England, as well as the creation of a statutory organisational duty of candour which was designed to promote greater transparency and accountability on the part of NHS bodies towards patients who had suffered harm in healthcare settings.[108] Avoidable deaths of patients arising from episodes of substandard healthcare have also acted as catalysts for examining the combination of both individual and systemic failings that led to such episodes. Recent reviews have emphasised the need to shift away from a no-blame culture in response to episodes of substandard health care, towards a focus on promoting a 'just culture'.[109] Fostering such a culture is aimed at creating a fairer, compassionate, and more accountable approach to patient safety,[110] as well as promoting improvements in quality and safety in healthcare settings at the local level.[111]

In NHS England, patient safety is viewed as central to the 'NHS's definition of quality in healthcare, alongside effectiveness and patient experience'.[112] There is a recognition that healthcare errors occur, but there is a need to focus on minimising their occurrence. The aim of NHS England's current patient safety strategy is to facilitate continuous improvements, building on the foundations of a safer culture and safer systems.[113] No specific targets have been set, but regular reporting mechanisms are provided for in line with the strategy, which is underpinned by three strategic aims:[114]

- improving understanding of safety by drawing intelligence from multiple sources of patient safety information (Insight);

- equipping patients, staff and partners with the skills and opportunities to improve patient safety throughout the whole system (Involvement); and

- designing and supporting programmes that deliver effective and sustainable change in the most important areas (Improvement).

---

[107] See e.g. Bill Kirkup, 'The Report of the Morecambe Bay Investigation', March 2015 (TSO 2015); Mazars Group, 'Independent Review of Deaths of People with a Learning Disability or Mental Health Problem in Contact with Southern Health NHS Foundation Trust April 2011 to March 2015', 16 December 2015; Gosport War Memorial Hospital, 'The Report of the Gosport Independent Panel', HC 1084, June 2018; 'Findings, Conclusions and Essential Actions From the Independent Review of Maternity Services at the Shrewsbury and Telford NHS Trust: Our Final Report', 30 March 2022 (HMSO 2022) (Ockenden Review).

[108] See Report of the Mid Staffordshire NHS Foundation Trust Public Inquiry, HC 947 (Chair: Mr Robert Francis QC) (TSO 2013). Part of the rationale for the statutory organisational duty of candour is to improve patient safety culture within the NHS, which is examined in more detail in Chapter 4.

[109] See e.g. Department of Health, 'Gross Negligence Manslaughter in Healthcare: The Report of a Rapid Policy Review' (Department of Health 2018) (Williams Review); General Medical Council, 'Independent Review of Gross Negligence Manslaughter and Culpable Homicide', June 2019 (Hamilton Review).

[110] For an overview of the principles underpinning the creation of a just culture in healthcare settings, see Sidney Dekker, *Just Culture: Restoring Trust and Accountability in Your Organization* (3rd edn, CRC Press 2016).

[111] See NHS England, 'Just Culture Guide', available at <https://www.england.nhs.uk/patient-safety/a-just-culture-guide/> accessed 12 January 2023.

[112] ibid., 6.

[113] NHS England and NHS Improvement, 'The NHS Patient Safety Strategy: Safer Culture, Safer Systems, Safer Patients', July 2019, available at <https://www.england.nhs.uk/patient-safety/the-nhs-patient-safety-strategy/> accessed 12 January 2023.

[114] ibid., 4.

Each of the strategic aims are underpinned by a series of specific actions to be achieved. It is estimated that continuous improvement in line with the strategic aims could produce the following outcomes from 2023/24 onwards:[115]

> Better incident reporting and response could save an extra 160 lives and £13.5 million. If boosting patient safety understanding and capability reduces harm by a modest 2%, an extra 200 lives and £20 million could be saved. Focusing improvement programmes on those areas where most harm is seen could save 568 lives and £65 million. This adds up to 928 lives saved and £98.5 million more available for care per year. It is not possible to quantify all the potential benefits, so this impact will likely be greater . . . In addition, the potential exists to reduce the claims provision related to neonatal brain damage incidents by around £750 million per year by 2025 (based on current prices).

In order to achieve these outcomes, the strategy recognises that it will be necessary to bring about a culture change, which moves away from fear and blame of NHS staff in relation to patient safety incidents. In line with a focus on promoting 'just cultures',[116] it recognises that while individual HCPs should be held to account for their actions, this needs to take place in a psychologically safe environment where they know 'they will be treated fairly and compassionately if things go wrong or they speak up to stop problems occurring'.[117] It also involves a recognition that HCPs 'operate in complex systems, with many factors influencing the likelihood of error. These factors include medical device design, volume of tasks, clarity of guidelines and policies, and behaviour of others.'[118] In the circumstances, both individual and systems factors should be taken into account in the pursuit of patient safety strategies.

In terms of implementation of the strategy, recent developments have included the appointment of over 700 patient safety specialists at NHS Trusts and independent healthcare services to provide leadership in the area, as well as to oversee and support patient safety activities across their respective organisations;[119] the publication of a new framework for involving patients in patient safety,[120] along with a major upgrade of the recording of patient safety incidents via the Learn from Patient Safety Events Service (LFPSE);[121] and the establishment of the Patient Safety Incident Response Framework (PSIRF) in August 2022. The PSIRF replaced the earlier Serious Incident Framework and will involve a new approach to how NHS bodies should respond to patient safety incidents for the purpose of learning and improvement.[122]

In 2022, the office of the Patient Safety Commissioner was established in response to the report of the Cumberlege Review. Formally known as the Independent Medicines and Medical Devices Safety Review,[123] the Review examined the response of NHS England to patients' reports of harm from drugs and medical devices. The Review panel spoke to over 700 affected individuals, held oral hearings, and received evidence from manufacturers,

---

[115] ibid., 6–7.   [116] ibid., 7.   [117] ibid., 8.   [118] ibid., 8.

[119] NHS England, 'Identifying Patient Safety Specialists', 26 August 2020, available at <https://www.england.nhs.uk/publication/identifying-patient-safety-specialists/> accessed 12 January 2023.

[120] NHS England, 'Framework for Involving Patients in Patient Safety 2021', available at <https://www.england.nhs.uk/patient-safety/framework-for-involving-patients-in-patient-safety/> accessed 12 January 2023.

[121] NHS England, 'The NHS Patient Safety Strategy, Strategy Implementation Updates', available at <https://www.england.nhs.uk/patient-safety/the-nhs-patient-safety-strategy/> accessed 12 January 2023.

[122] NHS England, 'Patient Safety Incident Response Framework (PSIRF)', available at <https://www.england.nhs.uk/patient-safety/incident-response-framework/> accessed 12 January 2023.

[123] 'First Do No Harm: The Report of the Independent Medicines and Medical Devices Safety Review', 8 July 2020 available at <https://www.immdsreview.org.uk/> accessed 12 January 2023.

clinicians, and other stakeholders. In its report, it identified a range of systemic issues in relation to how the NHS handled patient safety, finding it 'disjointed, siloed, unresponsive and defensive'.[124] This was combined with a dismissive attitude toward patients, underpinned by a reluctance in all parts of the healthcare system to collect evidence on potential harms; a lack of coordination that would allow HCPs and other health agencies to interpret and act on that information; and a culture of denial that failed to acknowledge harm and error, impeding learning and safety.[125] One of the Review's principal recommendations was for an independent Patient Safety Commissioner (PSC) to be appointed to address these concerns. The PSC would be:[126]

> a person of standing who sits outside the healthcare system, accountable to Parliament through the Health and Social Care Select Committee. The Commissioner would be the patients' port of call, listener and advocate, who holds the system to account, monitors trends, encourages and requires the system to act. This person would be the golden thread, tying the disjointed system together in the interests of those who matter most.

In response to the Review's findings and recommendations, the UK Government offered an apology on behalf of the NHS to the patients and families who had been affected by the specific case studies under examination by the review,[127] and accepted the Review's recommendation regarding the need for an independent PSC to be appointed with statutory responsibility to act as a champion of patient safety in England.[128]

In 2021, legislation was passed to create the PSC, as well as setting out a range of powers associated with the role. The PSC is an independent statutory office holder, funded by the DHSC and appointed by the SSHSC.[129] The Commissioner's core duties are to promote the safety of patients with regard to the use of medicines and medical devices, as well as to promote the importance of the views of patients and other members of the public in relation to the safety of medicines and medical devices.[130] The PSC's statutory functions include the power to make reports or recommendations and the power to request and share information with relevant persons.[131] The PSC will also be under an obligation to publish a set of principles to govern the way in which they carry out their core duties,[132] and will be required to take steps to consult patients and to ensure that patients are aware of their role.[133] Regulations will be made setting out further details about the appointment and operation of the Commissioner, which will be consulted on. Regulations may require the Commissioner to lay documents before Parliament and prepare reports. In combination, this means that the regulations could, for example, require the Commissioner to lay an annual report before Parliament and specify what that report should cover.[134] The expectation is that the PSC will be provider-neutral, able to exercise these powers in relation to both the NHS and the independent sector. It will enhance the work undertaken in

---

[124] ibid., ii.   [125] ibid., paras 1.18–1.19.

[126] ibid., ii. For a critical analysis of the findings from the Cumberlege Review, see Helen Haskell, 'Cumberlege Review Exposes Stubborn and Dangerous Flaws in Healthcare' (2020) 370 BMJ m30999.

[127] Department of Health and Social Care, Government Response to the Report of the Independent Medicines and Medical Devices Safety Review, 26 July 2021, available at: <https://www.gov.uk/government/publications/independent-medicines-and-medical-devices-safety-review-government-response> accessed 12 January 2023. With regard to patient reflections on the Cumberlege Review Report, see Department of Health and Social Care, 'The Independent Report of the Patient Reference Group: Response to the IMMDS Review Report', 21 July 2021, available at: <https://www.gov.uk/government/publications/the-independent-report-of-the-patient-reference-group-response-to-the-immds-review-report> accessed 12 January 2023.

[128] ibid.   [129] Medicines and Medical Devices Act 2021 (MMDA 2021), s 1(1).

[130] ibid., s 1(2).   [131] ibid., Sch 1, s 3.   [132] ibid., Sch 1, s 1.   [133] ibid., Sch 1, s 2.

[134] ibid., Sch 1, s 6.

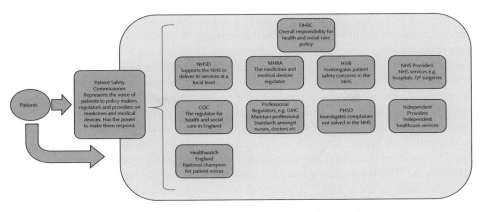

Figure 3.2 Patient Safety Commissioner and Representation of Patients' Voices

quality improvement, by focusing on the voice of patients and improvements to patient safety for medicines and medical devices.[135] The first PSC was appointed in mid-2022 and is in the process of establishing their office and plans in line with their statutory powers.[136] An overview of the way in which the PSC will liaise with other NHS bodies, but also contribute to ensuring that patients' voices and experiences are taken account of by such bodies, is set out in **Figure 3.2**.[137]

The Health Services Safety Investigations Body (HSSIB) has also been established as an independent statutory body which is responsible for conducting high-level investigations into qualifying patient safety incidents in NHS England, as well as the independent healthcare sector.[138] Qualifying incidents are defined as incidents that occur in England during the provision of healthcare services and have or may have implications for the safety of patients.[139] It will be a matter for the HSSIB to determine which qualifying incidents it will investigate, although this is subject to the SSHSC directing that an investigation be carried out in relation to a particular qualifying incident.[140] In addition to investigating qualifying incidents, the HSSIB is also responsible for promoting systems learning arising from the findings of its investigations through recommendations to be made in its reports.[141] Those NHS Trusts and independent healthcare services which are subject to HSSIB investigations will be required to respond to the report findings and recommendations within a specified period of time which must be set out by the HSSIB.[142]

---

[135] See Department of Health and Social Care, 'Factsheet: Patient Safety Commissioner', 25 January 2021, available at <https://www.gov.uk/government/publications/medicines-and-medical-devices-bill-overarching-documents/medicines-and-medical-devices-bill-patient-safety-commissioner> accessed 12 January 2023.

[136] Department of Health and Social Care, 'First Ever Patient Safety Commissioner Appointed', 12 July 2022, available at <https://www.gov.uk/government/news/first-ever-patient-safety-commissioner-appointed> accessed 12 January 2023.

[137] ibid.

[138] HCA 2022 (n 18), Part 4, s 109. For an overview of planned reforms in the area, see DHSC, Health and Care Bill: Health Services Safety Investigations Body, updated 10 March 2022 available at <https://www.gov.uk/government/publications/health-and-care-bill-factsheets/health-and-care-bill-health-services-safety-investigations-body> accessed 12 January 2023.

[139] HCA 2022, s 110(1).

[140] ibid., s 111 (1) and (2). However, the HSSIB will be required under s 112 to publish its criteria, processes and principles which will inform which qualifying incidents will be investigated.

[141] ibid., ss 110(2) and (3); see also ss 113 and 114 in relation to the provision of interim and final reports.

[142] ibid., s 116(3).

The plan is for the HSSIB to conduct investigations using a statutory 'safe space' approach, which prohibits unauthorised disclosure of protected material which form part of its investigations. This is to ensure that participants can provide information for the purposes of an investigation in confidence and therefore feel able to speak openly and candidly with the HSSIB. In particular, the draft reports of investigations are not admissible in proceedings to determine civil or criminal liability in respect of any matter; proceedings before any employment tribunal; proceedings before a regulatory body (including proceedings for the purposes of investigating an allegation); and proceedings to determine an appeal against a decision made in the previously referred to proceedings.[143] Protected material is any information, document, equipment, or other item which is held by the HSSIB, for the purposes of an investigation and has not already been lawfully made available to the public.[144] Unauthorised disclosure of such material, and obstruction of the HSSIB's investigations, have been criminalised in certain circumstances.[145]

The HSSIB also has new legal powers to enter and inspect premises in England, as well as to obtain information. This includes inspectors being able to inspect and seize documents, equipment, or other items at the premises.[146] In certain circumstances, an investigator may, with notice, require any person to answer questions or provide specified documents, equipment or items.[147] The HSSIB is required to cooperate with other arm's-length bodies which may also be conducting separate investigations into qualifying incidents.[148] To avoid logistical problems in this regard, the HSSIB will publish guidance on how this will work. It can also reach agreement with NHS bodies in Wales and NI to undertake investigations into qualifying incidents. Such investigations will be similar to the approach taken in England in that they will not involve the assessment or determination of blame or civil or criminal liability, 'but they will not benefit from protected information or other investigatory powers which apply to the HSSIB's investigation function'.[149]

One of the ALBs that may conduct work that overlaps with the HSSIB is the CQC. The CQC is the independent regulator of health and adult social care in England. It aims to ensure that health and social care services offer high quality care, as well as improve on the provision of such care where appropriate. It monitors, inspects, and regulates a range of health and social care services and publishes reports on its findings. It requires that certain fundamental standards are met by all registered persons (care providers and managers) registered with the CQC that carry on regulated activities.[150] It has a wide range of powers to take enforcement action requiring such services to implement improvements in line with the findings in CQC reports. Such powers include issuing requirement notices or warning notices to set out what improvements the care provider must make and by when; requiring that changes are made to a care provider's registration to limit what they may do; placing a provider under special measures, where they closely supervise the

---

[143] ibid., s 115 (draft reports) and s 117(1) and (2). Note that under s 117 (3)–(5), this can be overruled by the High Court in specified circumstances.

[144] ibid., s 122; although note under ss 123–125, as well as Sch 14, there are specified exceptions which would permit disclosure of protected material.

[145] ibid., s 121 (investigations).   [146] ibid., s 118 (powers of entry, inspection and seizure).

[147] ibid., s 119 (powers to require information).   [148] ibid., s 126.

[149] ibid., s 128; see also the HCA 2022's Explanatory Notes with regard to the operation of s 128 of the Act.

[150] See Health and Social Care Act 2008 (Regulated Activities) Regulations 2014 (Part 3) and the Care Quality Commission (Registration) Regulations 2009 (Part 4). See generally, Care Quality Commission, Legislation, updated May 2022, available at <https://www.cqc.org.uk/guidance-providers/regulations-enforcement/legislation> accessed 12 January 2023.

quality of care while working with other organisations to help them improve within set timescales. The CQC may also seek to hold a care provider to account for any identified failings by issuing cautions, fines, and conducting prosecutions where individuals are harmed or placed in danger of harm.[151]

Aligned with patient safety initiatives is work being conducted in the area of quality improvement, which has undergone successive policy and organisational reforms in recent years. A public body known as NHS Improvement had been responsible for overseeing quality improvement within NHS England, as well as independent healthcare services that provided NHS-funded care. However, NHS Improvement ceased to exist as of mid-2022, when a formal merger took place with NHS England. Many of its activities are now promoted through what is called the Improvement Hub, which is managed and maintained by NHS England's Sustainable Improvement Team. The Hub brings together improvement information, knowledge from a range of NHS organisations including NHS Improving Quality, the NHS Institute for Innovation and Improvement, the National Cancer Action Team, the National End of Life Care Programme, and NHS Diabetes and Kidney Care.[152] It also works with a range of other public bodies, including NICE, to facilitate quality improvements through guidance, standard setting and the establishment of indicators to measure outcomes that reflect the quality of care, or processes linked by evidence to improved healthcare outcomes.[153]

3.5 NORTHERN IRELAND

It is important to first provide a brief overview of NI's political and constitutional dynamics in order to understand the fragmented and at times uneven development of its health service, as well as why there have been challenges in relation to reforming the service in recent decades. NI is a devolved administration comprising six counties in the north-east of the island of Ireland. In 1921, two separate jurisdictions were formally established on the island. In 1922, the Irish Free State was founded, which subsequently became the Republic of Ireland in 1949, now more commonly known as Ireland. In contrast, NI remained part of the UK, governed through devolved arrangements which provided for an NI government and Parliament.[154] Although NI was formally created in 1921, its constitutional status, including whether it should remain part of the UK or form part of a united Ireland, was one of the factors in a violent sectarian conflict, colloquially known as 'The Troubles', which lasted for over 25 years in the closing decades of the twentieth century. The legacy of this conflict continues to impact local political and social arrangements in NI to the present date.[155] During this period, direct rule was imposed by the UK Government.

---

[151] Care Quality Commission, 'Taking Action', available at < https://www.cqc.org.uk/about-us/how-we-do-our-job/taking-action> accessed 12 January 2023.

[152] NHS England, 'The Improvement Hub', available at <https://www.england.nhs.uk/improvement-hub/> accessed 12 January 2023.

[153] National Institute for Health and Care Excellence, 'Quality Standards', available at <https://www.nice.org.uk/about/who-we-are/corporate-publications/the-nice-strategy-2021-to-2026> accessed 12 January 2023.

[154] For an overview, see **Mícheál** Ó Fathartaigh and Liam Weeks, *Birth of a State: The Anglo-Irish Treaty* (Irish Academic Press 2021).

[155] For an overview, see David McKittrick and David McVea, *Making Sense of the Troubles: A History of the Northern Ireland Conflict* (Penguin Books 2012).

In 1998, a peace accord known as the Belfast/Good Friday Agreement led to new devolved power-sharing institutions being re-established in NI.[156] These institutions include the NI Executive, which represents the devolved administration, and the NI Assembly, which is the devolved legislature. Over the past 25 years, power-sharing institutions have collapsed on several occasions; at the time of writing, this remains the situation. During these periods, senior NI civil servants take responsibility for the day-to-day running of government, but they can only act in line with policy directions set by the Executive when it was last in existence.[157] This has resulted in policy 'drift' and conflict-avoiding 'managerialism', adversely impacting on the ability to innovation and initiate ongoing reform of the health service.[158]

3.5.1 STRUCTURE AND ORGANISATION

In NI, the health service is known as Health and Social Care (HSC) and is responsible for a population of just over 1.9 million, representing around 3% of the total UK population.[159] It is a publicly funded healthcare system operated through primary, community, and hospital care, and is free at the point of access.[160] Unlike other health services in the UK, however, social care has been formally integrated with health care in NI since 1972.[161] At the time, this was done partly to address concerns about sectarian discrimination in local government, but there was also a recognition of the benefits of an integrated approach to meeting the full range of people's needs. The NI Department of Health has overall responsibility for the allocation of funding for health and social care.[162] The Strategic Planning and Performance Group (SPPG) in the Department is responsible for commissioning services, resource management, performance management, and service improvement for the HSC. It deploys and manages funds allocated by the Department and oversees the work of the six HSC trusts. It also works to identify and meet the needs of the local population through five Local Commissioning Groups (LCGs), which cover the same geographical areas as the HSC Trusts.[163]

Five HSC Trusts provide integrated health and social care services and are responsible for the day-to-day running of hospitals, health centres, residential homes, day centres, and other health and social care facilities. They are the Belfast HSC Trust, Northern HSC Trust, Southern HSC Trust, South-Eastern HSC Trust and Western HSC Trust. The sixth HSC Trust is the Northern Ireland Ambulance Service, which operates a Northern Ireland-wide service for people in need, see **Figure 3.3**.[164]

---

[156] See e.g. UK Government, Northern Ireland Office, 'The Belfast Agreement' GOV.UK, 10 April 1998, available at <https://www.gov.uk/government/publications/the-belfast-agreement> accessed 12 January 2023.

[157] Jess Sargeant, 'Northern Ireland: Functioning of Government Without Ministers', Institute for Government, 14 November 2022, available at <https://www.instituteforgovernment.org.uk/article/explainer/northern-ireland-functioning-government-without-ministers> accessed 12 January 2023.

[158] Greer (n 14) 19.

[159] UK Population Data, 'UK Population 2022,' available at <https://populationdata.org.uk/uk-population/> accessed 12 January 2023.

[160] Health and Social Care online, 'HSC Structure', available at <https://online.hscni.net/> accessed 12 January 2023.

[161] Health and Personal Social Services (Northern Ireland) Order 1972, Northern Ireland Orders in Council, 1972, No 1265 (N.I. 14).

[162] House of Commons and Northern Ireland Affairs Committee, 'Health Funding in Northern Ireland: First Report of Session 2019' (*House of Commons*, 2 November 2019), available at: <http://online.hscni.net/home/hsc-structure/> accessed 12 January 2023.

[163] Health and Social Care online, 'Our Work' available at: <http://www.hscboard.hscni.net/our-work/> accessed 12 January 2023.

[164] Health and Social Care online, 'Health and Social Care Trusts' <http://online.hscni.net/hospitals/health-and-social-care-trusts/> accessed 23 January 2023.

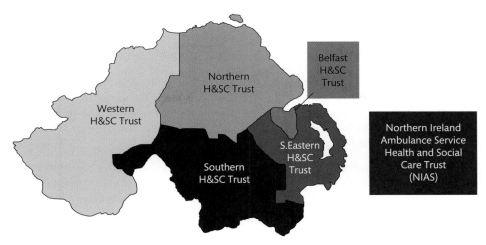

Figure 3.3 Organisational Structure of Health and Social Care (HSC) in NI[165]

Another key body is the Patient and Client Council (PCC), which is a regional body with local offices covering the geographical areas of the five HSC Trusts as noted. The objective of the PCC is to provide an independent voice for patients, clients, carers, and communities on health and social care issues.[166] The Business Services Organisation is responsible for the provision of a range of business support and specialist professional services to the whole of the health and social care sector (e.g. human resources, finance, legal services, procurement, digital technologies).[167]

It has long been recognised that NI's health and social care system is in need of reform. Over the past 25 years, at least seven system reviews have recommended major reforms to policy direction, organisational structure, workforce, and funding arrangements. There has also been a long-standing recognition that there was a need to reduce reliance on secondary care (hospitals), centralise specialist services, and focus more on public health prevention and redressing health inequalities.[168] However, ongoing political dysfunction created by successive collapses of NI's power-sharing institutions has meant that momentum has been lost with regards to moving forward with reform of the health and social care system.[169]

Most recently, organisational reform of the HSC has been proposed through the transition to an ICS, which bears many similarities to the model currently being implemented in England (though adapted for NI). The rationale for doing so is to respond to the pressures that the HSC has been under for some time to address the healthcare needs of the population, which is living longer with the increased risk of living with, and managing, multiple chronic conditions. Health inequalities are also significant in NI and it is recognised that a more comprehensive approach is needed to address such inequalities in

---

[165] Disclaimer: please note that the representation of HSCNI district boundaries is not exact.

[166] Northern Ireland Patient and Client Council <https://pcc-ni.net/> accessed 23 January 2023.

[167] Health and Social Care, 'Business Services Organisation' available at <https://hscbusiness.hscni .net/> accessed 12 January 2023.

[168] See e.g. Rafael Bengoa et al., 'Systems Not Structures—Changing Health and Social Care', 25 October 2016, available at <https://www.health-ni.gov.uk/publications/systems-not-structures-changing-health- and-social-care-full-report> accessed 12 January 2023.

[169] For an overview of NI's health and social care system and what reforms are needed, see Mark Dayan and Deirdre Heenan, *Change or Collapse: Lessons from the Drive to Reform Health and Social Care in Northern Ireland* (The Nuffield Trust 2019).

the context of providing health and social care services.[170] The impact of the Covid-19 pandemic has not only exacerbated these longstanding pressures on the HSC but further reinforced the need for a more integrated approach to delivering collectively on a range and of health and social care services.[171]

A key focus of the ICS will be to address the wider determinants of health and well-being through a population health approach. This will address the whole life course from prevention, early intervention through to treatment, and end of life care. A programme of work is underway to bring about the design, implementation, and delivery of the ICS, which is defined in the NI context as follows:

> A collaborative partnership between organisations and individuals with a responsibility for planning, managing, and delivering sustainable care, services and interventions to meet the health and well-being needs of the local population. Through taking collective action, partnerships will deliver improved outcomes for individuals and communities, and reduce inequalities.[172]

In NI, it will involve the following new structures:[173]

- *Area Integrated Partnership Boards* (AIPBs): these are comprised of representatives from health and social care representatives, the voluntary and community sectors, local government, and service users and carers. The AIPBs will be responsible for the planning and delivery of improved health and social care outcomes for the local population for which they are responsible. The AIPBs will be public facing, engaging people at a local level, and developing strong relationships with their respective communities.

- *Locality groups* will support AIPBs in assessing local population needs and the delivery of required health and social care interventions.

- *Regional ICS Executive* (RICSE) will comprise members from across the ICS and will enable other regional level bodies and the five area partnerships to work together. The RICSE will help develop the ICS culture and facilitate new ways of working in relation to integrated care planning and delivery, as well as ensuring that the ICS is clear and coherent in terms of roles and responsibilities.

In order to progress the new ICS, a Project Board was established in January 2021 to support the early phases of the project and ensure the timely development of all necessary policies, frameworks, and guidance to support the delivery of the objectives. This was followed up by the publication of an ICS draft framework document in June 2021. It envisages the ICS model as involving the delegation of decision-making and funding to local levels with the exception of regional and specialised services, and it will be underpinned by an outcomes-based accountability (OBA) approach. The OBA approach puts population health and the centre of policy and decision-making. It requires that

---

[170] See e.g. NI Department of Health, 'Health Inequalities Annual Report 2022', available at <https://www.health-ni.gov.uk/news/health-inequalities-annual-report-2022> accessed 12 January 2023.

[171] Northern Ireland Department of Health, 'Frequently Asked Questions – Future Planning Model: Integrated Care System', available at <https://online.hscni.net/our-work/integrated-care-system-ni/faqs-integrated-care-system-ni/> accessed 12 January 2023.

[172] See Northern Ireland Department of Health, Future Planning Model: Integrated Care System NI Draft Framework, June 2021; Northern Ireland Department of Health, 'Frequently Asked Questions' (n 169).

[173] ibid.

a desired set outcomes be identified for the NI population, with all agreed work, initiatives, and interventions undertaken within the ICS being focused on realising such outcomes.[174]

In early 2022, the HSC Board, which had previously been the statutory organisation which commissioned health and social care services for the population of NI, was dissolved,[175] although Local Commissioning Groups (LCGs) remain in existence.[176] The reason for the Board's dissolution was a recognition of the need to reform the approach taken to commissioning health and social care services in NI, involving a shift towards collaboration and partnership in the context of an ICS in order to better meet the needs of the NI population. The Board officially closed on 31 March 2022, with responsibility for its functions being transferred to the NI Department of Health. Since April 2022, such functions have been undertaken by the Strategic Planning and Performance Group (SPPG) within the Department as they work towards implementing the new ICS model. [177] In the second half of 2022, an ICS NI Steering Board was established to provide strategic leadership and oversight to the programme of work, together with an ICS NI Programme Board, which acts as a forum to facilitate senior managerial oversight with respect to the recommendations being proposed by the ICS NI Programme team.[178]

3.5.2 PATIENT SAFETY AND QUALITY IMPROVEMENT

The current plan for promoting quality and safety in health care is known as Quality Strategy 2020.[179] Originally launched in 2011, it was designed as a ten-year strategy to improve quality and safety in health care and is due to be renewed in the near future. Drawing on the seminal work of the United States Institute of Medicine on quality and safety in health care,[180] the Strategy defines quality as involving (i) *safety*: avoiding and preventing harm to patients from the care, treatment and support that is intended to help them; (ii) *effectiveness*: the degree to which each patient and client receives the right care (according to scientific knowledge and evidence-based assessment), at the right time, in the right place, with the best outcome; and (iii) *patient-focused*: patients are entitled to be treated with dignity and respect and should be fully involved in decisions affecting their treatment, care, and support.[181] In order to realise this vision of quality, there is a need to work towards five strategic goals. They include transforming the culture; strengthening the workforce; measuring the improvement; raising the standards; and integrating the care.[182]

As part of implementing the Quality 2020 Strategy, the Health and Social Care Quality Improvement hub (HSCQI) was established in 2019 under the auspices of the NI Public Health Agency. It operates a Quality Improvement (QI) Network, which provides supporting infrastructure for quality, improvement, and innovation across the NI health and

---

[174] ibid.   [175] See Health and Social Care Act (Northern Ireland) 2022, s 1(1).
[176] ibid. s 3.
[177] Health and Social Care Board, 'Health and Social Care Board Set to Close', 28 March 2022, available at < https://hscboard.hscni.net/health-social-care-board-set-close/> accessed 12 January 2023.
[178] Northern Ireland Department of Health, 'Integrated Care System (ICS) Northern Ireland', available at <https://online.hscni.net/our-work/integrated-care-system-ni/> accessed 12 January 2023.
[179] Northern Ireland Department of Health, 'Quality 2020', available at <https://www.health-ni.gov.uk/topics/safety-and-quality-standards/quality-2020> accessed 12 January 2023.
[180] See Institute of Medicine (US) Committee on Quality of Health Care in America, *To Err is Human: Building a Safer Health System* (National Academies Press 2000).
[181] Northern Ireland Department of Health, Quality 2020 (n 177).   [182] ibid.

social care system. Most recently, the HSCQI has published its strategy for the 2022–24 period.[183] As part of the strategy, it seeks to facilitate personal and public involvement and co-production for quality improvement; to promote equality and equity; and to focus on a population health approach, aimed at improving physical and mental health outcomes, promoting well-being and reducing health inequalities.[184] In addition to the strategic plans for improving quality and safety in health care identified above, other key initiatives include the established patient complaints and reporting system arising from treatment provided in the public and independent health and social care sectors,[185] as well the Northern Ireland Adverse Incident Centre (NIAIC), which operates under the auspices of the Department of Health. It is charged with safeguarding the health of patients and staff through management of a voluntary reporting and investigation system in relation to adverse incidents involving medical devices, non-medical equipment, plant and building elements, and for providing relevant safety guidance in relation to these items.[186]

Finally, the Regulation and Quality Improvement Authority (RQIA) operates as an independent body with responsibility for monitoring and inspecting the availability and quality of health and social care services in NI, as well as encouraging quality improvements where appropriate.[187] It registers and inspects a range of health and social care services, and conducts inspections which are based on minimum care standards.[188] While the RQIA does not have the legal powers to investigate individual complaints about health and social care services, if an individual does raise such concerns directly with the regulator, then it will inform the approach taken to the inspection or review activities.[189] In a review of the approach taken to quality and safety in health care in NI, it was recommended that the 'regulatory function' provided by the RQIA should be strengthened in relation to the provision of healthcare services. This would facilitate more routine inspections which could focus on 'areas of patient safety, clinical effectiveness, patient experience, clinical governance arrangements, and leadership'.[190] As an alternative, such inspections could be outsourced to the Scottish regulator, Healthcare Improvement Scotland, which could provide 'good opportunities for benchmarking'.[191] More generally, it was recognised that there were longstanding structural elements of the NI health and social care system 'that fundamentally damage its quality and safety', with a range of initiatives and responsibilities that interweave through various bodies in the NI health and social care system. In the circumstances, institutional reform was needed, given that existing arrangements operated 'against the interests of patients' and 'denied many twenty first century standards of care'.[192] It remains to be seen whether this will change under the proposed shift towards a new integrated care model, which is currently underway in NI.

---

[183] Health and Social Care Quality Improvement, Strategy 2022–24, available at <https://hscqi.hscni.net/about-hscqi/strategy-2022-24/> accessed 12 January 2023.

[184] ibid., 9.

[185] NI Direct, 'How to Complain or Raise Concerns About Health Services', available at <https://www.nidirect.gov.uk/articles/how-complain-or-raise-concerns-about-health-services> accessed 12 January 2023.

[186] Northern Ireland Department of Health, 'Introduction to Northern Ireland Adverse Incidents Centre (NIAIC)', available at <https://www.health-ni.gov.uk/articles/introduction-northern-ireland-adverse-incidents-centre-niaic> accessed 12 January 2023.

[187] The RQIA was established under the Health and Personal Social Services (Quality, Improvement and Regulation) (Northern Ireland) Order 2003.

[188] RQIA, 'What We Do', available at <https://www.rqia.org.uk/> accessed 12 January 2023.

[189] ibid.

[190] See Liam Donaldson et al., 'The Right Time—The Right Place' (Department of Health 2014), available at <https://www.health-ni.gov.uk/publications/right-time-right-place> accessed 12 January 2023.

[191] ibid., Rec 5.   [192] ibid., para 5.2.1; see also Rec 7.

3.6 SCOTLAND

For most of the twentieth century, Scotland enjoyed a significant degree of administrative independence from the UK Government, which was also reflected in the area of health.[193] Unlike NI and Wales, it was therefore more advanced in terms of asserting its independence in health policy and institutional arrangements, resulting in the establishment of the Scottish Board of Health in 1919, which was subsequently replaced by the Scottish Department of Health in 1929.[194] The creation of the NHS in Scotland in 1948 provided for a more uniform structure for services which had previously been provided by a combination of the Highlands and Islands Medical Service, local government, charities, and private organisations which in general were only free for emergency use.

Prior to the ushering in of new devolution arrangements in the late 1990s, health policy was substantively similar across the UK's health systems. There was a tendency to view Scottish health policy as a 'kilted' version of the English.[195] The origins of such views were to be found in the degree of centralised health policy and administrative control with the UK Government, which mainly operated with England in mind. While health policy may have been 'distinctive' in Scotland, it was nevertheless viewed from this centralised position as being 'distinctive at the margins'.[196] Since the late 1990s, however, health has become one of the most important policy areas devolved to Scotland under current constitutional arrangements.[197] As a result, the Scottish Government and Parliament have moved towards a more autonomous, distinctive approach to policymaking and regulation, aided by devolved powers in areas such as health. In recent times, a combination of both Brexit and the Covid-19 pandemic have further accelerated this approach.[198]

3.6.1 STRUCTURE AND ORGANISATION

NHS Scotland is a universal, publicly funded healthcare service that is offered free at the point of need for those who are ordinarily resident in in the UK. It currently manages the healthcare needs of 5.45 million people, accounting for just under 8% of the total UK population.[199] Since 2011, prescriptions filled in Scotland have been free of charge, and eye tests and dental check-ups are also free via NHS Scotland.[200] In support of a patient-centred approach, the Scottish Charter of Patient Rights and Responsibilities sets out what patients are entitled to when they use NHS services and receive NHS care in Scotland, as well as what patients can do when their rights have not been respected in such circumstances.[201] The Charter is a mix of rights and responsibilities that currently exist under law, and reflects what it is 'expected patients will do to help the NHS work

---

[193] UK Parliament, House of Lords, Select Committee on the Constitution, The Union and Devolution, 10th Report of Session 2015–16, HL Paper 149, published 25 May 2016, paras 18–20.

[194] Jacqueline Jenkinson, Scotland's Health 1919–1948 (Peter Lang 2002).   [195] Greer (n 14).

[196] ibid.   [197] ibid., 18.

[198] Scottish Government, 'After Brexit: The UK Internal Market and Devolution', 8 March 2021, available at <https://www.gov.scot/publications/brexit-uk-internal-market-act-devolution/> accessed 12 January 2023.

[199] UK Population Data, 'UK Population 2022,' available at <https://populationdata.org.uk/uk-population/> accessed 12 January 2023.

[200] Scottish Government, 'Help with Health Costs: Quick Guide - July 2022', available at <https://www.gov.scot/publications/quick-guide-help-health-costs-6/> accessed 12 January 2023.

[201] As set out in the Patient Rights (Scotland) Act 2011. Under the Act, the Scottish Ministers are required to publish a Charter setting out the rights and responsibilities of patients and other persons when receiving health care. Section 1(4) of the Act makes clear that nothing in the Charter gives rise to any new rights, imposes any new responsibilities, or alters in any way an existing right or responsibility.

effectively in Scotland and to help make sure it uses its resources responsibly'.[202] In addition, Health and Social Care Standards published by the Scottish Government came into effect on 1 April 2018 setting what is generally expected when persons use health, social care, or social work services in Scotland.[203] In setting out such standards, it is recognised that the outcomes relating to each of them may mean different things in different care settings.[204] The standards are grounded in the five core principles of dignity and respect, compassion, inclusiveness, responsive care, and support and well-being, and are set out in the following section.

Health and Social Care Standards in Scotland

1. I experience high quality care and support that is right for me.
2. I am fully involved in all decisions about my care and support.
3. I have confidence in the people who support and care for me.
4. I have confidence in the organisation providing my care and support.
5. I experience a high-quality environment if the organisation provides the premises.

Primary and secondary health care are integrated in Scotland. The provision of publicly funded health care is the responsibility of 14 geographically based local NHS boards (which are further subdivided into Health and Social Care Partnerships (HSCP)), seven national non-geographic special health boards, and many small contractors for primary care services.[205] Also known as 'territorial' health boards, these 14 NHS boards are responsible for the improvement of their population's health and for the delivery of front-line healthcare services. The boards operate differently, meaning there is variation in their size, role, function and governance arrangements. There are two types of health boards: (i) *health-only structures*, which are known as Community Health Partnerships (CHPs); and (ii) *integrated health and social care structures*, known as community health and care partnerships (CHCPs) or community health and social care partnerships (CHSCPs) (see **Figure 3.4**).[206]

In addition to the regional health boards, there are several NHS boards which operate across Scotland, providing specialist services. These include the following:[207]

- *Public Health Scotland*: responsible for public health (including national health protection) and, since April 2020, health education.

- *Healthcare Improvement Scotland*: responsible for improving quality of health and social care including quality assurance and improvement initiatives, providing quality assurance and facilitating the best use of health and social care resources.

---

[202] Scottish Government, 'Patient Rights and Responsibilities: Charter', updated 30 November 2021, available at < https://www.gov.scot/publications/charter-patient-rights-responsibilities-2/> accessed 23 January 2023.
[203] Scottish Government, Health and Social Care Standards: My Support, My Life, available at <https://www.gov.scot/publications/health-social-care-standards-support-life/> accessed 12 January 2023.
[204] The standards and outcomes set out in the Health and Social Care Standards have been developed as a result of two pieces of legislation, namely the Public Services Reform (Scotland) Act 2010, s 50; and the National Health Service (Scotland) Act 1978, s 10H.
[205] NHS Scotland Heath Board areas, reproduced for educational purposes only by kind permission of the Scottish Government, available at <https://www.gov.scot/publications/evaluation-attend-anywhere-near-video-consulting-service-scotland-2019-20-main-report/pages/4/> accessed 9 February 2023.
[206] Farrell and Frowde (n 31).   [207] ibid., 16.

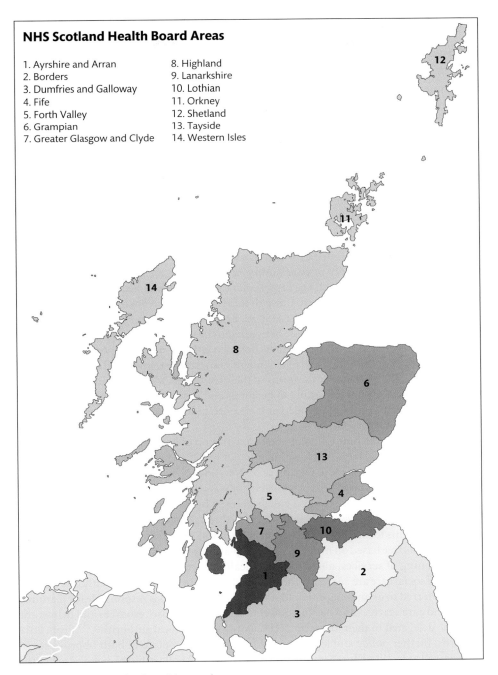

NHS Scotland Health Board Areas

1. Ayrshire and Arran
2. Borders
3. Dumfries and Galloway
4. Fife
5. Forth Valley
6. Grampian
7. Greater Glasgow and Clyde
8. Highland
9. Lanarkshire
10. Lothian
11. Orkney
12. Shetland
13. Tayside
14. Western Isles

Figure 3.4 NHS Scotland Health Board areas

Organisational structure of Scotland diagram reproduced for educational purposes only by kind permission of the Scottish Government.

- *Scottish Ambulance Service*: provides ambulance care to patients who need support to attend appointments, as well as assistance with transport for hospital admission, transfer and discharge.

- *The Golden Jubilee*: this board comprises a national hospital, research institute, innovation centre, and conference hotel. It focuses on healthcare innovation and is home to a range of specialist heart services.

- *State Hospitals Board for Scotland*: responsible for the secure psychiatric hospital at Carstairs, which provides high security services for mentally disordered offenders and others who pose a high risk to themselves or others.

- *NHS 24*: a telephone advice and triage service that cover the out-of-hours periods.

- *NHS Education for Scotland*: responsible for training and the e-library.

- *NHS National Services for Scotland*: Common Services Agency (CSA) which provides services and goods for the regional health boards.

There are also 32 local authorities which work closely with the regional NHS Boards to ensure the effective delivery of community health and social work services. This relationship is formalised through the representation of each local health authority on the board of each relevant NHS board, through local authority membership of all CHPs and joint accountability of CHCPs and CHSCPs, and through some joint appointments.[208] Unlike in England, there is no 'divide between purchasers of care and providers of health care'.[209] As a result, there are no contracts between boards and their operating divisions. Most primary care providers are independent contractors reimbursed for the services they provide to the NHS under the terms of their contracts. NHS boards directly employ, on a salaried basis, the staff working in hospitals and the community. They also manage, through CHPs, the contracts of independent contractors in primary care (GPs, dentists, and community pharmacists).

Since the 1990s, the promotion of better integration of health and social has been taking place on a gradual basis.[210] However, it took until 2016 for formal legislative integration of health and social care to take place.[211] New bodies, called Integration Authorities, were established and these were responsible for ensuring that the health and social care of local populations were organised collaboratively by NHS Scotland health boards and local authorities, with services being delivered through health and social care partnerships. Despite this formal attempt at integration, it was not a national health and care service which was free based on need.[212] Strategic planning of health and social care services, commissioning of services, and budgets of health boards and local authorities covering health and social care are currently the responsibility of new integration authority boards, usually referred to as an Integration Joint Board (IJB). The IJB is responsible for planning health and care services and has full power to decide how to use resources and deliver the services, delegated to them from the NHS boards and the local authorities.[213] From 2019 onwards, further policy and legislative reforms have taken place to both improve social care, as well as facilitate further integration initiatives.[214] Following the publication of the Feeley Review in 2021, it was recognised that current structures for social care had not fully delivered on the objective of facilitating integration of health and social care to date

---

[208] ibid., 16.   [209] ibid., 17, drawing on Greer (n 14) 19.   [210] ibid., 23.
[211] See Carers (Scotland) Act 2016, which was commenced through the Public Bodies (Joint Working) Scotland Act 2014.
[212] Farrell and Frowde (n 31) 31.   [213] ibid., 23–24.   [214] ibid., 34–35.

and it was recommended that a new National Care Service be established in Scotland.[215] This has now been carried through by the Scottish Government, with a bill to establish such a service currently before the Scottish Parliament.[216]

As previously mentioned in this chapter, health (and social) care are major areas of devolved competence in Scotland, and this is reflected in the prominence given to both in the organisation, policy, and legislative work of the Scottish Government. At Ministerial level, health care, public health, and social care is the responsibility of the Cabinet Secretary for Health and Social Care, as well as the Ministers for Mental Wellbeing and Social Care, and the Minster for Public Health, Women's Health and Sport. They are supported at senior management level by the Chief Executive for NHS Scotland and Director-General Health and Social Care, as well as the Chief Medical Officer.[217] Together they oversee several health and social care Directorates including Chief Nursing Officer, Chief Operating Officer NHS Scotland, digital health, health finance, health workforce, healthcare quality and improvement, mental health, population health, primary care, social care, and national care service development.[218]

In the latest published programme for government for 2022–23,[219] the Scottish Government has promised to eradicate waiting lists of over 18 months for most specialities for outpatients, waiting lists of over one year for in-patients/day cases, and waiting times in A&E within the NHS; provide funding to deal with the effects of long Covid-19 infection; open new national treatment centres; expand the number of early cancer diagnostic centres; publish new mental health and well-being and dementia strategies; provide a substantial investment to increase capacity and community health initiatives in relation to adult, children, and young people's mental health; introduce legislation to encourage people to make healthier food choices; appoint a women's health champion; improve access to and delivery of NHS gender identity services; and support legislation that will establish a new national care service for Scotland. In support of these initiatives, the Scottish Government has allocated a budget of £18 billion for health and social care in 2022–23, in recognition of the pressures that NHS Scotland as faced due to the Covid-19 pandemic, and well as part of Covid-19 recovery initiatives. As a result of the pandemic, the Government also recognised that more financial investment was required in social care, as well as in further integration of health and social care, which translates into a year-on-year 25% increase in social care spend for the next three years.[220]

[215] Scottish Government, Adult Social Care: Independent Review (Feeley Review), 3 February 2021, available at <https://www.gov.scot/publications/independent-review-adult-social-care-scotland/> accessed 12 January 2023.

[216] Once passed, the legislation will allow the Scottish Government to, inter alia, transfer health care functions from NHS Scotland, as well as social care responsibilities from local authorities, to the new National Care Service. See Scottish Parliament, National Care Service (Scotland) Bill, available at <https://www.parliament.scot/bills-and-laws/bills/national-care-service-scotland-bill> accessed 12 January 2023.

[217] See e.g. Scottish Government, Chief Executive of NHS Scotland and Director-General Health and Social Care, available at <https://www.gov.scot/about/how-government-is-run/civil-service/chief-executive-of-the-nhs-in-scotland/> accessed 12 January 2023.

[218] Scottish Government, 'Directorates', available at <https://www.gov.scot/about/how-government-is-run/directorates/ accessed 12 January 2023.

[219] Scottish Government, 'A Stronger and More Resilient Scotland: The Programme for Government 2022 to 2023', available at <https://www.gov.scot/publications/stronger-more-resilient-scotland-programme-government-2022-23/pages/3/> accessed 12 January 2023.

[220] Health and Social Care Alliance Scotland, 'Minister Lays Out Health and Social Care Spend in 2022-23 Scottish Budget', 16 December 2021. Note that Scottish health service expenditure, often referred to as the 'Cost Book', is also published on an annual basis. This is the only source of published costs information for NHS Scotland and provides a detailed analysis of where its resources are spent; see Public Health Scotland, 'Costs', available at <https://www.isdscotland.org/health-topics/finance/costs/> accessed 12 January 2023.

3.6.2 PATIENT SAFETY AND QUALITY IMPROVEMENT

In the first decade of the 2000s, the Scottish Patient Safety Programme (SPSP) was established to promote patient safety initiatives in Scotland, as well as address the problem of avoidable events causing harm to patients in healthcare settings. It represented the first time in the UK that a national quality improvement programme had been established to facilitate the safer delivery of healthcare. In 2007, the Scottish Patient Safety Alliance was established through a partnership between the Scottish Government, NHS Scotland, the Royal Colleges and other professional bodies, the Scottish Consumer Council, and the Institute for Healthcare Improvement (IHI).[221] One of the key activities of the Alliance was to extend patient safety initiatives across NHS Scotland, as part of the launch of the SPSP in 2007.[222] The rollout of quality improvement initiatives as part of the SPSP has extended across a range of specialities since its launch, and now includes acute adult care, mental health, primary care, maternity and children, healthcare associated infections, medicines, and the delivery of community health care in areas such as dentistry, pharmacy, and district nursing.[223]

In 2010, the Healthcare Quality Strategy for NHS Scotland was published, which sets out the approach to be taken for achieving an integrated vision of quality improvement for health and social care. It identified key priorities as caring and compassionate staff and services; providing clear communication and explanations about conditions and treatment; fostering effective collaboration between clinicians, patients and others; creating a clean and safe care environment; and offering continuity of care and clinical excellence.[224]

In 2011, Healthcare Improvement Scotland (HIS) was established. It now operates as the main body driving quality and safety in health care under the SPSP.[225] Quality improvement draws on the Excellence in Care Framework, which builds on four essential requirements: person-centredness; compassion; fundamentals of care; and communication, both verbal and written, with patients, their families, and between staff.[226] The Framework provides the foundation for promoting a culture of continuous improvement using a quality management systems approach.[227] HIS is also responsible for conducting inspections of NHS hospitals, as well as independent healthcare services across Scotland, as well as for the registration and regulation of such services. HIS inspections are designed to give NHS boards a proactive, assertive way to report evidence; create a methodology

---

[221] Note that the Institute for Healthcare Improvement (IHI) is a United States-based organisation that seeks to use improvement science to advance and sustain better outcomes in health and health care across the world, working in collaboration with a range of organisations to improve quality and safety in the delivery of health care on a systematic basis; see Institute for Healthcare Improvement, 'About IHI', available at <https://www.ihi.org/about/Pages/default.aspx> accessed 12 January 2023.

[222] Scottish Government, Healthcare Quality and Improvement Directorate, 'The Scottish Improvement Journey: A Nationwide Approach to Improvement', 20 April 2018, available at <https://www.gov.scot/publications/scottish-improvement-journey-nationwide-approach-improvement-compiled-2016-17/pages/4/> accessed 12 January 2023.

[223] ibid.

[224] Scottish Government, Healthcare Quality and Improvement Directorate, 'Healthcare Quality Strategy for NHS Scotland', 10 May 2010, available at <https://www.gov.scot/publications/healthcare-quality-strategy-nhsscotland/> accessed 10 January 2023.

[225] Healthcare Improvement Scotland, 'Safety Is at The Heart of Our Work', available at <https://ihub.scot/improvement-programmes/scottish-patient-safety-programme-spsp/> accessed 12 January 2023.

[226] Healthcare Improvement Scotland, 'Excellence in Care', available at <https://www.healthcareimprovementscotland.org/our_work/patient_safety/excellence_in_care.aspx> accessed 12 January 2023.

[227] ibid.

for analysing NHS board evidence that can validate, risk assess and identify targets for inspection; and to monitor NHS board improvement plans.[228] HIS also manages an 'ihub' which operates as an improvement resource and delivery agency for health and social care, including the SPSP.[229]

As noted previously, a Charter of Patient Rights and Responsibilities (Charter) was published in 2011.[230] The Charter sets out what patients are entitled to when they use and receive healthcare services in NHS Scotland, and what can be done where they consider that their rights have not been respected. The information in the Charter is divided into a number of areas, including patients' rights in relation to accessing and being provided with NHS services in Scotland; rights to communication and being informed about one's health care and services, as well as being involved in decisions about them; rights to privacy and confidentiality and to the protection of one's personal health information; and the rights of patients to provide feedback and submit complaints about treatment or care in line with NHS Scotland's complaints procedure.[231]

More recently, the Scottish Government has also moved forward to establish the office of the Patient Safety Commissioner for Scotland, mirroring similar developments in England arising from the publication of the Cumberlege Review report. Following an initial consultation on the role, a draft Bill was published to formally establish the role.[232] At the time of writing, the bill is currently under consideration by the Scottish Parliament.[233] It will cover all healthcare providers operating in Scotland, including the NHS and NHS-contracted and independent healthcare providers. The Commissioner will be responsible for bringing together patient feedback and safety data shared by NHS boards and HIS, to identify concerns and recommend actions as part of improving the patient safety landscape in Scotland. They will also be empowered to conduct formal investigations into potential systemic safety issues, with powers to require information be shared to make sure every investigation is fully informed.[234] The bill will likely become law in 2023, with the appointment of the first Commissioner taking place shortly thereafter.

3.7 WALES

In 1969, the Welsh NHS separated from the English NHS. Notwithstanding such separation, much of health policy and legislation that applied in Wales was generated by the UK Government. In the circumstances, there was a 'tendency to view Welsh health policy as a bilingual copy of English policy', essentially implementing UK health policy which

---

[228] Healthcare Improvement Scotland, 'Inspecting and Regulating Care', available at <https://www.healthcareimprovementscotland.org/our_work/inspecting_and_regulating_care.aspx> accessed 12 January 2023.

[229] Healthcare Improvement Scotland, 'ihub', available at <https://ihub.scot/> accessed 12 January 2023.

[230] Charter of Patient Rights and Responsibilities (n 199).

[231] Scottish Government, Healthcare Quality and Improvement Directorate, 'Charter of Patient Rights and Responsibilities—Revised: June 2022', 14 October 2022, available at <https://www.gov.scot/publications/charter-patient-rights-responsibilities-revised-june-2022> accessed 12 January 2023.

[232] Scottish Government, 'Patient Safety Commissioner Role for Scotland: Consultation', 5 March 2021 available at <https://www.gov.scot/publications/consultation-patient-safety-commissioner-role-scotland/pages/1/> accessed 12 January 2023.

[233] Scottish Government, 'Patient Safety Commissioner Bill Published', 7 October 2022, available at <https://www.gov.scot/news/patient-safety-commissioner-bill-published/> accessed 12 January 2023.

[234] Scottish Parliament, Patient Safety Commissioner for Scotland Bill, available at <https://www.parliament.scot/bills-and-laws/bills/patient-safety-commissioner-for-scotland-bill> accessed 12 January 2023.

had been 'designed with England in mind'.[235] From 1998, this began to change in light of political devolution, with health care and public health competence being devolved to Wales. With greater autonomy and independence to act in relation to health matters, the Welsh Government moved to reorganise local health boards, facilitating coordination with local government which has responsibility for primary care and commissioning from seven NHS trusts.[236] In addition, there was a shift from focusing on 'meeting targets and reducing waiting times in the NHS', although problems with primary care, delayed transfer of care, and poor quality hospital care have not magically disappeared as a result.[237] Nevertheless, the Welsh Government has been proactive in seeking to promote a range of public health initiatives, in addition to addressing health inequalities.[238] In relation to the former, Wales became the first UK jurisdiction to introduce deemed consent for deceased organ donation, which we discuss in more detail in Chapter 13. In relation to the latter, there was an increased focus on health inequalities, which involved addressing the social determinants of health impacting the Welsh population. This was subsequently translated into legislative form with a unique statutory duty being imposed on 'public bodies in Wales to think about the long-term impact of their decisions, to work better with people, communities and each other, and to prevent persistent problems such as poverty, health inequalities and climate change.'[239] Similarly to Scotland, Wales has also pursued an increasingly distinctive style to health policy and law in the wake of the combined impact of Brexit and the Covid-19 pandemic.[240]

3.7.1 STRUCTURE AND ORGANISATION

Similarly to the UK's other health services, NHS Wales is also a universal, publicly funded healthcare service that is offered free at the point of need for those who are ordinarily resident in the UK. It currently manages the healthcare needs of a population of 3.2 million, accounting for just over 5% of the total UK population.[241] It has been suggested that values such as solidarity, sustainability, and equality underpin the provision of health and social care in Wales.[242] These values can be observed across a range of policy documentation that sets out the principles and standards that inform and government the operation of NHS Wales. For example, the values that underpin its governance and accountability framework are grounded in a recognition that 'NHS organisations must be value driven, rooted in high standards of public life and behaviour':

- **Putting quality and safety above all else:** providing high-value evidence-based care for patients at all times.

- **Integrating improvement into everyday working** and eliminating harm, variation, and waste.

---

[235] Greer (n 14) 18.

[236] Mark Dayan and Sophie Flinders, 'How Well is the NHS in Wales Performing?', The Nuffield Trust, 9 June 2022, available at <https://www.nuffieldtrust.org.uk/news-item/how-well-is-the-nhs-in-wales-performing> accessed 12 January 2023.

[237] Greer (n 14) 22–23.   [238] Dayan and Flinders (n 234).

[239] Future Generations Commissioner for Wales, Well-being of Future Generations (Wales) Act 2015, available at <https://www.futuregenerations.wales/about-us/future-generations-act/> accessed 12 January 2023.

[240] John Harrington, Barbara Hughes-Moore, and Erin Thomas, 'Towards a Welsh Health Law: Devolution, Divergence and Values' (2022) 73(3) Northern Ireland Legal Quarterly 385.

[241] UK Population Data, 'UK Population 2022', available at <https://populationdata.org.uk/uk-population/> accessed 12 January 2023.

[242] See Harrington et al. (n 238).

- **Focusing on prevention, health improvement, and inequality** as key to sustainable development, wellness, and well-being for future generations of the people of Wales.

- **Working in true partnerships** with partners and organisations and with staff.

- **Investing in our staff** through training and development, enabling them to influence decisions and providing them with the tools, systems, and environment to work safely and effectively.[243]

This is also followed through the Health and Care Standards for Health Services in Wales, which were published in 2015.[244] The Standards are designed to be:

> implemented in all health care organisations, settings and locations, and by all teams and services. Every person in Wales who uses health services or supports others to do so, whether in hospital, primary care, their community or in their own home has the right to receive excellent care as well as advice and support to maintain their health.[245]

They also form part of the overall quality assurance system within the NHS in Wales. They are guided by the key principles of doing the right things well; knowing how well they are doing, being open and honest in all that they do, showing care, compassion, and commitment; and leading by example.[246] These principles feed into individual standards which are organised around the following themes: governance, leadership and accountability, staying healthy, safe care, effective care, dignified care, timely care, individual care, and staff resources.[247]

In terms of the structure for NHS Wales, it currently has seven health boards, three NHS Trusts and two special health authorities. With the 2009 reforms, the Welsh Government reorganised local health boards, facilitating coordination with local government which has responsibility for primary care and commissioning from seven NHS Trusts.[248] The health boards are responsible for planning and delivering NHS healthcare services in their areas, as set out in **Figure 3.5**. These services include dental, optical, pharmacy, and mental health. They are also responsible for improving physical and mental health outcomes, promoting well-being, reducing health inequalities across their respective populations, and commissioning services from other organisations to meet the needs of their residents.[249]

The three Welsh NHS Trusts are: (i) *Public Health Wales NHS Trust*, which is the national public health agency that works to protect and improve health and well-being and reduce health inequalities for the people of Wales; (ii) *Velindre University NHS Trust*, which provides specialist cancer services across South and Mid Wales through Velindre Cancer Centre and a national service through the Welsh Blood Service; and (iii) *Welsh Ambulance Services NHS Trust*, which provides a range of out-of-hospital, emergency, and

---

[243] NHS Wales, 'Shared Services Partnership, Values and Standards of Behaviour Framework', available at < https://nwssp.nhs.wales/a-wp/governance-e-manual/living-public-service-values/values-and-standards-of-behaviour-framework/> accessed 12 January 2023.

[244] Welsh Government, NHS Management, 'Health and Care Standards', 2 April 2015, available at <https://www.gov.wales/health-and-care-standards> accessed 12 January 2023; see also Health and Social Care (Community Health and Standards) Act 2003, s 47.

[245] ibid., 4   [246] ibid., 4–5.   [247] ibid., 7–35.   [248] Dayan and Flinders (n 234).

[249] NHS Wales, 'Organisation Structure of NHS Wales', available at <https://nwssp.nhs.wales/a-wp/governance-e-manual/knowing-who-does-what-why/organisation-structure-of-nhs-wales/> accessed 12 January 2023.

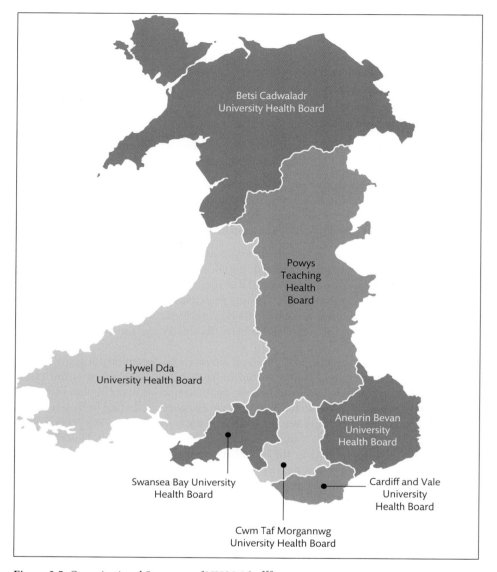

Figure 3.5 Organisational Structure of NHS Wales[250]

non-emergency services.[251] The two special health authorities are: (i) *Health Education and Improvement Wales* (HEIW), which is responsible for providing education, training, and development for the Welsh healthcare workforce; and (ii) *Digital Health and Care Wales,* which is responsible for designing and building digital services for health and care in Wales. Finally, there is the NHS Wales Shared Services Partnership (NSWWP) provides customer-focused support functions and services to NHS Wales.[252]

---

[250] ibid.
[251] NHS Confederation, 'About the NHS in Wales', 12 May 2021, available at <https://www.nhsconfed.org/articles/about-nhs-wales> accessed 12 January 2023.
[252] Welsh Government, 'NHS Wales Health Boards and Trusts', updated 4 May 2022, available at <https://www.gov.wales/nhs-wales-health-boards-and-trusts#section-48456> accessed 12 January 2023.

In terms of the recent performance of the Welsh NHS, the available evidence points to Welsh patients having longer waiting times than in the English NHS both in A&E as well as for surgical procedures across a range of medical specialities. However, the waiting times are less than in the NI health service. NHS Wales has a higher rate of treatable mortality than in England or NI, but around the same as in Scotland. There has been little progress in over a decade, with matters stalling over the last four years, with the Covid-19 pandemic no doubt being an exacerbating factor. It has been suggested that the reasons for poorer medical treatment times and health outcomes in Wales are attributable 'to the population being less healthy and needing more treatment' and there is empirical evidence available to support this view.[253] Clearly, Wales would benefit from greater financial investment in the delivery of its health and social care services, but it remains hamstrung by the Barnett formula for its annual budget, which does not accurately reflect the health demographics in Wales. To address the needs of the Welsh population, it has been estimated that Wales would needs at least a 10% higher allocation under the Barnett formula than Scotland and England, and 16% higher with an adjustment for health inequalities.[254]

The Welsh Government's current health strategy focuses on what is described as 'value-based, prudent health care' designed to make an impact on health and well-being throughout life. This is in line with the 'Quadruple Aim': namely, excellence in population health and well-being, personal experiences of care, best value from resources, and an engaged and committed workforce.[255] The plan sets out a long-term future vision of a 'whole system approach to health and social care', which is focused on health and well-being, and on preventing illness. It aims to ensure that the whole system is 'fit for the future', so that it can respond more quickly to future challenges and opportunities, which involves increased investment in digital technologies. The strategy also outlines 'common values for the whole system', in addition to employing ten design principles, which will translate its 'prudent healthcare philosophy and the central idea of the quadruple aim into practical tools which will help to align all of our transformation activity at every level'.[256]

Within the Welsh Government, there is a Minister for Health and Social Services, who is assisted by Deputy Ministers for Social Services and Mental Health and Wellbeing. Within the Welsh civil service, the Ministers are supported by the Director-General, Health and Social Services Group, who is also Chief Executive of NHS Wales. Other members of senior management include the Chief Medical Officer and the Chief Nursing Officer, as well as Directors for Health Protection, Vaccination, NHS Finance, Digital Transformation, NHS Workforce and Operations, Health and Wellbeing, and Social Care Officer for Wales and Social Services.[257] Health and social care remains a high priority for the Welsh Government, with over half of its total annual budget allocated in this area, which is 'by far the most important area for which Wales is responsible' under current devolution arrangements.[258] For the period 2023–24, it is estimated that health and social care services will be allocated a budget of £10.9 billion. However, it is recognised that additional funding allocations may need to be made to take account of the challenges currently facing NHS Wales, which has been exacerbated by the Covid-19 pandemic.[259]

[253] ibid.   [254] ibid.

[255] See Welsh Government, 'A Healthier Wales: Long Term Plan for Health and Social Care', last updated 8 November 2022, 4, available at <https://www.gov.wales/healthier-wales-long-term-plan-health-and-social-care> accessed 12 January 2023.

[256] ibid., 3.

[257] Welsh Government, 'Welsh Government Organisation Chart', September 2022, available at <https://www.gov.wales/welsh-government-organisation-chart> accessed 12 January 2023.

[258] Dayan and Flinders (n 234).

[259] BBC News, 'Welsh Government Budget: What Does It Mean for Me?', 13 December 2022.

It is also important to note that a Cooperation Agreement exists between the Welsh Ministers and the Welsh Parliament, which is based on a collective effort to develop a 'new politics—radical in content and co-operative in approach.'[260] They have committed to working together to realising the following initiatives relevant to health and social care. First, an expert group will be established to work on the development of a National Care Service, free at the point of need, continuing as a public service, with a view to implementing the plan by the end of 2023. This forms part of is part of an overall commitment to work towards better integration of health and social care and to promote parity of recognition and reward for health and care workers. Second, clearer referral pathways into NHS services will be implemented, which can help support young people in crisis or with urgent mental health or emotional well-being issues. Third, work will be undertaken to strengthen the rights of disabled people and tackle the inequalities they continue to face, underpinned by a commitment to the social model of disability.[261]

Building on the Cooperation Agreement, the Welsh Government has published a programme for government which focuses on the following policy initiatives to promote 'effective, high quality and sustainable healthcare', in line with the government's statutory commitment to promoting the future well-being of the Welsh population:[262]

- Provide medical treatments which have been delayed by the Covid-19 pandemic.
- Deliver better access to primary and secondary healthcare professionals, as well as reviewing patient pathway planning and hospice funding.
- Promote better integration of health and social care, including developing more than 50 local community hubs to co-locate front-line health and social care and other services. This is in addition to launching a new national social care framework.
- Prioritise investment in mental health, in particular child and mental health services.
- Keep prescriptions free in Wales.
- Establish an NHS National Executive.
- Focus on end-of-life care.
- Invest in and roll out new technology that supports fast and effective advice and treatments.
- Establish three new Intensive learning academies to improve patient experiences and outcomes.

In setting out its current programme, the Welsh Government recognises that the Covid-19 pandemic has had a significant adverse impact on the delivery of health and social care in Wales, and that additional financial investment and other resources are likely to be needed in the short to medium term to facilitate Covid-19 recovery for NHS Wales.[263]

---

[260] Welsh Government, 'The Co-operation Agreement 2021', 1, available at <https://www.gov.wales/co-operation-agreement-2021>accessed 12 January 2023.

[261] ibid., 3, 10.

[262] Welsh Government, 'Programme for Government Update', last updated 7 December 2021, available at <https://www.gov.wales/programme-for-government-update> accessed 12 January 2023.

[263] BBC News (n 257).

3.7.2 PATIENT SAFETY AND QUALITY IMPROVEMENT

In recent years, the Welsh Government has embarked upon a series of policy and legal initiatives in relation to quality and safety in health care in Wales. This has included the adoption of legislation to strengthen the duty of quality, as well as to establish a duty of candour, for the NHS in Wales.[264] In relation to the duty of quality, this provides that Welsh Ministers and local NHS health boards must exercise their functions in relation to the health service with a view to securing improvement in the quality of health services. In this respect, quality includes the effectiveness and safety of health services, as well as the experience of individuals to whom health services are provided. The Welsh Ministers are required to publish an annual report on the steps that they take to comply with the duty of quality, which will be laid before the National Assembly for Wales.[265] This duty is also extended to include local NHS health boards and trusts, as well as Special Health Authorities.[266] As part of discharging this new duty, the Welsh Government's Health and Care Standards must also be taken into account by relevant organisations.[267] In framing the duty of quality in this way, as well as creating a Citizen Voice Body (CVB) to ensure that patient voices are heard with respect to how best to delivery on quality and enhance patient safety,[268] emphasis has been placed on the importance of adopting a person-centred approach, which includes taking account of the patient experience, in determining the quality of a healthcare service.

In 2021, the new Welsh strategic framework for quality and safety in health care was published. It states that the combination of this new legislation, systems learning from recent healthcare scandals and the need to recover from the Covid-19 pandemic are the 'principal drivers' in the development of the new framework.[269] As part of the framework, healthcare organisations will be required to focus on meeting what has been described as the 'Quadruple Aim': namely, excellence in population health and well-being, personal experiences of care, best value from resources, and an engaged and committed workforce. Achieving such aims are to be in line with the commitment to value-based, prudent health care,[270] which in turn builds upon core values that underpin the NHS in Wales, such as putting quality and safety above all else.[271] Other initiatives that form part of the new framework include the creation of a new medical examiner service which is to be implemented across Wales, as part of a commitment to improving patient safety, as well as end of life care. The newly appointed medical examiners will independently examine all deaths that are not investigated by the coroner and will take account of any concerns expressed by family members. Where any potential issues are identified in relation to health care delivered to now deceased patients, then the examiners are required to pass this information on to NHS organisations for further review.[272]

---

[264] Health and Social Care (Quality and Engagement) Act 2020. See Chapter 4 for a more detailed examination as to how the duty of candour will operate in Wales once it is brought into force in 2023.

[265] ibid., s 2(2), inserting a new s 1A into the National Health Service (Wales) Act 2006.

[266] ibid., Part 2, ss 3–5, inserting new ss 12A, 20A and 24A into the National Health Service (Wales) Act 2006.

[267] Welsh Government, 'Health and Care Standards' (n 242).

[268] Health and Social Care (Quality and Engagement) Act 2020 (n 262) Part 4.

[269] Welsh Government, 'NHS Quality and Safety Framework: Learning and Improving', 17 September 2021, Foreword, available at <https://www.gov.wales/nhs-quality-and-safety-framework> accessed 12 January 2023.

[270] ibid.   [271] Welsh Government (n 253) 4.

[272] Welsh Government, 'NHS Quality and Safety Framework' (n 267), para 2.2.1.

Improvement Cymru, the Welsh national improvement support service for health care, will support the implementation of the new framework, focusing on the quality cycle across NHS organisations.[273] It has also published its own new strategy which is focused on supporting health and care organisations to redesign and continuously improve the service they provide; supporting a focus on reduction in avoidable harm and safety within systems of care; and sustainably building improvement capability within the health and care system.[274] In addition to the work undertaken by Improvement Cymru, there are other Welsh public bodies focused on patient safety and quality improvement. One such body is the NHS Wales Delivery Unit, which provides support with respect to patient safety, as well as the delivery of quality and safety in health care in NHS Wales. Within the Unit, there is a dedicated Quality and Safety team that provides leadership and support on incident reporting, learning from incidents and near miss events, compliance with patient safety solutions, and, where required, assurance reviews in NHS Health Boards and Trusts.[275] In addition, Healthcare Inspectorate Wales (HIW), the independent regulator of health care in Wales, undertakes inspection of NHS services, as well as regulating independent healthcare providers against a range of standards, policies, and laws, with a view to facilitating improvements.[276] Following inspections, HIW publishes reports that focus on the quality of the patient experience, the delivery of safety and effective care, and the quality of management and leadership.[277] It also has powers to escalate action requiring improvements, which is conducted via a service of concern process, where significant singular service failures have been identified, or where there are cumulative or systemic concerns regarding a service or setting.[278]

Mention should also be made of the Putting Things Right (PTR) programme, which is unique to Wales and is underpinned by legislation.[279] Introduced in 2011, PTR is a process that seeks to deal with complaints, clinical negligence claims, and patient safety incidents, which are collectively referred to as 'concerns'. It was originally established to promote a cultural change in NHS Wales in relation to dealing with things that go wrong in the provision of health care and to offer redress where harm had been caused to patient as a result.[280] It was hoped that the PTR process would 'streamline' the investigation of all concerns raised by patients, their families, and staff.[281] A three-person team currently oversees the process within NHS Wales, in addition to there being a dedicated point of contact in each NHS health board to facilitate the process at a local level.[282] While

[273] ibid., para 3.3.
[274] Improvement Cymru Strategy 2021–2026, 'Achieving Quality and Safety Improvement', available at <https://phw.nhs.wales/services-and-teams/improvement-cymru/about-us/improvement-cymru-strategy/> accessed 12 January 2023.
[275] NHS Wales, 'Delivery Unit, Patient Safety Wales', available at < https://du.nhs.wales/patient-safety-wales/> accessed 12 January 2023.
[276] Healthcare Inspectorate Wales, 'About Us', available at <https://www.hiw.org.uk/about> accessed 12 January 2023.
[277] Healthcare Inspectorate Wales, 'Inspect Healthcare', available at <https://www.hiw.org.uk/inspect-healthcare> accessed 12 January 2023.
[278] Healthcare Inspectorate Wales, 'Services Requiring Significant Improvement', available at <https://www.hiw.org.uk/services-requiring-significant-improvement> accessed 12 January 2023.
[279] See The NHS (Wales) Redress Measure 2008; NHS (Concerns, Complaints and Redress Arrangements) (Wales) Regulations 2011.
[280] NHS Wales, Cardiff and Vale University Health Board, 'Putting Things Right', available at <https://cavuhb.nhs.wales/patient-advice/concerns-complaints-and-compliments/putting-things-right/> accessed 12 January 2023.
[281] NHS Wales, Shared Services Partnership, 'Putting Things Right', available at <https://nwssp.nhs.wales/ourservices/legal-risk-services/areas-of-practice/putting-things-right/> accessed 12 January 2023.
[282] ibid.

admirable in its aims and objectives, there have been difficulties identified with the implementation of the PTR process.[283] These include inadequate resources within local NHS health boards to deal with the complaints being made to them; a defensive culture within the NHS in Wales in relation to responding to complaints; and institutional dysfunction with regards to investigation of complaints, including receiving prompt feedback from treating HCPs, and learning from complaints made. The Welsh Government has promised to reform the process in light of recommendations received for improvement.[284]

3.8 CONCLUSION

This chapter examined the governance of the health system in the UK. There are four health services, referred to collectively as the NHS, which operate in England and the devolved administrations of NI, Scotland, and Wales. Although the core values and principles that underpin the health services are broadly similar, their structures and organisational arrangements differ and are reflective of local healthcare policy and institutional cultures, as well as the need to focus on the (public) health needs of local populations. Over the past 25 years, the emergence of these distinctive approaches has been facilitated by political devolution arrangements in the UK, which have in turn become more pronounced in the wake of Brexit and the Covid-19 pandemic. Currently, the UK's four health services are facing significant challenges in delivering health and care to their respective populations as a result of the impact of the pandemic, with longer waiting times, an underpaid and demoralised health and care workforce, and growing health inequalities. Political leadership, as well as greater financial investment, are clearly needed to support Covid-19 recovery and to ensure that the UK's four health services remain fit for purpose in the twenty-first century.

FURTHER READING

1. Scott Greer, 'Devolution and Health in the UK: Policy and Its Lessons Since 1998' (2016) 118(1) Br Med Bull 16.

2. John Harrington, Barbara Hughes Moore, and Erin Thomas, 'Towards a Welsh Health Law: Devolution, Divergence and Values' (2022) 73(3) Northern Ireland Legal Quarterly 385.

3. Deirdre Heenan and Derek Birrell, *The Integration of Health and Social Care in The UK* (Palgrave 2018).

4. Caroline Redhead et al., 'Relationships, Rights and Responsibilities: (Re)viewing the NHS Constitution for the Post-Pandemic "New Normal"' (2023) 31(1) Medical Law Review 83.

5. May van Schalkwyk et al., 'Brexit and Trade Policy: An Analysis of the Governance of UK Trade Policy and What it Means for Health and Social Justice' (2021) 17 Globalization and Health 61.

---

[283] Response of the Public Services Ombudsman for Wales to the Welsh Government's Consultation on the Review of Concerns (Complaints) Handling within NHS Wales—'Using the Gift of Complaints', para 3.1.
[284] Welsh Government, 'Written Statement—A Review of Concerns (Complaints) Handling within NHS Wales—"Using the Gift of Complaints"—Next Steps', 24 November 2014, available at <https://www.gov.wales/written-statement-review-concerns-complaints-handling-within-nhs-wales-using-gift-complaints-next> accessed 12 January 2023. See also BBC News, 'NHS Wales: "No Blame Culture" Needed, Says Review', 2 July 2014, available at <https://www.bbc.co.uk/news/uk-wales-28113397> accessed 23 January 2023.

4

THE REGULATION OF HEALTH AND SOCIAL CARE PROFESSIONALS

4.1 INTRODUCTION

This chapter provides an overview of the regulation of health and social care professionals in the UK, with a focus on the work of the statutory professional regulators and their fitness to practise (FTP) procedures.* This is an increasingly important and visible layer of health and medical law and ethics, with high-profile outcomes of FTP panels, and appeals of those decisions, attracting media attention and scrutiny from patients, professionals, and members of the public. Professional guidance from the statutory regulators is often cited by the courts,[1] and has been scrutinised by public inquiries where there have been serious failures in care.[2]

The chapter will commence with an overview of the regulation of health and social care professionals in the UK, which will include consideration of the role and function of the Professional Standards Authority for Health and Social Care (PSA), the UK regulatory oversight body, and the ten statutory regulators that it oversees. While some discussions of this topic focus exclusively on the work of the General Medical Council (GMC) in relation to doctors, here we use the GMC's legislative regime as an example; an overview is also provided of key features of generic FTP proceedings. This provides the tools required to engage with the work of a variety of regulators and their respective statutory frameworks. Next, we focus on how regulators address concerns that are raised about their registrants. We consider the concept of 'impairment of fitness to practise', reflecting both on the roots of this concept, as developed by Dame Janet Smith in the Fifth Report of the Shipman Inquiry, and how this forward-looking test takes into account past actions, and has been applied by FTP panels.[3] Various case studies will be used by way of example to explore specific issues arising from FTP hearings, including those relating to criminal convictions, dishonesty, and sexual misconduct. Following this, we consider a current issue in professional regulation, namely the operation of the professional duty of candour which applies to all regulated health and social care professionals. In conclusion, this chapter provides some reflections on the future of professional regulation, including the impact and progress of longstanding calls for reform in this area.

* We are very grateful to Kisha Punchihewa and Simon Wiklund for their expertise and invaluable comments on this Chapter 4.

[1] *Montgomery* v *Lanarkshire Health Board* [2015] UKSC 11.

[2] UK Government, 'Report of the Mid Staffordshire NHS Foundation Trust Public Inquiry' (2013) HC 947.

[3] In this chapter we refer generically to fitness to practise 'panels'; some regulators use the terminology 'tribunal' or 'committee', and so we adopt this where appropriate.

4.2 AN OVERVIEW OF THE REGULATION OF HEALTH AND SOCIAL CARE PROFESSIONALS IN THE UK

To engage with the regulation of health and social care professionals in the UK it is necessary to first get to grips with the broad structure of this layer of health and medical law, which has been described variously as rigid and complex, and has evolved in a piecemeal fashion.

4.2.1 SETTING THE SCENE

To avoid confusion about the roles and functions in relation to the types of bodies and organisations that operate in this space, it is useful to begin by drawing a number of broad distinctions. The first distinction can be made as between the statutory regulators who operate at a *systems or organisational level* in health and social care, such as the Care Quality Commission (CQC),[4] and those that regulate at the *individual professional level*, such as the GMC. Clearly the work of both types of bodies impacts on the delivery of healthcare, but in different ways; in this chapter we focus on the latter.

To take the medical profession as an example, a second distinction exists as between the role of a body such as the GMC—a regulator whose statutory functions include ensuring that all doctors are registered with a licence to practise before they work in the UK[5]—and that of other bodies that support and/or represent medical professionals. Organisations that fall into the latter category include, for example: the medical royal colleges and faculties, such as the Royal College of Surgeons of Edinburgh, which are involved in the training and development of different specialities; trade unions, such as the British Medical Association, which support and negotiate on behalf of doctors and medical students; and defence organisations, such as the Medical Protection Society, which offers indemnity and advice. This brief description does not do justice to the varied scope of these different types of organisations, but is sufficient to make the point that the registration and licensing of doctors is a function that rests with the GMC. This position is mirrored across other professions which are subject to statutory registration.[6]

4.2.2 OCCUPATIONS AND JURISDICTIONS

Having focused on statutory regulation at the individual professional level, a second point that emerges from the preceding discussion is that this chapter so far has largely addressed the work of the GMC and how *doctors* are regulated and supported. However, there are other occupations within multidisciplinary health and care teams that the UK Parliament has also decided should be subject to statutory regulation. Indeed, in addition to the GMC, there are currently nine further statutory regulators (so, ten in total) that regulate a range of health and care professionals, and come within the remit of the oversight body, the PSA. These ten statutory regulators are set out in **Table 4.1**.

---

[4] The CQC is the independent regulator of health and social care in England. See CQC, 'About Us' (2022) available at <https://www.cqc.org.uk/> accessed on 05 August 2022.

[5] GMC, 'Registration and Licensing' (2022) available at <https://www.gmc-uk.org/registration-and-licensing> accessed on 08 September 2022.

[6] For example, consider the role of the Nursing and Midwifery Council (NMC), as opposed to the Royal College of Nursing and Royal College of Midwives.

Table 4.1 Ten statutory regulators that are overseen by the Professional Standards Authority

General Chiropractic Council (GCC)	General Pharmaceutical Council (GPhC)
General Dental Council (GDC)	Health and Care Professions Council (HCPC)
General Medical Council (GMC)	Nursing and Midwifery Council (NMC)
General Optical Council (GOC)	Pharmaceutical Society of Northern Ireland (PSNI)
General Osteopathic Council (GOsC)	Social Work England (SWE)

Some of these statutory regulators focus on a single occupation; for example, the GMC regulates doctors, the GCC regulates chiropractors, and the GOsC regulates osteopaths. Other bodies cover a number of related occupations, such as the GDC, which regulates dentists and dental care professionals, including dental hygienists, dental nurses, and dental technicians, among others. In further contrast, the HCPC regulates 15 different health, psychological, and care professionals, ranging from physiotherapists and para-medics, to speech and language therapists and operating department practitioners. These arrangements have evolved over time as new professions emerge or the risk profile of exist-ing professions change. For example, soon the GMC will also regulate two new groups of medical associate professions, namely physician associates and anaesthesia associates.[7]

It should also be noted that while the majority of the statutory regulators in **Table 4.1** cover the whole of the UK, this is not always the case. For example, while the GPhC regulates pharmacists and pharmacy technicians in Great Britain (England, Scotland, and Wales), the PSNI regulates pharmacists[8] in Northern Ireland. Further, and as its name suggests, the newest of the statutory regulators, Social Work England, only regu-lates social workers in England. In the other three countries of the UK, social workers must register with either the Scottish Social Services Council, Social Care Wales, or the Northern Ireland Social Care Council.[9]

4.2.3 A PIECEMEAL APPROACH, BUT WITH COMMONALITIES

Given the discussion so far in this chapter, it will come as no surprise that there is, at present, no single, coherent legal framework which sets out how each of the ten statutory regulators should operate. Rather, different pieces of primary[10] and secondary[11] legisla-tion have been enacted over time, in relation to each statutory regulator, that set out their respective governance structures and how they should carry out their functions. The cur-rent legal framework for the regulation of health and care professionals has been described by the Law Commission as 'fragmented, inconsistent and poorly understood'.[12] However, despite these variations between regulators, there are also a number of commonalities.

---

[7] At the time of writing, regulation is due to begin in the second half of 2024 at the earliest. See GMC, 'PA and AA Regulation Hub' (2022) available at <https://www.gmc-uk.org/pa-and-aa-regulation-hub> accessed on 08 September 2022.

[8] At the time of writing, pharmacy technicians are not regulated in Northern Ireland, unlike their coun-terparts in the rest of the UK.

[9] These regulators do not fall within the remit of the PSA and we touch on these only briefly here.

[10] For example, the Medical Act 1983.

[11] For example, the GMC, 'General Medical Council (Fitness to Practice) Rules Order of Council 2004)' (2004) available at <https://www.gmc-uk.org/-/media/documents/consolidated_version_of_FTP_Rules__as_amended_29Nov17_.pdf_72742310.pdf> accessed 07 September 2022.

[12] Department of Health and Social Care, 'Regulating Healthcare Professionals, Protecting the Public' (2022) available at <https://assets.publishing.service.gov.uk/government/uploads/system/uploads/attachment_data/file/978833/Regulating_healthcare_professionals__protecting_the_public.pdf> accessed 08 September 2022.

First, the position in relation to each of the occupations which are subject to statutory regulation is that professionals *must* have the necessary registration with the relevant regulator if they are to practise in the UK. Practising without being on the relevant register is a criminal offence. This stands in contrast to the position for those who work in health and social care in roles that are not subject to statutory regulation, such as practitioners of traditional acupuncture or counselling in the UK. Some professions that are not regulated by law can choose to join registers which are accredited by the PSA. However, this is not compulsory: in other words, professionals do so in order to demonstrate to those using the register (for example, members of the public who wish to find a practitioner) that they comply with certain quality standards, rather than because they are required to do so in order to practise in the UK.[13]

Second, while the precise wording differs, the over-arching objective of each of the regulators is to protect the public.[14] This objective is discharged through the regulators' work in four key areas.[15] These can be summarised as:

- setting the standards required for registration and practice;

- quality assuring education and training courses;

- maintaining a publicly accessible register of those who are entitled to practise in the relevant professions; and

- investigating concerns raised about those on their register and deciding whether they should be allowed to continue to practise without restriction (this area of work is often referred to as 'fitness to practise', or FTP, and is considered further in the next section).

Third, and as already alluded to, the ten statutory regulators each come within the remit of the PSA. In short, the PSA was established by statute by the National Health Service and Health Care Professions Act 2002[16] following the publication of the report of the public inquiry into children's heart surgery at the Bristol Royal Infirmary in 2001 (the Bristol Inquiry). The findings of the Bristol Inquiry, chaired by Professor Sir Ian Kennedy, concluded that there should be a unifying body to ensure that the relevant regulators serve the interests of the public and to provide a degree of consistency.[17] Today, the aim of the PSA is to protect the public by improving the regulation and registration of people who work in health and care. Its work falls into four main areas:

- reviewing the work of the regulators of health and care professionals against the PSA's own Standards of Good Regulation;[18]

- reviewing final FTP decisions to ensure that the outcome is sufficient to protect the public and to identify and share good practice via learning points. An outcome of

---

[13] For more information about accredited registers see Professional Standards Authority, 'What We Do – About Accredited Registers' (2022) available at <https://www.professionalstandards.org.uk/what-we-do/accredited-registers/about-accredited-registers> accessed 07 September 2022.

[14] For example, see Medical Act 1983, s 1A; Art 3(4) of the Nursing and Midwifery Order 2001.

[15] Professional Standards Authority, 'What We Do – About Regulators' (2022) available at <https://www.professionalstandards.org.uk/what-we-do/our-work-with-regulators/about-regulators> accessed 08 September 2022.

[16] Initially under another name, the Council for Healthcare Regulatory Excellence (CHRE).

[17] Secretary of State, 'The Bristol Royal Infirmary Inquiry' (2001) available at <http://www.bristol-inquiry.org.uk/final_report/index.htm> accessed 08 September 2022, Ch 25, para 75.

[18] Professional Standards Authority, 'What We Do – Our Performance Reviews' (2022) available at <https://www.professionalstandards.org.uk/what-we-do/our-work-with-regulators/read-performance-reviews> accessed 08 September 2022.

this may be that FTP decisions made by the regulators that do not protect the public are challenged in court;[19]

- accrediting organisations that register health and care practitioners in unregulated occupations,[20] and;

- giving policy advice to Ministers and others and encouraging research to improve regulation.[21]

In sum, the regulation of health and social care professionals is an area that spans a number of areas of work and engages with a wide range of stakeholders, including professionals and the public, as well as wider systems of health and care regulation and delivery. However, there are two areas that have attracted particular scrutiny over recent years.

The first can be addressed briefly and is in relation to maintaining a register, in order to assure the public that registered professionals have the training, skills, and experience to meet the standards that patients can expect. A key change in this area is that, for some professionals (such as doctors, nurses, and pharmacists) their initial registration is no longer indefinite in that it is also necessary for registrants to evidence, at regular periods, that their knowledge is up to date, that there are no concerns about their work, and that they provide a good level of care. This process is called revalidation[22] and it was first introduced for doctors by the GMC in 2012, having been consulted on as far back as June 2000.[23] However, a 2017 survey of over 1000 general practitioners and trainees indicated that 70% considered that this process was 'a time-consuming, box-ticking exercise which distracts from other learning'.[24] Some have argued that now is the time to consider whether the current system achieves its objectives, and so it remains to be seen how this process might evolve.[25]

The second area of the regulators' work that attracts significant public interest is their disciplinary function, i.e. their FTP processes. Only a small minority of healthcare professions will ever be involved in such processes, yet this consumes a large proportion of the regulators' budgets. We now consider this topic in more detail in the next section.

---

[19] Professional Standards Authority, 'What We Do – Decisions About Practitioners' (2022) available at <https://www.professionalstandards.org.uk/what-we-do/our-work-with-regulators/decisions-about-practitioners> accessed 08 September 2022.

[20] Professional Standards Authority, 'What We Do – Our Work with Accredited Registers' (2022) available at <https://www.professionalstandards.org.uk/what-we-do/accredited-registers> accessed 08 September 2022.

[21] Professional Standards Authority, 'What We Do – Improving Regulation' (2022) available at <https://www.professionalstandards.org.uk/what-we-do/improving-regulation> accessed 08 September 2022.

[22] This is distinct from Continuing Professional Development (CPD), though CPD is a component of revalidation.

[23] The King's Fund, 'Medical Revalidation—From Compliance to Commitment' (2014) available at <https://www.kingsfund.org.uk/sites/default/files/field/field_publication_file/medical-validation-vijaya-nath-mar14.pdf> accessed 08 September 2022.

[24] Pamela Curtis et al., 'Written Reflections in Assessment and Appraisal: GP and GP Trainee Views' (2017) 28(3) Education for Primary Care 141.

[25] Victoria Tzortziou Brown, Margaret McCartney, and Carl Heneghan, 'Appraisal and Revalidation for UK Doctors – Time to Assess the Evidence' (2020) 370 BMJ m3415.

4.3 FITNESS TO PRACTISE PROCEEDINGS

A key mechanism to ensure that regulators are able to discharge their objective to protect the public is their investigatory and decision-making function in circumstances where concerns are raised about a person on their register. As has already been established, the legislative frameworks differ as between the various regulators, though they share much in common.[26]

4.3.1 PURPOSE AND COMMON FEATURES

The purpose of FTP proceedings is, in its simplest terms, to protect the public from those who are not fit to practise. As we see later, this may be by reason of matters such as health, competence, conduct, criminal conviction or caution, and/or language proficiency. FTP processes may be distinguished from other routes through which individuals, such as patients, can seek civil redress, or professionals can be held accountable for their criminal actions (see Chapter 12).[27] The statutory regulators cannot force a registrant to apologise or deny them their liberty. They cannot order that compensation is paid, nor are FTP proceedings designed to punish registrants for past mistakes. Nonetheless, it is widely recognised that regulatory sanctions can have a punitive effect[28] and the process may be extremely stressful for those under investigation.[29] Until very recently little has been known about the impact of being a witness in FTP proceedings. However, research has been commissioned on this topic that seeks to explore this aspect further.[30]

Before turning to the specifics of *how* decisions with regard to FTP are made, it is worth briefly considering, in high-level terms, the processes and structures within which these decisions are made. As already established, the statutory framework varies between each regulator, and there are numerous inconsistencies with regard to the terminology that is used,[31] which makes it difficult to do so with great specificity. Nonetheless, it is possible to identify some generic features of FTP processes, which can assist in identifying the work of specific regulators, as set out in **Figure 4.1.** As we will see, case law can also help to shed light on how different aspects of these statutory processes should be interpreted.

Raising a Concern and Investigation

In summary, anyone can raise a concern about a registrant, including a member of the public, a patient, a colleague, an employer, or the police. Concerns could also arise from a media report. An initial filter may identify that some matters are not within the

---

[26] In this chapter we focus on FTP models based on the concept of 'impairment', although it should be noted that the model used by the General Osteopathic Council and the General Chiropractic Council is based on a test of 'unacceptable professional conduct'.

[27] In relation to the crucial differences between regulatory proceedings and criminal proceedings, see *The General Medical Council & Anor v Bramhall* [2021] EWHC 2109 (Admin), [43].

[28] *Bolton v Law Society* [1994] 2 All ER 486.

[29] See, GMC, 'Doctors who Commit Suicide While Under GMC Fitness to Practise Investigation' (2014) available at <https://www.gmc-uk.org/-/media/documents/internal-review-into-suicide-in-ftp-processes_pdf-59088696.pdf> accessed 08 September 2022 and GMC, 'GMC Publishes Report on Deaths During Investigations' (2022) available at <https://www.gmc-uk.org/news/news-archive/gmc-publishes-report-on-deaths-during-investigations> accessed 08 September 2022.

[30] Faculty of Wellbeing, Education and Language Studies, 'Witness to Harm, Holding to Account' (2022) available at <https://wels.open.ac.uk/research/witness-harm-holding-account> accessed 08 September 2022.

[31] A simple example is that while some regulators refer to the sanction of erasure, others refer to strike-off or removal.

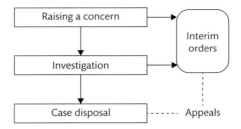

Figure 4.1 Some key features of a generic FTP processes

relevant regulator's jurisdiction (for example if they are not in relation to someone on their register)[32] and therefore can be closed quickly.[33] However, concerns that meet the regulator's threshold for action may be investigated in order to determine whether there is 'realistic prospect'[34] (i.e. one that is not remote or fanciful)[35] that the registrant's FTP is impaired. At present, this decision may be made by an Investigating Committee or by Case Examiners, depending on the regulator. Possible outcomes (again, depending on the regulator) include that the case may be closed (for example, with no further action, or with a warning given to the registrant, or undertakings offered by the registrant to the regulator) or referred on for further consideration.

Interim Orders

After an investigation has been opened, but before allegations have been proven, there may be some cases where it is appropriate to refer a case to a panel to consider whether it is necessary to put in place an interim order. The role of such a panel is not to make findings of fact, but rather to assess the risk posed by the registrant if they are allowed to continue in unrestricted practice while the investigation into their FTP is underway. To use the regulation of doctors as an example, the relevant test is whether the panel is 'satisfied that it is necessary for the protection of members of the public or is otherwise in the public interest, or is in the interests of a fully registered person, for the registration of that person to be suspended or to be made subject to conditions'.[36]

If an order is imposed, this will be time-limited and must be reviewed at regular intervals.[37] While there is no exhaustive list of the types of cases that will be suitable for consideration for interim measures, these may include those where there are serious concerns about a registrant's skills or conduct, concerns about intimate examinations or the maintenance of appropriate boundaries, or where a registrant's health poses a risk to patients or themselves.[38] The imposition of an interim order by a panel may be challenged by way of appeal to the relevant civil court.

---

[32] Note, however, that pre-registration conduct may be investigated in relation to a person who is on the register.

[33] The regulators may publish threshold criteria setting out matters which fall outside their jurisdiction or that will not be investigated.

[34] GMC, 'The Realistic Prospect Test' (2007) available at <https://www.gmc-uk.org/-/media/documents/DC4592_CE_Decision_Guidance___Annex_B___Realistic_Prospect_Test.pdf_25416411.pdf> accessed 08 September 2022.

[35] *Swain* v *Hillman* [2001] 1 All ER 91.   [36] Medical Act 1983, s 41A.   [37] ibid.

[38] These are some examples provided in the GMC's 'Guidance for Decision Makers on Referral to an Interim Order Tribunal (IOT)' (2021) available at <dc4593-interim-order-tribunal-referrals---ce-guidance-3799489.pdf (gmc-uk.org)> accessed 08 September 2022.

Case Disposal: Final Panel Hearings and Other Approaches

Where there is a realistic prospect that a registrant's FTP is impaired, the most serious cases may progress to a final panel hearing. Here, a wider range of sanctions are available, up to and including erasure from the register (available sanctions, and the terminology used, differ as between the regulators, depending on the substance of the allegations against the registrant).[39] Final hearings are usually heard by a specially constituted panel of the relevant regulator (so, for the NMC, their Fitness to Practise Committee; and for the General Dental Council, their Professional Conduct Committee). In contrast, the GMC's adjudicatory function is discharged by the Medical Practitioners Tribunal Service (MPTS) with the aim of providing some additional separation of the GMC's investigatory and adjudicatory functions. However, the MPTS remains a statutory committee of the GMC, and is accountable to the GMC Council and to the UK Parliament.[40]

Increasingly, regulators are also exploring other ways of disposing of cases without a final panel hearing. This can have the advantage of dealing with cases more quickly (which may benefit registrants and witnesses), and cost-effectively for the regulator, while still protecting the public. For example, the NMC provides that a consensual panel disposal may be appropriate where the registrant admits the facts of an allegation and agrees with the regulator that their FTP is impaired and on the appropriate sanction.[41] A key feature of current reform proposals (as addressed in more detail in section 4.7 below) is to make these powers of disposal available to case examiners at an earlier stage in the FTP process.

Appeals

Where an interim order is imposed, or certain sanctions are imposed by a final panel hearing, the registrant has the right to appeal the decision to the relevant civil court.[42] In addition, (though less common in practice), in circumstances where a final panel decision is not sufficient to protect the public, the PSA may refer a case for consideration by the relevant court.[43] In December 2015, the GMC was also given the power to appeal decisions of the MPTS where it considered them insufficient for the protection of the public, in relation to a finding, a penalty, or both. This right exists in tandem with the appeal rights of the PSA, and is not a power that has been bestowed on any of the other regulators. However, the GMC's right to appeal has not been without controversy. As is discussed further, the Williams Review has recommended that this should be revoked—a recommendation that has been accepted by the Government and is currently due to be actioned towards the end of 2023.

---

[39] For example, in respect of doctors, the MPTS may erase a doctor in any case except one that relates solely to the doctor's health and/or knowledge of English; see GMC. 'Sanctions guidance' (2018) available at <https://www.gmc-uk.org/-/media/documents/DC4198_Sanctions_Guidance_Feb_2018_23008260.pdf> accessed 09 September 2022, para 107. In contrast, the NMC's striking-off order 'can't be used if the [registrant's FTP] is impaired due to . . . their health, lack of competence or not having the necessary knowledge of English until they have been on either a suspension order **or** a conditions of practice order for a continuous period of two years.' See NMC, 'Striking-Off Order' (2020) available at <https://www.nmc.org.uk/ftp-library/sanctions/the-sanctions/striking-off-order/> accessed 08 September 2022.

[40] MPTS, 'Our Role' (2021) available at <https://www.mpts-uk.org/about/our-role> accessed 08 September 2022.

[41] NMC, 'Consensual Panel Determination' (2021) available at <https://www.nmc.org.uk/ftp-library/ftpc-decision-making/consensual-panel-determination/> accessed 08 September 2022.

[42] Depending on the registered address of the registrant this may be the Court of Session in Scotland, the High Court of Justice in Northern Ireland, or High Court of Justice in England and Wales.

[43] The power to do so is found in the NHS Reform and Health Care Professions Act 2002, s 29.

Case Law and a Note on Precedent Effect

Finally, although each regulator's FTP procedures operate within their own legislative framework, aspects of this will inevitably be disputed or open to interpretation. Some further assistance can be gleaned from a growing body of case law that has developed in this area. In short, the decisions of the final panels of the regulators (including the MPTS) have no direct precedent effect, meaning that any given FTP panel is not bound by its previous decisions. Such panels *are*, however, bound by decisions of the civil courts which hear FTP matters on appeal. Further, while the statutory frameworks for the various regulators differ, the case law that has emerged from the civil courts[44] applies across the regulators. In other words, just because a case was decided by the High Court in relation to an appeal of a decision of the NMC's Fitness to Practise Committee, the principles established can still apply to the other regulators (albeit that the exact detail of the underlying statutory framework might differ). This interplay between the framework provided for by legislation, and the role of case law in clarifying how this should be applied, is illustrated by the discussions that follow.

4.3.2 IMPAIRMENT OF FITNESS TO PRACTISE: AN 'ELUSIVE CONCEPT'

Statutory Framework

To use the GMC's statutory framework as an example, over the years a number of different phrases have been used to describe the circumstances in which steps may be taken by the regulator to restrict the practice of a registrant. These range from 'infamous conduct in a professional respect',[45] through 'serious professional misconduct',[46] to the present-day terminology of 'impairment of fitness to practise'.[47] The move to this 'new' approach to FTP was addressed in the findings of the Inquiry that was set up in the wake of the actions of the homicidal doctor, Harold Shipman, who was convicted in 2000 of the murder of 15 of his patients and the forging of a will.[48] The Shipman Inquiry (which ran from 2001 to 2005), was led by Dame Janet Smith and tragically found that Shipman had killed about 250 patients between 1971 and 1998.[49] Dame Janet's Fifth Report, published in December 2004, specifically addressed the role and processes of the GMC over this period. Among other matters, it was noted that the GMC's 'old' FTP procedures had 'failed in many respects to meet the reasonable expectations of patients and the public'.[50] Further, a feature of the 'new' approach introduced by the GMC was that this amalgamated what had previously been separate disciplinary procedures in relation to complaints about doctors' conduct, professional performance and ill health.[51] Instead, the relevant test became

[44] The vast majority of which are judgments of the Divisional Court of the High Court of Justice of England and Wales, but also from superior courts such as the Court of Appeal and the Supreme Court. In Scotland, the relevant Civil Courts are the Court of Session (Inner and Outer Houses) and the Supreme Court.

[45] Medical Act 1858.   [46] *Roylance v General Medical Council (No 2)* [2000] 1 AC 311, [330].

[47] Indeed, some of the misconduct case law which is still applicable predates the current impairment regime and relates to a time where the legal term was 'serious professional misconduct' as opposed to the simpler 'misconduct'.

[48] Department of Health, 'The Shipman Inquiry' (2006) available at <https://discovery.nationalarchives.gov.uk/details/r/C16350> accessed 08 September 2022.

[49] ibid.

[50] Department of Health, 'The Shipman Inquiry—The General Medical Council's "Old" Fitness to Practise Procedures' (2006) available at <https://webarchive.nationalarchives.gov.uk/ukgwa/20090809044228/http://www.the-shipman-inquiry.org.uk/5r_page.asp?id=4567> accessed 08 September 2022, para 10.

[51] Other improvements Dame Janet points to include: simplification of the preliminary stages of the process (para 134) and improved investigation of the facts of cases within the GMC's jurisdiction (para 135).

Table 4.2 The Medical Act 1983, section 35C

(2) A person's fitness to practise shall be regarded as 'impaired' for the purposes of this Act by reason only of

(a) misconduct;

(b) deficient professional performance;

(c) a conviction or caution in the British Islands for a criminal offence, or a conviction elsewhere for an offence which, if committed in England and Wales, would constitute a criminal offence;

(d) adverse physical or mental health;

(da) not having the necessary knowledge of English (but see section 2(4));

(e) a determination by a body in the United Kingdom responsible under any enactment for the regulation of a health or social care profession to the effect that his fitness to practise as a member of that profession is impaired, or a determination by a regulatory body elsewhere to the same effect.

Table 4.3 Guidance on impairment *(as formulated by Dame Janet Smith, Fifth Shipman Inquiry Report, Chapter 25, para 25.63)*

Is there one or more than one allegation of misconduct, deficient professional performance or adverse health and/or one or more than one report of a conviction, caution or determination which, if proved or admitted, might show that the doctor:

- has in the past acted and/or is liable in the future to act so as to put a patient or patients at unwarranted risk of harm; and/or
- has in the past brought and/or is liable in the future to bring the medical profession into disrepute; and/or
- has in the past committed a breach (other than one which is trivial) of one of the fundamental tenets of the medical profession and/or is liable to do so in the future; and/or
- has in the past acted dishonestly and/or is liable to act dishonestly in the future.

one of impairment of FTP on the basis of a number of specified grounds, as set out in **Table 4.2**. This meant that allegations of different types may be heard at the same time.

However, regardless of this and other developments, Dame Janet expressed continued concern that the term 'impairment of fitness to practise' was non-specific (a criticism also levelled against the previous terminology of 'serious professional misconduct'), and therefore called for further definition. She went on to consider the underlying reasons *why* a doctor's FTP might be impaired, and proposed that the test may be clarified in the terms set out in **Table 4.3**.

Case Law on Impairment

As the GMC's new regime bedded in (and similar regimes were introduced by other regulators), case law has helped to further clarify how impairment of FTP should be understood in this context. This has underlined that the emphasis is on *current* impairment, though this inevitably also requires considering past conduct.[52] As made clear by the case of *GMC* v *Meadow*:[53]

[52] *Cohen* v *GMC* [2008] EWHC 581 (Admin) and *Zygmunt* v *GMC* [2008] EWHC 2643 (Admin).
[53] [2006] EWCA Civ 1319.

the purpose of FTP procedures is not to punish the practitioner for past misdoings but to protect the public against the acts and omissions of those who are not fit to practise. The [Panel] thus looks forward not back. However, in order to form a view as to the fitness of a person to practise today, it is evident that it will have to take account of the way in which the person concerned has acted or failed to act in the past.[54]

As such, the decision-making process requires consideration of whether:

- the facts set out in the allegation are proved;
- those facts amount to the ground set out in the allegation (e.g. misconduct, as set out in **Table 4.2**); and
- in consequence, the registrant's fitness to practise is impaired.[55]

A further influential case in this area is *CHRE v NMC and Grant*.[56] This concerned a midwife who it was found had failed to provide appropriate assistance and support to a junior colleague, had subjected a junior colleague to bullying and/or harassment, and had failed to provide appropriate care to a patient who had been admitted for delivery of her baby who had died in utero. The registrant vigorously disputed the facts of the case but the majority of these were found proven. The panel subsequently moved to consider whether the midwife's FTP was impaired. They heard evidence in relation to a period of supervised practice undertaken by the midwife and a number of courses that she had undertaken. Ultimately, the panel found that the midwife's conduct, as established at the fact-finding stage, had been remediated and therefore that her FTP was not currently impaired.

This decision was appealed by the PSA's predecessor body on the basis that this it was unduly lenient. It was argued in particular that the panel had failed to give proper regard to the relevant public interest considerations, namely (i) the need for substantial weight to be given to the protection of the public, (ii) the maintenance of public confidence in the profession, and (iii) the upholding of proper standards of conduct and behaviour.[57] The appeal was upheld and provides an important reminder to panels that they do not only need to have regard to whether a registrant still poses a risk to members of the public but also to whether the need to uphold professional standards and public confidence in the profession would be undermined if a finding of impairment were not made, as was the case in *Grant*.[58]

So far, this chapter has focused on FTP processes and the decision-making framework, in order to orientate the reader within the sphere of professional regulation, and more specifically to the similar, yet distinctive, processes of each of the regulators. This working knowledge of these structures now allows for a deeper dive into the facts of a selection of some of the types of matters that the regulators consider. To do so we first consider matters relating to the conduct of Dr Bawa-Garba, a high-profile case which has had a significant impact on the regulatory landscape and raised issues, not least relating to the criminal charge of gross negligence manslaughter (GNM) and the relationship between systemic and individual failures in the regulatory context. This case can be contrasted with *Grant* in that the point at issue was not whether the doctor's FTP was impaired, but rather whether the appropriate sanction was suspension or erasure. Then we consider more generally the issues raised by two different types of serious cases, namely those that involve sexual misconduct and dishonesty.

---

[54] ibid., [32]; see also *Cheatle v GMC* [2009] EWHC 645(Admin), [22], which further elaborates on how the context of a doctor's behaviour must be examined.
[55] See, for example, ibid.   [56] [2011] EWHC 927 (Admin).   [57] ibid., [90].
[58] ibid., [101]; For cases that have applied the key case law in this see, for example, *PSA v (1) GMC (2) Uppal* [2015] EWHC 1304; *PSA v (1) HCPC (2) Roberts* [2020] EWHC 1906 (Admin). In both cases the PSA's appeal was not upheld.

4.4 THE CASE OF DR BAWA-GARBA

The facts relating to the case of Dr Hadiza Bawa-Garba can be briefly summarised as follows.[59] In February 2011, Dr Bawa-Garba was a junior doctor, specialising in paediatrics, who had recently returned from maternity leave. Together with two other members of staff, she provided care during the course of a 13-hour double shift to Jack Adcock, a six-year-old boy diagnosed with Down's Syndrome. Jack was brought to hospital and initially treated for a stomach bug and dehydration, and later with antibiotics for pneumonia. In fact, the Crown Court found that Jack was suffering with pneumonia, which caused his body to go into septic shock and resulted in heart failure and his death later that evening.[60]

A GNM prosecution was brought against Dr Bawa-Garba (and two other nurses who had provided care to Jack). The legal test in such cases is whether what the defendants did (or did not) do was 'truly exceptionally bad' and a direction to this effect was given to the jury hearing the criminal case.[61] The Crown's case against Dr Bawa-Garba relied on her failure to adequately assess and reassess Jack in light of obvious clinical findings and symptoms.[62] In Dr Bawa-Garba's defence it was noted, among other matters, that: a failure in the hospital's electronic computer system meant that blood test results were not delivered in the normal way and she was without the assistance of a Senior House Officer, and so she did not see these results until later in the day; staff shortages resulted in reliance on agency nursing staff, including her co-accused, Nurse Isabel Amaro,[63] who failed to properly observe Jack, and to communicate his deterioration while Dr Bawa-Garba was heavily involved in looking after other very sick children; she was not told by nursing staff that a crucial X-ray was ready for review; and that there was a delay in the administration of antibiotics she prescribed.[64] On 4 November 2015, Dr Bawa-Garba was found guilty of GNM at Nottingham Crown Court before Nicol J and a jury, and sentenced to two years' imprisonment, suspended for two years. Her application to the Court of Appeal (Criminal Division) for leave to appeal the Crown Court's findings was refused.[65]

Dr Bawa-Garba's conviction was subsequently considered by the GMC's MPTS. Unlike the case of *Grant*, there was no dispute that Dr Bawa-Garba's FTP was impaired by reason of her conviction. In their decision on 13 June 2017, the MPTS found that while her serious clinical failings had been remedied, and therefore she posed a low risk of future harm, a finding of impairment was required, to maintain public confidence in the profession and to promote proper professional standards and conduct. Moving to sanction the MPTS considered both mitigating factors, including the presence of multiple and systemic failures at the Trust, as well as aggravating factors, such as Dr Bawa-Garba's numerous and continued clinical failures, and concluded that a 12-month suspension order was appropriate, with a review.

---

[59] As taken from *R v Bawa-Garba (Hadiza)* [2016] EWCA Crim 1841 and *Bawa-Garba v General Medical Council [2018]* [2018] EWCA Civ 1879.

[60] *R v Bawa-Garba (Hadiza)* [2016] EWCA Crim 1841 [7].

[61] See, in contrast, the case of David Sellu in *Sellu v The Crown* [2016] EWCA Crim 1716 [156]. Here the direction to the jury on the issue of GNM was inadequate and, as a result, the conviction was unsafe and was quashed.

[62] *R v Bawa-Garba (Hadiza)* [2016] EWCA Crim 1841 [11].

[63] It should be noted that the NMC removed this nurse's name from the register following FTP proceedings.

[64] *R v Bawa-Garba (Hadiza)* [2016] EWCA Crim 1841 [17]–[18].   [65] ibid.

The GMC appealed the decision of the MPTS to the High Court of Justice (also referred to as the Divisional Court) on the basis that the sanction of suspension was not sufficient for the protection of the public. In particular, it was submitted:

(i) that the Tribunal had in effect allowed evidence of systemic failings to undermine Dr Bawa-Garba's personal culpability, and to do so even though those failings had been before the Crown Court which convicted her, and (ii) that remediation and personal mitigation were of too limited weight to satisfy the requirements of the public interest in upholding confidence in the profession.[66]

On behalf of Dr Bawa-Garba it was argued that 'The Tribunal had reached conclusions on the facts of remediation, mitigation and wider circumstances which were entirely open to it and should be respected.'[67] Ultimately, the Divisional Court decided that the appeal should be allowed and that the sanction of erasure should be imposed.[68] In particular it was noted that the criminal court had found that 'Dr Bawa-Garba's failures that day were not simply honest errors or mere negligence, but were truly exceptionally bad.'[69] Therefore, the MPTS's approach had fallen into error in that it 'did not respect the true force of the jury's verdict nor did it give it the weight required when considering the need to maintain public confidence in the profession and proper standards'.[70] In due course, this decision was appealed to the Court of Appeal, which came to a different conclusion.[71] The Appeal Court considered that the Divisional Court had adopted an impermissible approach, which effectively amounted to a presumption of erasure in such cases.[72] It was therefore found that the MPTS had been entitled to reach its evaluative judgment that suspension was the appropriate sanction.[73] As such, the MPTS's original sanction was restored.

Although this case was high-profile, these judgments serve as a stark reminder of the everyday complexities of FTP decision making.[74] This is in circumstances where events inevitably take place in the context of high-risk health (and social care) environments, where professionals work within multi-disciplinary teams, and individual and systemic issues may be interwoven. This case illustrates the devastating impact on patients and their families when things go wrong. However, Dr Bawa-Garba's case has also been described as 'unusual',[75] in circumstances where no other concerns had ever been raised about her practice and she continued to carry out clinical work up to the point of her GNM conviction. The issues raised by the case have certainly led to significant debate within and beyond the medical community. In particular, a review into GNM prosecutions against healthcare professionals in 2018, led by Professor Sir Norman Williams (known colloquially as the Williams Review), was commissioned by the then Secretary of State for Health to address 'great unease within the healthcare professions' as a result of a cases such as that of Dr Bawa-Garba. The Williams Review made a number of recommendations, as set out in **Table 4.4**, not least that the GMC should have its right to appeal cases removed, on the basis that this would 'help address mistrust that has emerged between the GMC and

---

[66] *General Medical Council* v *Bawa-Garba* [2018] EWHC 76 (Admin) [26].   [67] ibid. [29].
[68] ibid. [37].   [69] This being the legal test for GNM.   [70] *GMC* v *Bawa-Garba* (n 64) [38].
[71] *Bawa-Garba* v *General Medical Council* [2018] EWCA Civ 1879.   [72] ibid. [88].
[73] ibid. [97]–[98].

[74] For another case involving a GNM conviction of a healthcare professional (though here the conviction was subsequently overturned by the Court of Appeal), see *Rose* v *R* [2017] 3 WLR 1461. The optometrist was originally suspended by the General Optical Council, a decision that was challenged by the PSA: *PSA* v *(1) GOC (2) Rose* [2021] EWHC 2888 (Admin). The appeal was upheld and the optometrist was later struck off by the GOC. For further details on the GNM prosecution, see Chapter 12.
[75] ibid. [92].

Table 4.4 Summary of selected key recommendations from Williams Review

- Revised guidance to investigatory and prosecutorial bodies and a clearer understanding of the bar for gross negligence manslaughter in law to focus on those rare cases where an individual's performance is so 'truly exceptionally bad' that it requires a criminal sanction.
- Systemic issues and human factors will be considered alongside the individual actions of healthcare professionals where errors are made that lead to a death.
- Better support for bereaved families who should be provided with prompt, accurate and honest explanations following any untoward event which might have contributed to the death of a family member or loved one, and the opportunity to be actively involved throughout investigative and regulatory processes.
- The General Medical Council should have its right to appeal fitness to practise decisions by its Medical Practitioner Tribunal Service removed.
- The General Medical Council and General Optical Council will no longer be able to require registrants to provide reflective material when investigating fitness to practise cases.
- Concerns about the over-representation of Black, Asian, and Minority Ethnic healthcare professionals in fitness to practise procedures should be investigated, understood, and addressed.

the doctors that it regulates'.[76] Nonetheless, at the time of writing the necessary legislation is yet to be tabled by the Government and the GMC has continued to exercise their right to appeal.[77]

Following the Williams Review, further work has added to our understanding of some of the issues this raised. For example, in relation to concern about the over-representation of Black, Asian, and Minority Ethnic healthcare professionals in FTP procedures, a report commissioned by the GMC, 'Fair to Refer?', has addressed disparities between referrals of different groups of doctors to their regulator. This notes that the rate of referral to the GMC by employers of ethnic minority doctors was more than double that of white doctors.[78] Further, doctors whose primary qualification was obtained outside of the UK had a rate of referral by employers to the GMC that was 2.5 times higher than that of UK graduate doctors. The research demonstrates that there are 'risk factors' and 'protective factors' that may attach to doctors and could layer to create a cumulatively positive or negative impact, creating insider and outsider groups. Examples of risk factors include doctors being provided with inadequate inductions, working in isolated roles, or where doctors do not receive effective, honest, or timely feedback.[79] Action taken following this report includes the addition of new fairness checks on GMC referral forms as used by employers[80] and GMC reporting against targets to eliminate disproportionality in employer referrals by 2026.[81]

---

[76] ibid. [26].

[77] It has been reported that the Department of Health and Social Care will table legislation in the second half of 2023, at the same time as legislation that will introduce the statutory regulation of physician associates and anaesthesia associates. See Clare Dyer, 'GMC Set to Lose Power to Appeal Decisions by Medical Practitioners Tribunals' (2022) 378 BMJ o1875.

[78] GMC, 'Fair to Refer? Reducing Disproportionality in Fitness to Practice Concerns Reported to the GMC' (2019) available at <fair-to-refer-report_pdf-79011677.pdf (gmc-uk.org)> accessed 08 September 2022.

[79] See the full report for further examples and more detail.

[80] GMC, 'New Fairness Checks on Our Referral Form' (2021) available at <https://www.gmc-uk.org/responsible-officer-hub/news/new-fairness-checks-on-our-referral-form> accessed 09 September 2022.

[81] GMC, 'Equality, Diversity and Inclusion – Target, Progress and Priorities for 2022' (2022) available at <https://www.gmc-uk.org/-/media/documents/equality--diversity-and-inclusion--targets---progress-and-priorties_pdf-89470868.pdf> accessed 08 September 2022.

Following an Employment Tribunal finding of less favourable treatment by the GMC of a registrant on the grounds of race in 2021,[82] it seems likely that progress against these targets will be closely scrutinised. A more recent report by the BMA on delivering racial equality in medicine has pointed to the scale and impact of racism in healthcare and made a series of recommendation for organisational and institutional change.[83]

4.5 SEXUAL MISCONDUCT AND DISHONESTY

The analysis thus far has focused on different facets of a particular FTP case. However, now we move on to briefly consider two *types* of misconduct that are likely to fall at the more serious end of the spectrum, namely those that concern dishonesty or sexual misconduct. These are areas worthy of consideration in light of the case law that has been generated but also, on a more fundamental level, because of the questions they raise about what it means to be part of a regulated occupation, and the standards of professional and personal conduct that this entails.

4.5.1 DISHONESTY

It is perhaps trite to say that honesty is an essential quality for health and social care professionals to possess. However, this is particularly important where there is an imbalance of power between those who provide and receive care.[84] More specifically, honesty is necessary to justify the trust that patients and service users put in professionals, and to maintain public confidence in these professions more widely.[85] As such, honesty is a fundamental tenet of the health and social care professions, and *dis*honesty is specifically identified by Dame Janet Smith as something which might impair a registrant's FTP.[86] The first edition of 'Good Medical Practice' (GMP), issued by the GMC in 1995,[87] explicitly stated that: 'You must be honest and trustworthy'.[88] The importance of honesty and integrity are echoed and expanded on in the most recent edition of these ethical guidelines.

---

[82] Employment Tribunal, '*Dr O M A Karim v GMC*: 3332128/2018–Judgment with Reasons' (2021) available at <https://assets.publishing.service.gov.uk/media/60db0b898fa8f50ab2f55af7/Dr_O_M_A_Karim_v_GMC_3332128-2018_JR.pdf> accessed 09 September 2022. The GMC has announced that it intends to appeal this finding.

[83] BMA, 'Delivering Racial Equality in Medicine' (2022) available at <https://www.bma.org.uk/media/5745/bma-delivering-racial-equality-in-medicine-report-15-june-2022.pdf> accessed 09 September 2022.

[84] Ann Gallagher and Robert Jago, 'A Typology of Dishonesty – Illustrations from the PSA Section 29 Database' (2016) available at <https://www.professionalstandards.org.uk/docs/default-source/publications/research-paper/a-typology-of-dishonesty---illustrations-using-the-fitness-to-practise-database.pdf?sfvrsn=827d7020_6> accessed 08 September 2022.

[85] For example, see GMC, 'Domain 4: Maintaining Trust' (2013) available at <https://www.gmc-uk.org/ethical-guidance/ethical-guidance-for-doctors/good-medical-practice/domain-4---maintaining-trust> accessed 09 September 2022. para 65, 'You must make sure that your conduct justifies your patients' trust in you and the public's trust in the profession.'

[86] See Table 4.3.

[87] This was the first publication by the GMC that provided a 'positive statement about the standards of care patients should expect and doctors should work towards'. See GMC, 'Our History' (2022) available at <https://www.gmc-uk.org/about/who-we-are/our-history> accessed 09 September 2022.

[88] GMC, 'Good Medical Practice (1995)' (1995) available at <https://www.gmc-uk.org/-/media/documents/good-medical-practice-1995-55611042.pdf?la=en> accessed 08 September 2022.

A recent study found that there is some consistency across all of the statutory regulators' guidance to the effect that dishonesty is one of the types of misconduct that carries a 'presumption of seriousness'.[89] Nonetheless, this does not mean that all cases of dishonesty are alike, or that they are treated in the same way. Indeed, the same study found that:

> when it to comes to situating an act or omission on a spectrum of seriousness, there is variance within and between regulators. Analysis comparing cases with seemingly similar basic content in terms of the type of misconduct, looking across a series of dishonesty cases involving the falsification of documents, shows that these resulted in a wide range of sanction outcomes. Therefore, even in cases where there is a presumption of seriousness based on the type of misconduct involved . . . the outcome is shaped by the specific combination of factors in the individual case.[90]

Further, dishonesty may come in many forms.[91] Contrast, for example, withholding the truth (such as failing to disclose a previous conviction or an ongoing FTP investigation to a prospective employer) with deliberate mistruths (such as submitting false claims to a health insurer for payment). Other types of dishonesty may include matters such as impersonation, theft, fraud, and academic dishonesty.[92] Some of these types of dishonesty may occur outside of a registrant's *clinical* responsibilities and therefore not result in direct patient harm (for example, fraudulent claims for monies to a public body or insurer). However, such matters may still be considered serious in circumstances where institutions within healthcare should be able to trust in registrants' probity.[93] Indeed one factor that may indicate that erasure is an appropriate sanction is the presence of dishonesty, 'especially where persistent and/or covered up'.[94] However, as we come to next, the case law makes it clear that there is no presumption of erasure in cases of dishonesty.

Hassan v *General Optical Council*[95] (GOC) concerned the conduct of a student optometrist who had received a caution for misrepresentation by fraud when he was 18. The background was that the registrant had boarded a bus which his friend was driving and planned to crash so that the registrant could make a false insurance claim. The registrant was investigated by the police, pleaded guilty to the criminal offence and received a caution. Hassan did not declare this on a number of registration forms which requested such information, on the basis that he had thought that a caution (as opposed to a conviction) would not affect his practice as an optometrist. The registrant indicated that in discussion with his brother he later realised this was not the case and contacted the GOC to inform them of his caution. The FTP committee which heard his case was 'of the view that this is

---

[89]   Marie Bryce et al., 'The Concept of Seriousness in Fitness to Practise Cases' (2022) available at <https://www.nmc.org.uk/globalassets/sitedocuments/news/february-2022_concept-of-seriousness-in-fitness-to-practise-cases.pdf> accessed 09 September 2022, p 12.

[90]   ibid, p 12.

[91]   Indeed, the need to differentiate between different degrees of dishonesty has been addressed in case law. See *Watters* v *Nursing and Midwifery Council* EWHC 1888 (Admin); *Lusinga* v *Nursing and Midwifery Council* EWHC 1458 (Admin).

[92]   These examples and typologies of dishonesty are taken from Ann Gallagher and Robert Jago (n 84), p 25. In terms of the prevalence of certain types of dishonesty, this study further found that: 'Of the 151 cases reviewed the three most particular kinds of dishonest activities were firstly, failure to disclose convictions/ cautions to the regulator either upon registration or for the purposes of retention on the register (19 cases). Secondly, simple theft of identified monies, prescription pads and medication or drug paraphernalia (18 cases) and finally, receiving sick pay and salary from a second employer simultaneously (13 cases)'.

[93]   See, for example, MPTS, 'Sanctions Guidance' (2020) available at <https://www.mpts-uk.org/-/media/mpts-documents/dc4198-sanctions-guidance---16th-november-2020_pdf-84606971.pdf> accessed 09 September 2022, para 123; *Dr Shiv Prasad Dey* v *GMC* (Privy Council Appeal No.19 of 2001).

[94]   ibid., para 108.   [95]   [2013] EWHC 1887 (Admin).

a very serious dishonesty perpetuated by the untruthful applications to the GOC'[96] and, having considered the appropriateness of lesser sanctions in turn, the sanction of erasure was imposed. An appeal was subsequently brought by the registrant on a number of grounds, including that the legal advice provided by the committee has misdirected their decision. In particular, the committee were referred to case law from a different regulatory arena—namely the Solicitors' Disciplinary Tribunal—which it was argued 'gave the impression that there is a strong presumption that any finding of dishonesty should lead to striking off unless that presumption can be displaced by demonstrating some exceptional circumstances'.[97] Leggat J upheld the appeal and found that:

> Dishonesty encompasses a very wide range of different facts and circumstances. Any instance of it is likely to impair a professional person's fitness to practise and in that sense is a serious matter. But it is wrong in my view to approach the question of sanction on the basis that there is only a small residual category of exceptional cases where erasure would be a disproportionate sanction and then to ask whether there are any exceptional factors which take the instant case into that residual category.

Another key development in the case law relates to the correct test to be applied in order to determine whether an act is dishonest. The longstanding position until 2017 was that decisions should be made following the two-part approach in the criminal case of *R v Ghosh*,[98] which included an objective and a subjective element. It required consideration of, first, whether (objectively) what was done was dishonest by the standards of ordinary people. If not, the matter ended there. However, if the conduct *was* dishonest by those standards, then it was necessary to consider (subjectively) whether the registrant had to have realised that what they were doing was, by the standards of ordinary people, dishonest. If the answer to *both* questions was yes, then a finding of dishonesty would follow.

In what has been recognised as a substantial change in the law, this test has been disapproved by the more recent UK Supreme Court case of *Ivey v Genting Casinos (UK) Limited (t/a Crockfords Club)*.[99] In *Ivey*, Lord Hughes sets out a number of reasons why the second limb of *Ghosh*, in particular, is problematic. Among these are, first, that it is hard for decision makers to understand and apply, and, second, that 'the less the defendant's standards conform to what society in general expects, the less likely he is to be held . . . responsible for his behaviour'.[100] Now, following *Ivey*, the legal position is as follows:

> When dishonesty is in question the fact-finding tribunal must first ascertain (subjectively) the actual state of the individual's knowledge or belief as to the facts. The reasonableness or otherwise of his belief is a matter of evidence (often in practice determinative) going to whether he held the belief, but it is not an additional requirement that his belief must be reasonable; the question is whether it is genuinely held. When once his actual state of mind as to knowledge or belief as to facts is established, the question whether his conduct was honest or dishonest is to be determined by the fact-finder by applying the (objective) standards of ordinary decent people. There is no requirement that the defendant must appreciate that what he has done is, by those standards, dishonest.[101]

It is well established that the *Ivey* test ought to be applied in regulatory proceedings,[102] though the longer-term impact of this change in the law will remain to be seen. In addition, the preceding discussion demonstrates how interconnected professional regulation

---

[96] ibid. [20].   [97] ibid. [30].   [98] [1982] EWCA Crim 2.   [99] [2017] UKSC 67.
[100] ibid. [58].   [101] ibid. [74].
[102] The case of *GMC v Krishnan* [2017] EWHC 2892 (Admin) which was the first to be heard after the decision in *Ivey*.

is to other areas of law. Indeed, *Ivey* had nothing to do with healthcare—rather, it was a dispute between a professional gambler and a casino about whether he had been cheating (and therefore whether he was entitled to his winnings of around £7 million). Nonetheless, this UK Supreme Court judgment has significantly changed how FTP panels, and courts, will approach cases of dishonesty going forward.

A further connection that is increasingly being probed is that between dishonesty and publics' views on the standards that are expected of health and care professions. For example, a 2016 report commissioned by the PSA indicated that both members of the public and professionals could identify common aggravating and mitigating factors in dishonesty cases, and the majority recognised the fine judgments that must be made when balancing these.[103] A further finding was that both groups were intolerant of 'scapegoating' of junior members of staff where there were cultural factors in play and/or leadership failures.[104] Other research into promoting and maintaining public confidence in the medical profession,[105] commissioned by the GMC, has been relied upon in relation to a change in the GMC's guidance in relation to concerns involving low level dishonesty (and violence) to allow greater discretion on the action that can be taken to address these types of concerns.[106]

4.5.2 SEXUAL MISCONDUCT

A second type of serious case that may come within the FTP domain are those that relate to sexual misconduct by health and social care professionals. In common with the discussion of dishonesty, such cases may take place within or outside of a professional's clinical practice, and can 'encompass a wide range of conduct from criminal convictions for sexual assault and sexual abuse of children (including child sex abuse materials) to sexual misconduct with patients, colleagues, patients' relatives or others'.[107] Like dishonesty cases, those relating to sexual misconduct require decision makers to engage with questions in relation to a registrant's state of mind.[108] Some of the difficulties this may bring to the decision-making process are illustrated by the case of *Basson* v *General Medical Council*,[109] in which Mostyn J noted that: 'the state of a person's mind is not something that can be proved by direct observation. It can only be proved by inference or deduction from the surrounding evidence.'[110]

---

[103] Policis, 'Dishonest Behaviour by Health and Care Professionals: Exploring the Views of the General Public and Professionals' (2016) available at <https://www.professionalstandards.org.uk/docs/default-source/publications/research-paper/dishonest-behaviour-by-hcp-research.pdf?sfvrsn=cff17120_34> accessed 08 September 2022.

[104] ibid., p 59.

[105] GMC, 'Promoting and Maintaining Public Confidence in the Medical Profession' (2019) available at <https://www.gmc-uk.org/-/media/documents/promoting-and-maintaining-public-confidence-final-report_pdf-78744915.pdf> accessed 08 September 2022.

[106] GMC, 'Updates to our Guidance for Concerns Involving Low Level Violence and Dishonesty' (2021) available at <https://www.gmc-uk.org/responsible-officer-hub/news/updates-to-our-guidance-for-concerns-involving-low-level-violence-and-dishonesty> accessed 08 September 2022.

[107] MPTS (n 93) paras 149–159.

[108] For example, see the HCPC's guidance on this point, at HCPTS, 'Practice Note – Making Decisions on a Registrant's State of Mind' (2021) available at <https://www.hcpts-uk.org/globalassets/hcpts-site/publications/practice-notes/making-decisions-on-a-registrants-state-of-mind.pdf> accessed 08 September 2022.

[109] [2018] EWHC 505 (Admin).

[110] ibid. [17]. In *Basson* it was found that a male GP had inappropriately touched the leg of a female patient and made comments about the length of her skirt. The registrant's appeal of the sanction of a short 28-day suspension was rejected.

Further guidance on this point was offered in the case of *Haris* v *General Medical Council*[111] which was considered by the Court of Appeal. Here a doctor had appealed against the decision that there had been a sexual motivation for his intimate examination of two female patients. In doing so he had relied, among other matters, on evidence that he had no interest in a sexual relationship and described himself as asexual to a consultant forensic psychiatrist who gave evidence before the original tribunal. The Court of Appeal upheld the Divisional Court's finding of sexual motivation and noted that:

> the best evidence as to Dr Haris's motivation was his behaviour. As a matter of common sense, when a patient presents with pain in the upper back in consequence of a fall, there is no reason whatsoever for a doctor to examine her vagina, or to fondle her buttocks or breast. The behaviour was not just capable of being reasonably perceived to be overtly sexual, it *was* overtly sexual, and there is no other way in which it could have been perceived. A doctor, of all people, would have known that.[112]

This case, along with others,[113] demonstrates some of the issues that may face decision-makers when formulating allegations in relation to sexual misconduct and considering questions of sexual motivation during fitness to practise proceedings. Indeed, it has been suggested that fitness to practise panels may still 'struggle with the perceived "inherent unlikelihood" (as per *Re B* [2008] UKHL 35) of a sexual act being perpetrated against a patient by a member of the medical profession'.[114] Further, the decision in *Haris*:

> demonstrates in stark terms that even those Tribunals faced with overwhelming proven evidence of two strikingly similar sexual acts, will be tempted to find a way to deny the reality that professionals are human, fallible and capable of making bad decisions whether clinical or personal, in a professional context.[115]

As noted, as well as patients, sexual misconduct may also be directed towards others, such as colleagues. This is a persistent issue and may be closely related to what has been described as a 'culture of misogyny'[116] in medicine. A 2017 study indicated that among the professions examined, sexual misconduct was more prevalent 'as a misconduct amongst doctors, than any other profession'.[117]

More generally, the British Medical Association's report, 'Sexism in Medicine', which was published in 2021, stated that 91% of women doctors in the UK have experienced sexism at work and 42% felt that they could not report this. In addition, 31% of women and 23% of men who responded to the survey experienced unwanted physical conduct in their workplace, and 56% of women and 28% of men had received unwanted verbal conduct

---

[111] [2021] EWCA Civ 763.   [112] ibid. [37].

[113] See, for example, *Basson*; *General Medical Council* v *Jagjivan* [2017] EWHC 1247 (Admin); *PSA* v *HCPC and Wood* [2019] EWHC 2819 (Admin).

[114] 23 Essex Street, 'Professional Discipline & Regulatory Team Bulletin – Autumn 2020' (2020) available at <https://www.23es.com/wp-content/uploads/2020/11/Professional-Discipline-Regulatory-Team-Bulletin-October-2020.pdf> accessed 08 September 2022.

[115] ibid.

[116] Professional Standards Authority, 'Sexual Harassment and Assault in Health and Care: Getting the Regulatory Response Right' (2022) available at <https://www.professionalstandards.org.uk/news-and-blog/blog/detail/blog/2022/08/09/sexual-harassment-and-assault-in-health-and-care-getting-the-regulatory-response-right> accessed 08 September 2022.

[117] Rosalind Searle et al., 'Bad Apples? Bad Barrels? Or Bad Cellars? Antecedents and Processes of Professional Misconduct in UK Health and Social Care: Insights into Sexual Misconduct and Dishonesty' (2017) available at <https://pureportal.coventry.ac.uk/en/publications/bad-apples-bad-barrels-or-bad-cellars-antecedents-and-processes-o-2> accessed 08 September 2022, p 17.

related to their gender. An article published shortly after this survey states unequivocally that 'Surgery and surgical training have a problem with sexual harassment, sexual assault and rape'.[118] Numerous anonymous stories of sexism, sexual harassment, and sexual assault experienced by professionals (from a range of sources, including patients and colleagues) have been compiled and published by the Surviving in Scrubs campaign,[119] a common theme being fear around reprisals, resulting in conduct not being reported, or reported concerns not being taken seriously.

Taken together, this emphasises the complexity of this issue, which requires professionals and institutions to engage in uncomfortable discussions, to challenge the status quo, and to undertake sustained work to change workplace cultures. In relation to the role of statutory regulation, there are recent examples of cases where FTP panels' decisions have been successfully challenged on the basis that they were not sufficient for public protection and therefore did not fully reflect the seriousness of sexual misconduct at work, particularly when this is directed towards colleagues[120] and/or is verbal rather than physical.[121] One reason for this may be that this type of conduct is not seen as causing direct harm to patients, despite the 'positive association between a psychologically safe work environment and patient outcomes'.[122] Further, research has indicated that conduct such as this can normalise and lead to further, and potentially more serious, boundary crossing.[123]

As well as the PSA's work in this area, steps to address this issue have also been taken by the regulators, such as the GMC. For example, this includes the Embedding Learning from Sexual Abuse Cases programme of work,[124] and an ethical hub on the topic which provides, among other matters, guidance on identifying and tackling sexual misconduct.[125] Nonetheless, a recent article in *The Lancet* points to the need for more to be done by a range of stakeholders, and this is clearly an area where it is essential that there is sustained improvement over time.[126]

4.6 THE PROFESSIONAL DUTY OF CANDOUR

This chapter has already touched on some of the issues engaged by cases which relate to misconduct involving dishonesty. However, it would not be complete without mention of a related issue, namely the duty of candour—that is, the duty for health and social care professionals to be open and honest with patients when things go wrong.

---

[118] Simon Flemming and Ronald Fisher, 'Sexual Assault in Surgery: A Painful Truth' (2021) available at <https://publishing.rcseng.ac.uk/doi/pdf/10.1308/rcsbull.2021.106> accessed 08 September 2022.

[119] Surviving in Scrubs, 'We Are Surviving in Scrubs' (2022) available at <https://survivinginscrubsorg.wordpress.com/> accessed 08 September 2022.

[120] See, for example, the case of *PSA v (1) GMC and (2) Hanson* [2021] EWHC 588 (Admin).

[121] See, for example, the case of *PSA v (1) HCPC and (2) Yong* [2021] EWHC 52 (Admin).

[122] Jessamy Bagenal and Nancy Baxter, 'Sexual Misconduct in Medicine Must End' (2022) 399(10329) The Lancet 1030.

[123] Professional Standards Authority, 'Sexual Behaviours Between Health and Care Practitioners: Where Does the Boundary Lie?' (2018) available at <https://www.professionalstandards.org.uk/publications/detail/sexual-behaviours-between-health-and-care-practitioners-where-does-the-boundary-lie> accessed 08 September 2022; Rosalind Searle (n 117).

[124] GMC, '"Let's Start at Work"—Embedding Learning from Sexual Abuse Cases' (2021) available at <https://gmcuk.wordpress.com/2021/05/07/lets-start-at-work-embedding-learning-from-sexual-abuse-cases/> accessed 08 September 2022.

[125] GMC, 'Identifying and Tackling Sexual Conduct' (2022) available at <https://www.gmc-uk.org/ethical-guidance/ethical-hub/identifying-and-tackling-sexual-misconduct> accessed 09 September 2022.

[126] Jessamy Bagenal and Nancy Baxter, 'Sexual Misconduct in Medicine Must End' (2022) 399(10329) The Lancet 1030.

4.6.1 A BRIEF HISTORY

The development of the duty of candour in healthcare in the UK can crudely be separated into two periods of time, namely before and after the Mid Staffordshire NHS Foundation Trust Public Inquiry in 2013. This Inquiry, led by Robert Frances QC, uncovered the poor quality of care provided between 2005 and 2008 at the Trust's main hospital in Stafford. The Inquiry was prompted initially due to high mortality rates and the number of complaints received, and found:

> a culture of fear in which staff did not feel able to report concerns; a culture of secrecy in which the trust board shut itself off from what was happening in its hospital and ignored its patients; and a culture of bullying, which prevented people from doing their jobs properly.[127]

Among other matters, the Inquiry recommended that a 'statutory obligation should be imposed: On healthcare providers, registered medical and nursing practitioners to observe the duty of candour.'[128] This was in circumstances where, prior to 2013 there was a notable lack of a robust legal framework for the accountability of professionals and healthcare organisations. Indeed, serious failures in candour had previously emerged in relation to the negligent death (and post-death cover-up) of a child, Robbie Powell, in Wales in 1990, from a failure to diagnose and to treat Addison's disease.[129] This case highlighted a number of matters, including the absence of a legal duty of candour in healthcare.[130] The European Court of Human Rights found as follows:

> Whilst it is arguable that doctors had a duty not to falsify medical records under the common law (Sir Donaldson MR's 'duty of candour'), before *Powell v Boladz* there was no binding decision of the courts as to the existence of such a duty. As the law stands now, however, doctors have no duty to give parents of a child who died as a result of their negligence a truthful account of the circumstances of the death, nor even to refrain from deliberately falsifying records.[131]

4.6.2 TWO DUTIES OF CANDOUR

Following the Francis Inquiry, there have been a number of significant developments, both with regard to the introduction of (i) a *statutory organisational* duty of candour in England and Scotland, and work towards this in Wales and Northern Ireland; and (ii) the strengthening of the *individual professional* duty of candour for healthcare professionals (it is this professional duty that is the focus of this chapter). In particular, in 2014 a joint statement was issued by the statutory regulators explicitly encouraging their registrants to be candid, as set out in **Table 4.5**.[132]

---

[127] 'Report of the Mid Staffordshire NHS Foundation Trust Public Inquiry: Executive Summary' (London: The Stationery Office, February 2013) 10.

[128] UK Government (n 2), 75.

[129] Action Against Medical Accidents, 'Duty of Candour' (2014) available at <https://www.avma.org.uk/policy-campaigns/duty-of-candour/> accessed 7 January 2022.

[130] ibid.   [131] *Powell v The United Kingdom* (2000) 45305/99.

[132] GMC, 'Joint Statement from the Chief Executives of Statutory Regulators of Healthcare Professionals (2014) available at <https://www.gmc-uk.org/-/media/gmc-site-images/ethical-guidance/related-pdf-items/conflicts-of-interest/joint-statement-from-the-chief-executives-of-statutory-regulators-of-health-and-care-professionals.pdf?la=en&hash=A29836358B7C3AB3750A7CEAC6F49AEBC5C76C1D> accessed 08 September 2022.

Table 4.5 Joint statement from the Chief Executives of Statutory Regulators of Healthcare Professionals (2014)

Every healthcare professional must be open and honest with patients when something goes wrong with their treatment or care which causes, or has the potential to cause, harm or distress. This means that healthcare professionals must:

- tell the patient (or, where appropriate, the patient's advocate, carer or family) when something has gone wrong;
- apologise to the patient (or, where appropriate, the patient's advocate, carer or family);
- offer an appropriate remedy or support to put matters right (if possible); and
- explain fully to the patient (or, where appropriate, the patient's advocate, carer or family) the short and long term effects of what has happened.
- Healthcare professionals must also be open and honest with their colleagues, employers and relevant organisations, and take part in reviews and investigations when requested. Health and care professionals must also be open and honest with their regulators, raising concerns where appropriate. They must support and encourage each other to be open and honest and not stop someone from raising concerns.

Similar provisions can be found in the regulators' individual guidance to their registrants. For example, the GMC's current version of GMP (2013) touches on the duty of candour in various domains, and explicitly states that:

> You must be open and honest with patients if things go wrong. If a patient under your care has suffered harm or distress, you should: a. put matters right (if that is possible); b. offer an apology c. explain fully and promptly what has happened and the likely short-term and long-term effects.[133]

Both the organisational and individual duties of candour are fundamentally concerned with ensuring that when things go wrong with the care that is provided to patients or service users, the response of the relevant service provider/healthcare professional is open and honest. However, there are also important differences between how these duties operate, and what they require, as summarised in **Table 4.6**.

Therefore, the threshold for the activation of the *individual professional* duty of candour is *lower* than the various thresholds for the activation of the *statutory organisational* duty of candour. In other words, there may be circumstances in which the professional duty of candour applies but not the organisational duty.[134]

In sum, the space within which the duty of candour exists, that may once have been seen as notably absent of regulation, may now be characterised as a 'regulatory thicket', where different (individual and organisational) duties must be navigated and met. As such, the focus on the duties of candour has shifted away from the need for *more* regulation, and

---

[133] GMC, 'Domain 4' (n 85) para 55.
[134] Professional Standards Authority, 'A Tale of Two Duties (of Candour)' (2020) available at <https://www.professionalstandards.org.uk/news-and-blog/blog/detail/blog/2020/02/26/a-tale-of-two-duties-(of-candour)> accessed 08 September 2022.

Table 4.6 Duties of candour: key features

Statutory organisational duty of candour	Individual professional duty of candour
• Applies to organisations rather than individuals. However, individuals will inevitably be involved in managing and resolving incidents in order to discharge this duty. • Set out in legislation, which differs as between the four countries of the UK. • Applies in certain situations, defined in legislation as a 'notifiable safety incident' in England, an 'unintended or unexpected incident' in Scotland, and 'any unexpected or unintended harm that is more than minimal' in Wales, and prescribes certain steps that must be taken and records that must be kept.	• Applies to individuals rather than organisations. • Set out in individual ethical guidance issued jointly and individually by the statutory regulators. • Applies to all individual registrants 'when something goes wrong with . . . treatment or care which causes, or has the potential to cause, harm or distress'.

towards consideration of how existing regulation can better deliver on the promise of ensuring that healthcare professionals are open and honest with the people they care for when things go wrong.

4.6.3 IDENTIFYING AND TACKLING BARRIERS TO EMBEDDING CANDOUR

The PSA published an influential report on the progress of the regulators in embedding the duty of candour in 2019.[135] Among other matters, this report identified factors that could discourage or encourage candour. Although the focus was on the professional individual duty of candour, many of the barriers to candour that the report identifies concern workplace culture within the healthcare sector, and education and training needs, and therefore may be equally relevant to the statutory organisational duty of candour. These included:

- Toxic work environments—where there is a culture of blame or defensiveness.[136]

- Fear—including 'fear of litigation, fear of the regulator striking a professional off their register, or fear of public and media perceptions and the ensuing impact on a professional's livelihood.'[137]

- Timeliness—where heavy workloads and workforce shortages could limit the time that practitioners can spend with patients in order to have timely and meaningful discussions when something has gone wrong.[138]

[135] Professional Standards Authority, 'Telling Patients the Truth when Something Goes Wrong: Evaluating the Progress of Professional Regulators in Embedding Professionals' Duty to be Candid to Patients' (2019) available at <https://www.professionalstandards.org.uk/docs/default-source/publications/research-paper/telling-patients-the-truth-when-something-goes-wrong---how-have-professional-regulators-encouraged-professionals-to-be-candid-to-patients.pdf?sfvrsn=100f7520_4> accessed 08 September 2022.
[136] ibid., 13.   [137] ibid., 13.   [138] ibid., 14.

However, consideration was also given to how candour may be encouraged, for example through:

- Education and training—relating both to why candour is important and the communication skills required to have difficult conversations with patients.
- Whole sector response—to improve workplace environments, to increase engagement with frontline staff in order to listen to their concerns, and to set aside time for professionals to reflect upon experiences and discuss and review those experiences with peers.[139]

Events that followed the publication of this research, namely the impact of the Covid-19 pandemic, have exacerbated pressures on our healthcare systems. Nonetheless, candour remains more important than ever; it is not a 'nice to have', but rather a foundational part of providing safe and compassionate care. However, in order to embed candour as a cultural and behavioural change that sticks,[140] it is likely that this approach will include at least three facets. First, a patient-centred approach to ensure that the duty of candour (whether this is organisational or individual) does not become a matter of minimal compliance, or a 'tick box' exercise, but rather is a meaningful process between organisations, professionals, patients, and their families when things go wrong. Second, a focus not only on top-down regulation to deliver the duty of candour but also on skills, behaviours, processes, and cultures within healthcare that encourage candour at every level and remove barriers to being candid. And third, recognition that complex issues require multi-faceted solutions. Candour is undoubtedly a 'sector-wide' challenge, and getting this right will involve sustained and collaborative working over time between stakeholders, including healthcare providers, patient groups, charities, regulators, indemnifiers, and professional bodies, among others.

4.7 THE FUTURE OF PROFESSIONAL REGULATION

At various junctures in this chapter, references have been made to the inchoate and piecemeal nature of professional regulation, in part due to the silos in which it has developed over time. This lack of clarity and consistency has not gone unnoticed, and there have been various moves towards reform in this area, though progress may fairly be described as glacial.

Over ten years ago, the Law Commission set out to undertake a review of the UK law relating to the regulation of health care professionals, and social workers in England.[141] As a result, they produced a final report and draft Bill in April 2014, which set out a proposal for a new single legal framework for the regulation of all health and social care professionals. Some of the key recommendations related to new powers for the regulators

---

[139] ibid., 32.

[140] Dinah Godfree and Annie Sorbie, 'The Duty of Candour in Scotland – What we Heard from our 2021 Conference' (2021) available at <https://www.professionalstandards.org.uk/news-and-blog/blog/detail/blog/2021/11/02/the-duty-of-candour-in-scotland-what-we-heard-from-our-2021-conference> accessed 28 April 2022.

[141] Law Commission, Scottish Law Commission, and Northern Ireland Law Commission, 'Regulation of the Health Care Professionals'(2012) available at <https://s3-eu-west-2.amazonaws.com/lawcom-prod-storage-11jsxou24uy7q/uploads/2015/03/cp202_regulation_of_healthcare_professionals_consultation.pdf> accessed 08 September 2022.

to make their own rules, greater consistency across the regulators in the way that fitness to practise hearings are conducted, and enhanced duties on the regulators to consult the public and work collaboratively.[142] Such reforms were ambitious, and directed towards delivering greater consistency in some areas, where this was felt to be necessary in the public interest, and more autonomy to the regulators in others, where this was necessary to respond to the needs of different regulated professions. In response, the Government accepted a number of the Law Commission's recommendations, and committed to legislate, when parliamentary time allowed.[143]

Subsequently the government and devolved administrations published a consultation, 'Promoting professionalism, reforming regulation', which drew on many of the Law Commission's recommendations and aimed to deliver a more responsive model of professional regulation without the need for frequent legislative change.[144] The specifics of the regulators' responses to the consultation vary, but overall a sense of frustration can be detected, both with the current, outdated legislative regime, and the failure by successive governments to deliver promised changes.[145] The Government's response to the consultation again pledged specific changes, such as removal of the GMC's power of appeal (as recommended by the Williams Review), but also a more comprehensive legislative overhaul. Since that time reform of the current system of professional regulation has remained at the top of the political agenda. The Secretary of State for Health and Social Care committed to review the number of health and care professional regulators in order to 'bust bureaucracy',[146] and a White Paper on integration and innovation in health and social care specifically references the reform of professional regulation as a matter relating to 'Safety and Quality'.[147] This activity culminated in a consultation on more detailed policy proposals, 'Regulating healthcare professionals, protecting the public',[148] which was launched in March 2021 and closed in June 2021.[149] This covers a number of key areas, including FTP, where key proposals promote matters such as the

---

[142] Law Commission, 'Regulation of Health and Social Care Professionals' (2011) available at <https://www.lawcom.gov.uk/project/regulation-of-health-and-social-care-professionals/> accessed 08 September 2022.

[143] ibid.

[144] Department of Health and Social Care, 'Promoting Professionalism, Reforming Regulation' (2019) available at <https://www.gov.uk/government/consultations/promoting-professionalism-reforming-regulation> accessed 09 September 2022.

[145] UK Government, 'Regulating Healthcare Professionals, Protecting the Public' (2021) available at <https://www.gov.uk/government/consultations/regulating-healthcare-professionals-protecting-the-public> accessed 08 September 2022; see for example the GMC's response, 'GMC Response to Department of Health (England) Consultation: Supporting Professionalism, Reforming Regulation' (2020) available at <https://www.gmc-uk.org/-/media/documents/GMC_response_to_Department_of_Health__England__consultation_Supporting_professionalism_reforming_regulation.pdf_73271108.pdf> accessed 08 September 2022.

[146] Department of Health and Social Care, 'Busting Bureaucracy: Empowering Frontline Staff by Reducing Excess Bureaucracy in the Health and Care System in England' (2020) available at <https://assets.publishing.service.gov.uk/government/uploads/system/uploads/attachment_data/file/944045/20112020_Busting_Bureaucracy_FINAL_PDF_VERSION_.pdf> accessed 09 September 2022, for example, p19.

[147] UK Government, 'Integration and Innovation: Working Together to Improve Health and Social Care for All' (2021) available at <https://assets.publishing.service.gov.uk/government/uploads/system/uploads/attachment_data/file/960549/integration-and-innovation-working-together-to-improve-health-and-social-care-for-all-print-version.pdf> accessed 06 September 2022. See p 29, and then p 60 onwards.

[148] For a full list of the reports/inquiries reflected in the reforms, see Department of Health and Social Care, 'Promoting Professionalism, Reforming Regulation' (2019) (n 142), pp 2–4.

[149] UK Government, 'Regulating Healthcare Professionals, Protecting the Public' (2021) (n 143).

faster resolution of concerns, and more consistency as between regulations. More specifically, this includes a proposal that all regulators should use case examiners as part of their processes, and that case examiners should have a broader suite of measures available to them in order to conclude cases without a public hearing.[150] This includes a power to conclude a case with an 'accepted outcome' where the registrant accepts a finding of impairment and a sanction (with disputed cases proceeding to consideration by a fitness to practise panel).[151] A separate power for case examiners is also proposed to allow the imposition of an outcome on non-responding registrants.[152] Other proposals relate to the simplification of primary legislation to allow regulators to respond to changes more quickly. Both areas of reform have garnered some support, but also led to concerns being raised regarding the extent to which there will be effective oversight of both case examiner decisions and rule-making. This is in light of the need to maintain the 'public protection safety net' currently provided and to avoid major differences in ways of working emerging over time.[153]

At the time of writing, the outcome of the 2021 consultation is awaited. However, two general observations can be drawn from this whistle-stop tour of regulatory reform, as well as the content of this chapter overall. First, reform has been much debated in this area, but with very little progress in relation to the implementation of concrete legislative changes. Second, there has been a marked evolution away from a model of self-regulation of health and care professionals towards increasingly codified and complex statutory regulation, at least in part due to a number of national failures in regulation. However, increasingly there is evidence of a move back towards giving regulators more control and flexibility, for example with regard to the ability to deal with concerns without a hearing. In turn, this raises questions about how this can be achieved while ensuring that public protection is not compromised.

4.8 CONCLUSION

This chapter has provided an overview of the regulation of health and social care professionals in the UK. This has emphasised both commonalities and differences between the legislative frameworks and processes of the statutory regulators. The consideration of specific cases, as well as types of cases, has highlighted the wide range of individual and institutional actors engaged by the regulatory endeavour, which takes place within a complex system of health and social care. This is illustrated by the challenges of embedding the professional duty of candour. Going forward it now seems inevitable that there will be significant reform which will impact on how health and social care professions are regulated in the UK, and in particular on FTP processes. However this is resolved, progress will require careful scrutiny of how publics are protected and professionals are supported.

---

[150] ibid., paras 305–310.   [151] ibid., paras 311–315.   [152] ibid., paras 316–319.

[153] Professional Standards Authority, 'Response to Regulating Healthcare Professionals, Protecting the Public' (2021) available at <https://www.professionalstandards.org.uk/docs/default-source/publications/consultation-response/others-consultations/2021/authority-response-to-consultation-on-regulating-healthcare-professionals-protecting-the-public.pdf?sfvrsn=7a1a4920_4> accessed 09 September 2022.

FURTHER READING

1. Professional Standards Authority, 'Right Touch Regulation 2015' (2016), available at <https://www.professionalstandards.org.uk/publications/detail/right-touch-regulation-2015> accessed 09 September 2022.

2. Professional Standards Authority, 'Regulation Rethought' (2016), available at <https://www.professionalstandards.org.uk/publications/detail/regulation-rethought> accessed 09 September 2022.

3. Oliver Quick, 'Duties of Candour in Healthcare: The Truth, the Whole Truth, and Nothing but the Truth?' (2022) 30(2) Medical Law Review 324.

5

HEALTH RESOURCE ALLOCATION

5.1 INTRODUCTION

No resources are infinite. Even if a basic material is widely available, the costs of harvesting, treating, or assembling it impose restraint on its use; moreover, the labour required for distribution and exploitation of the finished product is also going to be limited. When it comes to medicine, it is clear that it is impossible to provide every form of therapy for everyone—some sort of selective distribution is inevitable even in the midst of the Secretary of State's duty to promote a 'comprehensive health service'.[1]

The massive technological advances of the last century have been such that, in the words of a leading article in *The Times*: 'genuinely world-class universal health care, free to all at the point of need, is no longer realistic'.[2] This does not mean universal basic health care is unachievable. As a leading article in *The Economist* put it: 'the goal of universal basic health care is sensible, affordable and practical, even in poor countries'.[3] A key consideration regarding the provision of 'world-class' health care, free to all at the point of need, is spending. As health care is, in the UK, free to all at the point of need, this becomes an acute issue. Costs of all types are rising, as is the average span of life.[4] Figures from the Office of National Statistics suggest that cohort life expectancy at birth in the UK is projected to reach 90.1 years for boys and 92.6 years for girls born in 2045.[5] As a result, people need treatment for longer and for more kinds of morbidities, ranging from mental to physical health and from short-term infections to longer-term degenerative conditions. In addition, patients and publics are better informed on medical matters than in times past and are better able to assimilate the information they are given. They have available at their fingertips a barrage of information on smartphone apps and the internet, albeit of varying quality, and, consequently, the choice of treatment is increasingly influenced

---

[1] NHS Act 2006, s 1.

[2] 'A Quiet Revolution: Co-Payments Are an Essential Part of the Future of the NHS' *The Times* (05 November 2008) p 2.

[3] 'Universal Health Care, Worldwide, is Within Reach' *The Economist* (26 April 2018) available at <https://www.economist.com/leaders/2018/04/26/universal-health-care-worldwide-is-within-reach> accessed 25 October 2022.

[4] The World Health Organization estimates that 73.4 years was the average life expectancy at birth of the global population in 2019. Updates can be found at The Global Health Observatory, 'Life Expectancy at Birth (Years)' (2022) available at <https://www.who.int/data/gho/data/indicators/indicator-details/GHO/life-expectancy-at-birth-(years)> accessed 25 October 2022.

[5] Office of National Statistics, 'Past and Projected Period and Cohort Life Tables: 2020-based, UK, 1981 to 2070' (2022) available at <https://www.ons.gov.uk/peoplepopulationandcommunity/birthsdeathsandmarriages/lifeexpectancies/bulletins/pastandprojecteddatafromtheperiodandcohortlifetables/2020baseduk1981to2070> accessed 25 October 2022.

by the patient's demands, with proportionate erosion of the doctor's discretion. Larger, structural forces also influence this relationship: doctors must be attuned to funding constraints in their surgery or hospital, and in turn surgeries and hospitals are constrained by resources from government or other funding sources.

Somehow, a compromise must be achieved between demand and supply. The distribution of scarce resources poses some of the more complex ethical problems of modern medicine and permeates every aspect of its provision. Indeed, we saw this most pronouncedly in the Covid-19 pandemic and the allocation of ventilators and provision of protective equipment and treatment for healthcare workers. These issues are not confined to the higher administrative echelons nor to the more esoteric departments of major hospitals. They do, indeed, arise—and are answered subconsciously—every time a GP signs a prescription form.

Such an example relates to the treatment of individuals. But the ethics of health service distribution can also be considered on a global scale; the problems arising at a national level occupy an intermediate position, albeit one which receives the most media attention and politicised debate.[6] We propose examining these as three distinct issues.

5.2 GLOBAL DISTRIBUTION OF RESOURCES

It is beyond question that the world's medical resources are distributed unevenly in both material and human terms. The money to buy the expensive tools and treatments associated with modern hospital medicine may not be available in lower- and middle-income countries and, often, the infrastructure with which to support patients throughout their illnesses may simply not exist. The Covid-19 pandemic and global economic recession following the pandemic has only exacerbated these challenges.[7] At the same time, there are inadequate facilities for the local training of doctors, who often must travel to obtain experience.[8] The result can be a vicious circle in which doctors accustomed to the sophisticated methods of higher-income countries return to their own countries, only to depart again dissatisfied with what they have found; permanent emigration of doctors and, in particular, nurses, adds to the problem. Even less morally acceptable is the practice in some higher-income countries of regarding lower- and middle-income countries as a ready supply of trained healthcare professionals when needed, only to withdraw their opportunities for employment when circumstances alter.

---

[6] See e.g., Michael Savage, 'NHS Crisis Caused by Tory Underfunding Not Covid, Say Doctors' *The Guardian* (26 June 2022) available at <https://www.theguardian.com/society/2022/jun/26/nhs-crisis-caused-by-tory-underfunding-not-covid-say-doctors> accessed 25 October 2022.

[7] See World Health Organization and World Bank, 'Tracking Universal Health Coverage: 2021 Global Monitoring Report' (2021), available at <https://www.who.int/publications/i/item/9789240040618> accessed 25 October 2022. The report found that the Covid-19 pandemic subsequently led to significant disruptions in the delivery of essential health services. Additionally, rising poverty and shrinking incomes resulting from the global economic recession are expected to increase financial barriers to accessing care and financial hardship owing to out of pocket health spending for those seeking care, particularly among disadvantaged populations. The report estimates that in 2017, the total population facing catastrophic or impoverishing health spending was estimated to be between 1.4 billion and 1.9 billion.

[8] Though this is changing somewhat with the rise of telehealth and mHealth training. See Judith McCool et al., 'Mobile Health (mHealth) in Low- and Middle-Income Countries' (2022) 43 Annual Review of Public Health 525.

All this occurs in the face of increasingly destructive public health emergencies of infectious disease such as Covid-19 and monkeypox, the effect of which is amplified by a shortage of public health resources. Requests are then made of higher-income countries for medical assistance in the form of rapid response and the supply of cheap drugs or containment strategies.[9] The response, such as it is, is not necessarily entirely altruistic. Along with the rapid rise of international travel, we have created ideal conditions for the spread of infectious diseases and any action taken at source may be a matter of self-preservation. Supply of medicines also, of course, comes at a price; while Western pharmaceutical companies might be well placed to ease the plight in developing countries, they also need to protect their markets. Therefore, the practice of buying drugs cheaply in one market for importation into lower-and middle-income countries in an attempt to address their public health crises has often been met by the strategic exercise of restrictive intellectual property rights by the manufacturers of the drugs. We saw this playing out in the Covid-19 pandemic, where attempts to waive intellectual property rights on Covid-19 vaccines met with fierce resistance by different stakeholders with vested interests in preserving the status quo,[10] although ultimately led to several companies agreeing to a patent pool for certain treatments.[11]

The tensions have been recognised by the World Trade Organization (WTO), which issued its Doha Declaration on the TRIPS Agreement and Public Health in November 2001 in an attempt to reach compromise and agreement on the issues. The Declaration stresses the importance of implementing international intellectual property agreements so as to promote access to medicines and to encourage the development of new ones. It also stresses that the Agreement on Trade-Related Aspects of Intellectual Property Rights (TRIPS) can and should be interpreted and implemented in a manner supportive of WTO Members' right to protect public health and, in particular, to promote access to medicines for all. Agreement on the TRIPS and medicines issue was eventually reached in August 2003, wherein member governments allowed for interim waivers under the TRIPS Agreement to permit a member country to export pharmaceutical products made under compulsory licences to least-developed and certain other member countries. The terms of the agreement, and indeed those of almost any kind of aid provided to countries in need, are, however, heavily politically influenced and as such are beyond the scope of our current discussion. Notwithstanding, the WTO has reported that 'Since the Doha Declaration was adopted, important developments in the WTO and elsewhere have already had a positive impact on access to medicines in developing countries. This includes making needed medicines available . . . at lower prices, enhancing international funding and using TRIPS flexibilities to leverage access to medicines'.[12] Others offer a less favourable account of progress to date.[13]

---

[9] See e.g., Bisi Bright et al., 'COVID-19 Preparedness: Capacity to Manufacture Vaccines, Therapeutics and Diagnostics in Sub-Saharan Africa' (2021) 17 Globalization and Health 24.

[10] Brink Lindsey, 'Why Intellectual Property and Pandemics Don't Mix' (The Brookings Institution, 03 June 2021) available at <https://www.brookings.edu/blog/up-front/2021/06/03/why-intellectual-property-and-pandemics-dont-mix/> accessed 25 October 2022.

[11] WIPO, 'Access to COVID-19 Treatments and the Medicines Patent Pool: Here's Why it Matters and How IP Makes it Possible' (17 November 2021) available at <https://www.wipo.int/policy/en/news/global_health/2021/news_0123.html> accessed 25 October 2022.

[12] WTO, 'Access to Medicines' (2022) available at <https://www.wto.org/english/thewto_e/coher_e/mdg_e/medicine_e.htm> accessed 25 October 2022.

[13] Brigitte Tenni et al., 'What is the Impact of Intellectual Property Rules on Access to Medicines? A Systematic Review' (2022) 18 Globalization and Health 40.

5.3 THE ALLOCATION OF NATIONAL RESOURCES

We come closer to personal significance when discussing resource allocation on a national scale and here, a mass of relevant literature has built up over the years—much of which admits the near impossibility of a wholly just solution. The primary problem, which is essentially political, is to establish what share of the national resources is to be allocated to health—and it is the open-endedness of claims to health care that leads to particular difficulties. Allocation of national resources is the responsibility of three main actors: the government (through taxation levels and funds allocation to health), public bodies that issue guidance to the health services on treatments (e.g. NICE), and commissioning groups (e.g. NHS Health Boards, integrated care boards) that consider the funding of treatments within their geographic remit. Although it is relatively protected, the budgetary allocation for the UK's health services as a whole cannot escape the reign of austerity that has affected the country since 2008 and which shows no sign of abating after 15 years.

Around £136.1 billion was spent on NHS England and NHS Improvement in 2021/22; on current spending plans, this includes £33.8 billion to respond to the Covid-19 pandemic by way of, inter alia, procuring personal protective equipment for staff, the vaccine and Test and Trace programmes, and improving the discharge process for hospital patients.[14] It is expected that NHS England's resource budget will rise to £162.6 billion in 2024-25.[15] By comparison, in Scotland, around £12 billion is allocated to the NHS for 2022/23, and a total of around £18 for the health and social care portfolio overall.[16] These may seem like astronomical figures dedicated to improving the health of the UK population, yet the healthcare services across the four nations are chronically underfunded, and the funding gap is increasing as the population ages.[17] The impression is that no matter how much money is allocated, claims can never be met in full. Having now reached the ripe age of 75 years, the NHS has become the paradigmatic socio-political sacred cow of the twenty-first century. Innumerable attempts to change its nature have been made but all have been restricted by the demands of the ballot box. Indeed, counter-political movements have occurred in the last few years to halt seemingly endless and fruitless reforms.[18]

Ideally, resource allocation within the country as a whole should provide equal access to health care for those in equal need; attempts have been made over the years to achieve this by systematically correlating the revenue given to the health authorities with their individual needs. A truly massive reorganisation was initiated by the Health and Social Care Act 2012,[19] which established the NHS Commissioning Board (NHS CB),[20] the function of which was, essentially, to assist the Secretary of State in the provision of services in accordance with the NHS Act 2006. The NHS CB operated under that name from 1 October 2012 until 1 April 2013 from when it has used the name NHS England.

---

[14] The King's Fund, 'The NHS Budget and How It Has Changed' (3 February 2022) available at <https://www.kingsfund.org.uk/projects/nhs-in-a-nutshell/nhs-budget> accessed 25 October 2022.

[15] NHS Confederation, 'Autumn Budget and Spending Review 2021: What You Need to Know' (27 October 2021) available at <https://www.nhsconfed.org/publications/autumn-budget-and-spending-review-2021> accessed 25 October 2022.

[16] Scottish Government, 'Scottish Budget 2022 to 2023' (09 December 2021) available at <https://www.gov.scot/publications/scottish-budget-2022-23/pages/5/> accessed 25 October 2022.

[17] BMA, 'NHS Funding Data Analysis' (2022) available at <https://www.bma.org.uk/advice-and-support/nhs-delivery-and-workforce/funding/nhs-funding-data-analysis> accessed 25 October 2022.

[18] See e.g., NHS Funding, 'Fund Our NHS' (2022) available at <https://nhsfunding.info/> accessed 25 October 2022.

[19] Complemented more recently by the Health and Social Care (Safety and Quality) Act 2015.

[20] Section 9, inserting s 1G into the National Health Service Act 2006.

More recently, on 1 July 2022, integrated care systems (ICSs) became legally established through the Health and Care Act 2022 and CCGs were closed down. In England, services are commissioned by the 42 integrated care boards (ICBs) overseen by NHS England on a regional and national basis.[21] They commission primary care, specialised services, and more particular services for prisons and the armed forces.[22] Space does not permit discussion of the position in the other health systems of the UK, for which the reader is referred to the links in this footnote (see also Chapter 3).[23]

Equity gives way to the dictates of demand when allocation at sub-regional level is considered. This inevitably involves choices, and the risk of inequitable decisions is high. The ethical control of resources must be strongly influenced, first, by the broad base of social representation on the allocation body and, second, on the willingness of the constituent members not to press their own interests too hard. The lay influence on the provision of services has always been regarded as being of major importance and this is now a central feature of operational practice, legal responsibility, and political commitment. Healthwatch England now exists on a statutory basis to act as a 'national consumer champion in health and care'. Its legal powers are designed to ensure that the consumer voice is heard 'by those who commission, deliver and regulate health and care services'.[24]

As to budgets, the ICBs exist with the function of arranging for the provision of health services in England.[25] In this role, they are required, inter alia, to secure continuous improvement in the quality of services provided to individuals, as well as to promote patient choice with respect to aspects of health services provided to them, and promote the involvement of patients, and their carers and representatives (if any), in decisions which relate to the prevention or diagnosis of illness in the patients, or their care or treatment.[26] Choices of action can never be easy—is it possible to decide the relative importance between, say, strict economy, the avoidance of suffering, or the prolongation of life? Given that there are similar populations in two groups, is it right to take their relative social conditions into consideration? And, if one considers only the medical parameters, how is one to identify the best route to the intended goal? There is a strong economic incentive to apply some sort of 'productivity test' in distributing the resources of society; the question is, 'Is it ethical to do so?' Analysis of the problem raises some stark questions and disturbing answers—particularly, perhaps, in relation to older age groups.

This immediately draws attention to one major difficulty encountered when any such evaluation is influenced by powerful public opinion—that the welfare of unproductive (that is, limited or non-tax paying) citizens is likely to be regarded as secondary to that of the productive; those with mental difficulties and the elderly are, in fact, in double jeopardy—not only may they be seen as less deserving of resources, but they are less likely to be invited to subscribe to the opinion-making process or be able to do so. Geriatric

---

[21] NHS England, 'Integrated care in your area' (2022) available at <https://www.england.nhs.uk/integratedcare/integrated-care-in-your-area/> accessed 25 October 2022.

[22] NHS England, 'Commissioned Services' (2022) available at <https://www.england.nhs.uk/commissioning/commissioned-services/> accessed 25 October 2022.

[23] For Scotland, NHS Scotland, 'NHS Scotland – How it Works' (2022) available at <http://www.ournhsscotland.com/our-nhs/nhsscotland-how-it-works> accessed 25 October 2022; for Wales, NHS Wales, 'NHS Wales Health Boards and Trusts' (2022) available at <https://gov.wales/nhs-wales-health-boards-and-trusts> accessed 25 October 2022; and for Northern Ireland, Department of Health, 'Home' (2022) available at <https://www.health-ni.gov.uk/> accessed 25 October 2022.

[24] Health and Social Care Act 2012, s 181 and the Healthwatch website: Healthwatch, 'Your Health and Social Care Champion' (2022) available at <https://www.healthwatch.co.uk/> accessed 25 October 2022.

[25] Health and Care Act 2022, s 21.   [26] ibid., s 25.

patients, it is said, would not and should not expect priority over younger patients. Which is true enough—but they *would* expect equal consideration.

It is probable that, so long as there is a restriction on resources, some principle of maximum societal benefit must be applied and that the individual's right to equity must, at least, be viewed in the light of the general need. In a way, this is inevitable in view of the government's dual objectives of patient satisfaction and prudent economic stewardship. Essentially, there are three potential measures of a free health service: comprehensiveness, quality, and accessibility. The realistic situation is that the goal of fully comprehensive, high-quality medical care that is freely available to all on the basis of medical need is unattainable in the face of steadily increasing costs—and the temptation is to lower one standard in favour of the other two.

The difficulties are formidable because what we are discussing at this level is essentially 'horizontal resource allocation', or priority setting between different types of service, which depends not so much on professional medical assessment and advice as on public opinion and on economic evaluation—and the former, at least, is a fickle measuring instrument. Not only can polls be grossly distorted by the way in which questions are put, but also opinion is subject to political and other extraneous influences—particularly that of the media, whose circulations depend on maintaining an aggressive and partisan attitude. However, the emphasis on explicitness—or transparency—in rationing strategies is an important pre-requisite and is evolving rapidly.

Despite the obvious difficulties in reaching any formula, we see it as self-evident that some form of cost evaluation in health care is essential at the resource-purchasing level, if only to ensure impartiality—pressure groups tend to be bad advocates from the point of view of society as a whole. We agree with those who believe that there are no intrinsic ethical barriers to applying economic considerations to health resource allocation. It should, rather, be accepted that without such control there is likely to be an unethical maldistribution of resources; as Williams once put it, anyone who says no account should be paid to costs is, in reality, saying no account should be paid to the sacrifices thereby imposed on others—and there are no *ethical* grounds for ignoring the effect of an action on other people.[27]

In addition, however, we must remember that there are more reasons than cost for limiting the availability of drugs and other treatments. A local health service may, for example, believe that a given therapy is useless and, accordingly, refuse to sanction its purchase. Such situations arise most commonly in relation to conditions for which there is, currently, no effective treatment. The result of leaving the adoption of a new drug to local opinion must, however, be an inequality of distribution which breeds consumer dissatisfaction. Alternatively, the nature of the condition itself may be questioned—is its alleviation a truly medical matter or is it one of 'lifestyle enhancement' only?[28] Here, we could place, for example, assisted reproduction and gender reassignment in the 'grey' area of the black to white scale where we are likely to get different answers from different local services. At the more extreme, we could consider the supply of sildenafil (Viagra) through the NHS.

---

[27] Alan Williams, 'Cost-Effectiveness Analysis: Is It Ethical?' (1992) 18 Journal of Medical Ethics 7.

[28] Several years ago, NHS England advised GPs and clinical commissioning groups to limit the prescribing of 18 'low value' treatments on the NHS with the aim of reducing costs and unwarranted variation. NHS England stated that it would save up to £141 m a year by restricting the prescribing of such treatments. See Gareth Iacobucci, 'NHS Advises GPs Not to Prescribe "Low Value" Drugs' (2017) 359 BMJ j5599. NHS England also proposed to stop routinely commissioning 17 procedures it considers 'unnecessary', unless a successful individual funding request (IFR) is made or when specific clinical criteria are met, again with the aim of reducing costs and unwarranted clinical variation across England. See Gareth Iacobucci, 'NHS Proposes to Stop Funding 17 "Unnecessary" Procedures' (2018) 362 BMJ k2903.

There are occasions when impotence—as opposed to sexual inadequacy—can be seen as a proper medical concern. But this is a far cry from supplying a drug with no intention other than to improve sexual performance. Consequently, the government foresaw an exceptional demand for sildenafil which could have had an adverse effect, both financial and health-wise, on the rest of the community; accordingly, it issued Circular no 1998/158 which advised doctors not to prescribe sildenafil and local health services not to support the provision of the drug at NHS expense other than in exceptional circumstances. The circular was, however, declared unlawful in the High Court in that its 'blanket' nature was interfering with doctors' professional judgements.[29] It has, in fact, long been apparent that the courts' inclinations will be to uphold the right of the *individual* patient to individual consideration in the face of attempted 'rationing', but only when it is agreed that it is the treatment of a recognisable *disease* that is in issue; indeed, it has been agreed that it is reasonable to allocate resources on the basis of clinical indications alone.[30]

More controversially, health services may be limited due to overtly political reasons. For example, the UK Supreme Court ruled in *R (on the application of A (A Child)) v Secretary of State for Health*[31] that it was not unlawful for the Secretary of State for Health in England to fail to exercise his power to require that abortion services be provided through the NHS in England to women ordinarily resident in Northern Ireland. In the majority judgment of Lord Wilson, Parliament's legislative scheme intended that separate authorities in the four nations of the UK were to provide free health services to those persons usually resident in that nation. The Secretary of State was entitled to respect local, devolved decision-making across the UK for provision of free health services. This included respecting 'the democratic decision of the people of Northern Ireland' not to make abortion services available free of charge and 'to have in mind the undeniable ability of Northern Irish women lawfully to travel to England and to purchase private abortion services there; and [the Secretary of State] was entitled to decide not further to alter the consequences of the democratic decision by making such services available to them free of charge under the public scheme in England for which he was responsible.'[32] The appellants submitted that the decision about whether to provide free abortion services to a group of women engaged their Article 8 and 14 rights under the European Convention on Human Rights (ECHR). The Court considered the fourfold test for justification for interference with a Convention right:[33]

(i) does the measure have a legitimate aim sufficient to justify the limitation of a fundamental right;

(ii) is the measure rationally connected to that aim;

(iii) could a less intrusive measure have been used; and

(iv) bearing in mind the severity of the consequences, the importance of the aim and the extent to which the measure will contribute to that aim, has a fair balance been struck between the rights of the individual and the interests of the community?

The majority found that the Secretary of State's decision was grounded in a legitimate aim, namely, 'to stay loyal to a legitimate scheme for health services to be devolved in the interests of securing local provision to residents in each of our four countries'.[34] It was

[29] *R v Secretary of State for Health, ex parte Pfizer Ltd* [1999] Lloyd's Rep Med 289; (2000) 51 BMLR 189.
[30] *R (on the application of Condliff) v North Staffordshire PCT* [2011] EWCA Civ 910.
[31] [2017] UKSC 41.   [32] ibid., [20].
[33] *R (on the application of Tigere) v Secretary of State for Business, Innovation and Skills* [2015] UKSC 57.
[34] *R (on the application of A (A Child)) v Secretary of State for Health* (n 31), [32].

rationally connected to the democratic decision reached in Northern Ireland. There was no measure available in the circumstances that would have intruded less on the Article 8 rights of Northern Irish women to respect for their private life. A fair balance had been struck between the rights of people who were UK citizens usually resident in Northern Ireland and who sought abortions in England, and the interests of the UK community as a whole. The difference in treatment was therefore justified and did not amount to discrimination. Lord Kerr, dissenting, argued that no legitimate aim existed for the interference with the Article 8 right to respect for private and family life.

Finally, it must, of course, be conceded that societies differ and, while some form of resource rationing is, as we believe, inevitable, no single system will be universally acceptable. Once it is established that the state is responsible, to a greater or lesser extent, for the health of *all* its citizens, the overall problem of the use of resources becomes that of balancing public demand against distributive justice. We believe that the imposition of some form of healthcare rationing is imperative in a free-for-all health economy. To do so, however, involves careful ethical analysis, to which we now turn, with particular reference to UK experience in recent years.[35]

5.4 HEALTHCARE ECONOMICS

The current approach in England and Wales rests on the National Institute for Health and Care Excellence (NICE).[36] As per the terms under the Health and Social Care Act 2012,[37] the core purposes of NICE have become preparation of standards on provisions of NHS services, public health services, and social care in England,[38] and provision of advice and guidance to the Secretary of State on any quality matter,[39] while having regard to (i) the broad balance of benefits and costs, (ii) the degree of need of persons, and (iii) the desirability of promoting innovation.[40] All of this, moreover, must be done 'effectively, efficiently, and economically'.[41]

'Best practice' in this context can be divided into three categories: clinical guidelines, recommendations as to audit and the appraisal of the clinical, and cost-effectiveness of new and existing health technologies. The last is, by far, the most important from this chapter's point of view. In this respect, NICE was initially hailed as a rational response to the existing situation, already outlined earlier, whereby individual health authorities determined whether, or in what circumstances, a given treatment would be provided—a system which had come to be popularly known as 'postcode prescribing'. Ideally, NICE's decisions were intended to be based on pure clinical need and efficiency, but, inevitably, they had to include consideration of what was best for the health service itself; as we have already seen, scientific value and social value judgements cannot be dissociated in a general taxation-funded service.

---

[35] For detailed work on the ethics and practice of rationing, see Greg Bognar and Iwao Hirose, *The Ethics of Health Care Rationing: An Introduction* (2nd edn, Routledge 2022); Andre den Exter and Martin Buijsen (eds.), *Rationing Health Care: Hard Choices and Unavoidable Trade-offs* (Maklu 2012). For a legal perspective, see Keith Syrett, *Law, Legitimacy and the Rationing of Health Care: A Contextual and Comparative Perspective* (CUP 2007).

[36] For Scotland, see the Scottish Medicines Consortium, which provides advice to NHS Scotland about the value for patients of newly licensed medicines. Scottish Medicines Consortium, 'Advising on New Medicines for Scotland' (2022) available at <https://www.scottishmedicines.org.uk/> accessed 25 October 2022.

[37] Health and Social Care Act 2012, s 232.   [38] ibid., s 234.   [39] ibid., s 236.

[40] ibid., s 233.   [41] ibid., s 233(2).

As a consequence, NICE was subject not only to commercial and political pressures but also to massive influence from the media—it becomes much easier to approve a new or expensive treatment than to refuse its use. Nonetheless, the importance of such an organisation to the health service is now well established and its decisions were unashamedly moulded to a large extent by their economic effect. At its simplest, this is a matter of deciding what increase in health is likely to accrue from the increased expenditure involved in introducing a new treatment—the so-called incremental cost-effectiveness ratio—and NICE's preferred measure of this is the cost per quality-adjusted life year (QALY). We discuss the concept of the QALY as applied to the individual going forward. Here, it need only be said that, having established for how long a new treatment offers an enhanced quality of life, a commissioning authority will estimate what extra cost this would involve individually and, by extrapolation, what effect this would have on the overall economy of a health service. We will see later that the definition, and use, of special reasons opens a can of worms. It has been suggested that it is not constitutionally appropriate for NICE to set thresholds, this being the function of the purse-holders—that is, Parliament. Rather it should be seeking the optimum threshold, incremental cost-effectiveness ratio, given the available expenditure.[42]

Be that as it may, a pattern has been well established but someone still has to pay the bill. The Darzi review of the health service[43] recommended that patients should, in future, have a legal right to all drugs approved by NICE if a doctor says they are clinically appropriate. The government, however, changed and the Darzi proposals were never implemented in full. Thus, the distribution of selected treatments still varies across the country. The legal position was summed up by the High Court in *R (on the application of Elizabeth Rose) v Thanet Clinical Commissioning Group*.[44] The claimant had been a long-standing sufferer of Crohn's disease and was due to receive chemotherapy which carried a high risk of making her infertile. Her request to access oocyte cryopreservation before the chemotherapy began was repeatedly turned down by her clinical commissioning group (CCG), and this judicial review was heard as a matter of urgency because her treatment could not be delayed for long. The core argument was that the CCG had unlawfully ignored NICE guidance from 2013 that cryopreservation in such cases be offered. Mr Justice Jay pointed to the obligation of the CCG under the NHS Constitution to make rational, evidence-based funding decisions, but equally noted that the regulatory regime under which NICE operates implicitly meant that recommendations in such cases do not have to be followed.[45] Notwithstanding, as a matter of general public law, citing *R v North Derbyshire Health Authority (ex parte Fisher)*,[46] the CCG must have due regard to

---

[42] Patricia Cubi-Molla, Martin Buxton, and Nancy Devlin, 'Allocating Public Spending Efficiently: Is There a Need For a Better Mechanism to Inform Decisions in the UK and Elsewhere?' (2021) 19 Applied Health Economics and Health Policy 635.

[43] Department of Health, 'High Quality Care for All: NHS Next Stage Review Final Report' (2008) available at <https://assets.publishing.service.gov.uk/government/uploads/system/uploads/attachment_data/file/228836/7432.pdf> accessed 25 October 2022.

[44] [2014] EWHC 1182 (Admin).

[45] The case involves a helpful discussion of the architecture of the regulatory regime, and in particular reg 5 (advice and guidance) which applied in this case; see National Institute for Health and Care Excellence (Constitution and Functions) and the Health and Social Care Information Centre (Functions) Regulations (SI 2013/259). Note, however, as the judge continued: 'This is in contrast to separate regulatory provisions relating to "technology appraisal recommendations" and "highly specialised technology appraisal recommendations", with which relevant health bodies such as CCGs must comply'; see Cubi-Molla, Buxton, and Devlin (n 42) para 22.

[46] (1998) 10 Admin LR 27.

national guidance such as that produced by NICE. In the event, the CCG's only reason for not following NICE was that it disagreed with its scientific basis; this was insufficient on its own and the associated policy was unlawful. Of course, being a judicial review, this did not mean that a differently formulated policy could not still deny the treatment, but the standing policy had to fail.

The legal position as described previously carries over into the work of ICBs. Specifically, it is required that each of the 42 ICBs adhere to the 'Clinical Commissioning Group Outcomes Indicator Set' developed by NICE,[47] and which provide comparative information for ICBs about the quality of health services and the associated health outcomes.[48]

As something of a quid pro quo, it is to be noted that NICE is also charged with advising as to what is known as disinvestment in the NHS—that is, in identifying those treatments that are no longer cost-effective or are no longer appropriate. This is clearly a logical counterpart to the duty of advising on what is the most effective way of delivering health care. Whether or not it makes any significant difference to the healthcare budget is, however, still undecided.[49] NICE can still be regarded as a brave attempt to rationalise, and nationalise, our health care allocation decision-making that will still be ongoing by way of the ICBs. But, in the end, the distribution of resources cannot escape the overall political mastery that characterises the NHS.

The question: 'What is NICE's, or its equivalent's, liability in the event that its advice is faulty?' is, so far as we know, as yet untested. Certainly, decisions are subject to judicial review, as we have seen already in this chapter, but this is of small consolation to the patient who sustains injury as a result of their doctor following the wisdom of the Institute, possibly against their better judgement. This aspect of the 'legitimacy' of the Institute was addressed in depth by Syrett[50] and the test is certainly a hard one, particularly in that an essentially scientific body is being asked to make what are often moral judgements within a pluralistic society. No NICE decisions are likely to please everyone and the role of the courts in enforcing 'reasonableness' becomes increasingly important. The question is, 'Is legal intervention to be welcomed or distrusted?'

5.5 THE LEGAL SITUATION

In much the same way, it is surprising that there have not been more actions brought by patients who feel that the Secretary of State has failed in their duty 'to require the Board to arrange, to such extent as it considers necessary to meet all reasonable requirements', broad provision as part of the health service.[51] But, on reflection, it is likely that

[47] Healthcare Financial Management Association, 'HFMA Introductory Guide to NHS Finance: Chapter 6: NHS Finance – The Role of Integrated Care Boards' (2022) available at <https://www.hfma.org.uk/publications/hfma-introductory-guide-to-nhs-finance> accessed 25 October 2022.

[48] NHS Digital, 'Clinical Commissioning Group Outcomes Indicator Set (CCG OIS)' (2022) available at <https://digital.nhs.uk/data-and-information/publications/statistical/ccg-outcomes-indicator-set#summary> accessed 25 October 2022.

[49] Sarah Garner and Peter Littlejohns, 'Disinvestment from Low Value Clinical Interventions: NICEly Done?' (2011) 343 BMJ d4519; Gaetano Calabrò et al., 'Disinvestment in Healthcare: An Overview of HTA Agencies and Organizations Activities at European Level' (2018) 18 BMC Health Services Research 148.

[50] R (on the application of A (A Child)) v Secretary of State for Health (n 31). See also Catherine Penny, 'Challenging Agency Guidance: What to do When NICE Gets it "Wrong"' (Manufacturing Chemist, 20 March 2020) available at <https://manufacturingchemist.com/news/article_page/Challenging_agency_guidance_what_to_do_when_NICE_gets_it_wrong/163425> accessed 25 October 2022.

[51] National Health Service Act 2006, s 3B.

the relative paucity of cases results from the extreme improbability of a successful outcome. A case has confirmed that:

> the obligation is limited to providing the services identified to the extent that NHS
> England considers that they are necessary to meet all reasonable requirements. This nec-
> essarily places a considerable amount of discretion (or judgement) in the hands of NHS
> England, not only as to the scope of the reasonable requirements and as to the services that
> it considers necessary to meet them, but also as to how it goes about its task.[52]

A further explanation, reiterated by the European Court of Human Rights (ECtHR), is
that nation states enjoy a wide margin of appreciation in determining how or whether to
allocate scarce resources involving social, economic, and healthcare policy.[53]

We are left, then, to consider the landmark decisions that exist. The classic action,
which set the tone for all later cases, is that of *Hincks*.[54] In that case, patients in an orthopaedic hospital sought a declaration that the Secretary of State and the health authorities
were in breach of their duty in that they had been forced to wait an unreasonable time for
treatment because of a shortage of facilities arising, in part, from a decision not to add
a new block to the hospital on the ground of cost. In dismissing the application, Wien J
said it was not the court's function to direct Parliament what funds to make available to
the health service, nor how to allocate them. The duty to provide services 'to such extent
as he considers necessary' gave the Minister a discretion as to the disposition of financial
resources. The court could only interfere if the Secretary of State acted so as to frustrate
the policy of the Act or as no reasonable Minister could have acted. Moreover, even if
a breach was proved, the Act did not admit of relief by way of damages. The case went
to appeal[55] where, as might be expected, the judgment turned on the interpretation of
'reasonable requirements'. Lord Denning MR considered this to mean that a failure of
duty existed only if the Minister's action was thoroughly unreasonable. It was further
thought that we should be faced with the economics of a bottomless pit if no limits in
respect of long-term planning were to be read into public statutory duties; the further the
advances of medical technology, the greater would be the financial burden placed upon
the Secretary of State.

However, health services, under whatever name, are required to balance their individual budgets, thereby bringing the decision-makers into closer contact with those affected.
Society, now in the guise of Local Healthwatch organisations, has a statutory place in the
process[56] and, as a corollary, is entitled to judicial review of decisions thought to have
been taken improperly. Nevertheless, attempts to extend this privilege to individuals
seeking improved access to treatment have foundered consistently on the rock of the reasonableness test inherent in the jurisprudence to date.

The paradigmatic case is that of *Walker*,[57] which concerned a baby whose surgery had
been postponed five times because of a shortage of skilled nursing staff. The trial judge,
Macpherson J, deprecated any suggestion that patients should be encouraged to think that

---

[52] *R (on the application of SB) v NHS England* [2017] EWHC 2000 (Admin), [18].

[53] *McDonald v United Kingdom* (2015) 60 EHRR 1. Note that the Court went as far as to point out that the
margin is particularly wide when resources are limited, citing *Osman v United Kingdom* [1999] 1 FLR 193;
(2000) 29 EHRR 245.

[54] *R v Secretary of State for Social Services, ex parte Hincks* (1979) 123 Sol Jo 436.

[55] *R v Secretary of State for Social Services, ex parte Hincks* (1980) 1 BMLR 93, CA.

[56] Health and Social Care Act 2012, s 181 amending Local Government and Public Involvement in Health
Act 2007, s 221.

[57] *R v Central Birmingham Health Authority, ex parte Walker* (1987) 3 BMLR 32, CA.

the court had a role in cases which sought to compel the authority to carry out an operation that was not urgent; and the Court of Appeal confirmed his refusal of the application for review. Within two months, the same health authority was involved in a comparable case, the only major difference being that the child was possibly in greater immediate danger.[58] Reiterating that, to be so unreasonable as to come within the jurisdiction of the court, the Authority would have had to make a decision that no reasonable body could have reached,[59] Stephen Brown LJ said:

> In the absence of any evidence which could begin to show that there was [such a failure] to allocate resources in this instance . . . there can be no arguable case . . . It does seem to me unfortunate that this procedure has been adopted. It is wholly misconceived in my view. The courts of this country cannot arrange the lists in the hospital . . . and should not be asked to intervene.

While expressing great sympathy with the parents, Stephen Brown LJ suggested that it might have been hoped that the publicity would bring pressure to bear on the hospital and there is no doubt that this effect could, and on occasion does, materialise—particularly in a lifesaving situation. Perhaps the most publicised relevant incident since then has been that of 'Child B', in which funding for an essentially ineffective treatment was refused.[60] In the words of the Chief Executive, who was, as the mouthpiece of the health authority, taken to be responsible for the decision: '[The] case took on a symbolic importance, helping people to grasp the reality that expectation and demand had now outstripped their publicly funded systems' ability to pay without regard to the opportunity cost.'[61]

Cases not explicitly involving resource-based decisions are likely to favour patients more, but not always. In *R (on the application of SB) v NHS England*,[62] the Administrative Court found that a decision of NHS England to refuse funding, on clinical effectiveness grounds, to treat a seven-year-old child who suffered from phenylketonuria (PKU) with a drug (Kuvan) which would alleviate his condition was irrational. NHS England's individual funding request (IFR) policy did not define the expression 'clinical effectiveness', and in the absence of a definition, the Court held that one would expect the expression to be interpreted in the way in which an ordinary clinician would understand it; a drug would be clinically effective if it achieved the intended clinical outcome in respect of the relevant condition. According to the Court, the evidence that Kuvan was clinically effective was overwhelming.

More recently, in the case of *R (on the application of Cotter) v NICE*, an 11-year-old girl suffering from PKU applied for judicial review of NICE's assessment of Kuvan.[63] The claimant sought to take Kuvan. In July 2018, NICE was asked by the Secretary of State for Health to assess Kuvan and to make a recommendation as to whether it should be provided by the NHS. NICE decided that the drug in question did not satisfy three of

---

[58] *R v Central Birmingham Health Authority, ex parte Collier* (6 January 1988, unreported).

[59] *Associated Provincial Picture Houses Ltd v Wednesbury Corpn* [1948] 1 KB 223 at 229.

[60] *R v Cambridge Area Health Authority, ex parte B (a minor)* (1995) 25 BMLR 5; revsd (1995) 23 BMLR 1, CA.

[61] Stephen Thornton, 'The *Child B* Case—Reflections of a Chief Executive' (1997) 314 BMJ 1838. Interestingly, reporting restrictions were lifted in order to facilitate a public appeal fund: *Re B (a minor)* (1996) 30 BMLR 10 1.

[62] [2017] EWHC 2000 (Admin).

[63] [2020] EWHC 435 (Admin). See also *Basma v Manchester University Hospitals NHS Foundation Trust* [2021] EWCA Civ 278, which held that decisions made by two consultants to deny a 10-year-old girl with type 3 spinal muscular atrophy the chance of treatment with a potentially life-changing drug were 'unlawful' and 'irrational'.

the seven criteria listed in its 2017 guidance on highly specialised technologies as necessary for an assessment under its Highly Specialised Technology (HST) process. It therefore decided to assess the drug under its standard Health Technology Appraisal (HTA) process. The claimant's case was that if the HST process had been used, the prospects of a positive decision being made in relation to the drug would have increased significantly. They submitted that NICE had erred in law in deciding to assess the drug under the HTA process. The claimant argued that it had misunderstood and misapplied its own guidance in failing to make use of the HST process. The Administrative Court refused the application, ruling that NICE had not erred in its choice of assessment method when considering whether to recommend that the NHS fund the new drug. The claimant conceded that not all technologies falling within the definition of 'highly specialised health technologies' had to be appraised under the HST procedure, and NICE was entitled to establish criteria to determine which health technologies were to be appraised under that procedure. As such, the seven criteria set out in the 2017 guidance were lawful. The ruling was upheld on appeal.[64]

A recent Court of Appeal decision also has affirmed that it is lawful for Clinical Commissioning Groups (CCGs, and now ICBs) to adopt a policy of offering a drug as a preferred treatment option to certain patients on the grounds that it is significantly cheaper than licensed alternatives; there is nothing inherently illegitimate in prescribing decisions being influenced by cost considerations where the evidence shows no differences in efficacy or safety.[65]

The Human Rights Act 1998 has provided an arena for the settlement of resource allocation cases. In practice, the Act has had surprisingly little impact on the provision of health services in the UK, and we have already noted that the ECtHR has confirmed that the margin of appreciation is particularly wide when resources are scarce. Nonetheless, it does, at the very least, require that decisions are made with regard to due process requirements and to claims to equality and proportionality. It is very unlikely that Article 2 ECHR, which protects the right to life, would ever provide an automatic entitlement to treatment in any particular case; it could, however, prevent the evolution of any policy which denied reasonable access to available resources. In 2006, a Ms Rogers did, in fact, challenge the refusal of her Primary Care Trust (PCT) to fund treatment of her early breast cancer with the currently unlicensed drug Herceptin; this was on the grounds, inter alia, that the refusal offended against Articles 2 and/or 14 ECHR.[66] An application for judicial review was refused at first instance. The Court of Appeal, however, considered that the Trust's *policy*—which involved withholding such treatment unless each patient concerned could demonstrate the existence of 'exceptional personal or clinical circumstances'—was irrational and, therefore, unlawful; Ms Rogers' personal problem was, as a result, not addressed—nor could it be in the context of a judicial inquiry.[67]

Interestingly, counsel for Ms Rogers and the court agreed that the case would have been very different had the Trust's policy been founded, at least in part, on budgetary considerations,[68] and this was demonstrated in the very comparable case of Ms Otley,[69]

---

[64] [2020] EWCA Civ 1037.   [65] *Bayer Plc v NHS Darlington CCG* [2020] EWCA Civ 449.

[66] *R (on the application of Rogers)* v Swindon NHS Primary Care Trust [2006] 1 WLR 2649.

[67] In the same vein, the court only ordered that the Trust should review its policy. See also *R (on the application of Gordon)* v Bromley NHS Primary Care Trust (2006) EWHC 2462 (Admin) for the importance of clarity in decision-making.

[68] At [58]; *R (on the application of Murphy)* v Salford PCT [2008] EWHC 1908 (case referred to Primary Care Trust on the grounds of inadequate consideration).

[69] *R (on the application of Otley)* v Barking and Dagenham Primary Care Trust (2007) 98 BMLR 182.

who was refused funding for treatment of her colorectal cancer with the unlicensed drug Avastin. Here, by contrast, the policy of the Trust—which included consideration of the 'impact of funding on the health of the whole population'—was assessed as being rational and sensible. Even so, Ms Otley's search for treatment was successful in that, first, the Trust's reasons for the *particular* exclusion were flawed and unlawful on *Wednesbury*[70] grounds and, second, that the proposed treatment would have required the allocation of only small resources. Unfortunately, the question of a breach of Article 2 ECHR was again not addressed directly.[71]

There is some evidence that these, and similar, cases have made their mark[72] insofar as, from 2009, NICE extended its customary QALY limit as to cost-effectiveness in the case of patients who are not likely to live for longer than 24 months and whose life will, as a result of treatment, be extended by at least three months.[73] We do, however, wonder if this apparent advance in patient care is not being bought at the expense of ethical principles. Whether it is right to approve exceptional expenditure *because* it will be, by definition, limited is, at least, arguable. In summary, whatever the reasoning employed, it has been said that, whether or not a patient is exceptional does not sit comfortably with the axiom that doctors should treat all patients with equal concern.[74] With which we would all agree—but it does nothing to *solve* the problem.

These ethical issues are seemingly becoming more pronounced and challenged in recent years. In 2020, there was a proposed judicial review challenge to the NICE Covid-19 guideline for clinical care; the guideline stipulated that all adults on admission to hospital, irrespective of Covid-19 status, should be assessed for frailty using the Clinical Frailty Scale (CFS) and that comorbidities and underlying health conditions should be considered. Upon concerns expressed by patient groups and threatened legal challenge, NICE amended the guideline so that the CFS was recommended to not be used for younger people, people with stable long-term disabilities, learning disabilities, autism, or cerebral palsy, and instead individualised assessment was to be recommended in all cases where the CFS was considered inappropriate.[75] And in 2021, NICE shelved guidance recommending 'graded exercise therapy' for those living with chronic fatigue syndrome (myalgic encephalomyelitis) following a threatened legal challenge and concerns expressed to the Institute by patients and health professionals.[76]

---

[70] *R* v *Central Birmingham Health Authority, ex parte Walker* (n 57).

[71] It has been held that a reasonable rejection of an IFR does not breach Art 8 of the Convention: *Condliff* (n 30). See also *R (Dyer)* v *The Welsh Ministers and others* [2015] EWHC 3712 (Admin), [17].

[72] For an exceptionally well-argued and described case where an appeal against refusal to finance an unapproved cancer treatment was successful, see *R (on the application of Ross)* v *West Sussex PCT* [2008] EWHC 2252.

[73] National Institute for Health and Clinical Excellence, 'Appraising Life-extending, End of Life Treatments' (2009) available at <https://www.nice.org.uk/guidance/gid-tag387/documents/appraising-life-extending-end-of-life-treatments-paper2> accessed 25 October 2022. See also Josien Bovenberg, Hannah Penton, and Nasuh Buyukkaramikli, '10 Years of End-of-Life Criteria in the United Kingdom' (2021) 24(5) Value in Health 691.

[74] Amy Ford, 'The Concept of Exceptionality: A Legal Farce?' (2012) 20(3) Medical Law Review 304.

[75] NICE, 'NICE Updates Rapid COVID-19 Guideline on Critical Care' (25 March 2020) available at <https://www.nice.org.uk/news/article/nice-updates-rapid-covid-19-guideline-on-critical-care> accessed 25 October 2022.

[76] Sarah Marsh, 'ME Exercise Therapy Guidance Scrapped by Health Watchdog Nice' (*The Guardian*, 28 October 2021) available at <https://www.theguardian.com/society/2021/oct/29/health-watchdog-nice-publishes-delayed-me-guidance> accessed 25 October 2022.

Three decades ago, Klein suggested that it was only a slight exaggeration to say that the demand for health care is just what the medical profession chooses to make it.[77] Which may well be so but, insofar as, in the event of a water shortage, one cannot make a pot of tea without tap water unless one takes the water from the coffee urn, it adds little to the solution of the *overall* problems. What the public needs is not so much a universally acceptable answer but, rather, honesty and openness in assessing the role of NICE and other resource allocation decision-makers; there is much to be said for the suggestion of an influential Member of Parliament that it be renamed the National Institute of Cost-Effectiveness and Rationing.[78] The first Triennial Review of NICE, published in July 2015, reported that the body is a 'respected, trusted, high-performing organisation'.[79] Most recommendations relate to increased efficiency within the organisation and between other bodies, and notably there is also a Recommendation to consider whether NICE should become the single expert body for clinical and cost-effectiveness appraisals, including the Cancer Drugs Fund and the Joint Commission on Vaccinations and Immunisation.[80] Whatever the logistics and operational considerations, the concentration of such power in the current body or an even larger body such as NICE does not detract from the central question which is, essentially, a matter of economics. The major *ethical* dilemma, however, centres on the consequently imposed limitations on the treatment of the individual and it is to that aspect that we now turn.

5.6 ALLOCATION OF RESOURCES FOR THE INDIVIDUAL

In discussing allocation of resources for treating an individual patient, we are faced with the patient who is actually at risk. Objectivity is no longer the main arbiter of treatment and is replaced by need—which, in a medical context, can be defined as existing 'when an individual has an illness or disability for which there is an effective and acceptable treatment'.[81] We should, therefore, first exclude from this discussion, and treat as a special case, the patient who is using a scarce resource but who is obtaining no benefit. The clearest example of this is one who is brain-damaged and is being maintained in intensive care. We believe that, once treatment is clearly of no avail, it is not only permissible but positively correct to discontinue heroic measures. Leaving that caveat aside, it has been abundantly clear throughout this discussion that access even to *effective* treatments will be limited by their cost—for a limited budget will provide only a limited number of treatment units—and effectiveness is a relative term. As a result, some form of differential treatment is enforced and, in turn, the assessment of relative needs involves value judgements.

How, then, are those judgements to be made? In practice, many urgent decisions are made instinctively and without the need for profound analysis. Moral agonising is largely reserved for the treatment of chronic, life-threatening diseases, not only because they offer the opportunity for analysis but because they attract the use of expensive

[77] Ran Klein, 'Dimensions of Rationing: Who Should Do What?' (1993) 307(6899) BMJ 309.
[78] E Harris, 'Cancer Treatments Need Rigorous Assessment' (*The Times*, 11 August 2008) p 27.
[79] Department of Health, 'Triennial Review of the National Institute for Health and Care Excellence' (2015) available at <https://www.gov.uk/government/consultations/nice-triennial-review> accessed 25 October 2022.
[80] ibid., Recommendation 5.
[81] Nick Bosanquet, 'A "Fair Innings" For Efficiency in Health Services?' (2001) 27(4) Journal of Medical Ethics 228.

resources and will consume these for a long time—at which point the dilemma involves not only the allocation of resources but also their withdrawal. The current position is that the only obligation of health services is to provide such therapy as is positively recommended by NICE; otherwise, individual ICBs are free to delineate those drugs or other aids that it will provide only in exceptional circumstances—essentially 'non-core' procedures which will be detailed in a local authority's policy. Application for treatment that is *not*, for whatever reason, routinely available through the NHS is submitted to the relevant ICB by the patient's doctor in the form of an individual funding request (IFR).[82] The request, of which there are some tens of thousands annually in England, is, then, usually referred to a multidisciplinary IFR panel. NHS England will only provide funding in response to an IFR if it is satisfied that the case meets the following criteria: 1) there is evidence that the patient presents with 'exceptional clinical circumstances'; 2) there is a basis for considering that the requested treatment is likely to be clinically effective for this individual patient; and 3) it is considered that the requested treatment is likely to be a good use of NHS resources.[83] The IFR panel's decision is subject to a series of appeals and, ultimately, to judicial review, with all that that implies in respect of clarity, reasonableness, and justice, the basic principle being that each case must be adjudged on its merits—a 'blanket' rule for the treatment of a disease is unlikely to be approved.[84]

In deciding whether to allocate certain resources for a particular individual, a cost–benefit analysis of some sort is inevitable, but care must be exercised in its application, particularly when we are dealing with potentially fatal situations. It needs no profound philosophical discourse to make one appreciate instinctively that it is right to deploy a helicopter to rescue a man on a drifting pleasure raft, despite the fact that his danger is of his own making, despite the expense, and despite the fact that the helicopter is designed to carry ten persons. The immediacy of the situation has placed a very high value on life which it would be immoral to ignore. The value cannot, however, be infinite—otherwise, faced with the choice of saving one man on a raft or ten people in a sinking dinghy, the grounds for any 'value choice' would be equal. Such choices must, however, be very rare in practice.

In the chronic situation, as exemplified by kidney dialysis, we are effectively confronted with a one-to-one choice between two individuals; at this point it might be possible to introduce a cost–benefit argument which takes the form of assessing the relative *societal* gain of saving one or the other. In practice, this would invoke the use of some formula such as 'earning capacity × (retiring age − actual age)'. Neither age nor income group should, however, be primary criteria regulating choice per se—it might be that the aged respond less well to treatment than do others[85] but that would be a different

---

[82] At the highest level see, NHS England, 'Commissioning Policy: Individual Funding Requests' (2017) available at <https://www.england.nhs.uk/publication/commissioning-policy-individual-funding-requests/> accessed 25 October 2022.

[83] ibid. It is worth noting that the IFR system in Wales was reformed in 2017. It is no longer necessary to provide evidence that the patient presents with 'exceptional clinical circumstances'; rather, there only must be evidence that a drug will bring 'significant clinical benefit' and that it represents 'reasonable value for money'. See NHS Wales, 'IPFR Policy' (2017) available at <http://www.wales.nhs.uk/sitesplus/documents/866/NHS%20Wales%20IPFR%20Policy%20-%20June%202017%20-%20Final.pdf> accessed 25 October 2022.

[84] Established in *R v North West Lancashire Health Authority, ex parte A, D and G* [2000] 1 WLR 977.

[85] Hence, say, the relative acceptability of denying in vitro fertilisation to older women: *R v Sheffield Health Authority, ex parte Seale* (1994) 25 BMLR 1.

consideration—and one which NICE was prepared to acknowledge, in that its major consultation document recommended that:

- health should not be valued more highly in some age groups rather than others;
- individuals' social roles, at different ages, should not influence considerations of cost effectiveness;
- however, where age is an indicator of benefit or risk, age discrimination is appropriate.[86]

Although this last passage is not easy to interpret, it clearly allows for some concern for the quality or expectation of life to be thrown into the therapeutic balance, as is discussed later.

The corollary to this line of thought is that scarce resources should be distributed on the basis of the basic merits of the recipients. This assessment is commonly taken to apply to the intrinsic worth to society of the individual subject—and we may look at this from the negative or positive aspect. First, such a method of selection inevitably discriminates against those who have some additional disability—whether this be physical or mental—which limits their perceived value in a societal sense; this group, however, is perhaps better included among those falling to be assessed under the 'medical benefit' test discussed later. The alternative, positive approach in the event of shortage of facilities for treatment is to select those who offer the greatest contribution to society now and in the future. In our view, allocation tests which attempt to distinguish the 'values' of citizens *qua* citizens are clearly beyond the capacity or function of the doctor—or, come to that, anyone—and the 'principle' can be dismissed out of hand.

The one basic merits-related issue which is most commonly raised is that of age. It is very widely held that the older a patient is, the less can they command equal opportunity in a competition for therapy. The reasons for this differ. Some will rely on the argument 'they've had their innings'[87]—but even this depends, to an extent, on their position in the batting order; others, more rationally, will point to the fact that results of treatment are generally better in the young than in the old—but simply because the results of coronary surgery are commonly more satisfactory in the middle-aged patient does not mean that surgery is not worthwhile in the 85-year-old. There is, moreover, a tendency to forget that not every therapy is effective for a full lifespan; it matters not whether the patient treated is aged 20 or 60 if we anticipate that the treatment will result in survival for no more than five years. We suspect that the reason underlying the common assumption is that those responsible for decision-making are below retiring age; it has been said, rightly, that there is often a wide discrepancy between the optimum solution of a problem from the perspective of society as a whole and that of the individual within that society.[88]

Some time ago, Lewis and Charny[89] tried, by means of an opinion poll, to establish the points at which the public would be prepared to accept age-based choices. While this was a praiseworthy effort which could, indeed, be copied in the future as the government-inspired lay participation in medical decision-making maintains momentum—e.g. by

[86] NICE, 'Social Value Judgements' (2005), Recommendation 6. This document has been superseded by NICE, 'Principles That Guide the Development of NICE Guidance and Standards' (2022) available at <https://www.nice.org.uk/about/who-we-are/our-principles> accessed 25 October 2022.

[87] An exceptionally lucid review of the model is provided by Michael Rivlin, 'Why the Fair Innings Argument is Not Persuasive' (2000) 1 BMC Medical Ethics 1.

[88] Phillip Lewis and Mikhail Charny, 'Which of Two Individuals Do You Treat When Only Their Ages Are Different and You Can't Treat Both?' (1989) 15(1) Journal of Medical Ethics 28.

[89] ibid.

way of Healthwatch—it is unlikely that a poll involving the elderly alone would reach the same conclusions. Harris's argument,[90] which sees the saving of life as the medical benchmark, is at its strongest when we are considering the use of QALYs as a parameter for the assessment of the disposal of scarce resources. The choice between a 20-year-old and an 80-year-old may be straightforward to the outsider. But, at the moment of decision, each patient values their life equally—and, as Harris, again, puts it:

> The age-indifference principle reminds us that the principle of equality applies as much in the face of chronological age or life expectancy or quality of life as it does to discrimination on the basis of gender, race, and other arbitrary features.[91]

Which is meat and drink to the moralist, but is far less digestible to the cash-strapped economist.

Clearly, the most widely acceptable criterion of selection would be that determined by medical benefit.[92] However, unless one is dealing with a recoverable condition, medical benefit is a relative matter; moreover, prognosis is, at best, uncertain. Medical benefit, although being an essential part of the equation, can never be more than an inspired supposition.

All basic merits-related models are, however, confrontational and we should not forget the alternative proposed by Daniels,[93] which is reminiscent of the standard legal approach to these questions in the UK and which certainly influences the policies of NICE. He advocated a fair, deliberative process of setting limits on difficult decisions where it is impossible to satisfy all parties; the process is typified by clear articulation of criteria for decision-making, transparency at every level, and an overall aim to reach decisions which are acceptable to all reasonable persons because the reasons—and values—behind them are at least understood, even if they are not agreed. This epitomises the search for justice in healthcare rationing,[94] and is clearly potentially relevant at each of the levels of resource allocation that we have identified; indeed, it seems to accord with current government policy[95] and with the attitude of the courts.[96] Justice must, however, be seen to be done and the majority would, we believe, agree that some form of structured distribution of facilities at micro-allocation level is essential even though equity and efficiency may be difficult to accommodate within the same design.[97]

Whatever principles are invoked to establish a fair and a preferred method of distribution of resources at individual patient level, it is impossible to exclude the health economist from decision-making even at the doctor–patient interface. Restricting the availability of expensive drugs inevitably raises questions of professional clinical independence—and, equally, promotes some polarisation of views. On the one hand, it has

---

[90] John Harris, 'Unprincipled QALYs: A Response to Cubbon' (1991) 17(4) Journal of Medical Ethics 185.

[91] John Harris, 'It's Not NICE to Discriminate' (2005) 31(7) Journal of Medical Ethics 373.

[92] As was also the implicit choice of the court in *Re J (a minor) (wardship: medical treatment)* [1993] Fam 15; [1992] 2 FLR 165.

[93] The seminal work is Norman Daniels, *Just Health Care* (CUP 1985); see, too, Norman Daniels and James Sabin, *Setting Limits Fairly: Learning to Share Resources for Health* (2nd edn, OUP 2008).

[94] An invaluable analysis was given by Richard Cookson and Paul Dolan, 'Principles of Justice in Health Care Rationing' (2000) 26(5) Journal of Medical Ethics 323.

[95] For a general overview, see Keith Syrett, 'Deconstructing Deliberation in the Appraisal of Medical Technologies: NICEly Does It?' (2006) 69(6) Modern Law Review 869.

[96] The suggestion that a patient was entitled to dictate their own treatment which was raised in the trial stage of *R (on the application of Burke)* v *General Medical Council* [2005] QB 424 was firmly refuted on appeal [2006] QB 273.

[97] For further discussion, see Alex Friedman, 'Beyond Accountability for Reasonableness' (2008) 22(2) Bioethics 101.

been said that to allow clinical problems to be resolved in financial terms is to condone 'the development by health economists of fairer methods of denying patients treatment'.[98] To which the economist would reply, 'The economic perspective is clear—to maximise health improvements from limited resources by targeting resources at those activities high in the cost-QALY league table'.[99]

It is up to society to define its objectives in an area where successful compromise is hard, if not impossible, to achieve. But, even if we allow the clinician responsibility for the allocation of their expertise unfettered by budgetary restrictions, they must consider the quality of the life they are extending and perhaps the greatest influence in this context over the last few decades has been the introduction of the concept of QALY, which we have already introduced at the national scale earlier.

5.6.1 QALY AND THE INDIVIDUAL

The principle of the QALY at this level is simple enough. A year of healthy life expectancy is scored as 1 and a year of unhealthy life as less than 1, depending upon the degree of reduction in quality; while death is taken as zero, a life considered to be worse than death can be accorded a minus score. The 'value' of treatment in terms of 'life appreciation' can then be assessed numerically. Thus far, however, QALYs as applied to the individual seem to be doing little more than expressing the intuitive findings of the competent clinician in a mathematical formula. And, therein lies the rub—for, at the individual level, the 'quality scoring' will still be founded on a 'best interests' assessment made by a third party and the paternalistic element in that assessment has been scarcely modified by the use of numbers. It is, therefore, apparent that, at this level, a QALY can only be properly evaluated with the patient's cooperation; it can then be used to decide between two possible treatments for the same condition. Used in this way, QALYs may actually augment the patient's autonomy by explicitly involving them in the process of shared therapeutic decision-making. Even so, a note of caution may be sounded, as it is not difficult to confuse the objectives. The easy phrase 'not clinically indicated' either may mean that the treatment is not considered to be of overall benefit to the patient or may imply an inappropriate allocation of resources. The distinction is conceptually important—the doctor and the patient may well be singing from different songbooks.

There are other more specific objections to QALYs as applied at the individual level. Clearly, they operate to the disadvantage of the aged; they measure only the end-point of treatment without considering the *proportional* loss or gain in the quality of life; and there are parameters other than simple health which need to be fed into the equation. Possibly the most important moral criticism is that the QALY sets no value on life per se. Harris considers that we should be saving as many lives, not life years, as possible—a proposition which simplifies the argument by removing it from the ambit of life-saving treatment which should, then, be apportioned only on a 'first come, first served' basis;[100] we also suggest that the customary use of the term 'life-saving', when what is really meant is 'death-postponing', can lead to false reasoning. What this view certainly does, however, is to emphasise that QALYs can never be used to compare the value of 'life-saving' therapies with those which are merely life-enhancing. Indeed, we may well wonder whether we have any right to pronounce on the quality of other people's lives and, hence, whether

---

[98] James Rawles and Kate Rawles, 'The QALY Argument: A Physician's and a Philosopher's View' (1990) 16(2) Journal of Medical Ethics 93.

[99] Alan Maynard, 'Ethics and Health Care "Underfunding"' (2001) 27(4) Journal of Medical Ethics 223.

[100] John Harris (n 91); John Harris 'NICE is Not Cost Effective' (2006) 32(7) Journal of Medical Ethics 378.

abstract formulae, whatever their nature, should ever be used to compare the management of individual persons or different disease states. We should be very careful lest we find that we have unwittingly written into the equation a constant such that individuals with lifelong disabilities are, by definition, possessed of less QALYs than those without such conditions.

In view of these criticisms, it is not surprising that alternatives to the QALY are sometimes sought. In this respect, there is much to be said for the alternative proposal of a 'discrete choice experiment' in which the attributes of a treatment—or those features of a treatment which influence the way in which the therapeutic outcome is achieved—are fed into its evaluation; in other words, the process as well as the outcome is taken into consideration.[101] The use of the word 'choice' indicates the importance attached to patient preference; research along these lines is, therefore, very much in line with current healthcare policies but, once again, we wonder if this is not just another example of using a slogan to describe good medical practice. Another suggestion has been for QALYs themselves to take a more inclusive, almost holistic, view of 'well-being' rather than medical benefit in making the assessment.[102]

In our view, much of the argument depends not so much on the theory of QALYs as on the conditions in which that theory should be applied. McKie and his colleagues, in a continuing debate with Harris, who is the main antagonist of the system,[103] saw QALYs as a sensitive and egalitarian method of distributing scarce resources among competing individuals.[104] We still doubt if they should be used in this way, as it perpetuates the fallacy that 'rationing' involves a conflict of interests. To say that 'the QALY approach is egalitarian because no one's QALYs count for more than anyone else's' takes no note of the fact that, when the chips are down, the QALYs available to each player are unequally stacked.[105] We believe they should be used only as a way of choosing between alternative *therapies*—either for general distribution, which is the function of NICE, or for the treatment of the individual patient, which is a matter of clinical judgement.[106]

5.6.2 THE RESPONSIBILITY OF THE INDIVIDUAL

No discussion of this type would be complete without a passing reference to the responsibility of the individual to avoid the need for medical resources and for the careful use of such resources as they are allocated.[107] The argument that prevention is better than

---

[101] Mandy Ryan, 'Discrete Choice Experiments in Health Care' (2004) 328(7436) BMJ 360 quoting Mandy Ryan and Shelley Farrar, 'Eliciting Preference for Healthcare Using Conjoint Analysis' (2000) 320(7248) BMJ 1530.

[102] Matthew Adler, 'QALYs and Policy Evaluation: A New Perspective' (2006) 6(1) Yale Journal of Health Policy, Law, and Ethics 1.

[103] John Harris, 'Would Aristotle Have Played Russian Roulette?' (1996) 22(4) Journal of Medical Ethics 209.

[104] John McKie et al., 'Double Jeopardy, the Equal Value of Lives and the Veil of Ignorance: A Rejoinder to Harris' (1996) 22(4) Journal of Medical Ethics 204.

[105] On the (non-) role of QALYs which seem to support death, see Stephen Barrie, 'QALYs, Euthanasia and the Puzzle of Death' (2015) 41(8) Journal of Medical Ethics 635; Jose-Luis Pinto-Prades et al., 'Valuing QALYs at the End of Life' (2014) 113 Social Science & Medicine 5.

[106] For amplification, see Karl Claxton and Anthony Culyer, 'Not a NICE Fallacy: A Reply to Dr Quigley' (2008) 34(8) Journal of Medical Ethics 598 following on Murieann Quigley, 'A NICE Fallacy' (2007) 33(8) Journal of Medical Ethics 465.

[107] For an interesting philosophical analysis, see Joar Fystro, Bjørn Hofmann, and Eli Feiring 'On the Person in Personal Health Responsibility' (2022) 23 BMC Medical Ethics 64. For an interesting empirical study in Norway, see Gloria Traina, Pål Martinussen, and Eli Feiring, 'Being Healthy, Being Sick, Being Responsible: Attitudes Towards Responsibility for Health in a Public Healthcare System' (2019) 12(2) Public Health Ethics 145–157.

cure has been widely popularised. No one would deny the importance of the theory at all levels but, equally, it is difficult to decide when friendly persuasion ceases and restriction of liberty begins. It follows that a good case can be made out for a right to choose to be unhealthy—and this not only on Kantian but also on utilitarian grounds, for every sudden death in late middle age that is prevented is potentially a long-term occupation of a bed in a psychogeriatric ward; it could well be that the quest for dementia that is inherent in many of the currently popular limitations on habit is remarkably cost-inefficient.

What does *not* follow is that there is a concomitant right to health resources when the consequences of that choice materialise. It seems that the public have little sympathy for the cavalier approach—in Williams's experience, the least unacceptable reason for discrimination in prioritisation was that the prospective patients had not cared for their own health.[108] In making such value judgements, however, the public are not constrained by principles of justice and professional ethics; the issue can certainly not be so easily dismissed by healthcare providers. For a fairly stereotypical example, we can look back on an interesting debate in the BMJ as to whether coronary bypass surgery should be offered to smokers.[109] The attitude of the surgeons was conditioned by the poor results obtained in smokers and the fact that they spent longer in hospital. Non-treatment could, therefore, be justified on the grounds that treatment of smokers deprived others of more efficient and effective surgery. An alternative medical view was that non-treatment of symptomatic patients is often less effective in terms of overall cost to society than is surgery, that there are many other 'self-inflicted' conditions which one would not hesitate to treat, and that, at least in some cases, smoking is an addictive disease which merits sympathy. A warning was also sounded that, in regarding those who have brought medical ills upon themselves as, somehow, less deserving, the doctor is coming perilously close to prescribing punishment. None of which addresses the powerful communitarian argument that such patients and those treating them are, in fact, acting anti-socially in that they are diverting resources which could be put to better uses in the context of the community as a whole. Could, then, limiting the treatment on offer to the irresponsible patient be regarded as good professional ethics?[110] In this respect, we might also take into account the prevalence of recidivism. Reports to the effect that 25% or more of those who have received a cardiac transplant will revert to smoking—and, in doing so, lose five years of life-gain—make depressing reading.[111]

The difficulty in using personal responsibility as a criterion controlling the use of scarce resources lies not so much in theory as in its practical application. It is rarely possible to attribute ill health solely to irresponsible behaviour; moreover, responsibility is by no means always a matter of free choice—it is almost always influenced to a greater or lesser extent by the socio-political and physical environment.[112] We see it as impossible

---

[108] Alan Williams (n 27).

[109] Martin Underwood and Jonathan Bailey, 'Should Smokers be Offered Coronary Bypass Surgery?' (1993) 306 BMJ 1047; 'Coronary Bypass Surgery Should Not be Offered to Smokers' at 1047; Matthew Shiu, 'Refusing to Treat Smokers is Unethical and a Dangerous Precedent' at 1048; Roger Higgs, 'Human Frailty Should Not be Penalised' at 1049; John Garfield, 'Let the Health Authority Take the Responsibility' at 1050.

[110] Although eschewing the precise problem outlined earlier, Margaret Brazier has made a trenchant case for the recognition of patients' responsibilities within a nationalised health service: Margaret Brazier, 'Do No Harm—Do Patients Have Responsibilities Too?' (2006) 65(2) Cambridge Law Journal 387.

[111] Phil Botha et al., 'Smoking After Cardiac Transplantation' (2008) 8(4) American Journal of Transplantation 866.

[112] A very useful discussion, including that of the principle of solidarity in a community, is provided by Alena Buyx, 'Personal Responsibility for Health as a Rationing Criterion: Why We Don't Like It and Maybe We Should' (2008) 34(12) Journal of Medical Ethics 871. See also Phoebe Friesen, 'Personal Responsibility Within Health Policy: Unethical and Ineffective' (2018) 44(1) Journal of Medical Ethics 53.

and undesirable to attempt a blanket response—whether it be all or nothing—to what is, in effect, an anti-social approach to social care. There seems no reason, however, why it should not be employed as one element in the distribution of resources in an egalitarian healthcare system.[113] We would accept the view that the patient should be offered the chance when a positive therapeutic advantage—albeit a less than ideal advantage—may be attainable, but that offer could properly be limited according to the limits of that advantage. NICE's Principle 9 ('Aim to reduce health inequalities') clarifies that as part of applying this principle:

> We do not alter our normal approach [to developing advice and guidance] because a condition may have been caused by the person's behaviour. But it may be appropriate to take behaviour into account if it is likely to continue and to make a treatment less clinically effective or cost effective.[114]

The solution to the problem thus comes down to the 'best interests' of the individual and we believe that this is the route that would be taken by the courts were such a case to be litigated—but the matter would, now, be more probably resolved on *Re S* standards[115] than by reliance on *Bolam*.

5.7 CONCLUSION

We appreciate that, at the end of this chapter, we have come to little in the way of firm conclusions. This chapter has emphasised that in any taxpayer-funded healthcare service that provides treatment free at the point of need, difficult resource allocation decisions necessarily must be made and allocation priorities must be established. This leads to a tension between maximising health and promoting health equity. Objective measures to ensure equitable, evidence-based decisions, as reflected by NICE guidelines and similar guidance and metrics (e.g. QALYs), have been developed over the past decades to present the picture of a level playing field. But broader, political issues such as adequate governing funding of the health service continue to play a front-and-centre role in the media and Parliamentary debate. The NHS, it seems, is in ever-present 'crisis', short of money and short of staff. This has ripple effects on the proper allocation of resources at the individual patient level. As ever, decisions are not wholly objective and evidence-based; value judgements and politics enter the frame and manifest in various ways. Gillon probably summed up the debate correctly when he implied that, provided resource allocation decisions are made taking into account fundamental moral values and principles of equity, impartiality, and fairness, and provided the bases for decision-making are flexible in relation to the times, then the underlying system is just and is likely to yield just results.[116]

---

[113] For a consideration of its introduction in Germany: Harald Schmidt, 'Personal Responsibility for Health—Developments Under the German Healthcare Reform 2007' (2007) 14(3) European Journal of Healthcare Law 241.

[114] NICE, 'Our Principles', (2022) available at <https://www.nice.org.uk/about/who-we-are/our-principles> accessed 25 October 2022, 31.

[115] *Re S (adult patient: sterilisation)* [2001] Fam 15; [2000] 3 WLR 1288, CA—the standard being the overall best interests rather than the medical assessment.

[116] Raanan Gillon, 'Justice and Allocation of Medical Resources' (1995) 291(6490) BMJ 266.

Alternatively, we can simply be stoical and acknowledge that: 'to live with circumstances that are unfortunate but not unfair is the destiny of men and women who have neither the financial nor the moral resources of gods and goddesses'.[117]

FURTHER READING

1. Victoria Charlton, 'NICE and Fair? Health Technology Assessment Policy Under the UK's National Institute for Health and Care Excellence, 1999–2018' (2020) 28(3) Health Care Analysis 193–227.

2. Victoria Charlton and Annette Rid, 'Innovation as a Value in Healthcare Priority-Setting: The UK Experience' (2019) 32(2) Social Justice Research 208–238.

3. Martin Gorsky and Gareth Millward, 'Resource Allocation for Equity in the British National Health Service, 1948–89: An Advocacy Coalition Analysis of the RAWP' (2018) 43(1) Journal of Health Politics, Policy and Law 69.

4. Simon McPherson and Ewen Speed, 'NICE Rapid Guidelines: Exploring Political Influence on Guidelines' (2022) 27(3) BMJ Evidence-Based Medicine 137–140.

5. Jonathan Anthony Michaels, 'Potential for Epistemic Injustice in Evidence-Based Healthcare Policy and Guidance' (2021) 47(6) Journal of Medical Ethics 417–422.

6. Keith Syrett, 'Courts, Expertise and Resource Allocation: Is there a Judicial "Legitimacy Problem"?' (2014) 7(2) Public Health Ethics 112–122.

7. Keith Syrett, *Law, Legitimacy and the Rationing of Health Care. A Contextual and Comparative Perspective* (CUP 2007).

---

[117] Hugo Engelhardt, 'Allocating Scarce Medical Resources and the Availability of Organ Transplantation' (1984) 311(1) New England Journal of Medicine 66.

6

HEALTH RESEARCH AND INNOVATION

6.1 INTRODUCTION

At one time, biomedical research using 'human subjects' proceeded almost as a routine. Researchers justified their activities as benefiting humankind, subjects were generally happy to oblige or be reasonably recompensed, and research was a manageable volume. Attitudes and conditions have changed in large part as a result of: (1) reactions against paternalistic medicine fuelled by an increasing concern for the rights of the individual; (2) the scope, power, and volume of investigations expanding greatly—there has been an explosion not only in the production of new therapeutic agents and in research and innovation more broadly in the biomedical sector, but also in control of the distribution of these agents; and (3) revulsion at the appalling depths which were plumbed in the genocidal era of World War II, when much valuable information was gathered at the cost of immense suffering.[1]

At base, modern research ethics codes appreciate the need for research involving humans, and accept that it can often only be accomplished with the 'informed' consent of participants, and in the case of populations deemed to be vulnerable, with heightened protections in place. Further, interpretation of the doctor's classic ethical position must be flexible. The Hippocratic Oath states: 'I will follow that regimen which . . . I consider for the benefit of my patients and abstain from whatever is deleterious and mischievous'. The absolutist could say that this precludes all experimentation on patients, yet it is clear that progress in medicine depends upon some form of trial in which the trialist is uncertain of the result—the so-called position of equipoise.[2] In allowing their patients to be involved, the primary clinical carer commits themselves to accepting a similar, more dubious, role. The commonest strategy adopted is that of the randomised control trial (RCT), which, in turn, provides the paradigmatic representation of the ethical problems in research. A balance determined by the interests of all the parties involved must be sought if the research is to be regarded as acceptable,[3] and we discuss that balance at length in the course of this chapter, including how it played out most recently in research over the course of the Covid-19 pandemic.

---

[1] The awareness of what had happened in labs and prison camps in Nazi Germany and Imperial Japan fortified a determination that medical research should never again be tainted by such callous disregard for individual rights, and it is this determination which led to the adoption of international codes on research ethics. See also David Rothman, *Strangers at the Bedside: A History of How Law and Bioethics Transformed Medical Decision Making* (Routledge 1991).

[2] Franklin Miller and Steven Joffe, 'Equipoise and the Dilemma of Randomized Clinical Trials' (2011) 364(5) New England Journal of Medicine 476.

[3] For a simplified overview, see Sarah Edwards et al., 'The Ethics of Randomised Control Trials from the Perspectives of Patients, the Public, and Healthcare Professionals' (1998) 317(7167) BMJ 1209.

In what follows, this chapter will trace the evolution of ethical codes and legal rules for conducting biomedical research. It then proceeds to look at the governance of biomedical research, the role of Research Ethics Committees, informed consent in the research context, and the importance of conducting biomedical research with integrity. It ends with an exploration of several cutting-edge areas in health research and innovation and in which the UK plays a leading role globally, in particular genomics (including gene editing), artificial intelligence, and brain organoids. Throughout, the chapter reflects on the limitations and strengths of a regulatory regime that enables (or thwarts) research into life-saving treatments and vaccines, as well as the importance of sharing data within and across organisations and institutions to address health emergencies.

6.2 THE EVOLUTION OF RULE-MAKING

The first internationally accepted ethical code was the Nuremberg Code, which was a direct consequence of the Nazi war crimes trials.[4] It was important, however, that the medical profession should publicly endorse (if not modify) the principles expressed in its ten clauses, so the Declaration of Helsinki—drawn up by the World Medical Association in 1964 and revised many times since—was subsequently adopted.[5] Many national authorities have attempted to explain or expand upon the basic principles established at Nuremberg, and important examples include the comprehensive set of guidelines issued by the Medical Research Council (MRC)[6] and Wellcome,[7] both leading funders of research in the UK.

In the European context, the Council of Europe's Additional Protocol to the Convention on Human Rights and Biomedicine, which specifically relates to biomedical research, was opened for signature in January 2005. It sets out the broad principles which govern research involving human participants—under which such research is justified only if there is no alternative of comparable effectiveness.[8] In the UK, the provisions of the 2001 EU Clinical Trials Directive have been implemented in domestic law in what we refer to as the 2004 Regulations.[9] These regulations remain in force following Brexit, but in 2022 the UK Government announced a consultation to change the UK clinical trial regulations via

---

[4] For a discussion of the problem of the significance of Nuremberg, see George Annas and Michael Grodin (eds.), *The Nazi Doctors and the Nuremberg Code: Human Rights in Human Experimentation* (OUP 1992).

[5] The latest version of the Declaration was agreed at the 64th WMA General Assembly, Fortaleza, Brazil, October 2013.

[6] The MRC produced some guidelines—MRC, 'Annual Report of the MRC: Responsibility in Investigations on Human Subjects' (1962–63)—before the Declaration of Helsinki. Since then, a stream of guidance has flowed from the MRC and UKRI, including the 'UKRI Policy on the Governance of Good Research Practice (GRP)' (2022) available at <https://www.ukri.org/about-us/mrc/our-policies-and-standards/> accessed 05 November 2022.

[7] See e.g. Wellcome, 'Responsible Conduct of Research' (2022) and 'Research Involving Human Participants Policy' (2021) both available at <https://wellcome.org/grant-funding/guidance/grant-funding-policies> accessed 05 November 2022.

[8] Council of Europe, 'Additional Protocol to the Convention on Human Rights and Biomedicine Concerning Biomedical Research' (2005) Art 5, available at <https://www.coe.int/en/web/conventions/> accessed 05 November 2022. Note that the Convention has not been ratified by the UK.

[9] Directive 2001/20/EC of 4 April 2001 relating to the implementation of good clinical practice in the conduct of clinical trials on medicinal products for human use, was implemented in the UK by the Medicines for Human Use (Clinical Trials) Regulations 2004 (SI 2004/1031), as amended by SIs 2006/1928, 2006/2984, and 2008/941.

the Medicines and Healthcare Products Regulatory Agency (MHRA), the medicines and medical device regulator in the UK.[10] The consultation noted that the aim is to 'update and strengthen the current clinical trial legislation' to, inter alia, 'remove obstacles to innovation, whilst maintaining robust oversight of the safety of trials' and 'streamline the regulation of clinical trials and reduce unnecessary burden to those running trials by embedding risk proportionality into the framework', yet while simultaneously aiming to 'ensure the legislation builds international interoperability so that the UK remains a preferred site to conduct multi-national trials'.[11] However, since at the time of writing, the 2004 Regulations remain in force, we refer to this legislation throughout the chapter.

The Directive's emphasis is on good clinical practice, which is defined as:

> a set of internationally recognised ethical and scientific quality requirements which must be observed for designing, conducting, recording and reporting clinical trials that involve the participation of human subjects. Compliance with this good practice provides assurance that the rights, safety and well-being of trial subjects are protected, and that the results of the clinical trial are credible.[12]

The Directive applies only to the conduct of clinical trials; other forms of research are unaffected.[13] Notably, it does not apply to non-interventional trials, i.e. those in which the recipient of the medicinal product is being treated in the normal way without assignment to treatment by way of an advance protocol.[14] Thus, Member States are only obliged to change their laws in respect of Clinical Trials of an Investigational Medicinal Product (CTIMPs). Despite this narrow application, the Directive's fundamental principles and its requirements for structural and regulatory changes to systems of research governance led the UK Government to overhaul its system of research regulation beginning in 2004. It did not take the opportunity, however, to ensure that CTIMPs and other types of research are subject to the same provisions.[15]

Various standard and novel interventions are now regulated at the EU level and in the near future, undoubtedly at the UK level, too, with some expected degree of regulatory divergence. Space does not permit a thorough review of these regimes, but it should be noted that many of the EU instruments now take the form of Regulations, which means

---

[10] MHRA, 'Consultation on Proposals for Legislative Changes for Clinical Trials' (2022) available at <https://www.gov.uk/government/consultations/consultation-on-proposals-for-legislative-changes-for-clinical-trials> accessed 05 November 2022.

[11] ibid.

[12] 2001 Directive, Art 1(2). A 'Clinical Trials Toolkit' is available to help researchers and others navigate the complex regulatory landscape, available at <https://www.ct-toolkit.ac.uk/> accessed 05 November 2022.

[13] For standards applicable in other research and clinical contexts, see: Regulations (EC) No 1901/2006 and 1902/2006 of the European Parliament and of the Council of 12 December 2006 on medicinal products for paediatric use; Regulation (EC) No 1394/2007 of the European Parliament and of the Council of 13 November 2007 on advanced therapy medicinal products and amending Directive 2001/83/EC and Regulation (EC) No 726/2004; Regulation (EU) 2017/745 of the European Parliament and of the Council of 5 April 2017 on medical devices; and Regulation (EU) 2017/746 of the European Parliament and of the Council of 5 April 2017 on in vitro diagnostic medical devices.

[14] See Directive 2005/28/EC of 8 April 2005, which joined such trials and laid down principles and detailed guidelines for good clinical practice as regards investigational medicinal products for human use, as well as the requirements for authorisation of the manufacturing or importation of such products.

[15] For criticism, see Jean McHale, 'Law, Regulation and Public Health Research: A Case for Fundamental Reform?' (2010) 63 Current Legal Problems 475, and Emily Jackson, *Law and the Regulation of Medicines* (Hart 2012).

they are of direct effect in Member States.[16] Our focus will be on clinical trials, the regime for which remains in a state of flux. The European Commission advanced a proposal for a Regulation in this area in July 2012, which was adopted in 2014. However, due to technical delays in developing the requisite online 'EU portal and database' for submitting clinical trial information, the Regulation did not take effect until early 2022. The 2014 Regulation articulates the general principle that a clinical trial may be held only if: (1) the rights, safety, dignity, and well-being of participants are protected and prevail over all other interests; and (2) it is designed to generate reliable and robust data.[17] The instrument also aims to streamline authorisation and reporting procedures.

The regulatory field of health research is now littered with actors, instruments, and amendments; following Brexit, we can expect an even more complex landscape. While both the EU and UK governments and funders promote 'responsible innovation', one of the ironies of this is that there may now be so many instruments, regulations, and guides that the system itself is standing in the way of good ethical research and innovation.[18] In this chapter, we consider the prevailing (and highly dynamic) regime that has evolved. But first, a definition of the subject.

6.3 CONDUCTING HEALTH RESEARCH

6.3.1 CORE DEFINITIONS AND DISTINCTIONS

While research and experimentation are commonly used interchangeably, we believe there is a distinction to be made. Research implies a predetermined protocol with a clearly defined endpoint. Experimentation involves a more speculative, ad hoc approach to an individual subject. The distinction is significant in that an experiment may be modified to take into account the individual's response; a research programme, however, ties the researcher to a particular course of action until such time as its general ineffectiveness is satisfactorily demonstrated.[19] Moreover, while the aim of experimentation is usually linked to the interests of the subject upon whom the experiment is being conducted—for example, the deployment of a last-chance experimental technique to improve the patient's diminishing health—the overall objective of research is to acquire generalisable knowledge which, by and large, has nothing directly to do with the health state or interests of research participants.[20] To these two terms we can add innovation, which means the deployment of various elements—discovery, invention, development, and adoption—to make something better. A recent UK Government white paper defines innovation as 'the creation and application of new knowledge to improve the world'.[21]

---

[16] Regulation (EU) No 536/2014 of the European Parliament and of the Council of 16 April 2014 on clinical trials on medicinal products for human use, and repealing Directive 2001/20/EC Text with EEA relevance.

[17] 2014 Regulation, Art 3.

[18] See list of relevant laws in biomedical research in Health Research Authority, 'UK Policy Framework for Health and Social Care Research' (2017), Appendix 2.

[19] For an excellent discussion which is not dated by its age, see Bernard Dickens, 'What is a Medical Experiment?' (1975) 113(7) Canadian Medical Association Journal 635.

[20] The current version of the UK's Policy Framework for Health and Social Care Research defines research as: 'the attempt to derive generalisable or transferable new knowledge to answer or refine relevant questions with scientifically sound methods': HRA, (n 18) para 3.01.

[21] Department for Business, Energy & Industrial Strategy, 'UK Innovation Strategy: leading the future by creating it' (July 2021) available at <https://assets.publishing.service.gov.uk/government/uploads/system/uploads/attachment_data/file/1009577/uk-innovation-strategy.pdf> accessed 07 November 2022, p 11.

Health research is a global, multibillion dollar industry involving funders and researchers from public, commercial, and joint enterprises. Research can be broadly categorised as *therapeutic*, which is aimed at improved treatment for the class of patients from which participants have been drawn, and as *non-therapeutic*, which is aimed at furthering scientific knowledge which may, eventually, have a wider application than patient care. This distinction makes little conceptual difference to the general requirements for ethical research. The mere fact that the research participant, being a patient at the time, may receive benefit does not mean that the programme can be undertaken unregulated by research codes—indeed, the fact that a relatively vulnerable group is involved emphasises the care with which the project should be monitored. Only the degree of risk to be permitted in proportion to the expected outcome is affected by the nature of the research.

It follows from this classification that research participants may be of four general types: individual patients; a group of patients suffering from one particular condition; patients who have no association with the disease or process under review but who are readily available; and, finally, healthy volunteers—a heterogeneous group which is of importance because it may involve other 'captive' populations, including the researchers themselves. It is also important to bear in mind that we can participate in health research without our even knowing it if our health data are accessed and used in population-based studies. While our physical integrity is not compromised in such cases, there can be a serious risk to our personal privacy, so this research must also be subject to ethical oversight and control.[22]

The logical implication of these categories of participants is that researchers should also be categorised. Thus, the individual patient is under the care of a doctor. Any experimental procedure or treatment is, therefore, performed on a care-associated basis, and while there may be difficulties in a hospital setting where 'care' is very much a team concept, the essential doctor–patient relationship is, and should be, maintained. But it cannot be said with reference to any of the other types of research participant that 'the health of my patient [and the singular noun is to be noted] is my first consideration'; consequently, the researchers should not normally include the patients' physicians. Even so, health professionals are expected to be involved whenever human participants are subject to biomedical research; the danger of non-medical trained researchers being non-comprehension of their participants' reactions. Thus, excluding health professionals would only be acceptable in the event that the researchers were their own experimental subjects. This categorisation of relationship is also important for the kinds of obligations owed between the parties, and, ultimately, the parameters of any liability. The 'pure' researcher–participant relationship is of a different nature to the doctor–patient relationship, and the standard of care owed in each will vary and depend on circumstances. Matters are complicated if these categories become blurred, but the best baseline rule should be that any clinical or quasi-clinical aspect of the relationship should be conducted according to the ethical principle, 'First Do No Harm'.

In *Walker-Smith* v *GMC*,[23] the court acknowledged the grey area between medical practice and research and suggested that the distinction is largely a matter of intent on the part of the responsible professional. Quoting the Royal College of Physicians, it was said:

The definition of research continues to present difficulties, particularly with regard to the distinction between medical practice and medical research. The distinction derives from the intent. In medical practice the sole intention is to benefit the individual

---

[22] The same is true of tissue samples removed from us, e.g. perhaps a biopsy has been removed during surgery and then retained for research purposes.
[23] [2012] EWHC 503 (Admin).

patient consulting the clinician, not to gain knowledge of general benefit, though such knowledge may incidentally emerge from the clinical experience gained. In medical research the primary intention is to advance knowledge so that patients in general may benefit; the individual patient may or may not benefit directly. Thus, when a clinician departs in a significant way from standard or accepted practice entirely for the benefit of a particular individual patient, and with consent, the innovation need not constitute research, though it may be described as an experiment in the sense that it is novel and un-validated.[24]

The importance of this legal statement lies in its regulatory implications. It suggests that it might fall largely to the medical profession to determine which regulatory regime—treatment or research—will govern their interventions with vulnerable patients. From the objective perspective, however, the overarching concern will be the nature and degree of any harms to which the person is likely to be subjected.

6.3.2 THE RISKS INVOLVED

All biomedical research involving human participants involves some risk, and it is the art of good investigation to minimise that risk. Having said that, normative and legal instruments such as the Declaration of Helsinki[25] and EU Clinical Trials Regulation[26] offer guidance. A risk–benefit analysis must be undertaken in each case and patients may be involved only when the benefit to them clearly outweighs the inconvenience, discomfort, or possible harm which the protocol may impose.

The question of whether healthy volunteers may ever be exposed to serious risks in the course of research is problematic. Paragraph 17 of the Declaration of Helsinki states that all medical research involving human subjects must be preceded by careful assessment of predictable risks and burdens to the individuals and groups involved in the research in comparison with foreseeable benefits to them and to other individuals or groups affected by the condition under investigation. At first blush it is difficult to see what benefits are involved in medical research that involves healthy volunteers, beyond perhaps the satisfaction of helping others. Certainly, a project would have to be of exceptional importance before a substantial risk to healthy volunteers would be acceptable. On the face of things, the Council of Europe's Additional Protocol (2005) allows more discretion in Article 6's direction in that research that does not have the potential to produce results of direct benefit to the health of the research participant may only be authorised if it 'entails no more than acceptable risk and acceptable burden for the research participant'; the emphasis appears to be more on risk-taking than on assessment of risk, but both are subjective exercises. What, for example, is one to say of the use of volunteers in potentially harmful research into the development of vaccines against diseases that may affect the community? One can interpolate a further question—at what stage does a prophylactic exercise directed against an unknown hazard become, or cease to be, a research project? The ethics depend on an uncertain amalgam of necessity, altruism, and courage, the contribution of each being difficult to quantify.

There will clearly be differing views as to which risks are justifiable; it is equally clear that there will be those who would accept risks of a very high order on communitarian grounds, and it is questionable whether they should be prevented from so doing. There

---

[24] ibid. [11]–[12].   [25] Paras 16–18.   [26] Especially Arts 6(1)(b) and 10 of the Regulation.

are, however, legal limits to the extent to which consent decriminalises the infliction of harm,[27] and it is interesting to speculate how far the consent of a volunteer to a dangerous medical experiment would serve as a defence to a charge of assault or homicide.[28] It may be that the interests of others are necessarily also in play. For example, the unknown risks of retroviruses spreading to the human population through xenotransplants would be reason enough to refuse all volunteers willing to make a personal sacrifice. When the threat of harm is only at the individual level, however, the choice to volunteer may be cast as one of the ultimate expressions of personal autonomy and pure altruism, and the rejection of such selfless acts becomes far more difficult to justify.

All of this was made tragically real in 2006 when six healthy volunteers at Northwick Park Hospital suffered extremely serious adverse reactions, including multiple organ failure, after participating in a first-in-human clinical trial of TGN412 (a new anti-inflammatory drug). The reactions were swift and entirely unanticipated and sent shock waves through the research community.[29] An Expert Scientific Group was set up to determine what went wrong and what lessons could be learned from the incident. Its report included 22 recommendations, many of which were focused on the establishment of a clearer evidence-base of risk before the transition to humans, and the vital importance of communication between researchers and regulatory authorities and between authorities on a worldwide basis.[30]

Ultimately, as to the running of risk, researchers should err on the side of caution; if different methods/sources indicate different estimates of a safe dose in humans then the lowest value should be taken as a starting point. The bottom line is that the decision to conduct a first-in-human trial in healthy volunteers or volunteer patients should be carefully considered and fully justified, taking into account all factors relevant to the safety of the subjects and the value of the scientific information that is likely to be obtained.[31] However, it is important to acknowledge that risk—voluntarily assumed or otherwise—is but one element of the overall regulation of ethical research.

6.3.3 GOVERNANCE OF THE RESEARCH UNDERTAKING

Approaches to research governance in many jurisdictions have been haphazard. In the UK, the first formal guidance on ethics review for NHS research ethics committees was only issued by the Department of Health in 1991,[32] and there was no legislation on human subject research until the adoption of the 2004 Clinical Trials Regulations. Responsibility for governance has been divided between England, Scotland, Northern Ireland, and Wales, with responsibility for the English system falling initially to the Central Office

---

[27] *A-G's Reference (No 6 of 1980)* [1981] 2 All ER 1057 (CA); *Smart v HM Advocate* 1975 SLT 65; *R v Brown* [1994] 1 AC 212.

[28] It is to be noted, however, that no such charges were brought in something of a cause célèbre at a noted US hospital: Julian Savulescu and Merle Spriggs, 'The Hexamethonium Asthma Study and the Death of a Normal Volunteer in Research' (2002) 28(1) Journal of Medical Ethics 3.

[29] Pamela Ferguson, 'Clinical Trials and Healthy Volunteers' (2008) 16(1) Medical Law Review 23.

[30] See also Adam Hedgecoe, 'A Deviation From Standard Design? Clinical Trials, Research Ethics Committees, and the Regulatory Co-Construction of Organizational Deviance' (2014) 44(1) Social Studies of Science 59.

[31] Department of Health, 'Expert Scientific Group on Phase One Clinical Trials: Final Report' (2006).

[32] Department of Health, 'Local Research Ethics Committees', HSG (91)5. NHS-based local research ethics committees can be found dating back to the 1960s, but their constitution and use were sporadic and lacking centralised control well into the 1990s.

for Research Ethics Committees (COREC) in 2000, then to the National Patient Safety Agency (from April 2005), and most recently to the Health Research Authority (HRA), from December 2011. The UK Ethics Committee Authority (UKECA), now under the HRA, has the task of establishing, recognising, and monitoring research ethics committees so as to ensure compliance with the 2004 Regulations.[33] And, while the 2004 Regulations relate only to CTIMPs, it is the intention of the Department of Health that their terms will be treated as covering all types of work carried out by research ethics committees (RECs). This leaves us with the rather odd legal position whereby the work of some RECs is covered by legal provisions (and the rules of liability), and that of others is governed by the stated will of a government department.

In 2017, the various Departments of Health issued a UK-wide 'Policy Framework for Health and Social Care Research', which sets out principles for good practice that those responsible for the management and conduct of all health and social care research in the UK are expected to meet.[34] In accordance with the Care Act 2014, the status of the Policy Framework is statutory guidance to which local authorities, NHS Trusts, and NHS Foundation Trusts in England must have regard.[35] Compliance with the Policy Framework by them and other health and social care providers also helps bodies that commission care to fulfil their legal duty under the Health and Social Care Act 2012 to promote the conduct of research. The Policy Framework lays out principles of good practice in the management and conduct of health and social care research that take account of legal requirements and other standards. These principles are designed to protect and promote the interests of patients, service users, and the public in health and social care research by describing ethical conduct and proportionate, assurance-based management of health and social care research. This is seen as crucial to support and facilitate high-quality research in the UK that has the confidence of patients, service users, and the public. The Policy Framework addresses areas as diverse as ethics, science, information, health, safety and employment, finance, and intellectual property. Here, we concentrate on the ethical dimension.

Given the crucially important nature of the ethical and personal issues at stake, the UK Health Departments require that research involving patients, their organs, tissues, or data must undergo prior independent scrutiny to ensure that ethical standards are met. Indeed, it is a criminal offence to commence a CTIMP without such prior approval.[36] The Policy Framework stresses that consent is the lynchpin to much ethically acceptable research, but also clarifies that explicit consent need not be sought in all types of research. This is framed within a principle of 'choice', which states that research participants should be 'afforded respect and autonomy, taking account of their capacity to understand'.[37] The Policy Framework's Appendix 2 details the full range of relevant legal provisions and regulations with respect to each area of research, and the similarities and differences in application across the UK of the legal requirements reflected in the Policy Framework.

Responsibility and accountability have become the watchwords of the modern research governance culture. The 2001 Directive requires that a 'sponsor' be named in each ethical review application, the sponsor being the body/person(s) with overall legal responsibility for the various elements of the conduct and management of the research, and the 2014 Regulation preserves this condition.[38] The UK Health Departments have rolled this out for all research undertaken in the context of the NHS or social care services.

---

[33] See Part II of the 2004 Regulations.   [34] Health Research Authority, Policy Framework (n 18).
[35] Section 111(6) and (7) of the Care Act 2014.   [36] 2004 Regulations, reg 49.
[37] Health Research Authority, Policy Framework (n 18), para 8.01.   [38] 2014 Regulation, Arts 5 and 45.

The Policy Framework also spends considerable time outlining the respective duties of those involved in research, such as researchers themselves, funders, health and social care providers, and research sites. Finally, the Policy Framework points to the need for adequate monitoring systems to ensure compliance with the Framework, and in the UK, the MHRA is the body responsible for receiving clinical trial reports. This is a legal obligation in respect of CTIMPs, but, once again, the UK Health Departments' policy is that appropriate systems of surveillance and reporting are to be implemented in respect of *all* research involving NHS patients.

6.3.4 RESEARCH ETHICS COMMITTEES (RECS)

As is perhaps clear from the previous section, Research Ethics Committees (RECs) are central to the research governance framework, but it is important to distinguish two major types of ethics committees. Clinical ethics committees have functions that extend beyond research and include therapeutic and prognostic decision-making. Common in the USA where they wield considerable power, they are being increasingly introduced elsewhere as an aid to ethical decision-making in a clinical setting. A number of clinical ethics committees now exist across the UK and in different settings—their role, however, differs from one institution to another.[39] Beyond this clinical setting, almost all universities conducting health research have established their own RECs to vet research being carried out under their name and that does not involve CTIMPs or NHS patients or service users.

'NHS RECs', set within the NHS under the auspices of UK Health Departments, are of a different genre. The composition of the 86 currently existing NHS RECs in the UK,[40] along with matters of procedure, are regulated by guidelines issued by the HRA, known as GAfREC.[41] Matters are overseen by the Research Ethics Service (RES, now under the auspices of the HRA)[42] in coordination with the Head Offices of the Research Ethics Services in the Devolved Administrations (i.e. Chief Scientist Office in Scotland, Health and Care Research Wales Ethics Service, and the Office for Research Ethics Committees Northern Ireland). Each of these are charged with delivering effective and proportionate governance.[43]

Under GAfREC, if REC review is required, then research may not begin until a favourable REC opinion has been obtained. Each REC should reflect the diversity of the adult population of society, with representation from hospital staff, general practitioners, and a sufficiently broad range of expertise so that the scientific and methodological aspects of proposals can be reconciled with the ethical implications. A quorum consists of at least seven members, and the REC must not normally exceed 18 members. It can, when indicated, seek the advice of specialist referees. At least one-third of the membership must be lay members, i.e. people who are not employed in health or care professions or whose

---

[39] See UK Clinical Ethics Network, 'Welcome to the UK Clinical Ethics Network' (2022) available at <https://www.ukcen.net/main> accessed 07 November 2022.

[40] Health Research Authority, 'REC Directory Page' (2022) available at <https://www.hra.nhs.uk/about-us/committees-and-services/res-and-recs/search-research-ethics-committees/> 07 November 2022.

[41] See Health Research Authority, 'Governance Arrangements for Research Ethics Committees: 2020 Edition' (2021) available at <https://www.hra.nhs.uk/documents/2472/GAfREC_Final_v2.1_July_2021_Final.pdf> accessed 07 November 2022.

[42] Health Research Authority, 'Research Ethics Service' (2022) available at <https://www.hra.nhs.uk/about-us/committees-and-services/res-and-recs/research-ethics-service/> accessed 07 November 2022.

[43] See Health Research Authority Regulations (SI 2011/2341) and Health Research Authority (Amendment) Regulations (SI 2012/1108).

primary professional interest is not health or care-related research. The inclusion of 'average citizens' might be seen as a necessary political gesture, but lay members may be better placed than professionals to appreciate the effects of different treatments on the day-to-day lives of patients, and their inclusion may therefore have practical advantages. One such member must be present in a quorum, as must one expert member. REC members must undergo both induction and ongoing training.

The HRA, as with its predecessors, has issued Standard Operating Procedures (SOPs),[44] which outline the kinds of factors to be considered by RECs. In the main, the considerations are very similar as between CTIMPs and other forms of research, although notable differences include (1) that approval for CTIMPs must also be given by the Medicines and Healthcare Products Regulatory Agency (MHRA), (2) sites to be used to conduct the trials must be subject to inspection and approval, and (3) an obligation of pharmacovigilance is imposed throughout the trial, such that any Suspected Unexpected Serious Adverse Reactions (SUSARs)[45] must be notified to the REC. More extensive and effective monitoring procedures are now in place, and chief investigators are expected to inform the REC of any Serious Adverse Events[46] within 15 days of it coming to their attention. The REC SOPs now also provide for ethical review and governance of research involving databases and human tissue, and communication with other regulators and review bodies.[47]

While as a strict matter of law the REC SOPs only carry weight in respect of CTIMPs, there are several reasons why undertaking medical research is effectively impossible without following them and receiving the necessary approvals. To begin with, it is not possible to use NHS patients or resources for an unapproved project.[48] Funding is also likely to be denied unless a REC's imprimatur is obtained, and the results of unapproved research are unlikely to be accepted for publication by reputable scientific journals. There are further pragmatic grounds compelling compliance with the guidelines, which clearly represent 'good professional practice'; for example, appeal to *Bolam* principles would be virtually unavailable in the event of misadventure associated with unapproved research— the *Bolitho* limitations would almost certainly apply.

The decisions of RECs are subject to judicial review in appropriate cases where the advice is illegal or discriminatory;[49] in the same way, a researcher frustrated by a REC could pursue a remedy by that route. Appeal mechanisms are also in place.[50] The aggrieved research participant may also seek redress, most obviously through an action against the

[44] See Health Research Authority, 'Standard Operating Procedures for Research Ethics Committees' (26 September 2022) available at <https://www.hra.nhs.uk/about-us/committees-and-services/res-and-recs/research-ethics-committee-standard-operating-procedures/> accessed 07 November 2022, which should be read in conjunction with reg 15 of the 2004 Regulations, which themselves outline the considerations a REC must undertake in preparing its opinion.

[45] The REC SOPs follow the 2004 Regulations in defining 'Suspected Serious Adverse Reaction'.

[46] The 2004 Regulations define this as an untoward occurrence that: (i) results in death; (ii) is life-threatening; (iii) requires hospitalisation or prolongation of existing hospitalisation; (iv) results in persistent or significant disability or incapacity; (v) consists of a congenital anomaly or birth defect; or (vi) is otherwise considered medically significant by the investigator.

[47] Sections 11, 12, and 14, respectively.

[48] The body conducting research is encouraged to submit its proposals to an NHS REC even when there is no NHS involvement.

[49] *R v Ethical Committee of St Mary's Hospital ex parte Harriott* [1988] 1 FLR 512 (Divisional Court).

[50] See REC SOPs, s 8.

researcher and sponsor.[51] Indeed, there is an obligation, as part of the ethical approval mechanism, to ensure that adequate compensation measures are available (as we discuss later). Beyond this, however, it could be argued that a relationship exists between the REC member and the research participant which is of sufficient proximity to give rise to a duty of care and that this might, in theory, lead to civil liability in a case where a REC member has failed to exercise due care in the scrutiny of a research proposal. This, however, has never been tested in a UK court, though a Canadian court found that a REC may be held liable for failing to adequately protect a research participant.[52] Furthermore, in the UK, the guidelines make it clear that the appointing authority (e.g. HRA in England, Health Boards in Scotland) will indemnify members of its RECs to relieve them of personal liability in respect of their opinions of the ethics of research.[53]

6.4 RANDOMISED CONTROLLED TRIALS

6.4.1 RANDOMISATION

Much of the best-regarded medical research involves an RCT.[54] The principle of RCTs is simple—in order to decide whether a new drug or treatment is better than an existing one, or is preferable to none at all, the new treatment is given to a group of patients or healthy volunteers and not given to another group as similar to the first as can be obtained. The subtleties of experimental design are critical to the success of the project because a badly conceived trial is fundamentally unethical, but even the best-designed RCT has its built-in moral problem: on the one hand, a relatively untried treatment which may do harm is being given to one group while, on the other, a treatment which may be of considerable benefit is being withheld from another. In one view, this is unacceptable on the grounds that it is ethically objectionable to withhold a treatment which it is believed would be beneficial to a patient; the doctor must do their best for the patient but the problem is to know what is best, and, in particular, to know whether the patient's recovery is being hindered by the restraints of the research protocol. The first essential for any RCT is, therefore, that it must provide its answer as rapidly as possible and it must be terminable as soon as an adverse effect becomes apparent (though statisticians may insist on evidence from many more cases—and possibly observed for longer—than physicians may feel is necessary).

When, then, should RCTs stop? At what point does the clinician say that the evidence of benefit is sufficient to justify the conclusion that a treatment does indeed do good? Conversely, at what point does the apparent emergence of an adverse effect dictate that the project be abandoned? The patient involved in such a trial will have been informed that they are possibly being denied a potential benefit—yet their consent will have been based on their trust that there is genuine scientific uncertainty. Once this uncertainty is resolved to the extent of a belief (on a balance of probabilities) that the treatment offers

---

[51] Those injured in the course of pharmaceutical trials may be compensated by the organisation sponsoring the trial.

[52] *Weiss* v *Solomon* (1989) 48 CCLT 280 (Que Sup Ct). See also Susan Zimmerman, 'Translating Ethics Into Law: Duties of Care in Health Research Involving Humans' (2005) 13(2–3) Health Law Review 13.

[53] In this regard, see *Noordeen* v *Hill* [2012] EWHC 2847 (QB), wherein a surgeon initiated proceedings against a REC member, and it was accepted that the Health Research Authority, as the body responsible for RECs, should be joined as a party given its responsibility for any costs which may be ordered against the member.

[54] See the classic text on the ethics of RCTs: Charles Fried, *Medical Experimentation: Personal Integrity and Social Policy* (OUP 2016) [1974].

clinical benefit, then it becomes questionable whether it can still be denied to some in a continuing quest for statistical significance.[55] In deciding this question, it is important that the researcher bears in mind the fundamental precept which governs ethical medical research: that one does not use patients as a means to a scientific end, but rather treats them as an end in themselves. Even so, the practical dilemma remains—the clinically orientated researcher stands to see their subsequent report criticised for want of scientific support, while the more scientifically minded one sleeps uneasily because they worry that their research has reached an inadequate conclusion. Well-designed trials should include plans for periodic analysis; there is also a good case to be made for an independent observer, or the REC, being responsible for monitoring the trial from this angle.

The regulatory framework must be assessed against these ethical parameters. We have already seen, for example, that before initiating a CTIMP, the sponsor(s) must obtain both a positive endorsement from a REC[56] and a Clinical Trial Authorisation (CTA) from the MHRA.[57] It is a criminal offence to do otherwise.[58] Monitoring research sites is part of the review process,[59] but, in general, a REC is not responsible in law for proactively monitoring research.[60] It does, however, have a duty to keep its favourable ethical opinion under review throughout the trial, especially in light of progress reports provided by the researchers, which are due annually.[61] A REC can review its favourable ethical opinion of a research project at any time,[62] and the REC may review its ethical opinion in light of concerns or challenges raised by patients, service users, carers, members of the public or patient organisations, researchers, etc. where these present relevant new information not originally considered by the REC and related to any of the following:

(a)   social or scientific value; scientific design and conduct of the study;

(b)   risks to the safety or physical or mental integrity of participants;

(c)   the competence or conduct of the sponsor or investigator(s);

(d)   the feasibility of the study;

(e)   the adequacy of the site or facilities;

(f)   suspension or termination of regulatory approval for the study; and

(g)   information provided to participants and documentation associated with the study.[63]

The principle of randomisation lies at the heart of clinical trials, and the ethical problems associated with them. It is almost impossible for health professionals not to have some preference when there is a choice of treatments.[64] For this reason, many doctors, especially within primary care, distrust the RCT for fear that the doctor–patient relationship will be jeopardised, and for concerns around informed consent. Suffice to say, the consent process has a profound effect on the patient's participation—refusal may be on simple

---

[55]   For an argument that medical ethics in the clinical and research contexts should not be conflated and that equipoise does precisely that, see Franklin Miller, 'Dispensing with Equipoise' (2011) 342(4) American Journal of the Medical Sciences 276.

[56]   The 2004 Regulations require that ethical review must normally occur within 60 days of receipt of an application: 2004 Regulations, reg 15.

[57]   REC SOPs, para 14.6.   [58]   2004 Regulations, reg 49.

[59]   REC SOPs, s 5.   [60]   See REC SOPs, s 10, for operational policy on research monitoring.

[61]   However, in the event of a SUSAR, the sponsor's obligation to report is enhanced: REC SOPs, paras 10.23–10.30.

[62]   REC SOPs, para 10.100.

[63]   REC SOPs, para 10.101. For suspensions of non-CTIMPs, see paras 10.121–10.134.

[64]   True 'equipoise' may be impossible to attain for many reasons; at best, it will be unusual. Perhaps we should be looking for genuine disagreement among experts, rather than genuine uncertainty.

utilitarian grounds, but is equally liable to stem from confusion. No RCT can be ethical unless the professionals genuinely disagree as to which treatment yields the best results. Given that the doctors are unsure, it may be difficult for the patient to solve what appears to be an insoluble problem. The result of the cumulative adverse factors is that accrual rates to important trials can be low. Researchers, therefore, use devices which circumvent the confrontation between clinicians and patient, and most of these involve some form of pre-selection—or 'pre-randomisation'—prior to discussion of treatment. There are specific ethical and practical objections to such manoeuvres, but it seems morally doubtful to use what is essentially a ruse to obviate an agreed ethical practice which is an integral part of the basic principles not only of the Declaration of Helsinki but also of all modern directives and guidelines. One must not, however, lose sight of the contrary view, namely that this is the penalty we have to accept if we wish to avoid a return to the dark ages when treatment was not determined by the scientific method.

One further feature deserves mention before we leave the subject of randomisation—that is the 'double-blind' technique. This form of research, which is virtually confined to drug trials, attempts to reduce subjectivity in assessment by keeping the assigned therapeutic groups secret not only from the patients but also from the physicians involved. This dictates that the patient's doctor cannot be the researcher; it also makes it implicit that the ethical justification of the trial is agreed by the 'caring' physicians involved, for they must have perfect equipoise if they are to join in the trial, and at the same time provide what is, to their mind, the 'best treatment' for their patients. This leads to some form of conscious pre-selection in that it may be, for example, necessary to exclude patients on the ground of the severity of their disease; the trial then becomes limited to establishing the effectiveness of a treatment for the milder forms of the disease and loses much of its validity. We find it hard to ethically justify many aspects of the 'double-blind' trial.

6.4.2 RESEARCH PARTICIPANTS AND INDUCEMENTS

Research participants may be 'healthy volunteers',[65] or they may be 'patients',[66] and within these broad categories they may belong to specific groups, such as adults with capacity, adults considered to lack capacity, minors, or pregnant and breastfeeding women.

There may be clear advantages to involving healthy volunteers but, by definition, their involvement must be limited to non-therapeutic research. It can be argued that their involvement is, a priori, unjustifiable, but we prefer the view that people have a right to exercise altruistic impulses, particularly in a society in which free health care is extended to all. Nonetheless, considerable caution is needed, particularly as to the repetitive volunteer who is prone to exploitation even if the researchers are unconscious of this. Motivation of the ever-ready volunteer takes several forms, some good and others less so, and, among these, the problem of recompense looms large. The 2004 Regulations proscribe incentives and financial inducements other than compensation in respect of

---

[65] And their use is not precluded by the Declaration of Helsinki (2013): see para 12.

[66] Medical research may be combined with medical care: Declaration of Helsinki (2013), paras 12 and 14. We doubt if this could be extended to using patients as if they were healthy; we believe that the use of persons who are already under stress, and who probably have a sense of obligation to the doctors, must bring such research close to unethical practice. In any event, non-therapeutic research in patients should be confined to a type which adds no extra burden—for example, through the use of existing blood samples. For what is, perhaps, the greatest example of the dangers of using patients in this way, see *Hyman v Jewish Chronic Disease Hospital* 206 NE 2d 338 (1965), where a group of hospital patients were injected with cancer cells as an active control for a group of cancer patients who were similarly treated.

minors and incapacitated adults.[67] It is probable that, given modern social conditions, few suitable volunteers would come forward in the absence of some inducement, but large payments are clearly unethical, so a reasonable balance must be set—if for no other reason than to satisfy the needs of randomisation.[68]

Generally, approaches to payment are cautious. The Additional Protocol to the Biomedicine Convention stipulates that the ethics committee must be satisfied that no undue influence, including that of a financial nature, will be exerted on persons to participate in research. In this respect, particular attention must be given to 'vulnerable or dependent persons'.[69] The Nuffield Council on Bioethics offers a taxonomy that distinguishes between (1) payment, (2) recompense (to include compensation and reimbursement), (3) reward (including remuneration), and (4) purchase.[70] Their intervention ladder then maps different kinds of financial involvement to the altruistic nature (or otherwise) of acts involving donation or participation in research. This signals the ethical significance of exchanges and transaction practices, leading possibly to a 'red flag' in cases tantamount to coercion. In the final analysis, however, they conclude that payment to healthy volunteers for first-in-human trials should be retained as ethically justified.[71] Similarly, the HRA's National Research and Ethics Advisors' Panel has opined that that while payments made to participants in phase I (i.e. first-in-human) trials must never be related to risk, it sympathises with the view that not to allow payments on the basis of risk would be unduly paternalistic in the absence of evidence that the participants' ability to provide valid consent would be compromised. They recommend that where payment is proposed, RECs should consider whether the payment is proportionate to the 'burden' imposed by the research.[72] Likewise, they find that payments to patients, in addition to reimbursement, for taking part in therapeutic research are permissible as they may serve to reduce the possibility of therapeutic misconception by highlighting that patients are being asked to take part in a research project rather than receive clinical treatment.[73]

The topic of inducement reintroduces the problem of populations who are special because of their easy access, malleability, etc. Students, particularly medical students, provide an example about whom there is little difficulty; they are of an age to make legally valid decisions, they may well have an active interest in the trial, and most educational establishments have stringent ethics committees to protect against repetitive use. Much the same could be said for the armed forces, who may be particularly vulnerable to improper research in war or when war threatens.[74]

---

[67] Parts 4 and 5 of Sch 1 to the 2004 Regulations. Otherwise, the matter would be considered by the responsible REC.

[68] *Cf.* Eleri Jones and Kathleen Liddell, 'Should Healthy Volunteers in Clinical Trials be Paid According to Risk? Yes' (2009) 339 BMJ 4142.

[69] Additional Protocol on Biomedical Research (2005), Art 12.

[70] Nuffield Council on Bioethics, 'Human Bodies: Donation for Medicine and Research' (2011) available at <https://www.nuffieldbioethics.org/publications/human-bodies-donation-for-medicine-and-research/guide-to-the-report> accessed 07 November 2022, para 2.44.

[71] See also Leanne Stunkel and Christine Grady, 'More Than the Money: A Review of the Literature Examining Healthy Volunteer Motivations' (2011) 32(3) Contemporary Clinical Trials 342.

[72] Health Research Authority, 'HRA Ethics Guidance: Payments and Incentives in Research' (2014) available at <https://s3.eu-west-2.amazonaws.com/www.hra.nhs.uk/media/documents/hra-guidance-payments-incentives-research.pdf> accessed 07 November 2022, paras 3.01, 3.04.

[73] ibid., para 5.02.

[74] See Efthimios Parasidis, 'Classifying Military Personnel as a Vulnerable Population' in I. Glenn Cohen and Holly Fernandez Lynch (eds), *Human Subjects Research Regulation: Perspectives on the Future* (MIT Press 2014). For ethics review of research involving soldiers and Ministry of Defence Research Ethics Committee (MoDREC) to review research involving the British Armed Forces or otherwise sponsored or funded by the Ministry of Defence, see REC SOPs, paras 1.29–1.31.

The use of prisoners is particularly controversial and exposes a range of ethical issues.[75] It is often felt that some advantage, even if only imagined, must accrue to the prisoner participant. Others feel that advantage may be so great as to induce the prisoner to volunteer for research which involves greater discomfort or risk than would be accepted by a free person, and which may compromise their inalienable right to withdraw from the trial. And, of course, prisoners could well resent protective attitudes on the grounds that it is their right to dispose of their bodies and to take such risks as they please. This could be the subject of lengthy debate but we suggest that the conditions in today's prisons are such that any process which provides some relief deserves a sympathetic evaluation, and many prisoners might be benefited through helping society.[76] Having said that, research on prisoners should be particularly rigidly controlled by RECs, which should always contain lay members with experience in criminology or penology.[77] Nowhere is it more important to observe the maxim 'the aims do not justify the means—the method must be judged in its own right'.

When comparing treatments, however, the use of patients is necessary. This is what the Declaration of Helsinki means by medical research combined with professional care, which is admissible 'only to the extent that this is justified by its potential preventive, diagnostic or therapeutic value, and if the physician has good reason to believe that participation . . . will not adversely affect the health of the patients who serve as research subjects'.[78] A clinical trial is rarely undertaken unless there is good reason to suppose that one therapy will show an advantage over others, and particularly over those currently accepted as the best available. The advantage need not be direct; it could be collateral in that the results of the method were not better but were achieved with less disfigurement or fewer side-effects. Anticipation of advantage is generally based on laboratory, or, where appropriate, animal experimentation, and while the view is occasionally expressed that the latter is less moral than is human biomedical research, it is still generally acceptable given that the conditions are controlled. The corollary, as we have already emphasised, is that an untried method must be immediately withdrawn if it is found to be positively deleterious, and the patients involved must be transferred, whenever possible, to an alternative regime. As already noted, there is a legal obligation to report early terminations of clinical trials to both the REC and the MHRA with full explanation for the decision.[79]

6.4.3 USE OF PLACEBOS

A placebo is an inert substance without pharmacological action. But in humans, the mere taking of a substance in a clinical or quasi-clinical setting may lead to subjective, or symptomatic, improvement; this is the 'placebo effect', which must be considered whenever a new drug or procedure is on trial. On the other hand, the trial drug may do more harm than inactivity; but, for psychological reasons, inactivity must involve apparent activity

---

[75] Article 20 of the Additional Protocol on Biomedical Research (2005) states: 'Where the law allows research on persons deprived of liberty, such persons may participate in a research project in which the results do not have the potential to produce direct benefit to their health only if the following additional conditions are met: (a) research of comparable effectiveness cannot be carried out without the participation of persons deprived of liberty; (b) the research has the aim of contributing to the ultimate attainment of results capable of conferring benefit to persons deprived of liberty, and (c) the research entails only minimal risk and minimal burden.'

[76] For more, see Anna Charles et al., 'Prisoners as Research Participants: Current Practice and Attitudes in the UK' (2016) 42(4) Journal of Medical Ethics 246.

[77] For the approach to research involving prisoners, see REC SOPs, s 1, Table B, and the provisions on Flagged RECs.

[78] Declaration of Helsinki (2013), para 14.   [79] 2004 Regulations, reg 31.

if the two regimens are to be properly compared. In either case, the controlled giving of a placebo necessarily involves the deception of patients, and this raises some complex issues.

The extreme position is that placebos offend against the fundamental rightness of fidelity. If there is patient resistance to the use of such controls, this should not be regarded as an excuse for further deception but rather as an indication that such experiments are unacceptable to society. To this one could reply that a poor experiment is a worse affront to society, and that the simple expedient is to leave out those who object—little is lost other than perhaps absolute numbers, and, as previously discussed, experimental volunteers are, by nature, already a selected group.

More practical objections are based on the effect of the experiment on patient care; the circumstances in which it is ethical to deprive a patient of treatment must be strictly regulated. It would, for example, be improper to use placebo controls when pain is a feature of the condition under treatment, despite the fact that some patients might derive benefit; many painkillers are available and can be used as reference substances. The basic circumstances in which placebo trials are ethical and (arguably) necessary include, first, when there is no alternative to the experimental treatment available—such as in the treatment of degenerative neural disease, though even here *some* form of pharmacologically active substance might well be thought preferable—and, second, when the effect of adding a new treatment to an established one is under study. In the majority of instances, however, the purpose of their use is to analyse the effect of a treatment on subjective symptoms rather than on organic disease.

The 2013 version of the Declaration of Helsinki has raised some interesting additional points around the use of placebos. Paragraph 33 states that the benefits, risks, burdens, and effectiveness of a new intervention must be tested against those of the best-proven intervention(s), except in the following circumstances:

- where no proven intervention exists, the use of placebo, or no intervention, is acceptable; or

- where for compelling and scientifically sound methodological reasons the use of any intervention less effective than the best proven one, the use of placebo, or no intervention is necessary to determine the efficacy or safety of an intervention; and

- the patients who receive any intervention less effective than the best proven one, placebo, or no intervention will not be subject to additional risks of serious or irreversible harm as a result of not receiving the best proven intervention.

It concludes that 'extreme care must be taken to avoid abuse of this option'.

This may seem trite and fairly easily accommodated within an ethical spectrum, but we have now been confronted with the extension of the placebo concept into surgery—and especially, although not exclusively, into surgery for those conditions in which symptoms and signs become intermingled, such as sham surgery in clinical trials for neurologic disease.[80] Essentially, we have here an RCT in which some patients are implanted but in which the control group's brains are untouched. Space does not permit further discussion, but on top of the philosophical difficulties involved in the acceptance of medicinal placebo therapy, we must now impose deceptive target imaging by way of magnetic resonance imaging, an anaesthetic, a scalp incision, and at least a token hole in the skull on a person who is to receive no additional therapy. Justification of the programme on utilitarian grounds is possible, but is certainly not easy.

---

[80] Sam Horng and Franklin Miller, 'Ethics of Sham Surgery in Clinical Trials for Neurologic Disease' in Jens Clausen and Neil Levy (eds), *Handbook of Neuroethics* (Springer 2015).

6.5 EXPERIMENTAL TREATMENT

Early in the chapter, we distinguished between research and experimentation—the latter being regarded as involving ad hoc and untried treatment applied to an individual with little more scientific basis other than expediency. It follows that we see medical experiments—as opposed to research—on human beings as being morally justified only in extreme conditions. Nonetheless, in practice, the Declaration of Helsinki supports the concept of experimental treatment.[81]

Unfortunately, the status of the experimental therapist has been uncertain since 1797, when Dr Baker was pilloried for introducing what remains the standard treatment for limb fractures.[82] The innovative doctor cannot depend upon *Bolam* if things go wrong since, by definition, no supportive body of medical opinion is available—the pioneer therefore seems alone in many senses. Perhaps a more accurate measure of how the pioneer will be judged, however, is to be found in the earlier Scottish case of *Hunter* v *Hanley*,[83] which was accepted in *Bolam* as laying down the correct test for assessing medical conduct which departs from the norm. As Lord Clyde stated, a mere deviation from ordinary professional practice is not necessarily evidence of negligence; indeed, it would be disastrous if this were so, for all inducement to progress in medical science would be destroyed. He went so far as to remark that, 'Even a substantial deviation from normal practice may be warranted by the particular circumstances'. If there *is* to be liability for deviation, it must be shown that:

1. there is a usual and normal practice;

2. practice was not adopted; and

3. the course that was adopted was one which no professional of ordinary skill would have taken had he been acting with ordinary care.

This is nothing more than an alternative formulation of the reasonableness test, and the sum and substance of the legal position, then, is that it will be for the court to ask in the circumstances of each case—drawing on medical opinion as it thinks fit—whether the deviation from established practice was reasonable for the patient at hand.[84]

The patient who has no other hope is surely entitled to grasp an outside chance and, given the fact that they believe it to be a genuine chance, the doctor is entitled, and perhaps obligated, to provide it. They must, however, *believe* that there is a chance—they cannot provide, nor can the patient consent to, treatment that is expected to result in serious bodily harm or death.[85] In this respect, the ruling in *Bolitho* (see Chapter 12) may be to the doctor's advantage; given the conditions envisaged, it could be relatively easy in the event of an action in negligence to convince a court that their decision was logical *in all the circumstances* of the case. In any event, and as specified in paragraph 37 of the Declaration of Helsinki, the informed consent of the patient is of paramount importance, not only in the context of experimentation but for all forms of research, and we return to this universally accepted precept in due course. But even where informed consent is not possible, highly experimental treatment may be legal in the right circumstances. As we have seen many times, in the absence of consent, the law in the UK falls back on the

---

[81] See Declaration of Helsinki, para 37.   [82] *Slater* v *Baker and Stapleton* (1797) 95 ER 860.

[83] 1955 SC 200; 1955 SLT 213.

[84] An excellent illustration is provided by *Hepworth* v *Kerr* [1995] 6 Med LR 139, in which an anaesthetist was found negligent for using an unnecessary and unvalidated hypotensive technique to provide a blood-free operating area. The patient sustained neurological damage.

[85] *A-G's Reference (No 6 of 1980)* [1981] 2 All ER 1057 (CA).

patient's 'best interests', and we have also noted the tendency of the courts to rely on the *Bolam* standard to help determine what those interests might be.

The joined cases of *Simms v Simms; A v A and another*,[86] which involved two teenagers in the advanced stages of variant Creutzfeldt-Jakob disease (vCJD), and more recently the case of *University College London Hospitals v KG*,[87] demonstrate how far the concept of best interests can be extended into the realm of unproven experiment. In the joined cases, both sets of parents sought declaratory relief to confirm that it would be lawful to undertake a highly experimental course of 'treatment' which had never been tested in humans, about which the risks and benefits were unknown, but which had shown some marginal varying success in mice, rats, and dogs in Japan (although higher doses in dogs often caused severe reactions and death). The 'last chance' nature of the case permeates the judgment—it was accepted by all that the children would not recover. Notwithstanding, the President of the Family Division, Lady Butler-Sloss, sought to apply the best interests test and held that this justified the attempt in light of medical evidence whereby no witness was willing to rule out the *possibility* that some benefit might accrue. She added further qualifiers, namely that, since the disease was progressive and fatal, and because there was no alternative treatment, and so long as there were no significant risks of increasing the suffering of the patient, then it would not be unlawful to attempt the treatment (even when the risks and benefits were largely unknown). Finally, she held that because there was some medical evidence that did not rule out a chance of benefit, she was content to assume that the *Bolam* test had been complied with. Tellingly, and echoing the words of Lord Clyde, she stressed that the *Bolam* test 'ought not to be allowed to inhibit medical progress',[88] in the circumstances there was a responsible body of sufficient expertise to satisfy its terms.

In the case of *KG*, the Court of Protection granted approval for University College London Hospitals NHS Foundation Trust to administer a novel treatment known as PRN100 to patient KG, who suffered from sporadic CJD. The treatment had never been tested on or administered to any person. However, Cohen J ruled that it was in KG's best interests to receive the treatment under a clinical plan to treat a small number of patients as part of their NHS care. It is worth noting that as part of his reasoning, Cohen J placed emphasis on the trust establishing an 'Oversight Committee' to facilitate the fulfilment of 'duties to promote and safeguard the health, well-being and rights of the patient'.[89] Cohen J noted that since PRN100 was not being given for the purposes of a research study, the hospital was not required to submit the proposal to a REC, but the Oversight Committee seemed to fulfil similar functions. Also of importance seemed to be that the unit at the hospital was a recognised world leader in the process which was to be undertaken.

In the end, it is difficult to tell what sort of guidance is offered by these cases; the extreme and rare nature of the circumstances set them apart and suggest that both the families and courts must have felt that 'doing something' was far better than 'doing nothing', a perfectly natural human response to tragic circumstances.[90]

---

[86] [2003] 1 All ER 669; [2003] 1 FCR 361.   [87] [2018] EWCOP 29.

[88] ibid. [48]. Note that the President followed her own ruling in similar cases: *An NHS Trust v HM* [2004] Lloyd's Rep Med 207; *EP v Trusts A, B & C* [2004] Lloyd's Rep Med 211.

[89] *KG* (n 87) [20].

[90] Something of an interesting contrast can be seen in *Re MM (a child) (medical treatment)* [2000] 1 FLR 224, wherein the court upheld the decision of a child's doctors to abandon what they regarded as foreign experimental treatment in favour of their own approach. *Walker-Smith v GMC* (n 23) confirms a reliance on the medical profession's own attitudes towards conduct in cases in the liminal spaces between research and therapy.

Ultimately, the balance between progress and patient interests remains a fine one and is not easily struck, though in recent years legislative efforts have been proposed to offer guidance. In 2014, Lord Saatchi proposed a Medical Innovation Bill that encouraged 'responsible innovation' in medical treatment by stipulating that it would not be 'negligent for a doctor to depart from the existing range of accepted medical treatments for a condition if the decision to do so is taken responsibly'.[91] The Bill was heavily criticised by the medical research community, as well as research charities and patient organisations, for encouraging irresponsible experimentation and producing nothing more than anecdotal 'evidence', at the potential expense of causing serious harm and suffering to patients. There was also concern that the Bill risked allowing negligent doctors to avoid liability.[92] The Bill did not make it past the first reading in the House of Lords and was terminated in the 2015–16 session.

More recently, the Access to Medical Treatments (Innovation) Act 2016, which is still not in force, aims to promote access to innovative medical treatments (including treatments consisting in the off-label use of medicines or the use of unlicensed medicines) by providing for (a) the establishment of a database of innovative medical treatments, and (b) access to information contained in the database. Under the Act, the Secretary of State may by regulations make provision conferring functions on the Health and Social Care Information Centre (now subsumed within NHS England) in connection with the establishment, maintenance, and operation of a database containing information about innovative medical treatments carried out by doctors in England and the results of such treatments.[93] Advocates for the Act believe it will encourage patients to volunteer to try innovative treatments and drugs, thereby building an evidence base around them and reducing the time it takes to bring them to market; critics argue that the Act adds nothing to already-existing legal frameworks that allow for innovative treatments for patients; that there is no compelling need for a new database; and that the legislation lacks details about the database's operation.[94]

6.6 RESEARCH AND INFORMED CONSENT

6.6.1 PRACTICAL CHALLENGES WITH CONSENT

The 'ideal' ethical research programme is one that can be based on free, autonomous participation by the participant, and this, in turn, depends upon 'informed consent'. The consent principles in relation to research and experimentation are similar to those governing treatment. However, most commentators would hold that the research participants' rights are, if anything, *greater* in the former situation than they are in the sphere of pure patient and treatment management, given the step into the unknown. The classic statement in law comes from the Canadian case of *Halushka* v *University of Saskatchewan*:

> In my opinion, the duty imposed upon those engaged in medical research, as were the appellants . . . to those who offer themselves as subjects for experimentation, as the

[91] UK Parliament, 'Medical Innovation Bill [HL]' (2015) available at <https://bills.parliament.uk/bills/1379> accessed 07 November 2022.
[92] José Miola, 'Bye-Bye Bolitho? The Curious Case of the Medical Innovation Bill' (2015) 15(2–3) Medical Law International 124.
[93] Access to Medical Treatments (Innovation) Act 2016, s 2(1).
[94] UKRI, 'MRC position statement on the Access to Medical Treatments (Innovation) Act' (2022) available at <https://www.ukri.org/about-us/mrc/our-policies-and-standards/position-statements/access-to-medical-treatments-innovation-act/> accessed 07 November 2022.

respondent did here, is at least as great as, if not greater than, the duty owed by the ordinary physician or surgeon to his patient. There can be no exceptions to the ordinary requirements of disclosure in the case of research as there may well be in ordinary medical practice. The researcher does not have to balance the probable effect of lack of treatment against the risk involved in the treatment itself. The example of risks being properly hidden from a patient when it is important that he should not worry can have no application in the field of research. The subject of medical experimentation is entitled to a full and frank disclosure of all the facts, probabilities and opinions which a reasonable man might be expected to consider before giving his consent.[95]

As *Halushka* suggests, the standard of information provided must certainly be that of the 'reasonable participant'—if not that of the actual participant—rather than that of the 'reasonable doctor'. Even so, there are many and varied difficulties which make it almost impossible to lay down hard and fast rules. These include the essential need for some measure of ignorance in the trial, the seriousness of the condition being treated, the psychology of individual patients, and the like. The complexity is such that some confrontation between the backroom and the coalface is almost inevitable.

It is widely agreed that the participant's consent must be based on five main lines of explanation:

(1) the purpose of the research;

(2) what is expected of the participant;

(3) the benefits to the subject and society;

(4) the risks involved, and;

(5) the alternatives open to the participant.[96]

But many questions arise. Who is to impart the information—the participant's physician or the researcher? Should the participant have the benefit of a 'friend' to interpret for them? Should there be confirmation of the consent procedure? It has been fairly widely mooted that, in fact, informed consent is a double-edged weapon—token consent may take the place of the genuine and relieve the researcher of responsibility. Might it not be better to burden the investigator with full responsibility rather than provide such a shield? Many of the US states have enacted 'informed consent statutes', some of which lay down specific disclosure requirements for particular procedures. In the same spirit, US courts, dealing with claims of inadequate information to research subjects, have tended to stress that there is a considerably higher burden of disclosure in cases involving non-therapeutic research than in therapeutic cases,[97] a view shared, as we have been, by a Canadian court in *Halushka*.[98] The difficulties are highlighted in 'care associated' research when, effectively, the doctrine of informed consent implies that the participant has to choose for themselves whether to accept an experimental treatment or to be randomised in a comparative therapeutic trial. The philosophical basis of personal autonomy is perfectly clear, but is the ideal end attainable in practice? Ought a patient to be told of a 'last chance' effort? Is the medically naive prospective participant capable of giving consent as required? Can they be expected to understand the risks when the medical profession itself is divided?

---

[95] *Halushka* v *University of Saskatchewan* (1965) 53 DLR (2d) 436 (Sask CA) [29].

[96] See also Sch 1, Pt 3 to the 2004 Regulations.

[97] E.g. *Whitlock* v *Duke University* 637 F Supp 1463 (NC, 1986); affd 829 F 2d 1340 (1987).

[98] See also Karine Morin, 'The Standard of Disclosure in Human Subject Experimentation' (1998) 19(2) Journal of Legal Medicine 157.

A real problem here is that doubts as to participants' ability to understand complex medical information can very easily result in the striking of an unacceptably paternalistic attitude. A further complicating factor arises when the risks are simply unknown. A case in point is the prospect of xenotransplantation trials and the unknown risks of animal-to-human transmission of pathogens. What is the participant to be told in such cases? An added complication, which cannot be resolved by consent alone, is whether the risks to the wider society of such trials are appreciated and can be mitigated.

Before leaving this topic, we should note that there have been growing arguments that consent—or the consent process—should be adapted to reflect the risks associated with the research, with less rigorous standards being applied to low-risk research.[99] Further, there remain unresolved problems associated with the use and status of consent forms, the latter of which remains unclear in the UK. It has been argued that greater attention must be paid within research governance frameworks to the research relationship and the preservation of trust through ongoing communication and consent as a relational process.[100]

6.6.2 RESEARCH INVOLVING PEOPLE WHO LACK CAPACITY

On one view, research (and experimentation) involving persons considered to lack capacity to provide the required consent should not be ruled out entirely because to do so would not only deprive them of an opportunity to engage in community-oriented beneficial activities to which they might have consented if able, but it would also mean that much research into the conditions from which these people suffer would simply be impossible.[101] In both circumstances, it is strongly arguable that a complete ban is unethical. By the same token, the vulnerability of such persons requires that special care is taken to protect them and their interests. In short, difficult ethical and legal problems arise in respect of those patients who cannot give a valid consent to participation in health research by virtue of their condition of capacity. Such participants might be involved in research provided certain safeguards were erected; these would be designed so to ensure that they are not subjected to appreciable risk or inconvenience and would include the agreement of relatives and/or that of some independent supervisory party. The required approval of an independent authority would cover those instances in which it was suspected that uncaring relatives had been thoughtless.

The Additional Protocol on Biomedical Research (2005) has addressed the matter of research on a person without the capacity to consent, stating that research can be undertaken if:

(1) the results of the research have the potential to produce real and direct benefit to his or her health;

(2) research of comparable effectiveness cannot be carried out on competent individuals;

(3) the research subject has been informed of his or her rights and the safeguards prescribed by law for his or her protection, unless this person is not in a state to receive the information;

---

[99] Danielle Bromwich and Annette Rid, 'Can Informed Consent to Research be Adapted to Risk?' (2015) 41(7) Journal of Medical Ethics 521.

[100] Graeme Laurie and Emily Postan, 'Rhetoric or Reality: What is the Legal Status of the Consent Form in Health-Related Research?' (2013) 21(3) Medical Law Review 371.

[101] This was expressly recognised in *Simms v Simms* (n 86) [57].

(4) the necessary authorisation has been given specifically and in writing by the legal representative or an authority, person or body provided for by law, and taking into account the person's previously expressed wishes or objections; and

(5) the person concerned does not object.[102]

Exceptionally, where condition (1) is not satisfied, research may be authorised if it has the aim of contributing 'to the ultimate attainment of results capable of conferring benefit to the person concerned or to other persons in the same age category or afflicted with the same disease or disorder or having the same condition' provided, at the same time, that the research entails only minimal risk and minimal burden for the individual concerned. It is this latter criterion, not the ultimate value of the research, that constitutes the benchmark.[103]

While the UK has not ratified the Biomedicine Convention (1997) nor signed the Additional Protocol (2005), the requirements of the prevailing regulatory framework reflect many of the terms of the Protocol. Moreover, they seek to apply both a principled and pragmatic approach to clinical trials involving incapacitated persons. As to principles, the 2004 Clinical Trials Regulations provide in Schedule 1, Part 5 that the following underpin research involving such persons:

(1) informed consent given by a legal representative to an adult considered to lack capacity in a clinical trial shall represent that adult's presumed will;

(2) the clinical trial has been designed to minimise pain, discomfort, fear, and any other foreseeable risk in relation to the disease and the cognitive abilities of the patient;

(3) the risk threshold and the degree of distress have to be specially defined and constantly monitored; and

(4) the interests of the patient always prevail over those of science and society.

The Regulations also lay down some 11 conditions for lawful research. In these, the subject's legal representative is central, and the same provisions regarding research involving persons with capacity apply equally to the representative of those considered to lack it.

The provisions of the Mental Capacity Act 2005 also address research involving adults considered to lack capacity to consent to it, but these explicitly exclude subjects involved in clinical trials (governed by the 2004 Regulations).[104] Briefly, the approach taken is that intrusive research is illegal unless the elements of the Act are complied with. The requirements are very similar save that, specifically, non-paid carers must be consulted as to the person's past (and likely present) views or wishes in respect of the research. Any indication, past or present, from the individual that they do not wish to participate must be respected. Importantly, however, and in contrast to the 2004 Regulations, the role of the carer is not to give or withhold their consent but rather 'to advise' on whether the person should take part in the research. The REC is the final approval authority.

The situation in Scotland in respect of research involving persons considered to lack capacity has been clear since the enforcement of the Adults with Incapacity (Scotland) Act 2000.[105] The necessary conditions almost exactly parallel those laid down in the

---

[102] Additional Protocol, Art 15. And see the Declaration of Helsinki, paras 28–30.

[103] See Alexander Friedman, Emily Robbins, and David Wendler, 'Which Benefits of Research Participation Count as "Direct"?' (2012) 26(2) Bioethics 60.

[104] Mental Capacity Act 2005, ss 30–34. The 2004 Regulations also apply to Scotland.

[105] Section 51, as amended.

Additional Protocol (2005) save that, in addition, authority for surrogate consent is specifically vested in a person appointed as the individual's guardian or welfare attorney;[106] where there is none appointed, power to consent lies with the individual's nearest relatives who have authority to act for the individual in the order that they appear in the list that is now provided in the Mental Health (Care and Treatment) (Scotland) Act 2003.[107]

The 2004 Regulations and Scottish legislation have been revised to allow adults considered to lack capacity to consent into trials in emergency situations.[108] The problem is that time may not permit the written consent of the appropriate person to be sought in circumstances where treatment to be given to such an adult as part of a trial must be given urgently. They can now be entered into a trial without the prior informed consent of a legal representative if, having regard to the nature of the trial and the particular circumstances of the case, it is necessary to take action for the purpose of the trial as a matter of urgency, but it is not reasonably practicable to obtain informed consent prior to entering the subject, and the action to be taken is carried out in accordance with a procedure approved by the REC. Consent must, however, be sought either from the participant themself (if they regain capacity) or from the legal representative as soon as is practicable thereafter. If such consent is not forthcoming, the participant must be withdrawn from the trial.

In 2018, the Scottish Government announced its intention to reform the Adults with Incapacity (Scotland) Act 2000, including the provision governing research (s 51); the consultation document indicated the Government's desire to favour an approach that focuses on greater inclusion of adults in research—whether they are considered to lack capacity or not.[109] We welcome such a change—provided this can be done responsibly and without incurring disproportionate risks—and note that such a change accords with recent legislative reform in other jurisdictions, including, for example, the Canadian province of Québec, which has moved away from a protectionist mode of research governance where persons considered to lack capacity are concerned.[110] However, five years later, as of the time of writing this edition, there is no indication of legislative reform forthcoming.

6.7 THE UNETHICAL RESEARCHER

All that has gone before has assumed that the researcher is acting in good faith with the interests of the profession and of the public at heart—and that includes assumption of the public-spirited objective of research, which is to produce generalisable knowledge to improve human health. Occasionally, however, concerns arise about non-intentional conduct of researchers that falls short of acceptable ethical standards, and, worse, intentional

---

[106] See too Scottish Government, 'Adults with Incapacity: Code of Practice for Medical Practitioners' (2010) available at <https://www.gov.scot/publications/adults-incapacity-scotland-act-2000-code-practice-third-edition-practitioners-authorised-carry-out-medical-treatment-research-under-part-5-act/> accessed 07 November 2022. Note the legal designation of a particular REC to oversee research with this group of participants: The Adults with Incapacity (Ethics Committee) (Scotland) Regulations 2002 (SSI 2002/190).

[107] Section 254(1)(b).

[108] The Medicines for Human Use (Clinical Trials) Amendment (No 2) Regulations 2006 (SI 2006/2984).

[109] Scottish Government, 'Adults with Incapacity (Scotland) Act 2000: Proposals for Reform' (2018) available at <https://www.gov.scot/publications/adults-incapacity-scotland-act-2000-proposals-reform/> accessed 07 November 2022. See also Scottish Government, 'Adults with Incapacity Reform' (2018) available at <https://consult.gov.scot/health-and-social-care/adults-with-incapacity-reform/> accessed 07 November 2022.

[110] Civil Code of Québec, Art 21 (2013).

conduct that ignores such standards, such as fraudulent behaviour and/or the publication of fraudulent studies.[111]

Doctors and researchers are under ongoing pressure, competitiveness is common, and the potential for lucrative commercial deals can all serve as temptations to act unethically. Even in the academic setting, those who publish attract more funding than those who do not; publishing impacts heavily on advancement, and academic impact is facilitated by 'being first', which can encourage premature reporting. All of this can lead to 'sloppy science' and/or deliberate falsification of results or suppression of truth. A critical danger is that the public, fed by the media, may be led to believe in therapeutic claims which are unsupported by the data, or they may be subjected to valueless or dangerous treatments. A further pressure is generated by the sometimes very different interests that are often asked to work in cooperation. While research, as we have suggested, has a very public ethos and objective, private interests are invariably at stake, and not all of them can be reconciled with the greater public good. In this respect, we must differentiate between two sets of actors—researchers and their funders. Researchers and funders must have a financial relationship, and clearly both the medical profession and society have a right to know how far this extends. Additionally, funders may have an interest in keeping unfavourable results out of the public domain. While this may not amount to outright public deception, there may be many reasons for a commercial enterprise to wish to protect its financial interests by questioning or disputing the value of research that goes against those interests.

Of course, the existence of the problems exposed by research integrity cases such as that of Dr Paolo Macchiarini[112] is appreciated within the medical and publishing world. The Committee on Publication Ethics (COPE) was founded in 1997 by journal editors as a medium through which to address their growing concern. COPE maintains a register of all cases reported to it since its inception, as well as a range of guidance.[113] It has produced guidelines and 'Core Practices' which are meant to provide greater clarity for researchers rather than merely adding to the already considerable morass of instruments with little practical effect. In 2006, the UK Research Integrity Office (UKRIO) was formed as an independent advisory body; it exists to promote good practice in addressing misconduct in research, and it has the support of government, research funders, and the industry regulators. While it has no statutory basis or disciplinary teeth, it has produced a 'Code of Practice for Research' to support researchers and research organisations in the conduct of research of the highest quality and standards.[114] The International Committee of Medical Journal Editors (ICMJE) also has articulated standards which demand, inter alia, extensive disclosure of competing interests before research results can be published.[115] The combined effect of these organisations and their guidance is that it should not be possible to publish one's research in a reputable medical journal unless the required details are provided.

[111] Ron Iphofen (ed), *Handbook of Research Ethics and Scientific Integrity* (Springer 2020); Adil Shamoo and David Resnik, *Responsible Conduct of Research* (4th edn, OUP 2022).

[112] John Rasko and Carl Power, 'Dr Con Man: the Rise and Fall of a Celebrity Scientist who Fooled Almost Everyone' *The Guardian* (01 September 2017) available at <https://www.theguardian.com/science/2017/sep/01/paolo-macchiarini-scientist-surgeon-rise-and-fall> accessed 07 November 2022.

[113] See COPE, 'Guidelines' (2022) available at <https://publicationethics.org/guidance/Guidelines> accessed 07 November 2022; and COPE, 'Core Practices' (2022) available at <https://publicationethics.org/core-practices> accessed 07 November 2022.

[114] UKRIO, 'Code of Practice for Research: Promoting Good Practice and Preventing Misconduct' (2022) available at <https://ukrio.org/publications/code-of-practice-for-research/1-0-introduction/> accessed 07 November 2022.

[115] ICMJE, 'Recommendations for the Conduct, Reporting, Editing, and Publication of Scholarly Work in Medical Journals' (2022) available at <https://www.icmje.org/recommendations/> accessed 07 November 2022.

Beyond these mechanisms, which are aimed at avoiding and reducing misconduct, the fraudulent researcher faces a variety of sanctions. First, there are powerful professional disciplinary procedures that can effectively end a scientific career, and cases are regularly investigated by the Association of British Pharmaceutical Industries (ABPI) and the General Medical Council (GMC). Indeed, Andrew Wakefield's fitness to practise medicine in the light of the allegations surrounding his MMR study was the subject of the longest-running disciplinary case of the GMC, and it ran at considerable cost both to Wakefield and to the GMC itself.[116] The researcher may also be criminally liable for fraudulently obtaining research funds, and civilly liable for any loss incurred by drug manufacturers. With respect to the criminal law, it is an offence to provide a REC with false or misleading information in a research application relating to a CTIMP.[117] And the REC SOPs make it clear where a REC receives information other than from the sponsor (or sponsor's representative) suggesting that a serious breach may have occurred in relation to an application for ethical review or the conduct of research, the information should be emailed to the HRA.[118] It will be for the HRA's Quality and Performance Manager to decide whether the information should be shared with other bodies, including the MHRA for clinical trials, so that the matter can be formally investigated if appropriate.[119] RECs have no power under the 2004 Regulations to suspend or terminate the Clinical Trial Authorisation or legally withdraw the ethical opinion given previously. However, the REC may review its opinion in the light of new ethical concerns following any new information received about the trial. It may also notify the MHRA that, if it had received the information with the initial application, its opinion of the trial would not have been favourable.[120]

The considerable increase in research regulation activity—and bureaucracy—in many countries has driven some researchers to pursue their work elsewhere, most notably to lower- and middle-income countries where research populations may be more accessible and programmes are subject to less intense scrutiny.[121] Notwithstanding this, the ethical imperatives surrounding research involving human beings remain, in essence, universal; the lack of local regulation, or of its enforcement, is no excuse for not respecting ethical fundamentals,[122] which clearly erect a hierarchy of values in this context: (i) the interests of medical research can never take precedence over the rights and interests of individual research subjects; and (ii) freedom of research must be preserved.[123]

Before leaving this issue, we should offer a word on experimentation. We have already referred to the fact that it can be difficult distinguishing courageous innovation from unethical experimentation—and, human nature being what it is, the answer often depends on the outcome. Moreover, we are left with the complex problem of whether information gained from frankly immoral research should be used for the general good—the classic examples being data obtained in the concentration camps of World War II. Wherever one stands on the issue, we must recognise that a not insignificant amount of medical knowledge today rests on the tainted history of past abuse.[124]

[116] David Rose, 'Case Against Dr Andrew Wakefield, who Linked MMR and Autism, to Cost Over £1m' *The Times* (16 March 2009). And see *Walker-Smith v GMC* (n 23).
[117] REC SOPs, paras 10.82–10.84; and 2004 Regulations, reg 49.
[118] REC SOPs, para 10.74.   [119] ibid., para 10.77.   [120] ibid., para 14.28.
[121] Adriana Petryna, *When Experiments Travel: Clinical Trials and the Global Search for Human Subjects* (Princeton University Press 2009).
[122] See e.g. Global Code, 'A Global Ethics Code to Promote Equitable Research Partnerships' (2022) available at <https://www.globalcodeofconduct.org/> accessed 07 November 2022.
[123] In this respect the Additional Protocol (2005), the 2001 EU Directive and its domestic manifestations, and the 2014 EU Clinical Trials Regulation are all in agreement.
[124] Doug Hickey et al., 'Unit 731 and Moral Repair' (2017) 43(4) Journal of Medical Ethics 270.

6.8 COMPENSATION FOR PERSONAL INJURY IN RESEARCH

A research participant who is injured in the course of research may resort to a claim for compensation under the law of tort. Such a route, of course, may prove to be difficult: researchers may have taken every precaution to avoid injury and there may therefore be no evidence of negligence. Although the odds against a plaintiff in such actions may not be as long as they once were, the research participant could still be in an uncertain situation, and it is, no doubt, for this reason that all modern governance frameworks on the management of research projects emphasise the importance of compulsory protection of participants against the possibility of mishap. Thus, the 2001 Directive and 2004 Regulations state that a clinical trial may only be undertaken if, inter alia, provision has been made for insurance or indemnity to cover the liability of the investigator and sponsor.[125] Before approving a proposal, NHS RECs must assure themselves that the sponsor and investigators will have appropriate insurance or indemnity cover for the potential legal liability arising from the research, and consider provision in proportion to the risk for compensation or treatment in the event of injury, disability, or death attributable to participation.[126] Of course, none of this guarantees the research participant adequate compensation should anything go wrong, and we suspect that most commentators would favour a form of no-fault compensation, but the answer lies in the hands of government.[127]

6.9 RESEARCH AND INNOVATION

The discussion thus far has proceeded on the assumption that research or experimentation will involve some direct intrusion into the physical integrity of the research subject—some form of bodily touching. However, this is by no means necessary for many forms of research, particularly epidemiological, which can be conducted without any need to involve the subject directly. Moreover, innovation at the interface of treatment and research increasingly makes use of technologies such as artificial intelligence and brain organoids. This section proceeds to look at use of human tissue and personal data, including genetic/genomic data, as well as the increasing use of artificial intelligence and brain organoids as an innovative practice in medicine.

6.9.1 HUMAN TISSUE AND PERSONAL DATA

Patient data and samples taken or given previously for unrelated purposes (such as treatment) are a source of potentially valuable medical research. On one view, the use of data in patient records or archived samples subjects the patient to no further discomfort, and it could be thought reasonable to pursue research in the name of the 'public good'. By the same token, there is a clear element of potential invasion of the patient's privacy in 'finding out things' about them without their consent, not to mention the sense of indignation, or

---

[125] 2001 Directive, Art 3(2)(f); 2004 Regulations, Part 2, s 14 of Sch 1.

[126] REC SOPs, para 3.43 and Annex F.

[127] Leslie Henry, Megan Larkin, and Elizabeth Pike, 'Just Compensation: A No-Fault Proposal for Research-Related Injuries' (2015) 2(3) Journal of Law and the Biosciences 645; Elizabeth Pike, 'Recovering From Research: A No-Fault Proposal to Compensate Injured Research Participants' (2012) 38(1) American Journal of Law & Medicine 7.

even outrage, that can be generated at the idea of using these 'personal' rudiments—again, without the proper authority to do so. It was precisely this reaction that provoked the investigations at Bristol and Alder Hey into the retention of body parts for 'research purposes'.[128]

The challenges here are manifold, not least because the 'call for consent' is not always realisable, nor is it necessarily desirable in some cases. For example, if a researcher wishes to examine tissue samples gathered many decades previously, is it reasonable to expect them to attempt to obtain consent from all the persons from whom the samples were taken, as persons may have moved, married, or died years before? The cost implications alone may make any such study non-viable *ab initio*. Another example relates to longitudinal studies, that is, those that propose to study persons over many years and usually by ongoing review of their medical records. Given that research generates new knowledge by its very nature, is it reasonable to require researchers to revisit these persons on a regular basis in order to obtain re-consent in the light of developments in the research?

A crude analysis of these examples might cast the core issue as one of pitting cost and convenience against consent. This would misconstrue the dilemma, which, in fact, arises from trying to force the issues into the consent paradigm—that is, from the belief that consent is 'the' answer to (all) ethical concerns. It must be remembered, however, that consent itself is a means to an end and that the real aim is to respect persons and their interests. Consent is but one means by which to achieve this. In this vein, the MRC has stated that existing collections of tissue samples, commonly known as biobanks, can be used for research even in the absence of consent provided the legal requirements are followed, the proposed use of samples (without consent) can be justified, use would be considered ethical and reasonable, the confidentiality of all donors and their associated health and research information is maintained, and an NHS REC has decided that use without consent is appropriate.[129] By the same token, the MRC reinforces the point that, in the first instance, the possibility of later research should be explained and appropriate consent obtained.[130]

This still leaves the problem of what is meant by 'appropriate consent', especially in the context of long-term studies,[131] and which in turn ought to be distinguished from securing a lawful basis to process personal data[132] and use confidential information.[133] Here, the MRC has stated that 'broad consent' is an acceptable concept whereby it is consent to future medical research projects which would have to be approved by a properly constituted research ethics committee.[134] Thus, we can see how the protectionist role of the REC

[128] Julie Kent and Ruud ter Meulen, 'Public Trust and Public Bodies: The Regulation of the Use of Human Tissue for Research in the United Kingdom' in Christian Lenk, Judit Sándor, and Bert Gordijn (eds), *Biobanks and Tissue Research: The Public, the Patient and the Regulation* (Springer 2011) 17–35.

[129] UKRI, 'Operational and Ethical Guidelines for Medical Research Council (MRC)-Funded Researchers Working with Human Tissue and Biological Samples' (2019) available at <MRC-0208212-Human-tissue-and-biological-samples-for-use-in-research.pdf (ukri.org)> accessed 07 November 2022, 10. The MRC proposes two approaches to 'reasonableness': 1. The stronger test—would a reasonable person have refused to allow their samples to be used, if you had asked them? 2. Would a reasonable person be distressed if they discovered that their samples had been used without their consent?

[130] MRC Guidelines, 10.

[131] This is, of course, the language of the Human Tissue Act 2004. For guidance from the Human Tissue Authority, see 'Code of Practice E: Research' (2017) available at <https://content.hta.gov.uk/sites/default/files/2020-11/Code%20E.pdf> accessed 07 November 2022.

[132] Jiahong Chen, Edward Dove, and Himani Bhakuni, 'Explicit Consent and Alternative Data Protection Processing Grounds for Health Research' in Eleni Kosta, Ronald Leenes, and Irene Kamara (eds.) *Research Handbook on EU Data Protection* (Edward Elgar 2022) 474–502.

[133] Edward Dove and Mark Taylor, 'Signalling Standards for Progress: Bridging the Divide Between a Valid Consent to Use Patient Data Under Data Protection Law and the Common Law Duty of Confidentiality' (2021) 29(3) Medical Law Review 411.

[134] MRC Guidelines, 11.

can be employed to circumvent some of the thornier issues surrounding specific consent. The REC SOPs detail the considerations and special procedures for approval of research involving databases and human tissue.[135]

6.9.2 GENETIC/GENOMIC RESEARCH AND GENE EDITING

It is becoming increasingly clear in the decades following the mapping of the human genome in 2000 (i.e. the unveiling of the complete genetic code of the human species) that a genetic component may well operate in many illnesses and conditions. The social, ethical, and legal implications which advances in genetics/genomics have for all of us expanded by the day; correspondingly, genetic considerations increasingly breathe new life into the study of medical jurisprudence.

Research and innovation over the last few decades now mean that access to genetic information through genetic testing is relatively cheap and easy but, as a result, this has given rise to serious concerns about access to, and the use of, test results. While the sensitivity of medical data is an issue of general concern which we address in the context of confidentiality in Chapter 11, matters are particularly complicated in the context of genetics because of certain features that are said to be particular to genetic information. First, a test result can have implications not only for the individual who has been tested (the 'proband') but also for blood relatives of that person who share a common gene pool—which came to the fore in the case of *ABC v St George's Healthcare NHS Trust*[136] (discussed in Chapter 11). Second, this information can have implications also for future relatives, in the sense that many genetic diseases pass vertically through generations and, thus, impact directly on reproductive decisions. Third, genetic test results can disclose a likelihood of future ill health in persons who are currently well. Fourth, because, in most cases, testing is carried out by analysing a person's DNA, genetic testing can be done at any stage from the cradle to the grave—and, indeed, either before or beyond. Thus, a foetus can be tested in utero for a condition such as Huntington's disease which might not manifest itself until middle age. Finally, underlying all of these factors is the perceived benefit which genetic testing can offer in the guise of predictability.

Advances in testing and screening constitute only one aspect of the progress which has been made in human genetics over recent decades. Perhaps more significantly from the scientific point of view, possibilities have opened up for *manipulation* of the genes of existing and future individuals. It has given rise to considerable bioethical debate. Gene therapy is one such form of manipulation and can be either somatic or germline. Somatic gene therapy is directed towards the remedying of a defect within the patient and involves the insertion of genetic material which will perform some function which the patient's own genetic material cannot achieve. Germline gene therapy can be visualised in two ways: the insertion of genetic material into the pre-embryo, which is pre-emptive treatment of the future being and their progeny, or as the insertion of a gene into the germ cells of an individual. The latter therapy has no direct bearing on the individual but is intended to ensure that any subsequent children are born with or without certain characteristics. The scientific techniques involved have spawned considerable—and emotional—debate; indeed, genetic engineering is one of the few modern medical technologies in which study of the moral aspects has preceded the practical realities.

---

[135] REC SOPs, ss 11 and 12, respectively.   [136] [2020] EWHC 455 (QB).

Trials involving gene therapy began in 1990 but suffered a real setback in 1999, when the first death attributable to the technique occurred.[137] Deaths in gene therapy trials can still happen, and occurred in both 2021[138] and 2022,[139] which prompt ongoing questions about the safety of this biotechnology.

In the UK, the Gene Therapy Advisory Committee (GTAC) is the research ethics committee with a specific remit to consider ethical approval of clinical trials involving gene therapy.[140] GTAC works with the HRA to deliver the safe exploration of gene therapies, while also seeking to deliver a proportionate and efficient review service. On a more practical level, the MHRA must approve all gene therapy products for market. The absorption of GTAC into the HRA has meant that it is now treated akin to other RECs, subject to 60-day approval times and more effective division of labour with four NHS RECs (three in England, one in Scotland) undertaking review under its auspices.

As one genetic biotechnology becomes absorbed into the mainstream, a new one surely emerges to take its place on the ethical stage. So it is with the prospect of somatic and germline *gene editing*, which arises with the development of new technology in the form of CRISPR-Cas9, an innovation that cuts and splices genetic material in much the same way found in nature.[141] With this possibility concerns have arisen about its actual uses, including the altering of embryo DNA (yet another form of gene therapy), and the creation of inter-species genomic material, giving a new twist to the chimera debate. Future uncertainties have led some to call for a moratorium on these techniques (arguing instead that current interventions should be explored fully first), while yet others reject this position in favour of a moral imperative to pursue such research, partly on the grounds that it could lead to an overall reduction in the number of embryos destroyed in the future.[142] This said, statements issued by two global summits on genome editing in 2015[143] and 2018,[144] as well

---

[137] Rick Weiss and Deborah Nelson, 'Teen Dies Undergoing Gene Therapy' *Washington Post* (29 September 1999) available at <https://www.washingtonpost.com/wp-srv/WPcap/1999-09/29/060r-092999-idx.html> accessed 07 November 2022; Meir Rinde, 'The Death of Jesse Gelsinger, 20 Years Later' (Distillations, 4 June 2019) available at <https://www.sciencehistory.org/distillations/the-death-of-jesse-gelsinger-20-years-later> accessed 07 November 2022.

[138] Alex Philippidis, 'Fourth Boy Dies in Trial of Astellas Gene Therapy Candidate' (GEN, 21 September 2021) available at <https://www.genengnews.com/news/fourth-boy-dies-in-trial-of-astellas-gene-therapy-candidate/> accessed 07 November 2022. See also Annalee Armstrong, 'Pfizer Reports Patient Death in Early-Stage Duchenne Gene Therapy Trial, Halts Enrollment' (Fierce Biotech, 21 December 2021) available at <https://www.fiercebiotech.com/biotech/pfizer-reports-death-patient-duchenne-trial-halts-enrolment> accessed 07 November 2022.

[139] Ned Pagliarulo, 'Novartis Reports Deaths of Two Patients Treated with Zolgensma Gene Therapy' (Biopharmadive, 11 August 2022) available at <https://www.biopharmadive.com/news/novartis-zolgensma-patient-death-liver-injury/629542/> accessed 07 November 2022.

[140] The Medicines for Human Use (Clinical Trials) Regulations 2004 (SI 2004/1031), reg 14(5). See more at Health Research Authority, 'Gene Therapy Advisory Committee' (18 May 2020) available at <https://www.hra.nhs.uk/about-us/committees-and-services/res-and-recs/gene-therapy-advisory-committee/> accessed 07 November 2022.

[141] Walter Isaacson, *The Code Breaker: Jennifer Doudna, Gene Editing, and the Future of the Human Race* (Simon & Schuster 2021).

[142] Compare Eric Lander et al., 'Adopt a Moratorium on Heritable Genome Editing' (2019) 567(7747) Nature 165 and Julian Savulescu et al., 'The Moral Imperative to Continue Gene Editing Research on Human Embryos' (2015) 6(7) Protein Cell 476.

[143] National Academies, 'On Human Gene Editing: International Summit Statement' (2015) available at <https://www.nationalacademies.org/news/2015/12/on-human-gene-editing-international-summit-statement> accessed 07 November 2022.

[144] National Academies, 'Statement by the Organizing Committee of the Second International Summit on Human Genome Editing' (2018) available at <https://www.nationalacademies.org/news/2018/11/statement-by-the-organizing-committee-of-the-second-international-summit-on-human-genome-editing> accessed 07 November 2022.

as a 2017 report from the US National Academies of Sciences, Engineering, and Medicine (NASEM),[145] and a 2018 report from the UK's Nuffield Council on Bioethics,[146] all trend towards cautious support of gene editing in limited circumstances and under certain conditions. Likewise, in 2021, the WHO's Expert Advisory Committee on Developing Global Standards for Governance and Oversight of Human Genome Editing promulgated recommendations on human genome editing for the advancement of public health, focusing on the governance and oversight of human genome editing in discrete areas, again taking a cautious but supportive approach.[147]

While *ex vivo* human germline gene editing is prohibited in the UK under the Human Fertilisation and Embryology Act 1990 (at least insofar as it is part of a fertility treatment for a woman) and in countries around the world,[148] the law is more permissive of somatic genome editing, which involves editing DNA in cells that are not eggs, sperm, or embryos and therefore are not heritable. We do think it only a matter of time, however, before the law moves to permit some form of germline gene editing as well, particularly with respect to serious monogenic disorders such as cystic fibrosis and Huntington's disease. Indeed, by the next edition of this textbook, we may find that the Human Fertilisation and Embryology Authority (HFEA) has issued one or more licences for research involving genome editing of human sperm, egg, or embryo cells. Moreover, we may find that additional law is created or existing primary legislation amended to cover existing gaps, including edits made to germline cells *inside* the human body (in vivo), which are not currently covered under the Human Fertilisation and Embryology Act 1990, but are indirectly covered by other regulations, such as those on clinical trials, gene therapy, and human tissues.[149]

For our part, we suspect the legal and policy response that emerges in the near future, both nationally and internationally, will once again fall back on safety and choice, subject to an initially cautious yet progressive approach that favours exploration. In this respect, this latest technological advance does little to advance our ethical or moral positions. We agree with our colleagues, however, that any such advance must be driven by the imperative to engage society widely and meaningfully in developing any genuinely defensible response.[150]

We note that much of the policy response to the prospect and the promise of genetics and genomics was laid down in the early days of debate in the 1990s. Many of the bodies that were initially set up to address the advent of the so-called 'New Genetics' have since been closed down or absorbed into other entities with far wider remits. We suspect this is as much to do with the growing realisation that there is less 'new' about genetics than

[145] National Academies, 'Human Genome Editing: Science, Ethics, and Governance' (2017) available at <https://nap.nationalacademies.org/catalog/24623/human-genome-editing-science-ethics-and-governance> accessed 07 November 2022.
[146] Nuffield Council on Bioethics, 'Genome Editing and Human Reproduction: Social and Ethical Issues' (2018) available at <https://www.nuffieldbioethics.org/publications/genome-editing-and-human-reproduction> accessed 07 November 2022.
[147] WHO, 'Human Genome Editing: Recommendations' (2021) available at <https://www.who.int/publications/i/item/9789240030381> accessed 07 November 2022.
[148] UK Parliamentary Office of Science and Technology, 'POST Note: Human Germline Genome Editing' (2020) available at <https://researchbriefings.files.parliament.uk/documents/POST-PN-0611/POST-PN-0611.pdf> accessed 07 November 2022.
[149] *ibid*.
[150] Courtney Addison and Samuel Taylor-Alexander, 'Gene Editing: Advising Advice' (2015) 349(6251) Science 935; Iñigo de Miguel Beriain, 'Should Human Germ Line Editing be Allowed? Some Suggestions on the Basis of the Existing Regulatory Framework' (2019) 33(1) Bioethics 105.

was first imagined, as it has anything to do with economic expediency. For the most part, this is to be welcomed. Having considered the policy and social issues that arise, much of the current debate returns us to age-old considerations about balances of rights and interests, scientific imperative against patient choice, and fundamental notions of justice (issues considered in depth in Chapters 1 and 2). The law's role here need not take on any special mantle to help us resolve the issues as and when they arise. Sadly, however, the spectre of abuse remains ever-present. The bioethical community was vexed by the news of the first human birth in China arising in November 2018 from the use of gene editing techniques undertaken by the rogue scientist Dr He Jiankui, who was subject to universal condemnation and sent to jail in China for three years.[151] The case reminds us of not only the importance of research ethics and integrity, not to mention adherence to law, but the at-times porous contours of responsible innovation in the realm of biotechnology.

6.9.3 ARTIFICIAL INTELLIGENCE

Space does not allow for comprehensive coverage of the legal and ethical issues regarding use of artificial intelligence in biomedicine, and indeed to do so faithfully would warrant a textbook all on its own.[152] In this chapter on health research and innovation, what we wish to cover are the basic elements of this increasingly important but fraught area.

Artificial intelligence can be defined as technologies and computer systems that do things on their own that would require intelligence and discernment if done by people. In the health context, a 2019 report published by NHSX noted the potential of AI to make a significant difference to health and care.[153] Many universities and companies in the UK are making significant investment and headway into creating Artificially Intelligent Systems (AIS) to carry out or augment health and care tasks (which could mean carrying out medical tasks traditionally done by professional healthcare practitioners), including inductive logic programming, robotic process automation, natural language processing, computer vision, neural networks, and distributed artificial intelligence. There is hope, given ongoing concerns about an ageing population and 'cash-strapped' health services, that AIS can lead to personalised NHS screening and treatments for cancer, eye disease, and a range of other conditions that ultimately reduce costs and save lives.

At the same, given the novelty and risks associated with this technology, in particular the 'black box' nature of much of AI development (e.g. the coding of algorithms) and concerns of transparency, fairness, bias, stigmatisation, not to mention liability, many recognise that in the health context, a standardised, ethically, and socially acceptable framework ought to be developed that fosters trust in this area and ensures risks are minimised. Indeed, the 2019 report highlighted that, worryingly, 'It is currently quite hit and miss whether or not developers seek ethical approval at the beginning of the development process with an almost 50/50 split between those that did and those that did not.'[154]

---

[151] Antonio Regalado, 'The Creator of the CRISPR Babies has Been Released From a Chinese Prison' (MIT Technology Review, 4 April 2022) available at <https://www.technologyreview.com/2022/04/04/1048829/he-jiankui-prison-free-crispr-babies/> accessed 07 November 2022.

[152] For a general overview, see Claire Thompson and Heather Morgan, 'Ethical Barriers to Artificial Intelligence in the National Health Service, United Kingdom of Great Britain and Northern Ireland' (2020) 98(4) Bulletin of the World Health Organization 293; Anto Čartolovni, Ana Tomičić, and Elvira Mosler, 'Ethical, Legal, and Social Considerations of AI-Based Medical Decision-Support Tools: A Scoping Review' (2022) 161 International Journal of Medical Informatics 104738.

[153] Ila Joshi and James Morley (eds), 'Artificial Intelligence: How to Get it Right' (NHSX, 2019) available at <https://transform.england.nhs.uk/documents/8/NHSX_AI_report.pdf> accessed 07 November 2022.

[154] ibid., p 22.

To this end, the Department of Health and Social Care has published 'A guide to good practice for digital and data-driven health technologies'[155] and more recently and on point, the NHS Artificial Intelligence Laboratory (NHS AI Lab), part of NHS England's Transformation Directorate (itself formerly known as NHSX) is currently developing a 'National Strategy for AI in Health and Social Care' for the responsible development, implementation, scaling, and monitoring of AI-driven technologies in the UK's health and adult social care systems.[156]

As seen in the recent UK Government policy paper, 'Data Saves Lives', the Government is keen to build a post-Brexit regulatory environment that promotes a 'proportionate, innovation-friendly regulation of AI technologies'.[157] As part of this, the Government's Office for Artificial Intelligence will set out in a future white paper how the Government intends to address the opportunities and risks arising from AI. Likewise, the NHS AI Lab is working with regulatory bodies such as the MHRA, the HRA, CQC, NHS Resolution, and NICE in helping to support the creation of a future 'robust regulatory framework for AI in health and care that supports innovation, and gives patients and clinicians confidence that AI products are safe and effective'.[158] Whether NICE is able to develop an evidence standard framework for digital health technologies, ensuring new technologies are effective and offer economic value, and one that the public and NHS patients broadly support, remains to be seen.

6.9.4 BRAIN ORGANOIDS

The human brain is commonly recognised as the most complex and under-discovered organ, and in turn neurological disorders are commonly recognised as the most complex and challenging to treat. A recent biotechnological development with promising potential for addressing neurological disorders and stimulating neuro-enhancement concerns cerebral organoids, otherwise known as brain organoids. These comprise artificially grown clumps of cells grown in vitro and created by culturing pluripotent stem cells, adult stem cells (stem cells taken from specific tissues), or somatic cells derived from human tissue in a three-dimensional rotational bioreactor, ultimately resulting in something that looks like a miniature brain.[159] Brain organoids present a more accurate model for studying the brain compared to existing cellular and animal models.

While promising in their potential for better understanding brain development and disorders—including malignant primary tumours in the central nervous system such as glioblastoma; neurodegenerative diseases such as motor neuron disease, Parkinson's disease, and Alzheimer's disease; and neurodevelopmental disorders such as microcephaly

---

[155] Department of Health and Social Care, 'A Guide to Good Practice for Digital and Data-Driven Health Technologies' (2021) available at <https://www.gov.uk/government/publications/code-of-conduct-for-data-driven-health-and-care-technology/initial-code-of-conduct-for-data-driven-health-and-care-technology> accessed 07 November 2022. The guide is an update to the 'Code of Conduct for Data-Driven Health and Care Technologies', first developed in 2019.

[156] NHS Transformation Directorate, 'The National Strategy for AI in Health and Social Care' (2022) available at <https://transform.england.nhs.uk/ai-lab/ai-lab-programmes/the-national-strategy-for-ai-in-health-and-social-care/> accessed 07 November 2022.

[157] Department of Health and Social Care, 'Data Saves Lives: Reshaping Health and Social Care with Data' (June 2022) available at <https://www.gov.uk/government/publications/data-saves-lives-reshaping-health-and-social-care-with-data/data-saves-lives-reshaping-health-and-social-care-with-data> accessed 07 November 2022.

[158] ibid.

[159] Nan Sun et al., 'Applications of Brain Organoids in Neurodevelopment and Neurological Diseases' (2021) 28 Journal of Biomedical Science 30.

and neuroinflammation—research and innovation involving brain organoids present several regulatory and ethical dilemmas.[160] On the ethical front, two issues in particular come to the fore: (1) whether brain organoids created in vitro have any kinds of consciousness which should be morally considered, and (2) how non-human animals with human-like brain functions resulting from the transplantation of human brain organoids should be treated.[161] The former issue in particular has generated a good deal of scholarship, raising queries about whether brain organoids can develop capabilities similar to human sentience such that they acquire moral status.[162] On the legal front, Lavazza and Pizzetti present the following hypothetical:

> Consider a neurobiology laboratory where brain organoids are grown with all the characteristics listed above: as said, the goal of the research is to make them more and more similar to a typical human brain. Indeed, one may well think that a human cerebral organoid shares some relevant features with a human being and cannot be treated as simple lump of biological material. Now, imagine that a researcher questioned the ethical correctness of such practices, on grounds that the brains thus created might have a glimpse of sentience (understood as the minimal degree of consciousness, i.e. the ability to experience basic phenomenal states such as pain and other sensations related to physical homeostasis, such as lack of vital resources). This researcher, unable to raise the case inside the laboratory, could go to the local police department or directly to the relevant judicial authority and report the fact that destructive experiments are being carried out on quasi-brains grown in a dish from human tissues.[163]

While there is no law, national or international, that regulates brain organoids per se, research and innovation in this biotechnological domain throws up a series of legal questions about brain death, right to life, and personhood. We do not have space to dwell on the ethical and regulatory specifics here, but our own view is that basic research into brain organoids for bona fide health purposes (i.e. for diagnosis and treatments) ought to be permitted, provided it is conducted in accordance with existing ethical standards and oversight mechanisms. At the same time, we agree with calls for an ethical framework that sets more stringent research restrictions for advanced brain organoids than for organoids that cannot plausibly possess consciousness.[164] This would accord with emerging empirical research, including recent patient interviews in the USA regarding organoid research and use.[165]

6.10 NEW APPROACHES TO RESEARCH GOVERNANCE

The plethora of legal instruments and official guidance which has invaded the sphere of medical research sadly does little to improve the most important relationship in the entire research enterprise—namely, that between researcher and research participant. For the

[160] Andrea Lavazza and Frederico Pizzetti, 'Human Cerebral Organoids as a New Legal and Ethical Challenge' (2020) 7(1) Journal of Law and the Biosciences lsaa005.

[161] Tsutomu Sawai et al., 'The Ethics of Cerebral Organoid Research: Being Conscious of Consciousness' (2019) 13(3) Stem Cell Reports 440.

[162] Nita Farahany et al., 'The Ethics of Experimenting with Human Brain Tissue' (2018) 556(7702) Nature 429; Dide de Jongh et al., 'Organoids: A Systematic Review of Ethical Issues' (2022) 13 Stem Cell Research & Therapy 337.

[163] Lavazza and Pizzetti (n 160).

[164] Julian Koplin and Julian Savulescu, 'Moral Limits of Brain Organoid Research' (2019) 47(4) Journal of Law, Medicine & Ethics 760.

[165] Juli Bollinger et al., 'Patients' Perspectives on the Derivation and Use of Organoids' (2021) 16(8) Stem Cell Reports 1874.

researcher, the foregoing discussion must seem like a bureaucratic nightmare from which they can only hope to wake unaffected. For the participant, the net result of all this 'protection' may simply be that there is more paperwork to read and sign. But, as the complexities of conducting research have increased, so too has sensitivity to the related ethical and social issues been heightened. A major driver behind the establishment of the HRA was to deliver 'proportionate governance'.[166] And there are now examples of research endeavours which are not content simply to follow the prescribed regulatory path, but which rather seek to adopt a more streamlined approach, especially in times of public health emergency, as well as an approach that engages more directly and more fully with the ethical, legal, and social issues (ELSIs) at stake. Indeed, the past several years and since the Covid-19 pandemic have to led to a significant flurry of white papers, policy papers, and independent reports that all aim to streamline regulation and inject greater proportionality into the system without compromising patient and participant safety, rights, and interests. In addition, from the bottom up, several organisations aim to embed ELSI into their core work. Three examples illustrate these points.

Genomics England was established in 2013 as limited company set up and owned by the UK Department of Health and Social Care. From 2013 to 2018, it ran the 100,000 Genomes Project (genomic analysis remains ongoing), which aimed to sequence 100,000 genomes from around 85,000 NHS patients affected by rare disease or cancer to drive insights and continued findings into the role genomics can play in healthcare.[167] The Project is seen by many as exemplar in involving the public in genomic research, including through its use of embedded ELSI scholars, focus groups and interviews with stakeholders, a participant panel as advisory group,[168] ongoing information dissemination, and interactive consent materials.[169] Similar active patient and public engagement approaches are seen in its current projects, including a pilot for a Newborn Genomes Programme, which aims to evaluate the feasibility and impact on the NHS of offering whole-genome sequencing for all newborns,[170] as well as the Diverse Data Initiative, which aims to reduce health inequalities and improve patient outcomes within genomic medicine.

Another example can be seen from recent UK Government policy papers and independent reviews regarding 'trusted research environments' (TREs) and 'secure data environments' (SDEs) in which health data can be safely and secured analysed to help drive research discovery. In its policy paper from 2022, 'Data Saves Lives', the UK Government stressed that the beneficial use of NHS data was at the forefront of combatting Covid-19 and the need to keep 'this momentum going, and apply it to the long-term challenges ahead of us, including tackling the Covid backlog and making the reforms that are vital to the future of health and care'.[171] This included use of a TRE for Covid-19 during that pandemic, which gave researchers across health and care the ability to review data at speed, streamlining research processes for quicker results while maintaining confidentiality.[172] It demonstrates the value and potential of secure data environments. As part of the this, the Government is committing to establish secure data environments as the default route

---

[166] See Health Research Authority Regulations (SI 2011/2341) and Health Research Authority (Amendment) Regulations (SI 2012/1108).

[167] Genomics England, '100,000 Genomes Project' (2022) available at <https://www.genomicsengland.co.uk/initiatives/100000-genomes-project> accessed 07 November 2022.

[168] Genomics England, 'The Participant Panel' (2022) available at <https://www.genomicsengland.co.uk/patients-participants/participant-panel> accessed 07 November 2022.

[169] Jack Nunn et al, 'Public Involvement in Global Genomics Research: A Scoping Review' (2019) 7 Frontiers in Public Health 79.

[170] For this programme, a Newborns Ethics Working Group has also been established.

[171] Department of Health and Social Care, 'Data Saves Lives' (n 157).   [172] ibid.

for NHS and adult social care organisations to provide access to their de-identified data for research and analysis. As the policy paper outlines:

> Secure data environments – a subset of which are known as trusted research environments – are a big step forward in how data can be accessed securely in a virtual setting. Analysis takes place within a secure online platform rather than data being shared and distributed.
>
> In secure data environments, access to data is granted to authorised researchers in a controlled and recorded manner. This will put an end to the routine sharing and distribution of healthcare data for research purposes. Users' interactions with the data will be recorded and monitored, and the information they can extract will be assessed and with personal identifiers removed. As no data that can be linked to an individual leaves the server, and all access to the data and analysis is monitored, we will greatly reduce the risk of data breaches or other misuse.
>
> We will be mandating the use of secure data environments for NHS data, and engaging with the public, both to demonstrate their inherent benefits and to understand any remaining concerns.[173]

The adoption of TREs was endorsed in the 2022 'Goldacre Review' led by Professor Ben Goldacre, and are seen by many as a best practice approach to data-driven research that protects the safety of the public's confidential data, while allowing professionals appropriate and proportionate access for research.[174]

A final set of examples comes from the Covid-19 pandemic. Multiple governance pathways were streamlined for research and innovation purposes during the pandemic; it remains to be seen the extent to which this becomes embedded practice or viewed as an emergency one-off exception to established rules and practices.

For example, in England, NHSX and NHS England (the two bodies have since merged) established the 'NHS COVID-19 Data Store', which brought together multiple data sources from across the health and care system in England into a single, secure location. As part of this, the UK Government used the Health Service (Control of Patient Information) Regulations 2002 (known as the 'COPI Regulations'; see Chapter 11) to issue time-limited notices requiring public sector organisations to share patient information to support the Covid-19 response. The Government has committed in the 'Data Saves Lives' policy paper to amending the 2002 COPI regulations 'in due course to facilitate timely and proportionate sharing of data—including, where necessary and appropriate, personal information—for the purposes of supporting the health and care system.' Whether this means establishing further exceptions to the common law duty of confidentiality, including in non-pandemic contexts, remains to be seen.[175]

As another example, the HRA and MHRA both streamlined their approval processes for clinical trials regarding vaccines and treatments for Covid-19, and the UK has been seen as a world leader here, becoming the first country in the world to approve any Covid-19 vaccine and the first country to approve a dual-strain vaccine specific to the Omicron variant that emerged in late 2021.[176] Specifically, the HRA and the devolved

---

[173] ibid.

[174] Ben Goldacre et al., 'Better, Broader, Safer: Using Health Data for Research and Analysis' (2022) available at <https://www.gov.uk/government/publications/better-broader-safer-using-health-data-for-research-and-analysis> accessed 07 November 2022.

[175] Department of Health and Social Care, 'Data Saves Lives' (n 157).

[176] James Gallagher, 'Covid: UK First Country to Approve Dual-Strain Vaccine' (BBC News, 15 August 2022) available at <https://www.bbc.com/news/health-62548336> accessed 07 November 2022; Rachel Elbaum and Alexander Smith, 'U.K. Becomes First Country to Approve Pfizer-BioNTech Covid-19 Vaccine' (NBC News, 2 December 2020) available at <https://www.nbcnews.com/news/world/u-k-becomes-first-country-approve-pfizer-biontech-covid-19-n1249651> accessed 07 November 2022.

administrations developed a fast-track process to review new studies for certain types of Covid-19 research studies and more broadly now, 'urgent public health reasons', used for Covid-19 studies, monkeypox, and studies affected by the war in Ukraine. It is claimed that reviews can be undertaken in as little as 48 hours.[177] The HRA liaises with the MHRA to ensure that the latter can expedite the review of the CTIMP. The HRA has also established a 'fast-track research ethics review' process, which became fully mainstreamed from August 2022. Researchers are able to request a fast-track research ethics review with one of the NHS RECs for global clinical and phase I trials for any disease area, and which is stated to be 'quicker than our usual review time'.[178] Moreover, a multi-agency initiative called 'RAPID C-19', and involving all four nations, was established to get treatments for Covid-19 to NHS patients quickly and safely; to date, as a result of the initiative, the NHS has given patients rapid access to nine different drugs to treat Covid-19. Its role in reviewing potential COVID-19 treatments is to be wound down in 2023 as NICE and other organisations move back to routine commissioning arrangements for Covid-19 treatments.[179]

For its part, in 2021 the MHRA established a 'Innovative Licensing and Access Pathway' (ILAP), which aims to accelerate the time to market of medicines, which include new chemical entities, biological medicines, new indications, and repurposed medicines. It comprises an Innovation Passport designation, a Target Development Profile, and provides applicants with access to a toolkit to support all stages of the design, development, and approvals process.[180] ILAP has been viewed as a successful way to fast-track approve medicines during the pandemic and build on tools the MHRA developing during Covid-19 clinical trials, including the Rapid Clinical Trial Dossier Pre-assessment tool and the Novel Methodology and innovative clinical trial design tool.[181]

Finally, it is worth reiterating that the clinical trials regulatory landscape as a whole is undergoing reform in the UK with the proposed legislative reform of the existing 2004 Regulations and which seeks to pivot away from EU regulatory frameworks,[182] and the reform ought to be situated with yet another recent policy, this one entitled 'Saving and Improving Lives: The Future of UK Clinical Research Delivery', endorsed

---

[177] Health Research Authority, 'Public Health Emergency Research' (2022) available at <https://www.hra.nhs.uk/planning-and-improving-research/policies-standards-legislation/public-health-emergency-research/> and 'COVID-19 Research' (2022) available at <https://www.hra.nhs.uk/covid-19-research/> accessed 07 November 2022.

[178] Health Research Authority, 'Fast-Track Research Ethics Review' (2022) available at <https://www.hra.nhs.uk/approvals-amendments/what-approvals-do-i-need/research-ethics-committee-review/fast-track-research-ethics-review-pilot/> accessed 07 November 2022.

[179] NICE, 'Research to Access Pathway for Investigational Drugs for COVID-19 (RAPID C-19)' (2022) available at <https://www.nice.org.uk/covid-19/rapid-c19> accessed 07 November 2022.

[180] Medicines and Healthcare products Regulatory Agency, 'Innovative Licensing and Access Pathway' (2022) available at <https://www.gov.uk/guidance/innovative-licensing-and-access-pathway> accessed 07 November 2022.

[181] Gail Francis et al., 'Regulators' Experience of Clinical Trials During the Covid-19 Pandemic (Part 3)—Looking Forward' (2022) available at <https://mhrainspectorate.blog.gov.uk/2022/02/18/regulators-experience-of-clinical-trials-during-the-covid-19-pandemic-part-3-looking-forward/> accessed 07 November 2022. See also Medicines and Healthcare products Regulatory Agency, 'MHRA Guidance on Coronavirus (COVID-19)' (2022) available at <https://www.gov.uk/government/collections/mhra-guidance-on-coronavirus-covid-19> accessed 07 November 2022.

[182] MHRA, 'Consultation on Proposals for Legislative Changes for Clinical Trials' (n 10).

by all four nations' health departments, and which sets out the 'UK vision to unleash the full potential of clinical research delivery to tackle health inequalities, bolster economic recovery and to improve the lives of people across the UK'.[183]

6.11 CONCLUSION

As noted in *Richmond Pharmacology Ltd* v *Health Research Authority*,[184] health research and innovation are governed by a 'complex web of regulatory provisions [from] EU Directives and domestic legislation', and while this case pre-dated Brexit, there is little reason to think the post-Brexit health research regulatory environment will be 'un-webbed' and streamlined to such a degree as we witnessed for some of the research undertaken during the Covid-19 pandemic. Moreover, significant regulatory divergence from the EU will only drive up transaction costs for multinational pharmaceutical companies, technology companies developing AI, and other organisations that conduct research at sites across the globe; many of these organisations prefer regulatory harmonisation to regulatory divergence, even if it means 'more efficient' processes in one jurisdiction compared to another.

This said, recent and ongoing efforts to reform the setting are attempting to create a more holistic framework that is more closely aligned to the concepts of proportionality, engagement, accountability, and transparency such that responsible research and innovation can be encouraged; undoubtedly, more work remains to be done, particularly in areas at the cutting edge, such as germline gene editing and brain organoids, where risks and ethical issues have only begun to be charted. Regulators have not yet succeeded, but nor can they be chastised for failing. The HRA was criticised in *Richmond Pharmacology* for supplying to users, via its website, material that is 'so ambiguous as to the expression of its scope as to mislead'.[185] A 2018 House of Commons Science and Technology Committee report on clinical trials transparency[186] expressed disappointment that half of clinical trials in the UK remain unreported (including those sponsored by Public Health England) and that the HRA has not effected significant change despite being explicitly responsible for 'promoting research transparency' as part of its statutory objectives since 2014. The report noted that there are currently no sanctions imposed on sponsors or investigators who fail to comply with HRA rules, or even on those who fail to respond to the HRA when their non-compliance is queried. The report recommended the HRA should introduce a system of sanctions to drive improvements in clinical trials transparency, such as withdrawing a favourable ethics opinion or preventing further trials from taking place, and also recommended that the Government consult specifically on whether to provide the HRA with the statutory power to fine sponsors for non-compliance.

The HRA and other health research regulators have made improvements in the past few years, in large part spurred on by the Covid-19 pandemic and nudges from government

---

[183] Department of Health and Social Care, The Executive Office (Northern Ireland), The Scottish Government, and Welsh Government, 'Saving and Improving Lives: The Future of UK Clinical Research Delivery' (March 2021) available at <https://www.gov.uk/government/publications/the-future-of-uk-clinical-research-delivery/saving-and-improving-lives-the-future-of-uk-clinical-research-delivery> accessed 07 November 2022.

[184] [2015] EWHC 2283 (Admin).   [185] ibid. [86].

[186] House of Commons Science and Technology Committee, 'Research Integrity: Clinical Trials Transparency' (2018) available at <https://publications.parliament.uk/pa/cm201719/cmselect/cmsctech/1480/148007.htm> accessed 07 November 2022.

to facilitate research discovery and innovation. Such improvements cannot only be top-down, however, nor broadly accepted by society in the absence of their support. Thus, if further reform in the areas of engagement, accountability, and transparency can be achieved, it will not only assist researchers but also better protect and promote the interests of society *qua* potential research participants. Efforts continue to make the UK 'a great place to do health research, to build confidence and participation in health research, and so improve the nation's health'.[187]

FURTHER READING

1. Edward Dove, *Regulatory Stewardship of Health Research: Navigating Participant Protection and Research Promotion* (Edward Elgar 2020).

2. Peter Feldschreiber, *The Law and Regulation of Medicines and Medical Devices* (2nd edn, OUP 2022).

3. Rhiannon Frowde, Edward Dove, and Graeme Laurie, 'Reconciling Fragmented Sectors of Health Research Regulation: Toward an Ecosystem of Processual Regulation' (2022) 11(9) Humanities and Social Sciences Communications 11.

4. Isabel Fletcher et al., 'Co-production and Managing Uncertainty in Health Research Regulation: A Delphi Study' (2020) 28(2) Health Care Analysis 99.

5. Graeme Laurie et al., *Cambridge Handbook of Health Research Regulation* (CUP 2021).

6. Nuffield Council on Bioethics, 'Genome Editing: An Ethical Review' (Nuffield Council on Bioethics 2016).

---

[187] Health Research Authority, 'About Us' (2022) available at <https://www.hra.nhs.uk/about-us/> accessed 07 November 2022.

7

PUBLIC HEALTH

7.1 INTRODUCTION

As we illustrated in Chapter 3, medical practice encompasses more than a simple, private doctor–patient relationship and a relationship between a patient and any healthcare professional that attends to their clinical needs. Not only is our experience of medicine now more of an encounter with a system (e.g. a GP surgery with a number of doctors and allied health professionals, one or more hospital visits at different sites) than a one-on-one, enduring relationship with one professional across our lifespan, we also come to experience health and medicine through its larger community-orientated functions. We and the state have a collective interest in the well-being of individuals and communities, and we both have obligations to protect and promote this. The state, in particular, has a basic duty, grounded in the social contract and the demands of the human rights regime, to protect its citizens from harm. From a health perspective, this means protecting individuals and communities from the ravages of disease, both communicable and non-communicable.[1] As such, the health profession, together with a range of public bodies, must be heavily involved in what can be termed 'public health'.

This public role nuances the health professional's private relationships, necessitating a consideration of how our concepts of medical ethics are altered when engaged in public health supporting measures,[2] which tend to fall into two overlapping categories: health promotion and health protection (or disease control and prevention). We have touched on this already in Chapter 1's discussion of public health ethics. There is much that we can do to promote our own health for the sake of ourselves and others: we can eat healthily, exercise, avoid tobacco, and be sparing in our consumption of alcohol. We must also acknowledge, however, structural limitations that can make this a challenge for many people in the UK due to the social determinants of health, such as the cost-of-living crisis, lack of access to affordable housing and healthy foods, and absence of free time to exercise; moreover, a healthy lifestyle can only help so much in the face of a highly transmissible, airborne communicable disease such as SARS-CoV-2. When our state of health slips out of our control, or if it becomes a threat to others, then personal action can be superseded

---

[1] Communicable disease is a disease spread from one person to another or from an animal to a person. All communicable diseases are infectious, yet not all infectious diseases are communicable: some infectious diseases may not spread to other people (e.g. tetanus). Non-communicable disease is a disease not transmitted through contact with an infected or afflicted person; it is instead caused by various genetic, physiological, environmental, and behavioural factors. Non-communicable diseases include cancer, cardiovascular diseases, chronic respiratory diseases, and diabetes.

[2] See generally Nuffield Council on Bioethics, 'Public Health: Ethical Issues' (2007) available at <https://www.nuffieldbioethics.org/publications/public-health> accessed 08 November 2022; John Coggon, *What Makes Health Public? A Critical Evaluation of Moral, Legal, and Political Claims in Public* Health (CUP 2012); John Coggon, Keith Syrett, and Adrien Viens, *Public Health Law: Ethics, Governance, and Regulation* (Routledge 2016).

or supplemented by the need for government action aimed at protecting the community, even when this entails inference with our individual rights. The important relationship in public health, then, is less that of doctor and patient than that of citizen and state, and the many actors in between.

The role of law and policy in public health is to police the boundaries of these relationships, and to ensure that reasonable justifications for state actions that encroach on individual rights are offered and are well founded—a function that is complicated by the fact that threats to public health can appear quickly and with potentially devastating regional and global effects. For example, the outbreaks of H1N1 influenza in Mexico in 2009,[3] Ebola in West Africa in 2014, Zika in the Americas in 2015–16, the Kivu Ebola epidemic in 2018–20, Covid-19 globally since early 2020, and monkeypox globally since mid-2022, have been declared 'public health emergencies of international concern' (PHEICs) by the World Health Organization (WHO), with coordinated efforts following therefrom.[4] The importance of legal preparedness, therefore, cannot be overstated, and action is required at each of the national, regional, and international levels.

This chapter focuses in particular on the issues of public health law within the UK. Public health law is subject to multiple meanings, but we define it broadly as the corpus of laws, regulations, and polices designed to identify and address the health of populations. Coggon, Syrett, and Viens similarly define public health law as 'a field of study and practice that concerns those aspects of law, policy, and regulation that advance or place constraints upon the protection and promotion of health (howsoever understood) within, between, and across populations'.[5] We can contrast public health law, which has a more national or country-specific orientation, with global health law, which Gostin and Taylor define as:

> a field that encompasses the legal norms, processes, and institutions needed to create the conditions for people throughout the world to attain the highest possible level of physical and mental health. The field seeks to facilitate health-promoting behaviour among the key actors that significantly influence the public's health, including international organizations, governments, businesses, foundations, the media, and civil society. The mechanisms of global health law should stimulate investment in research and development, mobilize resources, set priorities, coordinate activities, monitor progress, create incentives, and enforce standards. Study and practice of the field should be guided by the overarching value of social justice, which requires equitable distribution of health services, particularly to benefit the world's poorest populations.[6]

Much of public health law necessarily has a normative focus, actively seeking to protect health at a broad population level, rather than at an individual, clinical level, and emphasising health protection and promotion rather than treatment of disease. This does not mean, however, that public health law is always designed in ways we would

---

[3] On 11 June 2009, the WHO declared H1N1 to be the first influenza pandemic in 41 years.

[4] A 'public health emergency of international concern' (PHEIC) is a legal term defined in the WHO's International Health Regulations 2005 as 'an extraordinary event which is determined to constitute a public health risk to other States through the international spread of disease and to potentially require a coordinated international response'. This definition implies a situation that is: serious, sudden, unusual, or unexpected; carries implications for public health beyond the affected state's national border; and may require immediate international action.

[5] Coggon, Syrett, and Viens (n 2), p. 17.

[6] Lawrence Gostin and Allyn Taylor, 'Global Health Law: A Definition and Grand Challenges' (2008) 1(1) Public Health Ethics 53.

normatively label 'good'; laws in this field may well be misguided and have negative consequences for population health, including laws that may exacerbate stigma and existing vulnerabilities.

We begin our discussion with the most serious public health event the UK has faced since the 1918 influenza pandemic—Covid-19—and the numerous legal and regulatory responses that emerged in the days, weeks, and months following its emergence, and the controversies these have engendered.

7.2 COVID-19: UK PUBLIC HEALTH UNDER THREAT

The coronavirus disease 2019 (Covid-19) pandemic is, as of the time of writing this edition, an ongoing global crisis caused by the SARS-CoV-2 virus (severe acute respiratory syndrome coronavirus 2), itself a variation of the SARS-CoV-1 virus that caused global havoc from 2002–04.[7] Covid-19 was first formally identified in December 2019 in Wuhan, China; declared a PHEIC by the WHO on 30 January 2020; and then declared a pandemic on 11 March 2020.[8] As of the time of writing, the global death toll approached 7 million people[9] (by some estimates, it is significantly higher in the tens of millions[10]). In the UK, it is estimated that over 225,000 people have died;[11] no doubt, as the disease is expected to become endemic, the number will continue to climb between this edition of the textbook and the next.[12] Following the WHO declaration of a pandemic, governments around the world responded in a variety of ways, and to varying degrees of success, to protect their populations and stop the spread of the virus, which has proved, over the years, to be significantly challenging given its highly transmissible airborne nature.

7.2.1 LEGAL AND REGULATORY PREPAREDNESS AND RESPONSES

Given the UK's geographic position and London's global interconnectedness, it is unsurprising that Covid-19 hit the country with force beginning in March 2020, even if it was likely circulating across the country in the few months prior to widespread diagnostic

---

[7] Communicable diseases have varying rates of transmissibility and case fatality; some may be low-incidence, high-consequence pathogens; others may be high-incidence, low-consequence pathogens. SARS-CoV-1 was less transmissible than SARS-CoV-2 but had a higher case fatality rate; about 9% of all patients with confirmed SARS-CoV-1 infection died and with a significantly higher rate among the elderly. (The related respiratory virus of MERS-CoV has an even higher case fatality rate of around 34% but is not highly transmissible.) SARS-CoV-2 is highly transmissible and appears to have a case fatality rate of around 1% among all people infected with the virus. It is estimated that seasonal flu has a case fatality rate of approximately 0.1% to 0.2%. See Yousef Alimohamadi et al., 'Case Fatality Rate of COVID-19: A Systematic Review and Meta-Analysis' (2021) 62(2) Journal of Preventive Medicine and Hygiene E311.

[8] WHO, 'WHO Director-General's opening remarks at the media briefing on COVID-19 – 11 March 2020' (2020) available at <https://www.who.int/director-general/speeches/detail/who-director-general-s-opening-remarks-at-the-media-briefing-on-covid-19---11-march-2020> accessed 08 November 2022.

[9] Our World in Data, 'Coronavirus Pandemic (COVID-19)' (2023) available at <https://ourworldindata.org/coronavirus> accessed 14 January 2023.

[10] The Economist, 'Tracking Covid-19 Excess Deaths Across Countries' (2021) available at <https://www.economist.com/graphic-detail/coronavirus-excess-deaths-tracker> accessed 14 January 2023.

[11] UK Government, 'UK Coronavirus Dashboard' (2023) available at <https://coronavirus.data.gov.uk/details/deaths> accessed 14 January 2023.

[12] Our World in Data, (n 9).

testing. Yet national pandemic preparedness was underwhelming, as was the initial response of 'locking down' early on and curbing major superspreading events such as a Six Nations Rugby match, the Cheltenham Festival, and a Liverpool vs Atlético Madrid football match, where in each, tens of thousands of people attended and spread the virus. As some of us have noted elsewhere,[13] the UK did have a pandemic response plan in place—but this was much more evident on paper than in reality. It had been known for some time that the UK faced limitations of preparedness for a highly transmissible airborne virus such as influenza or SARS. For example, significant weaknesses in the UK's emergency preparedness, resilience, and response (EPRR) plan were highlighted in 2016, yet no significant remedial steps were taken before the advent of Covid-19.[14] The simulation exercise carried out by NHS England in October 2016, 'Exercise Cygnus', was conducted under the auspices of Public Health England and modelled an influenza pandemic; the leaked report showed that the exercise found that the NHS in England would collapse from a lack of resources and that a shortage of ventilators and capacity for disposal of the deceased would present serious challenges. The NHS's surge capacity was shown to be of serious concern, with a shortage of personal protective equipment (PPE) and ICU beds. Much of this, as is now well known, came to fruition in the UK during the first few months of the pandemic, and early Government missteps and delays likely contributed to a significant number of casualties. We suspect, too, that the devolution of public health responsibilities to Scotland, Northern Ireland, and Wales had not been stress-tested prior to Covid-19, and this may have contributed to early confusion about the scope of responsibilities between the UK Government and Westminster, and the devolved administrations across the three nations. Whatever the underlying contributing factors were, it has been recognised by many observers that the UK's initial response to the pandemic was poor. It also severely strained the health service: for much of 2020, the health services across the four nations were at their breaking point and many healthcare professionals lacked the resources needed to adequately treat the number of seriously ill patients. Special triage guidelines were developed to help clinicians determine who to treat first and under what conditions.[15]

After some delay, the state eventually spang into action. As responsibility for legal and practical responses to health, including matters of public health and health protection, is a devolved matter, the Coronavirus Act 2020,[16] which quickly entered into effect in March 2020, conferred powers to take emergency action in response to the pandemic to the UK Government and to the devolved administrations. For example, the Act enabled

---

[13] Rhiannon Frowde, Edward Dove, and Graeme Laurie, 'Fail to Prepare and you Prepare to Fail: The Human Rights Consequences of the UK Government's Inaction During the COVID-19 Pandemic' (2020) 12(4) Asian Bioethics Review 459.

[14] Paul Nuki and Bill Gardner, 'Exercise Cygnus Uncovered: The Pandemic Warnings Buried by the Government' *The Telegraph* (28 March 2020) available at <https://www.telegraph.co.uk/news/2020/03/28/exercise-cygnus-uncovered-pandemic-warnings-buried-government/> accessed 08 November 2022.

[15] See e.g. Scottish Government, 'Coronavirus (COVID-19): Guidance on Critical Care Management of Adult Patients' (2021) available at <https://www.gov.scot/collections/coronavirus-covid-19-guidance/> accessed 08 November 2022; Scottish Government, 'COVID-19 Guidance: Clinical Advice' (2020) available at <https://www.gov.scot/collections/coronavirus-covid-19-clinical-guidance-for-health-professionals/> accessed 08 November 2022.

[16] It should be noted that numerous statutory instruments were passed dealing with a variety of matters, including restrictions on travel and movement. These included The Health Protection (Coronavirus, Restrictions) (England) Regulations 2020 (SI 2020/350) and The Health Protection (Coronavirus, Restrictions) (No. 2) (England) Regulations 2020 (SI 2020/684), which were made under the Public Health (Control of Disease) Act 1984 rather than the Coronavirus Act 2020. Similar statutory instruments were passed in Scotland, Wales, and Northern Ireland.

discretionary powers to limit or suspend public gatherings, to detain individuals suspected to be infected by Covid-19, and to increase the available health and social care
workforce (including by way of bringing back recently retired individuals, and streamlining the process for foreign training health and care workers to practice in the country).
The UK Government recognised the measures as 'extraordinary', meaning they would
not apply in normal circumstances. For this reason, the legislation was time-limited to
two years, and indeed the Act was formally repealed in March 2022, although several provisions were revoked early in July 2021 and others were extended for six months beyond
the two-year period. We discuss later in this chapter the Civil Contingencies Act 2004,
which makes provision about civil contingencies, including epidemics. There was some
debate as to why the UK Government did not rely on its existing provisions; it appears
the Government was concerned about legal challenges to its invocation, as it is designed
to address sudden, unanticipated events rather than the gradual onset of an epidemic or
pandemic. Several scholars have questioned this interpretation of the Act.[17]

For its part, the Scottish Government passed the Coronavirus (Scotland) Act 2020 in
April 2020 and the Coronavirus (Scotland) (No. 2) Act 2020 in May 2020 to regulate
the devolved response to Covid-19, which in particular made adjustments to the law on
evictions to protect those renting their homes during the outbreak; made adjustments
to criminal procedure, and to other aspects of the justice system, to ensure that essential
justice business could continue to be disposed of throughout the outbreak; and made a
range of provision designed to ensure that business and public services could continue
to operate effectively. As of the time of writing, the Coronavirus (Scotland) Act 2020 and
Coronavirus (Scotland) (No. 2) Act 2020 are no longer in effect.[18]

In June 2022, the Scottish Parliament passed the Coronavirus (Recovery and Reform)
(Scotland) Act 2022, which seeks to help Scotland recover from the pandemic and ensure
greater resilience against future public health threats. Among other things, it effects
changes in 35 specific legislative areas, many of which originated in the temporary
Scottish and UK Covid-19 legislation, and includes reforms related to permanent public
health protection powers under the Public Health Etc. (Scotland) Act 2008, similar to
those which already exist in England and Wales, increased protection for private rented
tenants facing evictions, and a temporary extension of some changes in the justice system
to help manage the backlog of court cases arising from the pandemic.

7.2.2 SOCIAL AND POLITICAL EFFECTS

The aforementioned legal and regulatory responses have generated several social and
political effects, not to mention ethical and legal concerns, and the UK has been no outlier here. As in many other countries, a significant segment of the population expressed
alarm, some with respect to the perceived slow and chaotic response to the pandemic,
and others with respect to the perceived disproportionate curtailment of personal liberty during the pandemic,[19] including ongoing lockdowns that closed almost all public

[17] House of Commons Public Administration and Constitutional Affairs Committee, 'Parliamentary
Scrutiny of the Government's handling of Covid-19, Fourth Report of Session 2019–21' (10 September 2020)
available at <https://committees.parliament.uk/publications/2459/documents/24384/default/> accessed
08 November 2022.
[18] For more information, see Scottish Government 'Coronavirus (COVID-19) legislation' (2022) available at <https://www.gov.scot/collections/coronavirus-covid-19-legislation/> accessed 08 November 2022.
[19] Under the European Convention on Human Rights, individuals enjoy a right to liberty under Art 5.
However, states can impose measures to detain persons for the prevention of the spreading of infectious diseases.

services and shops and restricted travel outside one's home or council area. Concern was also raised about rules governing one's conduct to help protect others from SARS-CoV-2 infection, specifically through covering one's nose and mouth with a face covering. Lord Sumption, a former Justice of the Supreme Court, was a prominent critic of Covid-19 restrictions regulations in the UK,[20] as were several backbench Conservative Party Members of Parliament, who feared then-Prime Minister Boris Johnson went too far with the restrictions and for too long. Lockdown and anti-mask protests sprung up across the UK during 2020 and 2021, at the height of the pandemic, although it is debatable the extent to which they had any impact on the application of the existing or newly creating public health laws.

Of greater concern, in our view, than sporadic protests against perceived infringements against personal liberty, has been the disproportionate impact of the pandemic on those most vulnerable in UK society. The UK is not an outlier here, either—sadly this has been seen across multiple countries[21]—but it is worth emphasising that numerous empirical studies have shown that ethnic minority healthcare workers[22] and society more generally in this country have felt the brunt of pandemic more severely than others, not just directly through exposure to the virus itself, but also indirectly in terms of lost employment, eviction, and access to public services.[23] In the midst of longer-term, macrostructural economic challenges (in part due to Brexit, in part due to global events), we fear that this will only lead to widening gaps of inequality in our society and long-term health consequences that may take years to overcome through public health law and structural reforms.

In 2021, Prime Minister Boris Johnson agreed to a public inquiry into the pandemic, focusing on the UK Government's handling of the crisis.[24] After some delay, it is now expected that the inquiry will start taking full evidence in 2023; yet even before it began, inquiry costs already exceeded £85 million and it is expected to become the most expensive in British history, exceeding the Bloody Sunday Inquiry of 2000–10.[25] It may well be

---

[20] Jonathan Sumption, 'You Cannot Imprison an Entire Population' *The Spectator* (17 May 2020) available at <https://www.spectator.co.uk/article/jonathan-sumption-you-cannot-imprison-an-entire-population-> accessed 08 November 2022; Jonathan Sumption, 'We Are so Afraid of Death, No One Even Asks Whether This "Cure" is Actually Worse' *The Sunday Times* (05 April 2020) available at <https://www.thetimes.co.uk/article/coronavirus-lockdown-we-are-so-afraid-of-death-no-one-even-asks-whether-this-cure-is-actually-worse-3t97k66vj> accessed 08 November 2022.

[21] See e.g. Gunagxiao Hu et al., 'Assessing Inequities Underlying Racial Disparities of COVID-19 Mortality in Louisiana Parishes' (2022) 119(27) Proceedings of the National Academy of Sciences e2123533119; Lydia Navarro-Román and Gustavo Román, 'The Devastating Effects of the COVID-19 Pandemic Among Ethnic Minorities, Migrants, and Refugees', in Mustapha El Alaoui-Faris, Antonio Federico, Wolfgang Grisold (eds.), *Neurology in Migrants and Refugees* (Springer 2021) 153–163.

[22] Christopher Martin et al., 'Risk Factors Associated with SARS-CoV-2 Infection in a Multiethnic Cohort of United Kingdom Healthcare Workers (UK-REACH): A Cross-Sectional Analysis' (2022) 19(5) PLoS Medicine e1004015.

[23] Daniel Morales and Sarah Ali, 'COVID-19 and Disparities Affecting Ethnic Minorities' (2021) 397(10286) The Lancet P1684; Kirti Chaudhuri et al., 'How Susceptible is the Black and Ethnic Minority (BAME)? An Analysis of COVID-19 Mortality Pattern in England' in Mousumi Dutta, Zakir Husain, and Anup Sinha (eds.), *The Impact of COVID-19 on India and the Global Order: A Multidisciplinary Approach* (Springer 2022) 151–167.

[24] Robert Booth, 'Johnson Says Public Inquiry into Covid will Begin This Parliament' *The Guardian* (11 May 2021) available at <https://www.theguardian.com/world/2021/may/11/boris-johnson-public-inquiry-into-covid-begin-this-parliament> accessed 08 November 2022.

[25] Emilio Casalicchio, 'UK COVID Inquiry Bill Tops £85M Before Hearings Begin' *Politico* (20 August 2022) available at <https://www.politico.eu/article/uk-covid-inquiry-bill-tops-85m-before-hearings-begin/> accessed 08 November 2022.

years before the inquiry releases its report and a thorough accounting of what went wrong and what went right is laid bare before the public.

Despite this less-than-rosy portrayal of the UK's response to the pandemic, we now turn to discuss more a positive development and an example of some success, namely the development and distribution of vaccines to protect against Covid-19, as well as the nature of vaccination law and policy in the UK more generally.

7.3 VACCINATION

A powerful tool in the state's arsenal to protect and promote population health is vacci-nation, both of animals (e.g. to protect against foot-and-mouth disease) and of humans. The goal of vaccination is not only to protect an individual against harm from a spe-cific disease but also to achieve 'herd immunity'. If a large proportion of the population have immunity to or significant protection against a particular disease, those people are unlikely to contribute to its transmission and chains of infection are more likely to be disrupted. This in turn slows, stops, or even eradicates the disease, thereby providing 'herd immunity' (or indirect protection) to those who are not immune. The more infec-tious a disease, the greater the population immunity needed to ensure herd immunity.[26] Measles, for example, is highly contagious and one person with measles can infect up to 18 other people, thus requiring that around 95% of people need to be immune in order for the wider group to have herd immunity.[27] Vaccine hesitancy, both among parents of child and adults themselves, can significantly affect the ability of a country to achieve herd immunity to a given disease.

7.3.1 COVID-19 VACCINES

While the UK has been roundly criticised for its initially slow response to the pandemic in March 2020, it has been generally praised for its swift fast-tracking of multiple vac-cines against Covid-19 through streamlined regulatory approvals, which is discussed in Chapter 6. Indeed, the UK was the first country in the world to provide emergency use authorisation for a safe, effective Covid-19 vaccine, namely the Pfizer-BioNTech vaccine, which was granted on 2 December 2020, only seven months after the start of clinical trials.[28] On 8 December 2020, Margaret Keenan became the first person in the world to be given the vaccination as part of a mass vaccination programme;[29] there-after, the UK executed what many consider to be an efficiently run mass vaccination programme due to the NHS's logistical strengths in reaching local communities. Over the course of 2021 and 2022, the UK approved five vaccines for use: Pfizer-BioNTech,

---

[26] For more information, see the excellent report from the House of Commons Library: Elizabeth Rough, 'UK Vaccination Policy: Research Briefing' (2022) available at <https://researchbriefings.files.parliament. uk/documents/CBP-9076/CBP-9076.pdf> accessed 08 November 2022.

[27] Priya Joi, 'What is Herd Immunity?' (2020) available at <https://www.gavi.org/vaccineswork/what-herd-immunity> accessed 08 November 2022.

[28] We note that China and Russia had already approved their own Covid-19 vaccines prior to December 2020, but neither waited for the immunisations to complete the final round of tests in people before granting approval.

[29] BBC News, 'Covid-19 Vaccine: First Person Receives Pfizer Jab in UK' (8 December 2020) available at <https://www.bbc.com/news/uk-55227325> accessed 08 November 2022.

Oxford-AstraZeneca, Moderna, Janssen and Novavax, four of which require two doses for maximum protection. The UK was the first major European economy and first G20 member to vaccinate 50% of its population with at least one dose, and to provide boosters to 50% of the population.[30] Subsequently, the UK has become one of the more Covid-19 vaccinated countries in the world[31] and more recently in 2022, approved a bivalent Moderna vaccine (Spikevax) that targets both the original strain and the first Omicron variant (BA.1), which emerged in 2021.[32]

Much of the success story regarding the development and roll-out of vaccines can be seen as a reflection of the UK Government's belief that vaccines are the first line of defence against a virus that we must learn to 'live with' for some time. In its 2022 guidance, for example, the Cabinet Office wrote:

> Vaccines have enabled the gradual and safe removal of restrictions on everyday life over the past year, and will remain at the heart of the Government's approach to living with the virus in the future.
>
> . . .
>
> The Government expects that the population's defences against new variants will continue to strengthen as immunity increases through advances in vaccine technology and repeated exposure to the virus.[33]

This also reflects, we noted in Chapter 6, a more general post-Brexit push for a streamlined regulatory environment for clinical trials and life sciences research, making the UK an attractive environment in which to conduct ground-breaking research that leads to further scientific and medical breakthroughs, in both public health and in biomedicine. The UK Government has in particular spotlighted its support of the life sciences industry in the UK to develop vaccines, such as the AstraZeneca Covid-19 vaccine, which was developed with the University of Oxford and which also first received regulatory approval for emergency use authorisation in the UK. The UK Government has invested hundreds of millions of pounds for UK life sciences manufacturing as part of the 'Global Britain Investment Fund' to support investment into the UK economy, while the Vaccine Taskforce, set up in April 2020 to drive forward the development, procurement, and production of a Covid-19 vaccine as quickly as possible, has invested in facilities at the UK Health Security Agency's Porton Down site to increase the UK's capacity to test the efficacy of vaccines against emerging variants.[34]

The Joint Committee on Vaccination and Immunisation (JCVI),[35] an independent expert advisory committee first established in 1963, has played a key role in providing advice to governments on deploying vaccinations. The JCVI has advised on, inter alia, the decision to offer vaccination to all 5–11-year-olds and further vaccinations (boosters)

---

[30] Cabinet Office, 'COVID-19 Response: Living with COVID-19' (2022) available at <https://www.gov.uk/government/publications/covid-19-response-living-with-covid-19/covid-19-response-living-with-covid-19> accessed 08 November 2022.

[31] As of the time of writing, it is estimated that 88% of the over-12 UK population is fully vaccinated. See Office of National Statistics, 'Coronavirus (COVID-19)' (2022) available at <https://www.ons.gov.uk/peoplepopulationandcommunity/healthandsocialcare/conditionsanddiseases> accessed 14 January 2023.

[32] James Gallagher, 'Covid: UK First Country to Approve Dual-Strain Vaccine' (BBC News, 16 August 2022) available at <https://www.bbc.com/news/health-62548336> accessed 08 November 2022.

[33] Cabinet Office (n 30).   [34] ibid.

[35] UK Government, 'Joint Committee on Vaccination and Immunisation' (2022) available at <https://www.gov.uk/government/groups/joint-committee-on-vaccination-and-immunisation> accessed 08 November 2022.

for people who are most vulnerable to Covid-19. While the UK Government has stated that it has procured enough doses of vaccine to anticipate a wide range of possible JCVI recommendations, it remains to be seen whether further bivalent or multivalent vaccines and periodic boosters will be needed in the coming years. Regardless, we hope that one of the core lessons learnt from the Covid-19 pandemic is the need to implement a variety of long-term contingency plans, properly take up recommendations from planning exercises, and embed resilience to ensure adequate protection is in place to secure population health and to respond quickly in an emergency, particularly a highly transmissible communicable disease.

7.3.2 VACCINATION: MANDATORY VERSUS VOLUNTARY

Across Europe, countries take a different approach to vaccination. Some mandate vaccination for standard childhood immunisations, such as polio, mumps, pertussis, and tetanus (e.g. France, Italy, Poland, Czech Republic, Croatia), whereas others, including the UK, the Netherlands, Spain, and Austria, take a voluntary approach. The UK's current routine immunisation schedule provides protection against 14 infections, including measles, meningococcal disease, and polio. Most vaccinations are given during childhood but some are aimed at adults, such as vaccination against seasonal influenza, where those aged 65 years and older are eligible in the UK, and shingles, where those aged 70-79 years are eligible in the UK.[36]

Voluntary vaccination of adults is standard, and only in exceptional cases is mandatory vaccination implemented,[37] and always with controversy, given the concern about infringement of bodily integrity and autonomy interests. This was seen, for example, in the Covid-19 pandemic. Under public health legislation in the UK, governments are not empowered to implement health protection regulations that include provision requiring a person to undergo medical treatment, which includes vaccination and other prophylactic treatment.[38] This accords with fundamental principles of medical law and ethics, namely that an adult person, outside of limited exceptions, cannot be compelled to undergo medical treatment.

This said, indirect means of requiring vaccination are sometimes enacted. The UK Government passed the Health and Social Care Act 2008 (Regulated Activities) (Amendment) (Coronavirus) Regulations 2021, which required all people working in a care home, regardless of their role and the age of the residents, to be fully vaccinated against Covid-19 as a condition of employment. The Government then took steps to extend this to other social care workers and healthcare staff[39] under the Health and Social Care Act 2008 (Regulated Activities) (Amendment) (Coronavirus) (No. 2) Regulations 2022, with the mandatory vaccination requirement due to come into force 12 weeks after the regulations were made to allow time for employees to be vaccinated. However, after significant

[36] UK Health Security Agency, 'The Complete Routine Immunisation Schedule from February 2022' (2022) available at <https://www.gov.uk/government/publications/the-complete-routine-immunisation-schedule/the-complete-routine-immunisation-schedule-from-february-2022> accessed 08 November 2022.

[37] For example, Slovakia requires persons living in social care facilities and persons living or working in an area with increased risk of infection to be vaccinated against seasonal influenza.

[38] See e.g. Public Health (Control of Disease) Act 1984, s 45E.

[39] Department of Health and Social Care, 'Making Vaccination a Condition of Deployment in the Health and Wider Social Care Sector' (2021) available at <https://www.gov.uk/government/consultations/making-vaccination-a-condition-of-deployment-in-the-health-and-wider-social-care-sector> accessed 08 November 2022.

backlash from the health worker community, the plans were scrapped.[40] Even if there is no specific mandate for an individual to be vaccinated against Covid-19, many no doubt came to discover that freedom to travel internationally and access many services around the country and globally was *de facto* contingent on showing proof of vaccination (by means of a so-called 'vaccine passport', raising ethics and human rights concerns[41]), if not proof of a recently negative Covid-19 test, although by late 2022, many countries relaxed their requirements for proof of vaccination to travel and to access a variety of services.

Vaccines, like any form of medical treatment, are not risk-free, and some are riskier than others. The European Court of Human Rights has recently emphasised the moral obligation of states to ensure redress for injuries arising from vaccination. In *Vavřička and Others* v *the Czech Republic*,[42] the Court considered the compatibility of compulsory childhood vaccination in a country (the Czech Republic) with the European Convention on Human Rights (ECHR). The Court affirmed the legality of mandating childhood vaccination, finding that the public health interest in achieving herd immunity from contagious diseases outweighed the individual right to private life, and that the Czech law contained sufficient provisions for the exemption of those with medical or religious reasons for not receiving vaccination. The Court also affirmed, however, the importance of the availability of adequate compensation for those who suffer harm. We now turn to cover the UK's scheme for this.

7.3.3 VACCINE DAMAGE PAYMENT SCHEME

In the UK, under the Vaccine Damage Payments Act 1979, a Vaccine Damage Payment Scheme has existed whereby individuals 'severely disabled' as a result of vaccination against a number of diseases may receive a one-off tax-free payment of £120,000 (this does not exclude individuals from seeking legal action to claim compensation).[43] The Scheme covers vaccination against, inter alia, Covid-19, pertussis, rotavirus, rubella, and mumps. The Scheme covers individuals vaccinated before their 18th birthday, unless the vaccination was against certain diseases such as Covid-19, poliomyelitis, seasonal influenza, and human papillomavirus.[44] Disablement includes both mental or physical disablement and is based on medical evidence from the doctors or hospitals involved in the individual's treatment. It is worked out as a percentage, and 'severe disablement' means at least 60% disabled, although how *exactly* a percentage is arrived at remains something of a bit of guesswork, and the justice of awarding payment only upon reaching this threshold has not been without controversy for settling Covid-19 claims, among others.[45] As Goldberg notes, the concept of severe disablement derived from pre-World War II industrial injuries and war pensions schemes; its application to public health and vaccination can be

---

[40] HC Deb 1 March 2022, vol 709.

[41] See e.g. Tasnime Osama, Mohammad Razai, and Azeem Majeed, 'Covid-19 Vaccine Passports: Access, Equity, and Ethics' (2021) 373 BMJ n861; Ana Beduschi, 'Taking Stock of COVID-19 Health Status Certificates: Legal Implications for Data Privacy and Human Rights' (2022) Big Data & Society, available at <https://journals.sagepub.com/doi/full/10.1177/20539517211069300> accessed 08 November 2022.

[42] App Nos 47621/13, 3867/14, 73094/14, 19306/15, 19298/15, and 43883/15, 8 April 2021.

[43] See also Jacqui Wise, 'Covid-19: UK Makes First Payments to Compensate Injury or Death From Vaccines' (2022) 377 BMJ o1565.

[44] UK Government, 'Vaccine Damage Payment' (2022) available at <https://www.gov.uk/vaccine-damage-payment> accessed 08 November 2022.

[45] Rachel Schraer, 'Vaccine Damage Payment Scheme: The Battle for Compensation' (BBC News, 23 June 2022) available at <https://www.bbc.com/news/health-61898694> accessed 08 November 2022.

called into question.[46] There have been growing calls to reform the legislation,[47] and in one case, a private member's Bill was tabled in 2021–22 to establish an independent review of disablement caused by Covid-19 vaccinations and the adequacy of the compensation offered to persons so disabled, although it did not make to a second reading in the House of Commons.[48]

We turn now to discuss public health at a broader level, namely from health protection to promotion. Here, we explore at international and national levels how the law may be designed to improve the health of the community.

7.4 HEALTH PROMOTION: IMPROVING THE HEALTH OF THE COMMUNITY

7.4.1 GENERAL AND INTERNATIONAL CONTEXT

Even with respect to communicable disease, and recognising the structural limitations noted previously, there is much that we can do to promote our own health for the sake of ourselves and our significant others, and indeed for the community. Both the state and the community—our local council, our neighbourhood, our immediate neighbours—have an interest in encouraging us to make decisions that support health and productivity. States and local governments now take much more interest in the health of their citizens. This may simply be a matter of sound social investment, or it may be an economics-driven policy designed to avoid greater and longer-term costs dealing with a chronically ill population. Either way, states spend vast sums of money trying to persuade or coerce their citizens into healthier lifestyles through a variety of mechanisms, from laws to information campaigns to invisible 'nudges' that promote certain desirable (healthy) behaviours.

Despite pursuing legitimate state objectives of educating and encouraging the public in good health practices, these programmes can be controversial, given the retreat from paternalism and the rise of autonomy, but also due to the potential for stigmatising certain communities. To what extent, for example, is it justifiable for a government to require the wearing of seatbelts? Or to discourage the use of cars in inner cities through charging schemes? Or to tax salt and sugar?[49] Or to broadcast graphic posters targeting smokers? And what about state action aimed at promoting the future health of children? Has the government the right to control meals taken to school in the interests of an anti-obesity programme? The state is at a double disadvantage. Not only is the focus on individual rights and protections greater now than ever before, which makes such programmes politically charged, but many public health issues—whether of a health promotion or health protection character—are agnostic to national borders, making individual state action ineffective or potentially counterproductive in any event.

---

[46] Richard Goldberg, 'Vaccine Damage Schemes in the US and UK Reappraised: Making Them Fit for Purpose in the Light of Covid-19' (2022) 42(4) Legal Studies 576.

[47] ibid. See also Duncan Fairgrieve et al., 'In Favour of a Bespoke COVID-19 Vaccines Compensation Scheme' (2021) 21(4) The Lancet Infectious Diseases P448.

[48] Covid-19 Vaccine Damage Bill (Bill 44 2021–22, House of Commons, Session 2021–22) available at <https://bills.parliament.uk/bills/2926> accessed 08 November 2022.

[49] BBC News, 'Salt and Sugar Tax for England to be Ruled Out' (11 June 2022) available at <https://www.bbc.com/news/uk-61767847> accessed 08 November 2022.

Consider tobacco, a worldwide industry with powerful protagonists. Tobacco is esti-mated to have killed some 100 million people in the twentieth century—more than AIDS, tuberculosis, and malaria combined—and it remains a significant cause of preventable deaths, accounting for more than 8 million deaths and costing the global economy $1.4 trillion each year.[50] As such, it is one of the health issues for which states have taken international legal action. The Framework Convention on Tobacco Control 2003 (FCTC), adopted by consensus by the World Health Assembly, is legally binding in 182 ratifying countries, covering more than 90% of the world population.[51] According to Article 3, the FCTC's objective is to protect people, including future generations, from the social, environmental, economic, and health consequences of tobacco consumption and expo-sure. Its guiding principles include provision of good public information (something the industry long stymied), building cooperation, and promoting civil society engagement.[52] The FCTC addresses demand reduction through pricing and taxation,[53] tobacco ingredi-ents,[54] packaging, labelling, education, advertising,[55] and illicit trade,[56] and it tackles the critical issue of promoting viable alternatives for tobacco farmers, workers, and sellers.[57]

Of course, as a framework convention, it provides only the regulatory bones, which must be fleshed out through domestic law and policymaking. Some states have been more proactive than others in monitoring and enforcing compliance.[58] Bearing the aforemen-tioned guidance in mind, therefore, one might still ask what measures can and should states take in relation to tobacco nationally/locally? There are no examples of outright bans on tobacco production, distribution, and sales. Rather, states have taken a range of steps to reduce consumption, including the banning of smoking in public places. But are such bans appropriate,[59] and what about when they are not uniformly enforced?[60] And what other measures might states take, and how might they need to coordinate?

7.4.2 UK CONTEXT

As public health programmes reach deeper into our private lives, the subtlety with which they are promoted may increase as well. In the UK, the establishment of the Behavioural Insights Team in the Cabinet Office in 2010 was heralded as a more

---

[50] WHO, 'WHO Report on the Global Tobacco Epidemic 2021: Addressing New and Emerging Products' (2021) available at <https://www.who.int/publications/i/item/9789240032095> accessed 08 November 2022.

[51] WHO, 'WHO Framework Convention on Tobacco Control: Parties' (2022) available at <https://fctc.who.int/who-fctc/overview/parties> accessed 08 November 2022.

[52] ibid., Art 4.   [53] ibid., Art 6.   [54] ibid., Art 9.   [55] ibid., Arts 10–13.

[56] ibid., Arts 15–16.   [57] ibid., Arts 17–18.

[58] Heikki Hiilamoa and Stanton Glantz, 'Implementation of Effective Cigarette Health Warning Labels Among Low and Middle Income Countries: State Capacity, Path-Dependency and Tobacco Industry Activity' (2015) 124 Social Science & Medicine 241.

[59] See e.g. Health Act 2006; The Smoke-free (Premises and Enforcement) Regulations 2006 (SI 2006/3361); and Health (Tobacco, Nicotine etc. and Care) (Scotland) Act 2016.

[60] It could be argued that, since smoking is a powerful anxiolytic, banning it entirely at a mental health institution is a rights infringement of persons compulsorily detained, despite being good public health medicine. This was the view taken by the UK Supreme Court in *McCann* v *The State Hospitals Board for Scotland* [2017] UKSC 31, which held that the State Hospitals Board for Scotland's decision to implement a comprehensive smoking ban at a state hospital through a prohibition of having tobacco products, as well a search and confiscation regime, was unlawful under domestic law because it did not comply with the Mental Health (Care and Treatment) (Scotland) Act 2003 and the Mental Health (Safety and Security) (Scotland) Regulations 2005, and consequently infringed the appellant's rights under Art 8 of the European Convention on Human Rights.

libertarian form of paternalism in encouraging citizens to act in their own health interests.[61] Behavioural insights work on the basis of evidence from psychology and behavioural economics to understand better how people make choices and to influence them accordingly.[62] The paradigm example is placing salads and other healthy options in the front sections of a buffet on the understanding that people tend to fill their plates with what they first see.[63]

While such so-called 'nudge' policies and practices are thought to be a more acceptable and effective form of public health promotion,[64] they still represent, for many, a questionable exercise of paternalism by the 'nanny state'.[65] Their legitimacy turns largely on perspective—is one's own health simply a matter of individual choice, or do we owe a responsibility to ourselves and to others to ensure that we remain as healthy as possible? The communitarian will favour the latter; the libertarian will tend towards the former. This, however, might have significant implications regarding access to health care in the face of scarce resources—is the smoker less entitled to coronary bypass surgery than the non-smoker?[66] For now, we need only note that states take more interest in their public's health than ever before and this means that, when set against the unprecedented rise in autonomy, the tensions inherent within public health law are more acute than ever before.

The idea of 'facilitating choice' and encouraging 'self-responsibilisation' is certainly more palatable than 'manipulative behaviour' and fits within a neoliberal ethos of enabling personal choice and responsibility within the confines of market logic, but to the extent that choice is predicated on information, and responsibility contingent on structures that facilitate equitable access, one of the biggest challenges for governments is ensuring that misinformation does not become the primary driver for citizens' behaviour and resources are adequately implemented to promote equality and equity. The UK, as with many countries, has a long way to go. To take the issue of misinformation, the BSE (bovine spongiform encephalopathy) and MMR (measles, mumps, and rubella) controversies have put into stark relief the need for health agencies to pay as much attention to assessing public perceptions about risk and communication as they do to investigating hazards and controlling exposures.

The MMR controversy related to the perceived risks associated with the vaccine, which was introduced in the UK in 1988. A fear developed that it caused autism in children.[67]

---

[61] The Behavioural Insights Team has since spun out of the Cabinet Office and is now fully owned as a subsidiary company of the British charity Nesta.

[62] Department of Health, 'Choosing Health: Making Healthier Choices Easier' (2004) available at <https://webarchive.nationalarchives.gov.uk/ukgwa/+/dh.gov.uk/en/publicationsandstatistics/publications/publicationspolicyandguidance/dh_4094550> accessed 08 November 2022.

[63] Cabinet Office, 'Applying Behavioural Insight to Health' (2010) available at <https://www.gov.uk/government/publications/applying-behavioural-insight-to-health-behavioural-insights-team-paper> accessed 08 November 2022; Christopher Robertson, I. Glenn Cohen, and Holly Lynch (eds.), *Nudging Health: Health Law and Behavioral Economics* (Johns Hopkins University Press 2016).

[64] Richard Thaler and Cass Sunstein, *Nudge: The Final Edition* (Allen Lane 2021).

[65] Andreas Schmidt and Bart Engelen, 'The Ethics of Nudging: An Overview' (2020) 15(4) Philosophy Compass e12658; Loni Ledderer et al., 'Nudging in Public Health Lifestyle Interventions: A Systematic Literature Review and Metasynthesis' (2020) 47(5) Health Education & Behavior 749.

[66] For discussion, see Chapter 5.

[67] The original Wakefield paper, since retracted by *The Lancet*, was heavily criticised as unsound: see Kreesten Madsen et al., 'A Population-Based Study of Measles, Mumps and Rubella Vaccination and Autism' (2002) 347(19) New England Journal of Medicine 1477; and Hideo Honda et al., 'No Effect of MMR Withdrawal on the Incidence of Autism: A Total Population Study' (2005) 46(6) Journal of Child Psychology and Psychiatry 572. Dr Wakefield was struck off the medical register: General Medical Council, 'Fitness to Practise Panel Hearing, 24 May 2010, Andrew Wakefield, Determination of Serious Professional Misconduct' (2010). A colleague also involved had his registration reinstated: *Walker-Smith v GMC* [2012] EWHC 503.

This provoked a crisis of confidence among British parents, many of whom began to refuse to vaccinate their children. Matters came to a head—in the courts at least—with *Re C (welfare of child: immunisation)*,[68] in which two estranged fathers sought court orders to ensure that their children were inoculated, despite the mothers' disagreement. The Court of Appeal confirmed the trial judge's approach, which was to consider the best interests of the children, first, from the medical, and then, from a non-medical perspective. Sedley LJ stated that such an approach could admit a variety of possibilities, including support for a parental view that medical intervention was not appropriate. In the instant cases, however, the scientific evidence relied upon by the mothers to demonstrate the dangers of the vaccine was held to be unreliable. In contrast, the effectiveness of the vaccine was shown to be high and side effects rare.[69] Orders were issued that the children should be vaccinated.[70]

The decision may be contrasted with that of the Irish Supreme Court in *North Western Health Board* v *W (H)*,[71] in which the Court considered an action brought by a local health board against parents who had refused a 'heel prick' test for their son—a simple blood test aimed at screening for some treatable conditions, including phenylketonuria (PKU).[72] Though a routine practice for all newborns, the parents resisted because of the 'assault' on their son that the prick would represent. The Supreme Court upheld the right of the parents to refuse, relying on the Irish constitutional right to 'family autonomy' which, it was held, should be protected against undue interference by the state. As in the English courts, the notion of the child's best interests was a central consideration; the difference came in how, and by whom, these were to be determined.[73]

There is, also, a wider social interest to be gained from the long-term storage and use of the cards upon which these blood spots are kept—so-called Guthrie cards or bloodspot cards. In the UK, these have now been kept for almost 60 years (since the mid-1960s), beginning at a time when informed consent was anathema, in particular with respect to long-term storage of the cards for research purposes. Can or should such collections be used for the public good, their social value lying in their being a research resource and (more controversially perhaps) a forensic tool? The issues are manifold and the answers to the questions raised are far from obvious, but their existence raises once again the delicate balance between individual and collective interests that arises in health promotion programmes.[74]

Ultimately, these cases demonstrate important points, including the extent of parental rights over their children, to which we shall return. For present purposes, they illustrate

---

[68] [2003] 2 FLR 1095 (CA). For more, see Emma Cave, 'Adolescent Refusal of MMR Inoculation: F (Mother) v F (Father)' (2014) 77(4) Modern Law Review 630.

[69] For comment, see Kath O'Donnell, '*Re C (Welfare of Child: Immunisation)*: Room to Refuse? Immunisation, Welfare and the Role of Parental Decision-Making' (2004) 16(2) Child and Family Law Quarterly 213.

[70] There are many cases in which parental disagreement over vaccination has come before the courts, which consistently consider the welfare of the child(ren), the risk of the vaccine, and the relationships within the family: *Re B (a child: immunisation)* [2003] 2 FCR 156 (CA); *C* v *A (a minor)* [2011] EWHC 4033 (Fam); *F* v *F (MMR Vaccine)* [2013] EWHC 2683 (HC); *Re SL (permission to vaccinate)* [2017] EWHC 125 (Fam).

[71] [2001] IESC 70.

[72] PKU is a genetic metabolic disorder which—if detected early—can be avoided by simple dietary changes; otherwise, victims can suffer profound disability.

[73] For commentary, see Graeme Laurie, 'Better to Hesitate at the Threshold of Compulsion: PKU Testing and the Concept of Family Autonomy in Eire' (2002) 28(3) Journal of Medical Ethics 136.

[74] For more, see Graeme Laurie, Kathryn Hunter, and Sarah Cunningham-Burley, *Guthrie Cards in Scotland: Ethical, Legal and Social Issues* (Scottish Government 2013).

that there is often no clear line between health promotion and health protection measures, and it is the extent to which any given measure can be classified under the latter heading—at least at the community level—that determines the degree of paternalistic or coercive state interference that is involved. Whether it is justified must, then, be argued on the particularities of the case; as demonstrated, any intervention that interferes with individual human rights can be justified only when it can be shown to be a necessary and proportionate response to the harm that is to be avoided.

7.5 HEALTH PROTECTION: HANDLING THREATS TO THE COMMUNITY

7.5.1 GENERAL AND INTERNATIONAL CONTEXT

The health landscape is ever-changing. Tuberculosis (TB), once considered to be under control, has persisted in lower- and middle-income countries[75] and is increasing in prevalence, killing some 1.5 million people globally per year. Even polio, once thought forever eliminated in the US and the UK, reappeared in 2022.[76] While lower respiratory infections (e.g. from TB) remain the world's most deadly communicable disease, alongside malaria and HIV/AIDS, the prospect of virus transfer to humans from other species (zoonoses) has increased, and is highlighted by variants of SARS (severe acute respiratory syndrome), and by swine and avian flu. Continued environmental destruction and encroachment in forests and areas of wildlife around the globe exacerbate this risk with each passing year. Risks are also potentially exacerbated by the prospect of xenotransplantation (using animal organs or tissues) and bioterrorism (the deliberate release of biological agents). In short, the health interests of the community can sometimes be so strong—or the threat to its health so great—that even compulsory action against the bodily integrity and freedoms of individuals can be defended.

However, public health measures should not be taken as a form of unqualified utilitarianism whereby the public good must always necessarily trump individual freedoms. Rather, robust health protection programmes should always require the state to justify every measure and intervention, the interventions should be 'proportionate' and 'necessary' in the circumstances (i.e. no other reasonable means are available to achieve the same justifiable ends), and there should be full respect for the rights of individuals who are not implicated in the immediate health threat.[77] For example, state agencies must remain bound by confidentiality law and data protection measures (discussed

---

[75] The WHO states that in 2020, the 30 high TB burden countries accounted for 86% of new TB cases. Eight countries account for two-thirds of the total, with India leading the count, followed by China, Indonesia, the Philippines, Pakistan, Nigeria, Bangladesh, and South Africa. See WHO, 'Tuberculosis' (2022) available at <https://www.who.int/news-room/fact-sheets/detail/tuberculosis> accessed 08 November 2022.

[76] CDC, 'Polio Elimination in the United States' (2022) available at <https://www.cdc.gov/polio/what-is-polio/polio-us.html> accessed 08 November 2022; Jim Reed and Philippa Roxby, 'Polio Virus Detected in London Sewage Samples' (BBC News, 22 June 2022) available at <https://www.bbc.com/news/health-61896411> accessed 08 November 2022.

[77] The human rights dimension of detention for people living with infectious disease was addressed in *Enhorn* v *Sweden* (2005) 41 EHRR 30. Sweden was found to be in violation of its obligations under the ECHR, not because it had legalised measures to detain people who posed a risk to others, but because these measures had not been deployed as a last resort. Sweden had failed to strike a fair balance between the need to ensure that infection (HIV) did not spread and the applicant's right to liberty.

in Chapter 11).[78] To reiterate, health risks threaten us as a local, national, and global community, not merely as individuals. Responsive state agencies exist in most jurisdictions, but responses often cannot simply be local. International efforts and coordination are essential to effective strategies. The WHO's International Health Regulations 2005 (IHR)[79] establish 'an agreed framework of commitments and responsibilities for States and for WHO to invest in limiting the international spread of epidemics and other public health emergencies while minimising disruption to travel, trade and economies'.[80] Notwithstanding, while acknowledging that the WHO and the IHR may play an important role in surveillance and outbreak reporting, and in providing a framework for tackling a public health emergency, as is often the case in international law, there is little that can be done against a refractory state; effective action must begin and be maintained at the state level.

7.5.2 UK CONTEXT

Major reforms to public health powers have occurred, as seen most pronouncedly in the discussion concerning Covid-19.[81] One particularly important reform prior to the pandemic was the abolition of the Health Protection Agency, a UK-wide body whose remit was to anticipate, identify, and respond to infectious disease threats and other health dangers. It was abolished by s 56 of the Health and Social Care Act 2012, with the aim of providing more transparent, responsible, and accountable service in public health. The result is that legal and practical responses to infectious diseases remain divided along jurisdictional lines within the UK, with responsibility in Northern Ireland falling to the Public Health Agency (established in 2009), in Wales to Public Health Wales (established in 2009), in Scotland to Public Health Scotland, itself established in April 2020,[82] and in England until recently Public Health England, established in 2013 to bring together public health specialists from more than 70 organisations. As we noted, it is not yet clear whether such division across the four nations has led to a seamless interoperation for protecting the UK's health in the face of immediate dangers.

In the midst of the Covid-19 pandemic, the UK Government established the UK Health Security Agency (UKHSA) as an executive agency, sponsored by the Department of Health and Social Care, charged with protecting the population from the impact of infectious diseases, chemical, biological, radiological and nuclear incidents, and other health threats. Its jurisdiction extends only to England. There was initial confusion about whether UKHSA's establishment meant Public Health England's abolishment, although

---

[78] See e.g. Public Health England, 'COVID-19 Privacy Information' (2021) available at <https://www.gov.uk/government/publications/phe-privacy-information/covid-19-privacy-information> accessed 08 November 2021.

[79] WHO, 'International Health Regulations (2005) Third Edition' (2016) available at <https://www.who.int/publications/i/item/9789241580496> accessed 08 November 2022.

[80] For comment on the role of the WHO, see Shawn Harmon, 'International Public Health Law: Not so Much WHO as Why, and Not Enough WHO and Why Not?' (2009) 12(3) Medicine, Health Care, and Philosophy 245.

[81] The Health and Social Care Act 2012 reformed the law for England and Wales, with further change imposed under the Public Health (Wales) Act 2017, while in Scotland the law is found in the Public Health etc. (Scotland) Act 2008. Northern Ireland has amended its Public Health Act (Northern Ireland) 1967 over the years, but has become rather outdated. In 2015, the Department of Health undertook a consultation for the review of the Public Health Act (Northern Ireland) 1967. As of the time writing, and in part due to ongoing political challenges in the Northern Ireland Assembly, no public health legislation reform has occurred.

[82] Prior to this, Health Protection Scotland exercised public health functions on behalf of the Scottish Government.

it is now clear that Public Health England has indeed been disbanded, with UKHSA holding functions related to health protection and the Office for Health Improvement and Disparities holding functions related to health promotion, although the boundaries between improvement and protection are hardly watertight and the change has not been without controversy.[83] Within UKHSA sits the Joint Biosecurity Centre, a scientific body that advises the UK Government and provides evidence-based, objective analysis to inform local and national decision-making in response to Covid-19 outbreaks. The JBC is expected to continue to function even after the Covid-19 pandemic is declared over.

Despite the plethora of public health bodies now operating across the four nations, all make an effort to coordinate regularly and relatively well to ensure a consistent approach and effective communication of any emerging public health threat.[84] It is hoped that such a joined-up approach will persevere long after the Covid-19 pandemic subsides.

As noted earlier in this chapter, the Civil Contingencies Act 2004 continues to have UK-wide application. It modernised the law to reflect contemporary emergencies (e.g. terrorist threats, environmental degradation, and pandemics),[85] and imposes on authorities the responsibility of assessing risks and making plans for the assessment, mitigation, and prevention of emergencies.[86] It was considered to be the key piece of legislation that governs legal authority to act in a 'true' emergency (although, as noted, this was not the statute seen as fit for purpose to address Covid-19), empowering authorities and other actors to intervene in response thereto, but it is crucial to note that the Act offers emergency powers only as a last resort, and only when existing legislation is insufficient to respond to the situation in an effective way.[87] This means that, first, we must consider existing public health laws.

The prevailing public health legislation in England is the Public Health (Control of Disease) Act 1984, as amended, which establishes general rules and broad powers for the state, including Justices of the Peace in response to reports by a local authority's 'Proper Officer'. These powers are exceptionally wide as regards both 'persons' and 'things', and, as to the former, run from admission to hospital, through attending training sessions, to abstaining from specified work. Associated regulations specify both the diseases of interest and the powers available to control them.[88] In doing so, they categorise diseases as 'notifiable'; a notifiable disease is one which a registered medical practitioner is legally bound to report to relevant authorities or face summary conviction and fine.[89] Indeed, the most important feature of the Act, from the point of view of the doctor–patient

---

[83] ITV News, 'Boss "Sorry Beyond Words" After Details on Public Health England's Future Leaked' (17 August 2020) available at <https://www.itv.com/news/2020-08-17/boss-sorry-beyond-words-after-details-on-public-health-englands-future-leaked> accessed 08 November 2022; Gabriel Scally, 'The Demise of Public Health England' (2020) 370 BMJ m3263.

[84] See e.g. UK Health Security Agency, 'Agency Agreement Between the Secretary of State for Health and Social Care and the Devolved Administrations Relating to the Joint Biosecurity Centre' (2020) available at <https://ukhsaexchange.kahootz.com/JBCDAGovernance/view?objectId=109130085> accessed 08 November 2022; UK Health Security Agency, 'Participation of the Devolved Administrations in the Joint Biosecurity Centre' (2020) available at <https://ukhsaexchange.kahootz.com/JBCDAGovernance/view?objectId=109130277> accessed 08 November 2022.

[85] Civil Contingencies Act 2004, ss 1 and 19.   [86] ibid., s 2.   [87] ibid., ss 21 and 23.

[88] See the Health Protection (Local Authority Powers) Regulations 2010 (SI 2010/657), the Health Protection (Part 2A Orders) Regulations 2010 (SI 2010/658), and the Health Protection (Notification) Regulations 2010 (SI 2010/659).

[89] The list of notifiable diseases for England is set out in the Public Health (Control of Disease) Act 1984, as amended, and its associated regulations, particularly the Health Protection (Notification) Regulations 2010/659, and for Scotland in Sch 1 of the Public Health etc. (Scotland) Act 2008. For Wales, see Health Protection (Notification) (Wales) Regulations 2010/1546. For Northern Ireland, see Sch 1 of the Public Health Act (Northern Ireland) 1967.

relationship, is the statutory obligation to notify authorities about the existence of certain diseases as they occur. In addition to being the lynchpin on which the control of infectious disease depends, it has obvious significance for confidentiality in medical practice, which is discussed in detail in Chapter 11. (Note that local authorities may, themselves, add to the list of notifiable diseases.) Whereas questions remained as to whether the old legislation applied to pandemic influenza or other new and emerging conditions, the amended 1984 Act under section 45A defines a public health threat broadly: 'Any reference to infection or contamination is a reference to infection or contamination which presents or could present significant harm to human health.'

As this Act and its Regulations make clear, effective health protection for the community depends on a number of factors which include early detection, rapid and effective intervention and control, and ongoing surveillance. Central to these is the proper flow of information between those responsible for implementing the public health agenda. In the present context, the Health and Social Care Acts 2008 and 2012 in England and the Public Health etc. (Scotland) Act 2008 can be contrasted. The English legislation does little more than empower the Minister to make such regulations as they see necessary to cover a multitude of potential public hazards, and in doing so, they may incorporate international agreements or arrangements such as recommendations from the WHO. The rationale behind the provisions is to allow the Minister to take action according to the circumstance prevailing at the time rather than in respect of a predetermined set of conditions. The interests of the individual are preserved so far as is compatible with public safety—in general, any action taken must be proportionate to the risk involved. In particular, regulations may not include provisions requiring an individual to undergo medical treatment—including immunisation—nor may health protection regulations create an offence punishable by imprisonment.

We could also bring an ethical evaluation to bear on these and other legal measures. For example, the Nuffield Council on Bioethics has highlighted the importance of precaution when dealing with threats to public health.[90] It references a European Commission Communication on the precautionary principle, which identifies five elements for consideration when developing responses to public health emergencies:

- scientific assessment of risk, acknowledging uncertainties and updated in light of new evidence;
- fairness and consistency;
- consideration of costs and benefits of actions;
- transparency; and
- proportionality.[91]

The Nuffield Council prefers the term 'precautionary approach' in addressing public health threats and advocates an intervention ladder which offers a way of thinking about possible government action and appreciating the associated consequences for civil liberties. This ranges across options from 'doing nothing' and monitoring a situation, to 'enabling choice', 'guiding choice', 'restricting choice', and, ultimately to 'eliminating choice'. As the intervention becomes more intrusive, so the need for justification becomes more compelling; indeed, some of our University of Edinburgh colleagues

---

[90] Nuffield Council on Bioethics, (n 2).
[91] European Commission, 'Communication from the Commission on the Precautionary Principle' COM (2000) 1.

have argued that a Civil Liberties Impact Assessment should accompany all contingency plans with particularly close attention paid to the points at which escalation of action will take place.[92]

7.5.3 DISEASE NOTIFICATION (HIV/AIDS)

Many lessons for the future are to be learned from experiences of the past and present and, to this extent, it still remains valid to consider the legal responses to one of the greatest public health threats of modern times before Covid-19 appeared, namely infection with the Human Immunodeficiency Virus (HIV).[93] HIV/AIDS emerged in the UK in 1981, but as with many countries, was likely circulating among the population for some years prior.[94] The virus attacks the human immune system, leaving the individual exposed to any number of opportunistic diseases. In 2021, some 38.4 million people worldwide were living with the virus, some 1.5 million people became newly infected with HIV, and some 650,000 people died from AIDS-related illnesses. On a more hopeful note, in 2021, some 28.7 million people were accessing antiretroviral therapy, meaning 75% of all people living with HIV were accessing treatment, and new HIV infections have been reduced by 54% since the peak in 1996, while AIDS-related deaths have been reduced by 68% since the peak in 2004.[95]

The hysteria which met the advent of HIV/AIDS has calmed as a result of public education campaigns and the development of antiretroviral drugs which can significantly slow the progress of the disease, but significant public health issues remain; in particular, over access to those drugs, most especially in developing countries. Numerous countries also continue to impose restrictions on entry, stay, residency, and access to adequate care for people living with HIV, all of which contributes to the continuing stigma associated with the disease.[96] HIV/AIDS is paradigmatic modern pandemic affecting humanity on a global scale and a precursor to what we witnessed with the Covid-19 pandemic. Its spread has been greatly facilitated by modern travel, the absence of a cure makes the prospect of infection particularly significant, and ignorance and misunderstanding about the disease and its pattern of spread led to calls for draconian measures to be taken against affected groups (including against groups thought to be at 'high risk').

[92] Graeme Laurie and Kathryn Hunter, 'Mapping, Assessing and Improving Legal Preparedness for Pandemic Flu in The United Kingdom' (2009) 10(2) Medical Law International 101.

[93] HIV is a virus that attacks the immune system leaving it incapable of dealing with further assault. Acquired Immune Deficiency Syndrome (AIDS) refers to a state when the individual's immune system is compromised beyond a certain degree. There is international disagreement about the point at which AIDS should be diagnosed; recent trends are away from the use of the term altogether. For more on legal responses, see James Chalmers, *Legal Responses to HIV and AIDS* (Hart 2008).

[94] Marie Leoz et al., 'The Two-Phase Emergence of Non Pandemic HIV-1 Group O in Cameroon' (2015) 11(8) PLoS Pathogens e1005029.

[95] UNAIDS, 'Global HIV & AIDS statistics — Fact sheet' (2022) available at <https://www.unaids.org/en/resources/fact-sheet> accessed 08 November 2022.

[96] *Kiyutin v Russia* [2011] ECHR 439 (violation of Arts 8 and 14 for refusal of residence permit to HIV-positive foreigner); *AB v Russia*, App No 1439/06, Judgment 14 October 2010 and *Logvinenko v Ukraine*, App No 13448/07, Judgment 14 October 2010 (inadequate medical assistance to detainees); *Centre of legal resources on behalf of Valentin Campeanu v Romania*, App No 47848/08 (insufficient medical treatment for an HIV-positive person with a mental disability).

Although HIV/AIDS dominated headlines and captured public attention over decades, HIV has never been treated as notifiable in the UK.[97] The reasoning behind this decision reveals one of the fundamental tensions associated with notification of diseases—that is, that its compulsory nature effectively requires practitioners to breach patient confidentiality, albeit under strict and defined conditions of disclosure.[98] Concern with HIV infection has traditionally related not to the nature of the disease itself—which is less easily spread than hepatitis, much less an airborne communicable disease such as SARS-CoV-2, and constitutes a lesser threat to global health,[99] but rather to the extensive social stigma that surrounded it. The fear was that patients would perceive a forced breach of their confidentiality as a significant threat to their interests and would not return for care; in turn, other infected persons might refuse to come forward. Thus, health authorities would be left with no effective means by which to monitor the disease. We see, then, that this policy was originally justified on both private and public grounds. It has not been borne out in practice, however, with labs and clinics voluntarily passing on statistics (on an anonymous basis) to authorities.

Even so, the case of HIV/AIDS illustrates the sensitivity of the situation when a new disease emerges and we are uncertain as to what we are dealing with. A major difference between HIV/AIDS and something like H1N1 or SARS-CoV-2 is that HIV is actually difficult to spread, whereas the latter viruses can be passed easily through casual contact. In terms of legal preparedness, the question is: should the law provide specifically for measures to address the particular nature of a particular condition, or should it set up a framework of action which empowers relevant agents to act in response to emergencies? Each approach has its pros and cons, and UK legislation is something of a synthesis.

7.6 HEALTH PROTECTION: THE CRIMINAL LAW

Discussion of the state's protection role in public health would be incomplete without mention of the role of the criminal law—rules may be considered ineffective in the absence of penalties for their transgression. In most circumstances, disease transmission is not a matter of choice; it is not, therefore, something that can rightly be subject to deterrence. But this is not always true. A person with TB may be the unfortunate victim of nature, but what if they wantonly transmit the bacillus to another through conscious intimate contact? Such considerations will apply particularly to sexually transmitted infections (STIs), which require unique circumstances for their transmission—circumstances which can be brought about, or avoided, through individual action. It is therefore meaningful to consider STIs as a prime example when discussing whether the criminal law has a role to play in encouraging people to behave responsibly in respect of public health.

---

[97] Specific legislation for HIV/AIDS was introduced in the AIDS (Control) Act 1987, which required regular reporting by a health authority on the incidence of HIV/AIDS within its area. This is not the same as notification, which requires the reporting of the name, age, sex, and residence of each infected person. The Act was repealed in Scotland by the Public Health etc. (Scotland) Act 2008, Sch 3 and in England and Wales by the Health and Social Care Act 2012. The AIDS (Control) Act 1987 did not extend to Northern Ireland.

[98] For discussion of a case of HIV disclosure in Ireland, see Andrea Mulligan, 'Patient Confidentiality and Disclosure of HIV Status: Disentangling the Entitlement to Disclose From the Duty to Warn' (2021) 29(4) Medical Law Review 688.

[99] Hepatitis B is 100 times more infectious than HIV, and, according to the WHO, as of 2019, an estimated 296 million people worldwide are living with hepatitis B and 58 million people worldwide are living with hepatitis C. See World Health Organization, 'Fact sheets' available at <https://www.who.int/newsroom/fact-sheets> accessed 14 January 2023.

The landmark English case was *R v Clarence*, in which a husband with gonorrhoea infected his wife knowing that he had the condition.[100] Clarence was prosecuted—and convicted—under sections 20 (inflicting grievous bodily harm) and 47 (inflicting bodily harm) of the Offences Against the Person Act 1861. There was no suggestion that he intended to infect his wife. It was accepted that she would not have consented to sexual intercourse had she known the truth. His convictions were, however, overturned, largely on the grounds that (i) prosecution depends on some direct and intentional wounding to the victim (not present in the case of reckless infection), and (ii) consent of a wife to sexual intercourse was a given in the absence of fraud as to the nature of the act in question or as to the identity of the actor. This precedent stood for more than a century and distorted the jurisprudence as a result. Thankfully, it is now overturned.[101]

There have been a number of attempts in Commonwealth jurisdictions to circumvent the evidential difficulties left by *Clarence*,[102] but the jurisprudence has been inconsistent. The first successful prosecution for reckless transmission of HIV in the UK is the unreported Scottish case of *Kelly v HM Advocate*,[103] where the relative flexibility of Scots law allowed for a charge of 'culpably and recklessly engaging in sexual intercourse to the danger of a woman's health and life'.[104]

The essential legal issues for reckless transmission were laid out in *R v Dica*,[105] and this still represents the current legal position in England and Wales. This case involved the prosecution under section 20 of the Offences Against the Person Act 1861 of an HIV-positive defendant for having infected two partners. This route, as we have seen, has caused logical and doctrinal problems because (i) there is no 'assault' on the victim in the sense of physical violence to the victim's body, and (ii) authority suggested that consent to such an 'assault' was irrelevant for criminal purposes.[106] But here the court held that so long as all the other elements of a section 20 offence were present, infection with disease could constitute a crime. Moreover, consent is only irrelevant in circumstances where there is actual intention to harm; in cases involving recklessness, the consent of the victim to running the risk of infection could be a complete defence. The central issue is not consent to sexual intercourse but rather consent to run a known risk by engaging in unprotected sexual intercourse.

R v Konzani[107] confirmed that the nature of the consent in question is informed consent, and that a genuine, albeit mistaken, belief that a partner has consented to sexual intercourse will allow the defence to operate. This may turn, for example, on whether a diagnosis of HIV has been confirmed. *Konzani* has been criticised, however, for not

---

[100] (1889) 22 QBD 23.

[101] The 'given' as to intra-marital consent to sexual intercourse was rejected in *R v R* [1992] 1 AC 599. For Scotland, see *Stallard v HM Advocate* 1989 SCCR 248. For consent in HIV infection generally, see *R v Konzani* [2005] 2 Cr App R 14. On the difficulties, see Lisa Cherkassky, 'Being Informed: The Complexities of Knowledge, Deception and Consent When Transmitting HIV' (2010) 74(3) Journal of Criminal Law 242.

[102] The New South Wales Crimes Act 1900, s 36, as amended, includes an offence of causing grievous bodily disease. The moral obligations are, of course, a distinct matter: Richard Bennett, Heather Draper, and Lucy Frith, 'Ignorance is Bliss? HIV and Moral Duties and Legal Duties to Forewarn' (2000) 26(1) Journal of Medical Ethics 9.

[103] (2001) High Court of Justiciary, Glasgow, 23 February. See BBC News, 'HIV Case Man Jailed for Five Years' (16 March 2001) available at <http://news.bbc.co.uk/2/hi/uk_news/scotland/1223845.stm> accessed 08 November 2022.

[104] See also *HM Advocate v Mola* 2007 SCCR 124 (elements that must be shown in determining someone's recklessness towards infecting their partner with a sexually transmitted disease).

[105] [2004] 3 All ER 593.   [106] *Clarence* (n 100) and *R v Brown* [1994] 1 AC 212.

[107] [2005] 2 Cr App R 14.

accepting that engaging in unprotected sex might, in itself, be seen as consent for the purposes of the defence.[108] While this and other cases send clear messages about personal responsibility,[109] questions remain as to where the line between intention and reckless-ness should be drawn.[110] In *R v Golding*,[111] a case of reckless transmission of herpes, the Court reiterated that a person with an STI who has sexual intercourse with a partner, not intending deliberately to infect her, but knowing that she is unaware of his condition, may be guilty of recklessly inflicting grievous bodily harm, and there is no necessity for an assault to have been committed. Ultimately, the prosecutor bears a responsibility to decide which messages to send to the community for adjudication.[112]

More recently, the case of Daryll Rowe is the first in the UK involving prosecution for intentionally infecting others with HIV (or indeed any STI). Rowe was convicted in England in 2017 on five counts of causing grievous bodily harm (GBH) with intent and five of attempted GBH with intent for deliberately trying to infect ten men (of whom five became HIV-positive) and was jailed for life with a minimum term of 12 years.[113] He was also convicted in Scotland in 2018 for culpable and reckless conduct for deliberately try-ing to infect four men with HIV, one of whom contracted the virus; he was sentenced to eight years in prison, served concurrently with the life sentence given to him in England, in addition to being placed on the sex offenders register for life.[114] Rowe's appeal of his conviction in England was dismissed; in the judgment, the Court of Appeal found the CPS guidance to prosecutors to be 'full, fair and thorough',[115] and that:

> the [CPS] policy makes clear that much as anyone may sympathise with someone diagnosed with the HIV infection, including this applicant, they cannot knowingly and deliberately spread the virus to others. Their sexual partners deserve the protection of the law and pro-tection from infection with a disease that may have lifetime consequences for them.[116]

For many who question the role of the criminal law in the transmission, exposure, and non-disclosure of STIs,[117] Rowe may well be seen as the 'limit case' in which the criminal

---

[108] Matthew Weait, '*R v Konzani*: Knowledge, Autonomy and Consent' (2005) Criminal Law Review 763, 765; Samantha Ryan, 'Reckless Transmission of HIV: Knowledge and Culpability' (2006) Criminal Law Review 981.

[109] In Canada, see *R v Mabior* [2012] SCC 47 (relevance of viral loads and of testimony that partners would not have consented to intercourse had they known of HIV status). In the USA, see *United States v Gutierrez*, No 13–0522, 23 February 2015, USCA (Armed Forces) (aggravated assault against defendant not sustainable because chance of infection too low to constitute likelihood of death or grievous bodily harm).

[110] Margaret Brazier, 'Do No Harm: Do Patients Have Responsibilities Too?' (2006) 65(2) Cambridge Law Review 397. On the effect of consent in the context of contact sports, see *R v Barnes* [2005] 2 All ER 113.

[111] [2014] EWCA Crim 889. See also *R v Peace Marangwanda* [2009] EWCA Crim 60, in which the defendant pleaded guilty to reckless transmission of gonorrhoea to two minors as a result of poor hygiene, as opposed to sexual contact. This decision has been criticised for its apparent acceptance of a duty to protect against disease transmission in the absence of awareness of the risk of transmission.

[112] Crown Prosecution Service, 'Intentional or Reckless Sexual Transmission of Infection' (2014); Scottish Prosecution Service, 'Prosecution Policy on the Sexual Transmission of Infection' (2014).

[113] *Daryll Rowe* (Unreported) Lewes Crown Court 15 November 2017. See also BBC News, 'Daryll Rowe Jailed for Infecting Men with HIV' (18 April 2018) available at <https://www.bbc.com/news/uk-england-sussex-43807662> accessed 08 November 2022.

[114] *HMA v Daryll Rowe* (Unreported) 4 May 2018. See also BBC News, 'Daryll Rowe Admitted Infecting Men with HIV in Edinburgh' (4 May 2018) available at <https://www.bbc.com/news/uk-scotland-edinburgh-east-fife-44003613> accessed 08 November 2022.

[115] *R v Rowe (Daryll)* [2018] EWCA Crim 2688, [50].   [116] ibid. [51].

[117] Samantha Ryan and Matt Phillips, 'HIV Disclosure—Professional Body Guidelines, the Law and the Boundaries of Medical Advice' (2021) 29(2) Medical Law Review 284.

law has a rightful role to play where intent to transmit is established, given the particularly heinous behaviour and callous disregard shown to others' health. Others, however, who argue that HIV should not be exceptionalised as an STI, and STI transmission, whether reckless or intentional, should be treated as a public health matter alone, may continue to criticise the extant legal framework in the UK and many other countries.[118]

7.7 DOCTORS, HEALTH, AND PUBLIC SECURITY

Political violence is all around us and the doctor cannot wholly dissociate themself from this; society occasionally demands questionable practices from its doctors. An international attempt to define their position can be found in the Declaration of Tokyo,[119] last revised in 2016, which shows well the difficulties of operationalising ethical codes—definitions of principle can only be interpreted in the mind of the individual. The Declaration's first guideline states:

> The physician shall not countenance, condone or participate in the practice of torture or other forms of cruel, inhuman or degrading procedures, whatever the offense of which the victim of such procedures is suspected, accused or guilty, and whatever the victim's beliefs or motives, and in all situations, including armed conflict and civil strife.[120]

But who is to define a degrading procedure? Is it self-evident that the well-being of an indiscriminate terrorist bomber is as valuable as that of his potential victim? Given that unethical physiological measures are used in detention and interrogation,[121] might it not be that a doctor's presence, although disapproving, could be to the benefit of the subject? And, one might ask, by what right can the doctor command complete clinical independence when, in some circumstances, they may be ignorant of the widespread affect their decision may have on others?[122] The motivation of the Declaration of Tokyo is impeccable in condemning the excesses of politically motivated punishment and torture, but it fails in its general purpose because it was drafted with that rather narrow end in view.[123]

There has always been something of an uneasy truce between doctors and the police as to confidentiality. The anxiety engendered here has been summed up:

> Although doctors in general wish to cooperate with the police, they must be sure that any information divulged in confidence will not be used in court unless they are aware at the time of interview that that information might be so used.[124]

---

[118] Matthew Weait, 'Limit Cases: How and Why We Can and Should Decriminalise HIV Transmission, Exposure, and Non-Disclosure' (2019) 27(4) Medical Law Review 576.

[119] The spirit of the Declaration of Tokyo is also expressed in the United Nations Declaration of Human Rights, Art 5 and, domestically, in the Human Rights Act 1998, Sch 1, Art 3 which allows for no derogation.

[120] World Medical Association, 'WMA Declaration of Tokyo – Guidelines for Physicians Concerning Torture and Other Cruel, Inhuman or Degrading Treatment or Punishment in Relation to Detention And Imprisonment' (2016) available at <https://www.wma.net/policies-post/wma-declaration-of-tokyo-guidelines-for-physicians-concerning-torture-and-other-cruel-inhuman-or-degrading-treatment-or-punishment-in-relation-to-detention-and-imprisonment/> accessed 08 November 2022.

[121] For which there is considerable evidence: Derek Summerfield, 'Fighting "Terrorism" with Torture' (2003) 326(7393) BMJ 773.

[122] Sophie Arie, 'Doctors Need Better Training to Recognise and Report Torture' (2011) 343 BMJ d5766.

[123] Peter Polatin, Jens Modvig, and Therese Rytter, 'Helping to Stop Doctors Becoming Complicit in Torture' (2010) 340 BMJ c973.

[124] The problem is discussed further in Chapter 11.

At times, medical authorities will agree access arrangements to govern requests from the police for sight of patient information,[125] but the default position, both with respect to physical samples and patient data, is that an appropriate court order should be sought and served before any access is given.

However, the impact of human rights law has to be fed into such equations, as demonstrated by *S and Marper v United Kingdom*.[126] Here the European Court of Human Rights held that the blanket policy in England and Wales of retaining DNA profiles and samples indefinitely when taken from persons without their consent and who had not been convicted of a crime was an unjustified breach of their human rights. Mere retention, even without use, was held to be an interference with the right to respect for private life because of the possible implications that future uses could have for individuals. While a lawful policy for obtention and retention could be developed, it must be proportionate to the pressing social need under scrutiny (pursuant to the three-part test articulated previously). As a result of *Marper* and other cases, the Protection of Freedoms Act 2012 was enacted. It should ensure that more than a million innocent persons' samples and data are removed from the database, and that future samples taken on arrest for a minor offence are destroyed where there is no charge or conviction.[127] Since then, it has been held that the police policy of retaining indefinitely materials and data obtained from adults convicted of a recordable offence, though an interference with Article 8 ECHR, was, bearing all factors in mind, both justified and proportionate, and within the margin of appreciation extended to domestic authorities.[128]

The professional relationship between doctors and the police in England and Wales is, to a large extent, dictated by the Police and Criminal Evidence Act 1984. As regards confidentiality, the British Medical Association (BMA)—and other interested groups— succeeded in protecting medical records from the powers of police search by having them classified as 'excluded material'.[129] The doctor, however, remains the holder of the records and is entitled to disclose them if they so wish;[130] on the other hand, in the absence of a court order, they may withhold them even in the face of serious crime.[131] Quite clearly, the law and the professions will, when possible, take a pragmatic approach which includes consideration of the community's interests.[132] As to searches, the BMA agreed with those politicians who regarded the legal permit to make searches as 'an

---

[125] NHS England, 'Transformation Directorate – Sharing Information With the Police' (2022) available at <https://transform.england.nhs.uk/information-governance/guidance/sharing-information-with-the-police/> accessed 08 November 2022.

[126] *S and Marper v United Kingdom* (2009) 48 EHRR 50.

[127] For more serious offences, those charged but not convicted will have samples retained for three years with a single extension period of two further years (on application to a district judge): Part 1 of the 2012 Act, amending Part 5 of the Police and Criminal Evidence Act 1984.

[128] *Re Gaughran's Application for Judicial Review* [2015] UKSC 29.

[129] Police and Criminal Evidence Act 1984, ss 11 and 12.

[130] *R v Singleton* [1995] 1 Cr App R 431. Section 29 of the Data Protection Act 1998 permits the use or disclosure of 'personal data' for the purposes of prevention or detection of crime or the prosecution or apprehension of offenders without observing the normal formalities of the Act (such as informing the subject of any such use or disclosure).

[131] *R v Cardiff Crown Court, ex parte Kellam* (1993) 16 BMLR 76. Evans LJ made this ruling 'with considerable reluctance'.

[132] In *HM Advocate v Kelly* (2001)—an unreported Scottish High Court case of reckless exposure to HIV infection—the police were allowed to breach the anonymity and confidentiality of a research project involving prisoners in order to trace the strain of virus involved. Sheila Bird and Andrew Leigh Brown, 'Criminalisation of HIV Transmission: Implications for Public Health in Scotland' (2001) 323(7322) BMJ 1174; James Chalmers, 'The Criminalisation of HIV Transmission' (2002) 28(3) Journal of Medical Ethics 160.

oppressive and objectionable new statutory power [which was] a serious affront to a person's liberty'.[133] Many others would consider hard drug peddling, with its potential catastrophic effect on people of all ages, as being a crime which merits draconian preventive methods. In the event, the 1984 Act retained the legal right of the authorities to ask for an intimate search, and/or for the taking of an intimate sample, but stipulated that the latter must be performed by a medical practitioner or a registered nurse.[134] This is now modified further by the provisions of the 2012 Act, discussed earlier.

7.8 CONCLUSION

While the human rights paradigm has been important to public health (and medical law more generally), at least from a constitutive perspective, it has not led to social justice being fully realised. Public health practice has been accused of leaving unaltered the marginalisation of women's health, ethnic minorities, those living in deprived areas of the UK, not to mention the health of those in developing countries.[135] We saw how the Covid-19 pandemic disproportionately impacted those from already-marginalised communities in the UK. We also saw some examples of UK-wide success, such the development and roll-out of Covid-19 vaccines. This chapter explored how the pandemic led to both the temporary use of emergency public health powers, as well as in some cases the permanent creation of new bodies, powers, and policies to better address future public health emergencies, as well as to better promote the UK population's health over the coming years. These are necessarily political exercises that engender deep questions about the role of the state and the appropriate balance to be struck between the betterment of collective health and respect for individual autonomy and liberty. Some have argued that public health is in need of a greater, more principled, theoretical, and moral foundation if it ever hopes to meet practical needs while also realising human rights and achieving global health justice.[136] In the UK, our concern is that disproportionate weight will be accorded to individualistic notions of autonomy and concepts of self-responsibilisation, which undermine public health actions and collective well-being, not to mention the role of solidarity, charity, and goodwill in our society. Autonomy is undoubtedly an important consideration, but it remains just one value of several that underpins and informs this discipline, especially in public health. As this chapter has shown, collective interests and more communitarian values must also enter the fray.[137]

---

[133] William Russell, 'Intimate Body Searches—For Stilettos, Explosive Devices, et al.' (1983) 286 BMJ 733.

[134] Section 62(9) as amended by the Criminal Justice and Police Act 2001, s 80. There have been a number of amendments to the 1984 Act which include increased powers of the police to retain samples and records in certain circumstances even if the donor was acquitted. These have survived a challenge: *R (on the application of S) v Chief Constable of South Yorkshire* [2004] 4 All ER 193 (HL). Comparable powers are available in Scotland under the Criminal Procedure (Scotland) Act 1995, ss 18 and 19 or by obtaining a sheriff warrant. Further amendments, similar to those in England, are contained in the Criminal Justice (Scotland) Act 2003, Part 8.

[135] Marie Fox and Michael Thomson, 'Realising Social Justice in Public Health Law' (2013) 21(2) Medical Law Review 278.

[136] Jennifer Prah Ruger, 'Good Medical Ethics, Justice and Provincial Globalism' (2015) 41(1) Journal of Medical Ethics 103; Angus Dawson, 'Ebola: What it Tells us About Medical Ethics' (2015) 41(1) Journal of Medical Ethics 107.

[137] Richard Ashcroft, 'Could Human Rights Supersede Bioethics?' (2010) 10(4) Human Rights Law Review 639.

FURTHER READING

1. Rebecca Brown, Hannah Maslen, and Julian Savulescu, 'Against Moral Responsibilisation of Health: Prudential Responsibility and Health Promotion' (2019) 12(2) Public Health Ethics 114–129.

2. John Coggon, 'Lord Sumption and the Values of Life, Liberty and Security: Before and Since the COVID-19 Outbreak' (2021) 48(10) Journal of Medical Ethics, 779–784.

3. John Coggon, *What Makes Health Public? A Critical Evaluation of Moral, Legal, and Political Claims in Public Health* (CUP 2012).

4. Patrick Diamond and Martin Laffin, 'The United Kingdom and the Pandemic: Problems of Central Control And Coordination' (2022) 48(2) Local Government Studies 211–231.

5. Nicola Glover-Thomas, 'The Vaccination Debate in the UK: Compulsory Mandate Versus Voluntary Action in the War Against Infection' (2019) 7(1) Journal of Medical Law and Ethics 49–73.

6. Nick Phin, 'Public Health Scotland – the First Year: Successes and Lessons' (2021) 51(S1) Journal of the Royal College of Physicians of Edinburgh S34–39.

7. John Coggon, Keith Syrett, and Adrien Viens, *Public Health Law: Ethics, Governance, and Regulation* (Routledge 2016).

8

CONSENT TO MEDICAL TREATMENT

8.1 INTRODUCTION

Based on the strong moral conviction that everyone has the right of self-determination with regard to their body, the common law has long recognised the principle that every person has the right to have their bodily integrity protected against invasion by others.[1] Only in certain narrowly defined circumstances may this integrity be compromised without the individual's consent—as where, for example, physical intrusion is involved in the carrying out of lawful arrest. In general, however, a non-consensual touching by another may—subject to the principle *de minimis non curat lex*—give rise to a civil action for damages or, in theory at least, constitute a criminal assault.[2] Consent from the patient can render physical invasion lawful, but the reality of such consent may be closely scrutinised by the law and is subject to policy limitations. For example, consent will not normally render legitimate a serious physical injury.

Theory, then, is quite simple—the reality is somewhat different. Much jurisprudence in common law countries has focused on the issue of consent and, as a result, the so-called doctrine of 'informed consent' has assumed a significant role in the medical negligence debate. As a general rule, medical treatment, including physical examination, should not proceed unless the doctor has first obtained the patient's consent.[3] This may be expressed or it may be implied, as it is when the patient presents themself to the doctor for examination and acquiesces in the normal routine.

In this chapter, we consider the contours of consent in relation to medical treatment. We begin by focusing on the function of consent and the consequences of failing to obtain it. We then consider what constitutes informed consent for the purposes of medical treatment, with a focus on the nature of information which must be disclosed to a patient to secure this. Finally, we address circumstances where medical treatment may proceed even in the absence of consent.

---

[1] This is also a human rights issue: per *YF v Turkey* [2004] 39 EHRR 34, the physical and psychological integrity of the person is protected by Art 8 European Convention on Human Rights (ECHR), and compulsory medical intervention is an interference with this right irrespective of whether 'consent' has been obtained. It falls, therefore, to the state to justify any such interference under Art 8(2).

[2] In practice, this is unlikely, although possible, particularly when the supposed assault includes an element of indecency or maliciousness. See e.g. *R v Manish Shah* [2020] EWCA Crim 1676.

[3] 'Physical contact which is generally acceptable in the ordinary conduct of daily life' will not constitute an offence. See *Collins v Wilcock* [1984] 3 All ER 374 [376].

8.2 THE FUNCTION OF CONSENT

At a basic level, it is a patient's consent which allows medical treatment to proceed, both from a legal and ethical perspective. Concerning the latter, consent is intended to ensure that what happens to a patient's body is in line with their autonomous wishes, and reflective of the choices they have made.

Legally, failure to obtain such consent entitles the patient to sue for damages for the battery that is committed. As such, consent also functions as a defence to a bodily invasion. It is also possible to base a claim in negligence, the theory being that the doctor has been negligent in failing to obtain appropriate consent (and this is discussed in detail going forward; see also discussion in Chapter 12). A lack of consent may also constitute an interference with a patient's human rights and, as such, may give rise to claims under the Human Rights Act 1998. As the European Court of Human Rights stated in *Pretty v UK*:

> In the sphere of medical treatment, the refusal to accept a particular medical treatment might, inevitably, lead to a fatal outcome, yet the imposition of medical treatment, without the consent of a mentally competent adult, would interfere with a person's physical integrity in a manner capable of engaging the rights protected under Article 8.1 of the [European Convention on Human Rights].[4]

An action for battery (or assault in Scots law) arises when the claimant (or pursuer) has been touched in some way by the defendant and when there has been no consent, express or implied, to such touching. All they need establish in such an action is that the defendant (or defender) wrongfully touched them; it is unnecessary to establish some form of loss as a result of it, although the degree of harm suffered can speak to the measure of award the claimant will receive. The motive of the aggressor is irrelevant; it does not matter whether the touching is designed to 'help' the person. This broad definition means that every touching of a patient by way of medical treatment is potentially a battery, as classically expressed by Cardozo J:

> Every human being of adult years and sound mind has a right to determine what shall be done with his own body; and a surgeon who performs an operation without the patient's consent commits an assault.[5]

By contrast, in an action based in negligence, the claimant/pursuer must establish (1) that the defendant/defender wrongfully touched them, and (2) that the negligence of the defendant in touching them without consent has led to the injury (for which damages are sought). Usually, the injury is related to the manifestation of an inherent risk in the medical procedure itself. As discussed further, it may be significantly difficult to demonstrate factual causation in the latter case, and, for this reason, the action for battery/assault may be the easier option for the claimant/pursuer. The measure of damages recoverable will also be different. All direct damages are recoverable in battery, whereas only those which are foreseeable and for which it is fair and just to compensate may be recovered in an action for negligence. Thus, an unforeseen medical complication arising from the procedure in question may give rise to something for which damages are recoverable in battery but not in negligence.

An action for battery/assault is appropriate where there has been no consent at all to the physical contact in question. An obvious example would be if a patient has refused

---

[4] *Pretty v UK* (2002) 66 BMLR 147 (ECtHR) [63].
[5] *Schloendorff v Society of New York Hospital* 105 NE 92 (NY 1914).

to submit to a procedure but the doctor has, nevertheless, gone ahead in the face of that refusal. Two historic Canadian cases illustrate the typical circumstances. Actions for battery were sustained in *Mulloy v Hop Sang*,[6] where the claimant's hand was amputated without his consent, and in *Schweizer v Central Hospital*,[7] where the claimant had consented to an operation on his toe, but the surgeon performed an operation on his back. Apparent in both cases is that what the doctor *actually* did was quite unconnected with the procedure to which the patient had consented. Therefore, they lay within the courts' policy of restricting battery actions to acts of unambiguous hostility. However, it is not necessary for the claimant/pursuer to prove that the defendant acted with 'hostility'. Rather, the patient must prove that the defendant/defender doctor carried out a medical treatment or procedure involving intentional contact with the patient without their valid consent (or that of another person authorised by law to consent on their behalf) or other lawful authority.[8]

A claim based on negligence is apt when consent has been given to an act of the general nature of that which is performed, but there is a flaw in this consent, meaning it had not been given to certain features of the act (for example, where the patient was not made aware of a particular risk). In *Chatterton v Gerson,* the Court emphasised that an action for trespass to the person is inappropriate once the patient is informed in 'broad terms' of the nature of the procedure and consent is given; an action for negligence is the proper remedy if there is a failure to disclose risks.[9] However, this does not mean an action in assault or battery is entirely irrelevant to health and medical law. Indeed, where a healthcare professional undertakes the agreed procedure but acts outwith the terms of a given consent, they may be liable to action in assault. For example, surgeon Simon Bramhall was convicted of two counts of assault because he marked his initials on the transplanted livers of two patients with an argon beam coagulator.[10]

Equally, where dishonesty is involved in securing consent, an action in assault or battery may also be appropriate. Those who pose as a qualified medical practitioner and elicit consent on this basis will be guilty of criminal assault.[11] A qualified practitioner who deceives patients may similarly be guilty of an offence. In *Appleton v Garrett*,[12] the High Court awarded both exemplary and aggravated damages against a dentist who had actively deceived patients as to their need for treatment over a number of years. Any consent offered by the patients was vitiated by the fraudulent misrepresentation of the defendant doctor. The Court held that information had been deliberately withheld and the defendant had acted throughout in bad faith, making an action in battery, rather than in negligence, appropriate. Similarly, in *R v Paterson*, the Court of Appeal made clear that because the doctor knew that the treatment he advised and undertook on his patients was one that no responsible body of breast surgeons would have advised (i.e. did not accord with the *Bolam* standard), he had deceived his patients as to the true position and vitiated their consent to the procedures.[13] This having been said, there need not be a nefarious purpose behind the touching for an assault to be committed.[14] However, only notional damages are likely to be awarded in such cases in recognition of the affront to bodily integrity that the unauthorised touching represents.

---

[6] [1935] 1 WWR 714.   [7] [1974] 53 DLR (3d) 494.   [8] *Re F* [1989] 2 All ER 545.
[9] [1981] QB 432.
[10] *The General Medical Council and another v Simon Bramhall* [2021] EWHC 2109 (Admin).
[11] See *R v Tabassum* [2000] Lloyd's Rep Med 404; *R v Melin (Ozan)* [2019] EWCA Crim 557. On the role of deception, see *R v Jheeta (Harvinder Singh)* [2008] 1 WLR 2582.
[12] (1995) 34 BMLR 23.   [13] [2022] EWCA Crim 456, [33].
[14] *B v NHS Hospital Trust* [2002] 2 All ER 449. £100 in token damages was awarded.

8.3 STANDARDS OF CARE AND INFORMED CONSENT

Having set out the basics of consent, we now turn to the elements of 'informed consent', where much discussion centres in this area. The concept of informed consent remains a classic example of the importation of a healthcare philosophy from the United States, but its journey has, in fact, been remarkably slow. Its first mention in the English courts seems to have been as late as 1981,[15] whereas the seed was sown in the United States in the 1957 case of *Salgo*.[16] Here, the Court concluded that the doctor had a duty to disclose to the patient 'any facts which are necessary to form the basis of an intelligent consent by the patient to the proposed treatment'.[17] It is perhaps unfortunate that the original terminology 'intelligent consent' was replaced, in a later passage related to therapeutic privilege, by:

> In discussing the element of risk, a certain amount of discretion must be employed consistent with full disclosure of facts necessary to an *informed* consent. [Emphasis added.][18]

Informed consent introduced a new element to medical treatment. It is no longer a simple matter of consent to a technical assault; consent must now be based on a knowledge of the nature, risks, consequences, and alternatives associated with the proposed therapy.

8.3.1 WHAT INFORMATION NEEDS TO BE DISCLOSED?

Looked at from the ethical point of view, the matter is again one of self-determination.[19] A person should not be exposed to a risk of harm unless they have agreed to run that risk. And, importantly, they cannot properly agree to—or make a choice between—risks in the absence of relevant factual information. The twin problems to be resolved are, therefore, (1) by what general standard should the information be judged and, within that, (2) to what extent must or should particular details be divulged?

The general standards available are conveniently described as the 'patient standard' and the 'professional standard'. Beginning with the patient standard, this can be further divided into subjective or objective versions. The first involves a purely subjective judgement—that is, what would that particular patient have considered to be adequate information? The extreme of this school of thought would hold that, faced with a rational patient, the doctor must reveal all the relevant facts as to what they intend to do. It is not for them to determine what the patient should or should not hear. Such a standard is clearly open to the abuse of hindsight; it would be only too easy for a patient, once they have suffered damage, to allege that they would not have given their consent to a procedure when, in reality, they may well have been quite prepared to do so, even with full knowledge of the risks entailed. The subjective standard is weighted overwhelmingly in favour of the claimant and has not been adopted by UK courts.

The objective patient standard, often called the 'prudent patient' test, considers how much information the 'reasonable patient' would wish to know. This, as with all objective tests, has the disadvantage of being potentially unfair to the claimant. There may be

---

[15] *Chatterton* (n 9).
[16] *Salgo v Leland Stanford Junior University Board of Trustees* 317 P 2d 170 (Cal, 1957).
[17] ibid. (Bray J).   [18] ibid.
[19] For stringent criticism from the ethical perspective, see Neil Manson and Onora O'Neill, *Rethinking Informed Consent in Bioethics* (CUP 2007).

222 CONSENT TO MEDICAL TREATMENT

specific circumstances that are unique to the individual and it may well be that because of these, they genuinely would wish to know certain potential effects treatment would have on them. To apply the objective standard might, then, be equally unsatisfactory: 'if it is Utopian to think one must concentrate on the particular patient, the law should surely be aiming at Utopia'.[20] The prudent patient test has practical value in that judges are, themselves, potential patients, and therefore can assess the standard at first hand rather than by proxy. Yet at the same time, this potentially introduces the element of personal prejudice.

A third compromise position possibility exists. The court may opt for an objective approach but qualify it by investing the hypothetical reasonable patient with the relevant special peculiarities of the individual claimant. In this way the edge is taken off the objective test, while the pitfalls of the purely subjective approach are avoided. Obviously, there must be some assessment of whether risk is or is not significant but, apart from the exclusion of irrelevant material, the patient should be as fully informed as possible so that they can make up their mind in the light of all the relevant circumstances.

As further elaborated later in this chapter, the UK Supreme Court judgment in *Montgomery* v *Lanarkshire Health Board* has now established that the law of consent to medical treatment follows this third approach:

> An adult person of sound mind is entitled to decide which, if any, of the available forms of treatment to undergo, and her consent must be obtained before treatment interfering with her bodily integrity is undertaken. The doctor is therefore under a duty to take reasonable care to ensure that the patient is aware of any material risks involved in any recommended treatment, and of any reasonable alternative or variant treatments. The test of materiality is whether, in the circumstances of the particular case, a reasonable person in the patient's position would be likely to attach significance to the risk, or the doctor is or should reasonably be aware that the particular patient would be likely to attach significance to it.[21]

In the subsequent case of *Thefaut* v *Johnston*, the Court noted that doctors must communicate material risk to patients, including reasonable alternatives or variants; the test of materiality comprises a mixture of subjective and objective elements:

> It is common ground between counsel in the present case that the test is a mixture of the subjective and the objective. Logically, and as a matter of policy, it cannot be wholly subjective because this would engage liability in favour of a patient who was irrational or wildly eccentric yet genuine. The test whether '. . . in the circumstances of the particular case, a reasonable person in the patient's position would be likely to attach significance to the risk', combines subjectivity with objectivity.[22]

Rather than 'bombarding the patient with technical information which 'they could not be expected to grasp', the Supreme Court in *Montgomery* emphasised the importance of 'dialogue' between the doctor and patient, requiring a discussion of risks and benefits of the proposed treatment, as well as the reasonable alternatives.[23] Picking up on this point in *Thefaut,* Green J went on to observe:

> No doubt, in this day and age, dialogue can occur, for example, face to face, or by skype, or over the phone. A patient who suffers from a disability or who is abroad may engage in a perfectly adequate 'dialogue' via electronic means. The issue is not so much the <u>means</u>

---

[20]   Kenneth Norrie, 'Informed Consent and the Duty of Care' [1985] Scots Law Times 289.
[21]   *Montgomery* v *Lanarkshire Health Board* [2015] UKSC 11 [87].
[22]   *Thefaut* v *Johnston* [2017] EWHC 497 [54].   [23]   *Montgomery* (n 21) [90].

of communication but its <u>adequacy</u>. Mr Peacock used the apt expression 'adequate time and space' to describe the characteristics of a 'dialogue' that satisfied the test in law . . . The second point arising from paragraph [90] is the need to de-jargonise communications to ensure that the message is conveyed in a comprehensible manner.[24][Emphasis in original]

This third compromise approach to the patient standard most fully satisfies the requirements of self-determination but can be criticised on the grounds that it leaves little scope for the exercise of clinical judgement by the doctor. It is for this reason that even those most dedicated to patient autonomy will allow the doctor—in certain circumstances— the 'therapeutic privilege' to withhold information which would merely serve to distress or confuse the patient.

The concept of therapeutic privilege was also imported from the US by the House of Lords in *Sidaway*[25] and remains valid under qualified terms following *Montgomery*, as per Lord Kerr and Lord Reed:

> The doctor is however entitled to withhold from the patient information as to a risk if he reasonably considers that its disclosure would be seriously detrimental to the patient's health. The doctor is also excused from conferring with the patient in circumstances of necessity, as for example where the patient requires treatment urgently but is unconscious or otherwise unable to make a decision. It is unnecessary for the purposes of this case to consider in detail the scope of those exceptions . . . [I]t is important that the therapeutic exception should not be abused. It is a limited exception to the general principle that the patient should make the decision whether to undergo a proposed course of treatment: it is not intended to subvert that principle by enabling the doctor to prevent the patient from making an informed choice where she is liable to make a choice which the doctor considers to be contrary to her best interests.[26]

GMC and British Medical Association guidance (see **Table 8.1**) similarly advises that therapeutic privilege should be treated with a high degree of caution.

The concession applies only to specific items selected by the doctor for specific reasons. It does, however, go beyond the alternative approach to disclosure of information—that

Table 8.1 Professional guidance on the use of therapeutic privilege

General Medical Council[27]	*British Medical Association*[28]
In very exceptional circumstances you may feel that sharing information with a patient would cause them serious harm and, if so, it may be appropriate to withhold it. In this context 'serious harm' means more than that the patient might become upset, decide to refuse treatment, or choose an alternative. This is a limited exception and you should seek legal advice if you are considering withholding information from a patient.	There is some limited scope for doctors to withhold information where they have a reasonable belief that providing the information would cause the patient serious harm. The Supreme Court has made clear, however, that this exception should not be abused; it is designed to protect patients from serious harm, not to prevent them from making a choice the doctor considers to be contrary to their best interests.

[24] *Thefaut* (n 22) [58]–[59].
[25] *Sidaway* v *Board of Governors of the Bethlem Royal Hospital* [1985] AC 871.
[26] *Montgomery* (n 21) [88], [91].   [27] GMC, 'Decision Making and Consent' (2020), para 15.
[28] BMA, 'Seeking patient consent toolkit' (2019), 8.

is, one based solely on the professional standard. Here, counselling and informing are regarded as an integral part of clinical management; the extent and detail of the information supplied is a matter for decision by the doctor, subject to the same standard of duty of care as when prescribing or operating. It follows that, whichever standard is adopted, litigation based on inadequate information must be undertaken in the tort or delict of negligence.[29] Any difference lies in the test to be applied. Given a patient standard, the quality of information will be judged from the viewpoint of the prudent—or, in one formulation, the particular—patient; under the professional standard, it will be that of the prudent doctor.

The choice between a 'patient standard' and a 'professional standard' is a difficult one for the healthcare professional. There must be respect for the patient's legitimate interest in knowing to what they are subjecting themselves but, at the same time, there may be cases where a paternalistic approach is appropriate. In addition, the practicalities of the situation must be borne in mind. Although it might be ethically desirable for patients to be as fully informed as possible, the time spent in explaining the intricacies of procedures could be considerable, particularly if a doctor is expected to deal with remote risks. It has also long been pointed out that adherence to a professional standard provides a coherent body of principles;[30] courts that are subject to this standard are, therefore, at least less likely to be inconsistent in their adjudication of disputes.

A final point about the nature of the doctrine of informed consent relates to patient understanding. The focus of the concept is on information given to the patient, which is provided with the objective of furthering their autonomy. But the consequent implication is that all a doctor needs do to fulfil their duty of care is provide that information. Such a narrow interpretation ignores consideration of the patient's ability to assimilate and analyse the information they receive.[31] If it is not also part of the doctor's duty to ensure at least a degree of understanding on the part of the patient, they can discharge their duty by offering information in a way that results in no enhancement of the patient's autonomy—the ethical basis of the doctrine is, accordingly, undermined. An overly technical explanation of a procedure might involve lots of information, but equally may do little to advance autonomous decision-making.

Take consent forms, for example. It is a fallacy to make consent forms longer and more detailed in an attempt to meet the requirements of the law, for at least two reasons. First, this is likely to hinder rather than promote patient understanding, and second, because a signed consent form has, in any case, no binding validity. It merely serves as *some* evidence that consent has been obtained, but this can always be rebutted if contrary evidence demonstrates that the patient was uncomprehending and did not truly provide their voluntary assent. This was confirmed by *Williamson* v *East London and the City Health Authority*.[32] The surgeon maintained that she had explained that an extensive breast operation might be likely, but the claimant did not accept that she was told this before the operation. The form that was signed related to silicon replacement but was subsequently altered to read 'Bilateral replacement. Breast prosthesis. Right subcutaneous mastectomy'. There was no evidence that the patient had re-signed the form or initialled the amendments. The judge was satisfied that, on the balance of probabilities, the surgeon did not properly or sufficiently explain her intention to alter the operation.

---

[29] See Chapter 12 for a more detailed discussion of the conduct of clinical negligence litigation.

[30] Christopher Newdick, 'The Doctor's Duties of Care Under *Sidaway*' (1985) 36 Northern Ireland Legal Quarterly 243.

[31] Matthew Falagas et al., 'Informed Consent: How Much and What do Patients Understand?' (2009) 198(3) American Journal of Surgery 420; Tomasz Pietrzykowski and Katarzyna Smilowska, 'The Reality of Informed Consent: Empirical Studies on Patient Comprehension—Systematic Review' (2021) 22 Trials 57.

[32] (1998) 41 BMLR 85.

Table 8.2 GMC Guidance on decision-making and consent: Finding out what matters to a patient

---

16. You must listen to patients and encourage them to ask questions.

17. You should try to find out what matters to patients about their health—their wishes and fears, what activities are important to their quality of life, both personally and professionally—so you can support them to assess the likely impact of the potential outcomes for each option.

18. You must seek to explore your patient's needs, values and priorities that influence their decision making, their concerns and preferences about the options and their expectations about what treatment or care could achieve.[33]

The appropriate conclusion to draw from this is that consent must be seen as a process of communication and not as a one-off event. It requires a 'partnership' between the doctor and patient in reaching a decision that is right for the patient in their circumstances—a process that is now seen as 'shared decision-making'.[34] This largely reflects the tenor of detailed guidance from the Department of Health and Social Care,[35] the BMA,[36] and the GMC[37] as to what patients should be told in order to obtain valid consent, with the latter guidance illustrated in **Table 8.2**.

8.3.2 THE STANDARD OF CARE CASES

The UK Supreme Court ruling in *Montgomery* confirmed that doctors have a legal duty to advise patients of any material risks involved in a recommended treatment, and also of any reasonable alternative treatments.[38] The law in the UK has, however, not always given a clear steer on what is legally required of doctors. Whatever standpoint one takes on information disclosure, a decision of some court can be found which will endorse one's preferred approach. Within the Commonwealth, there are decisions ranging from the endorsement of the deliberate medical lie, to the acceptance of the extreme patient-orientated approach which emphasises complete disclosure of risk. Nevertheless, it is worth reiterating the reasons given in favour of a shift from the professional standard to the patient standard as set out in an US case in which the onus was transferred.[39] These included:

   (i) that conditions other than those that are purely medical will influence the patient's decision;

  (ii) that following the whim of the physician is inconsistent with the patient's right to self-determination; and

 (iii) that the professional standard smacks of anachronistic paternalism.

---

[33] ibid. paras 16–18.

[34] Erica Spatz, Harlan Krumholz, and Benjamin Moulton, 'The New Era of Informed Consent: Getting to a Reasonable-Patient Standard Through Shared Decision Making' (2016) 315(19) Journal of the American Medical Association 2063.

[35] Department of Health and Social Care, 'Reference Guide to consent for Examination or Treatment' (2nd edn) (04 August 2009) available at <https://www.gov.uk/government/publications/reference-guide-to-consent-for-examination-or-treatment-second-edition> accessed 01 September 2022.

[36] BMA (n 28).   [37] GMC (n 27).   [38] *Montgomery* (n 21).

[39] *Largey* v *Rothman* 540 A 2d 504 (NJ 1988). The prudent patient standard was set in *Canterbury* v *Spence* 464 F 2d 772 (DC 1972).

In addition, the court in *Largey* specifically ruled out the criticism that the patient standard obliges the doctor to list every possible complication of the proposed procedure.

The starting point for the UK position is found in the complementary cases of *Hunter v Hanley*[40] in Scotland and *Bolam v Friern Hospital Management Committee*[41] in England, both of which continue to define the essence of 'technical clinical negligence' as we outline in more detail in Chapter 12. For the purposes of the present discussion, the reader need only remember the key *Bolam* dictum: 'a doctor is not negligent if he acts in accordance with a practice accepted at the time as proper by a responsible body of medical opinion'.[42]

Since actions based on lack of consent to medical treatment should be taken in the tort or delict of negligence, it follows that any argument as to what needs to be disclosed in UK medical practice hinges upon whether the *Bolam* principle applies to diagnosis and treatment *and* to the giving of information. For a prolonged period, its applicability was upheld by the UK courts in this area,[43] and the 'acid test' came in the seminal House of Lords decision in *Sidaway*.[44] This concerned a neurosurgeon who had omitted to warn his patient of the 1–2% intrinsic risk of damage to the spinal cord associated with the surgical procedure that he had advised. Although the surgery was performed with proper care and skill, the inherent risk materialised and the claimant suffered injury as a result. A 4:1 majority held that the *Bolam* standard (or a somewhat modified version thereof) was the appropriate legal test, and that the surgeon had acted in accordance with a responsible body of medical opinion when withholding information about the risks involved prior to obtaining Mrs Sidaway's consent to the operation.

Lord Diplock pointed out that the doctrine of 'informed consent' had never formed part of English law, and that disclosure of risks may alarm patients and deter them from undergoing treatments that are—in the expert opinion of the doctor—in their best interests. Decisions on whether to advise patients of inherent risks and the way in which such warnings should be put constituted an exercise of professional skill and judgement, just as any other part of the doctor's comprehensive duty of care to the individual patient. Expert medical evidence should therefore be used to determine the standard of care regarding the provision of information. Others within the majority were prepared to alter the existing law in certain respects. Thus, Lord Bridge held:

> A judge might, in certain circumstances, come to the conclusion that the disclosure of a particular risk was so obviously necessary to an informed choice on the part of the patient that no reasonably prudent medical man would fail to make it.[45]

While Lord Templeman considered that:

> The court must decide whether the information afforded to the patient was sufficient to alert the patient to the possibility of serious harm of the kind in fact suffered.[46]

Lord Scarman, however, delivered what was effectively a dissenting judgment in which he indicated that: 'it was a strange conclusion if our courts should be led to conclude that our law . . . should permit doctors to determine in what circumstances . . . a duty arose to warn'. He found great merit in the US case of *Canterbury v Spence*,[47] in which it was held that, while medical evidence on this matter was not excluded, it was the court which

---

[40] 1955 SLT 213.   [41] [1957] 2 All ER 118.   [42] ibid. (McNair J) [122].
[43] *Chatterton* (n 9); *Hills v Potter* [1983] 3 All ER 716.   [44] *Sidaway* (n 21).
[45] ibid. [900].   [46] ibid. [903].   [47] *Canterbury* (n 39).

determined the extent of, and any breach of, the doctor's duty to inform. Information includes providing a warning. In the Australian case of *F v R*, King CJ specifically instructed that the doctor's duty extends not only to disclosing any real risks in the treatment but also to warning of any real risk that the treatment may prove ineffective.[48]

Two specific aspects of the information issue were confirmed as a result of *Sidaway*. The first is that risks of a certain magnitude must be disclosed. Following *Canterbury*, a risk could be defined as 'material' if a reasonable person in the patient's position, if warned of the risk, would be likely to attach significance to it. Similarly, it is material if the doctor is or should reasonably be aware that the particular patient, if warned of the risk, would be likely to attach significance to it.[49] Quite what that means in relation to chance is impossible to assess and, indeed, generalisations may be *inappropriate* because the test relates to the circumstances of the particular case. Moreover, significance in this field is a function not only of incidence but also of severity; as to incidence, it was agreed in *Sidaway* that a risk of 10% of a stroke resulting—as was established in *Reibl v Hughes*[50]—was one which a doctor should have provided a warning; but non-disclosure was considered proper in Mrs Sidaway's case when the risk of damage to the spinal cord was of the order of 1% or less. We have to admit to some concern that odds longer than 100:1 might be regarded as immaterial in the eyes of the law.[51] A great deal will, however, hang on the *patient's* requirements as expressed by way of questioning and through genuine communication.

Second, *Sidaway* confirmed a legal basis for the 'therapeutic' or 'professional' privilege to withhold information that might be psychologically damaging to the patient. This, again, follows the direction in *Bolam*, in which the judge said in his charge to the jury:

> You may well think that when a doctor is dealing with a mentally sick man and has a strong belief that his only hope of cure is submission to electroconvulsive therapy, the doctor cannot be criticised if he does not stress the dangers, which he believed to be minimal, which are involved in the treatment . . .[52]

As noted, this principle continues to receive judicial recognition[53] and is accepted by the GMC as good medical practice in certain limited circumstances.[54]

It is also clear from *Sidaway* that, by way of exception to this rule, there must be particularly good reasons, which the doctor would have to justify, for failing to answer such questions put to them by the patient puts and, indeed, there may be a strict obligation to do so. Thus, Lord Bridge held in relation to what has since been dubbed the 'reactive duty', albeit obiter, that:

> When questioned specifically by a patient of apparently sound mind about risks involved in a particular treatment proposed, a doctor's duty must, in my opinion, be to answer both truthfully and as fully as the questioner requires.[55]

Elsewhere we have Mason CJ: 'The fact that the patient asked questions revealing concern about the risk would make the doctor aware that this patient did, in fact, attach significance to the risk'[56]—and, hence, affect its materiality; it was certainly this fact which served to turn a 1:14,000 chance of blindness into a risk which it was found negligent not to disclose in the Australian case of *Rogers v Whittaker*.

---

[48] *F v R* (1983) 33 SASR 189. [49] *Rogers* v *Whittaker* (1992) 109 ALR 625 [634] (Mason CJ).
[50] (1980) 114 DLR 3d 1. [51] King JC accepted 200:1 as not being material in *F v R* (n 48).
[52] [1957] 2 All ER 118 [124]; [1957] 1 WLR 582 (McNair J) [590]. [53] *Montgomery* (n 21) [91].
[54] GMC (n 27), para 15. [55] [1985] AC 871 [898]. [56] *Rogers* (n 49) [82].

The House of Lords' approach in *Sidaway* was subject to strong criticism. Reliance on the *Bolam* standard—even with some modifications—appeared paternalistic and increasingly untenable in the face of the current universal acceptance of a patient's right to decide on their own treatment, as evidenced in guidance from the UK Department of Health and the GMC. While appearing to lag behind other jurisdictions,[57] a gradual but definite shift away from the *Bolam* standard in disputes over information disclosure was also occurring in the lower courts in the UK. In *Smith v Tunbridge Wells Health Authority*,[58] for example, the failure of a consultant surgeon to inform a 28-year-old man of impotence and bladder dysfunction following an operation to treat rectal prolapse was held to be negligent, despite medical support for the decision. Indeed, it was considered that disclosure of the risk was the *only* reasonable course of action.

Of particular significance was the Court of Appeal decision in *Pearce v United Bristol Healthcare NHS Trust*,[59] in which an action in negligence was brought by a couple whose child died in utero almost three weeks overdue. The mother had pleaded with the consultant two weeks after her delivery date either to induce the birth or to carry out a Caesarean section, but he advised against it, citing the high risks of induction and the long time for recovery from Caesarean section. He did not disclose the risks of fetal death in the womb as a result of delay in delivery. In deciding whether the consultant was negligent in this regard, the Court endorsed *Sidaway* as the law and accepted *Bolam* as the relevant test, but also followed Lord Bridge's caveat concerning the need to warn of 'significant risks'. Lord Woolf MR considered that Lord Templeman's views in *Sidaway* best summed up the position, whereby the patient was entitled to such information as was needed to make a balanced judgement in the circumstances. Yet Lord Woolf only generated hope in half-measure, for he went on to apply his test to the facts of the case. In doing so, he concluded that there was no 'significant risk' because: 'The doctors called on behalf of defendants did not regard that risk as significant; nor do I'. Moreover, he stated that the consultant could not be criticised when dealing with a distressed patient for not informing her of 'that very, very small additional risk'—one in the order of 0.1–0.2%.[60] In this sense, the risk was 'small' in statistical terms. Even so, there is little doubt that the tenor of debate surrounding these matters was veering to the side of the patient and their right to choose.

Birch v University College London Hospital NHS Foundation Trust concerned a patient who had been informed accurately of the risks involved with catheter angiography and had consented to the procedure, after which she suffered a stroke. The claimant argued that her treating doctor had been negligent in failing to inform her of an alternative, non-invasive procedure with lower or no risks—namely an MRI scan.[61] After expressing concern about the continuing uncertain nature of the law on standards of disclosure in relation to risks associated with medical treatment, Mr Justice Cranston stated:

> If patients must be informed of significant risks it is necessary to spell out what, in practice, that encompasses. In this case the defendant informed the patient of the probabilities, the one per cent, and the nature of the harm of this risk becoming manifest, the stroke. But these were the objectively significant risks associated with the procedure which was performed, the catheter angiogram. Was it necessary for the defendant to go further and to inform Mrs Birch of comparative risk, how this risk compared with that associated with other imaging procedures, in particular MRI? . . . [I]n my judgment there

[57] ibid.; *Reibl* (n 50).   [58] [1994] 5 Med LR 334.   [59] [1999] ECC 167.   [60] *ibid* [174].
[61] [2008] EWHC 2237 (QB).

will be circumstances where consistently with Lord Woolf MR's statement of the law in *Pearce* ... the duty to inform a patient of the significant risks will not be discharged unless she is made aware that fewer, or no risks, are associated with another procedure. In other words, unless the patient is informed of the comparative risks of different procedures, she will not be in a position to give her fully informed consent to one procedure rather than another.[62]

Much of the fate of informed consent was sealed by the House of Lords' decision in *Chester* v *Afshar*.[63] The consensus in the case was that the doctor had not fulfilled his duty to warn the claimant of a low risk inherent in the surgical procedure, which appeared to signify support for patient autonomy. Yet the House of Lords gave the issue of informed consent surprisingly brief treatment; the ruling did not explicitly alter the standard of care and questions regarding the exact threshold level of risk that would trigger the duty to warn were left unanswered.

Further clarity, and a more evident shift away from the *Bolam* standard in risk disclosure, was brought by the ruling in *Montgomery* v *Lanarkshire Health Board*.[64] In this case, a clinical negligence claim was brought by the claimant against her consultant obstetrician in relation to her antenatal care. The claimant had diabetes and was of short stature. As her baby was likely to be larger than average in size, the risk of shoulder dystocia occurring during a vaginal delivery was estimated to be of the order of 9–10%. The claimant had not been apprised of this fact or advised of the alternative of a Caesarean section. In her obstetrician's opinion, providing this information was unnecessary as the likelihood of a grave problem for the baby resulting from shoulder dystocia during vaginal delivery was very small. The risk of a brachial plexus injury in cases of shoulder dystocia was put at around 0.2% and the risk of cerebral palsy at under 0.1%. Furthermore, the obstetrician held the view that it was not generally in the interests of pregnant women to have Caesarean sections.

During labour, the risk of shoulder dystocia materialised and the baby was deprived of oxygen due to compression of the umbilical cord, resulting in serious permanent disabilities. The claim was subsequently brought in Scotland. The Outer House of the Court of Session rejected the contention that there had been a breach of the duty to inform, and this position was upheld on appeal to the Inner House. After close analysis, both Courts held that neither *Pearce* nor *Chester* signified a change in the law as set out by the majority in *Sidaway*. This meant that the relevant rule to be applied was the *Bolam* standard, unless the proposed treatment entailed a substantial risk of grave adverse consequences— in which case there was a legal duty to inform. Applying that test to the facts at hand, it was held that there was no duty to warn the patient of the very small risk of the grave outcome that unfortunately manifested. Furthermore, the claimant had not made any specific enquiries herself as to the risks entailed. The doctor's duty to give full and honest answers was not triggered merely by the expression of general concerns.

On a further appeal, the UK Supreme Court saw the case differently. The position of the majority in *Sidaway* was considered to be 'unsatisfactory', in that it subsumed the doctor's duty to advise the patient of the risks of proposed treatment under the *Bolam* test. Such an approach failed to take account of important social changes that had occurred in the dynamics of the doctor–patient relationship since *Sidaway*. Patients were now widely regarded as persons holding rights, rather than as the passive recipients of the care of the

---

[62] ibid. [74] (Cranston J).
[63] [2004] UKHL 41. Discussed in further detail regarding causation and in Chapter 12.
[64] *Montgomery* (n 21).

medical profession. GMC guidance advocated supporting patient autonomy in medical decision-making. Furthermore, the important legal development of the Human Rights Act 1998 put increased focus on the extent to which the common law reflects fundamental values. In considering these and other factors, the Supreme Court was unanimous in rejecting the continued application of the *Bolam* test in this context.

Subject to refinements by the Court of Appeal in *Pearce* v *United Bristol Healthcare NHS Trust* and the High Court of Australia in *Rogers* v *Whitaker*, the view expressed by Lord Scarman in *Sidaway* now prevails, with the nature of the duty described as being: 'a duty to take reasonable care to ensure that the patient is aware of any material risks involved in any recommended treatment, and of any reasonable alternative or variant treatments.'[65]

The Supreme Court clarified three more matters. First, assessment of materiality of risk cannot be reduced to percentages. It involves a variety of factors besides statistical probability, including the nature of the risk, the effect which its occurrence would have upon the life of the patient, the importance to the patient of the benefits sought to be achieved by the treatment, the alternatives available, and the risks involved in those alternatives. The assessment, therefore, depends on the context and the patient's characteristics. Second, the discharge of the duty to provide information entails a dialogue between doctor and patient so that the patient is able to exercise autonomy in a meaningful way. Bombarding the patient with technical information that they cannot reasonably be expected to grasp is not consistent with this approach. Third, as discussed, while a 'therapeutic privilege' subsists, it is a limited exception, that should not be abused. It is subordinate to the principle that the patient should make the decision whether to undergo a proposed course of treatment; it is not intended to subvert that principle by enabling the doctor to prevent the patient from making an informed choice where they are liable to make a choice which the doctor considers to be contrary to their best interests.

While *Montgomery* gives clear directions to doctors that they must disclose 'material risks' to patients when obtaining consent to treatment, the legal category of 'material risks' remains ambiguous and something of a black box. Perhaps wisely, the Supreme Court has eschewed setting a specific percentage threshold above which risks must be disclosed. At the coalface in healthcare settings, however, the resulting legal uncertainties could prompt doctors to disclose even low inherent risks associated with treatments so as to avoid possible clinical negligence claims.

8.3.3 POST-*MONTGOMERY* CASE LAW

The ratio in *Montgomery* has been applied in number of subsequent cases which cast some light on the risks that will be regarded by courts as material, as well as the way other contextual factors are taken into account. These cases indicate that the *Bolam* test is alive and well when considering aspects of consent to treatment. In *Duce* v *Worcestershire Acute Hospitals NHS Trust*,[66] the claimant underwent a total abdominal hysterectomy and bilateral salpingo-oophorectomy to relieve the symptoms of heavy and painful periods. Following the surgery, she suffered neuropathic post-operative pain and claimed that the doctor had negligently failed to warn her of the risk of developing chronic post-surgical pain (CPSP). At trial, the judge found that the doctor had not been negligent, and, in any event, causation had not been established. The claimant appealed, alleging in part that the judge had failed to consider whether the risk of CPSP was 'material' as per the test in *Montgomery*.

[65] ibid. [87].   [66] [2018] EWCA Civ 1307.

The Court of Appeal noted that the Supreme Court in *Montgomery* highlighted the importance of patient autonomy and the patient's entitlement to make decisions as to whether to incur risks of injury inherent in treatment. That entitlement was held to be 'a fundamental distinction between, on the one hand, the doctor's role when considering possible investigatory or treatment options and, on the other, her role in discussing with the patient any recommended treatment and possible alternatives, and the risks of injury which may be involved.'[67] The former role was said to be 'an exercise of professional skill and judgment: what risks of injury are involved in an operation, for example, is a matter falling within the expertise of members of the medical profession', but the latter role was not so limited, as one cannot leave 'out of account the patient's entitlement to decide on the risks to her health which she is willing to run (a decision which may be influenced by non-medical considerations)'.[68]

The Court held that the application of *Montgomery* involved a two-stage approach: (1) the risks that were (or should have been) known to the clinician, which is a matter falling within the expertise of medical professionals; and (2) whether the patient should have been told about such risks by reference to whether they were material, which is a matter for the court to determine and is therefore not the subject of the *Bolam* test and not something that can be determined by reference to expert evidence alone.[69] The Court rejected the complaint, on the basis that the 'reason that the judge did not address the issue of materiality is that he had found the claim failed at the first hurdle: proof that gynaecologist were or should have been aware of the relevant risks, which is a matter for expert evidence.'[70] The Court went on to state that the 'reasoning is consistent with the *Montgomery* approach—a clinician is not required to warn of a risk of which he cannot reasonably be taken to be aware.'[71]

In *Mills v Oxford University Hospitals NHS Trust*,[72] it is clarified that doctors must advise as to alternative treatments in addition to the risk involved in the treatment proposed, and when a treatment is seen as innovative, the patient must be informed of this. In this case, the claimant underwent brain surgery and suffered a haemorrhage during the course of the operation, which caused him to suffer a stroke in the left anterior cerebral artery territory. The surgical technique—minimally invasive endoscopically assisted technique—was considered novel, still in its evolution, and not well established. The claimant brought a clinical negligence claim for damages, alleging in part that the consultant neurosurgeon employed by the defendant Trust had failed to take reasonable care to ensure that the claimant was aware of the material risks involved in the proposed procedure and/or of any reasonable alternative or variant treatments (in this case, microscopically assisted resection). The court concluded that although the consultant neurosurgeon did not perform the surgery negligently, he breached his duty of care by (a) not offering microscopically assisted resection as an alternative option and (b) not explaining the comparative risks and benefits of these alternative surgical techniques—including, and importantly, that this technique was novel and not well established. The court went on to note that these risks were material and ought to have been disclosed to the patient during the consent process.[73]

Richards and colleagues extend this analysis in the context of innovative treatment to argue that not only do doctors have a duty to disclose material risks to patients, including the novelty and unknown-ness of any innovative treatment, but also a duty to disclose the

---

[67] *Montgomery* (n 21) [83].   [68] ibid. [84].
[69] See also *Kennedy v Frankel* [2019] EWHC 106 (QB).   [70] *Duce* (n 66) [42].
[71] ibid. [43].   [72] [2019] EWHC 936 (QB).   [73] ibid. [201], [203].

rationale underpinning the innovation, which must be unambiguously clinical, to avoid what they term 'trespass by technology'. This term relates to situations in which consent may be vitiated when a doctor fails to inform the patient that the treatment is new and, potentially, also lacks a clear evidence base as to its clinical benefit. The authors indicate it may arise in situations in which a doctor has motivations other than purely clinical considerations behind the provision of any innovative treatment, such as personal and financial profit.[74] The authors argue that while untested in the courts to date, this concept applies well-established trespass principles and is consistent with existing law around medical trespass.

Within the context of information disclosure about alternative treatments, the *Bolam* test is the appropriate standard to be applied. In *Malik v St George's University Hospitals NHS Foundation Trust*, the claimant underwent emergency spinal surgery. The surgery was executed without criticism and the spinal cord was successfully decompressed; however, the claimant's recovery was slow and incomplete. The surgeon recommended further revision decompression surgery, which unfortunately left the claimant with an incomplete paraparesis (i.e. partial paralysis in the legs). As part of the complaint of negligence, an issue was raised as to whether non-surgical alternatives should have been offered and whether the claimant was given the opportunity to give informed consent for the revision surgery. His Honour Judge Blair QC applied a *Bolam* gloss, finding that 'a responsible, competent, and respectable body of skilled spinal surgeons would have reasonably concluded that there were no reasonable alternative treatments available in the context of the parameters and discussion'.[75]

This would suggest that in assessing what is a reasonable alternative, as part of the duty to take reasonable care to ensure a patient is aware of any material risks involved in any recommended treatment, the Court will apply the *Bolam* test, namely would any reasonable body of medical practitioners in that particular field have been aware of and considered reasonable alternative treatments in the case in question. This is the position adopted in Scotland, per the Inner House decision in *McCulloch v Forth Valley Health Board*. In this case, the Court held:

> *Montgomery* was about advising of the risks associated with a proposed course of action, which would of course include the risks if that course of action were not adopted. It does not follow that where a doctor concludes that a course of treatment is not a reasonable option in the circumstances of the patient the duty under *Montgomery* nevertheless arises . . . where the doctor has rejected a particular treatment, not by taking on him or herself a decision more properly left to the patient, but upon the basis that it is not a treatment which is indicated in the circumstances of the case, then the duty does not arise. The doctor may of course, have made an error, but if so the consequences of that error, and an assessment of whether there was negligence, would be assessed on the standard *Hunter* v *Hanley* basis.[76]

---

[74] Bernadette Richards, Mark Taylor, and Susannah Sage Jacobson, 'Consent and Innovation—Embracing the Unknown and Empowering the Patient' in Bernadette Richards, Mark Taylor, and Susannah Sage Jacobson (eds.), *Technology, Innovation and Healthcare: An Evolving Relationship* (Edward Elgar 2022). See also their discussion of the Australian case of *Dean v Phung* [2012] NSWCA 223, in which Basten JA set out four broad principles of trespass drawn from the relevant case law.

[75] *Malik v St George's University Hospitals NHS Foundation Trust* [2021] EWHC 1913 (QB) [93].

[76] *McCulloch v Forth Valley Health Board* [2021] CSIH 21 [40].

Whether this approach aligns with the patient autonomy ethos of *Montgomery* remains an open question.[77]

For its part, the GMC guidance stresses patient autonomy in decision making and consent. It advises doctors that while it would not be reasonable to share every possible risk of harm with a patient, the doctor is expected to tailor the discussion to each individual patient, guided by what matters to them, and share information in a way they can understand.[78] To that end, doctors are expected usually to disclose three categories of risk to patients, each of which may be considered material to the patient:

1. recognised risks of harm that the doctor believes *anyone* in the patient's position would want to know. The doctor is expected to know these already from their professional knowledge and experience;

2. risks of harm and potential benefits that the patient would consider significant for any reason. These will be revealed during the doctor's discussion with the patient about what matters to them; and

3. any risk of serious harm, however unlikely it is to occur.[79]

8.3.4 CAUSATION AND INFORMED CONSENT

Demonstrating that informed consent has not been obtained is not, in and of itself, sufficient to demonstrate negligence; information disclosure cases often turn on the question of causation, and it is this we now turn to discuss. For a claim to be successful, a patient must demonstrate that had they been warned of the risk, they would not have consented to run it, and therefore because they did not know about the risk, the harm (the materialisation of the risk) has been caused by a negligent failure to disclose. The hurdles in demonstrating this are manifold. It may, for example, simply be a question of witness credibility. In both *Smith v Salford Health Authority*[80] and *Smith v Barking, Havering and Brentwood Health Authority*,[81] the courts refused to accept that the claimants would not have proceeded with the respective medical treatment had they been informed of the risks. To be clear, these are not examples of the courts accusing witnesses of lying; rather it is the courts' assessment of the 'facts' of the case that the patients would, on the balance of probabilities, have proceeded with the treatment, even if they had been told of the relevant material risks.[82] Rougier J summed up the situation well when he said: 'It is not integrity which is in question but objectivity.'[83] Or, as a Californian court had it: 'Subjectively he may believe [he would have declined treatment] with the 20/20 vision of hindsight but we doubt that justice will be served by placing the physician in jeopardy of the patient's bitterness and disillusionment.'[84]

In the UK, the complexities have been demonstrated only too well in the House of Lords' decision in *Chester v Afshar*.[85] In this case, the claimant was being treated by the defendant surgeon for serious back pain and failed to disclose a low (1–2%) but serious

---

[77] For a commentary, see Zahra Jaffer and Ruby Reed-Berendt, 'Defining the Boundaries of *Montgomery*: A Scottish Approach' (2022) 38(2) Journal of Professional Negligence 105. As of the time of writing, permission to appeal the case has been granted by the UK Supreme Court.

[78] GMC (n 27), para 22.   [79] ibid., para 23.   [80] (1994) 23 BMLR 137.

[81] [1994] 5 Med LR 285.

[82] See also *Markose v Epsom & St Helier NHS Trust* [2004] EWHC 3130 (QB). For a Scottish equivalent, see *Murray v NHS Lanarkshire Health Board* [2012] CSOH 123.

[83] *Gregory v Pembrokeshire Health Authority* [1989] 1 Med LR 81 [86].

[84] *Cobbs v Grant*, 104 Cal Rptr 505 (1972).   [85] *Chester* (n 63).

risk of nerve damage and paralysis inherent in the surgery to be performed to address such pain. This manifested itself and the patient sued in negligence claiming that had she been informed of the risk, she would not have gone ahead with the operation when she did.[86] However, it was not established at trial, and indeed the claimant did not argue, that she would never have undergone the surgery (and so never have run the risk).[87] Moreover, it was accepted that the risk in question was a constant: it was an integral part of the operation in question; it was irrelevant who performed it or when. Thus, a very important issue arose as to whether it could meaningfully be said as a matter of law that the surgeon *caused* the patient's harm.

Lords Hoffmann and Bingham were adamant and emphatic in their rejection of the claimant's case. For Lord Bingham, the claimant had not met the basic requirements of the 'but for' test—she had not shown that *but for* the failure to warn she would never have undergone surgery.[88] Lord Hoffmann stated, quite simply, that there was no basis on which the claimant could succeed in line with the ordinary principles that applied in the tort of negligence, and he was not convinced that a special rule was needed in the instant case.[89] But it was precisely on this last point that the three remaining members of the bench took issue with their colleagues.[90] While each acknowledged that, indeed, there could not be recovery on the 'standard rules', they argued, variously, that policy, justice, or the particular nature of decisions relating to one's health and well-being called for a departure from those rules. Most significantly, common to their arguments was the view that these negligence actions are essentially concerned with protecting the patient's right to choose—that is, their autonomy. They pointed out that each of their Lordships in *Sidaway* recognised this as the basic legal interest at stake; Lord Walker went as far as to emphasise the importance of the growth of autonomy-based arguments in recent decades as the basis for justifying an outcome in the claimant's favour in the instant case.[91]

Notwithstanding the judgment, however, it does not appear that we are moving towards the recognition of a new tort of infringement of autonomy.[92] This was discussed in the case of *Diamond v Royal Devon and Exeter NHS Foundation Trust*,[93] which also demonstrated the complexities in establishing causation.[94] In this case, the claimant sued in clinical negligence arising out of spinal fusion surgery and subsequent identification and repair of a post-operative abdominal hernia. The patient claimed that, inter alia, the surgeon who performed the abdominal repair failed to obtain informed consent from the patient prior to proceeding with a mesh repair of the hernia. At trial, the judge found the claimant's surgeon to be in breach of duty by reason of his failure to inform the patient of the risks that the mesh repair would present in the event she became pregnant. However, the judge also concluded that, had the claimant had been so informed, she would have chosen to proceed with the mesh repair, which in fact took place.

[86] The breach of the requisite standard of care requiring that the information should have been disclosed was not in doubt.
[87] This contrasts with *Montgomery* (n 21), in which the claimant was able to establish on the balance of probabilities that had she been warned of the risks of shoulder dystocia, she would have requested a caesarean section.
[88] *Chester* (n 63) [8].   [89] Ibid. [32].
[90] A lot of support was drawn from the Australian decision in *Chappel v Hart* [1999] 2 LRC 341; (1998) 72 ALJR 1344, which dealt essentially with the same issue and where there was also division of opinion among the justices.
[91] *Chester* (n 63) [92].
[92] This question was explored in greater detail in John Kenyon Mason, *The Troubled Pregnancy* (CUP 2007). For an argument against recognising such a tort, see Craig Purshouse, 'Liability for Lost Autonomy in Negligence: Undermining the Coherence of Tort Law?' (2015) 22 Torts Law Journal 226.
[93] [2019] EWCA Civ 585.   [94] This is discussed in further detail in Chapter 12.

At the Court of Appeal, the issue turned on consent and any injury or damage caused thereby. It was argued by the appellant that the trial judge had wrongly applied a test of 'rationality' to her decision-making process. Further, the authorities of *Chester* and *Montgomery* supported the proposition that a fundamental purpose of the requirement for properly informed consent was to ensure that respect is given to a patient's autonomy, dignity, and right to self-determination. Such a right included the choice to make decisions that others, including the court, might regard as unwise, irrational, or harmful to their own interests. Conversely, the respondent Trust argued that that the judge did not apply a rationality test in the sense of imposing on the appellant the actions of a hypothetical rational person. Rather, the judge weighed the evidence appropriately and reached a finding of fact about the decision which the appellant would have made as to her preferred method of surgery, if properly advised.

In the leading judgment, Nicola Davies LJ found that the issue of causation defeated the patient's appeal. Her evidence, to the effect that she would not have elected to undergo the mesh repair had she been fully informed of the risks, was not accepted. The Court held that the trial judge had been scrupulous in his assessment of the patient and of her evidence and had considered the clinical facts in the context of her character and circumstances. He had found that the patient genuinely believed that she would have opted for the suture repair had she been provided with the relevant information and that her evidence accorded with that honestly held belief, but that it did not follow that that belief would have been the position at the material time. Thus, he had not applied a single test of 'rationality' to the causation issue. In view of the surgeon's clear opinion as to the non-viability of the suture repair, the evidence before the judge had provided a proper basis for the finding of fact which he made:

> The judge's approach, coupled with his assessment of the appellant [patient] and her evidence, was detailed, nuanced and insightful. It was an assessment that was properly open to him to make on the evidence before the court. The judge met the requirement set out in *Montgomery* in that he took account of the reasonable person in the patient's position but also gave weight to the characteristics of the appellant herself. He did not apply a single test of 'rationality' without more to the issue of causation. No valid criticism of the judge's approach, still less his assessment of the factual evidence can be made. There is no basis for this court to find that there was a material error of law or that a critical finding of fact was made for which there is no evidential basis.[95]

Two aspects are worth highlighting in this judgment. First, as argued by some commentators, the Court appears to have mistakenly applied the materiality test (which is the test to apply in determining a breach of the duty of disclosure, measured by the materiality in both its objective and subjective limbs) to the issue of causation, which deploys the subjective test and is determined by asking and answering the hypothetical question of what the *particular* patient would have done, had they been given the information to which they were entitled.[96] It does not in fact appear the trial judge applied a 'rationality' test, even though this is what the patient argued on appeal and what the Court of Appeal agreed with; rather, the trial judge correctly applied a subjective test,[97] holding

---

[95] ibid. [22].

[96] Joanna Manning, 'Oh What an Unholy Mesh! *Diamond v Royal Devon & Exeter NHS Foundation Trust* [2019] EWCA Civ 585' (2019) 27 Medical Law Review 519.

[97] An approach, we note, that UK and Australian courts have long taken, in contrast with Canadian courts, which since *Reibl v Hughes* have applied a modified objective test. But see Michael Jones, *Medical Negligence* (6th edn, Sweet & Maxwell 2021) at para 7–099, who argues the difference in practice may be smaller.

that patient would have agreed to a mesh repair, given the surgeon's firm advice, and this decision was supported by the fact that it would have been objectively rational in the circumstances, and as the trial judge put it: 'Ms Diamond was not someone who would act irrationally.' Given that in *Montgomery*, the Supreme Court dealt with the question of causation entirely on the basis of the evidence about what *the claimant* would probably have done had she been informed about the material risks, we consider *Diamond* to be an outlier in the informed consent and causation cases. In our view, causation in these types of cases continues to turn not on what a reasonable person in the patient's position would have done, but rather whether the specific individual patient would have proceeded with treatment, if appropriately warned of the risks.

On the question of a new tort of infringement of autonomy, the Court confirmed that breach of the duty of disclosure does *not* create a stand-alone right to damages for infringement of autonomy. As Davies LJ put it, 'It is accepted that the issue has now been determined in *Shaw* v *Kovac* ... and *Duce* v *Worcestershire Acute Hospitals NHS Trust* ... The appellant must show that the breach of duty has caused her to suffer injury.'[98] It remains to be seen whether the Supreme Court or Parliament will ever take up the mantle and recognise the loss of autonomy as on the part of a patient as the basis for recovery of compensation in a clinical negligence action.

8.4 LAWFUL TREATMENT IN ABSENCE OF CONSENT

As mentioned earlier in this chapter, medical treatment should not proceed unless the doctor has first obtained the patient's consent. There are, however, limited circumstances in which a doctor may be entitled to proceed without this consent.

Essentially, these can be subsumed under the heading of 'non-voluntary treatment', which has to be distinguished from 'involuntary treatment'. The latter implies treatment against the patient's expressed wishes; the occasions on which this would be ethical are, indeed, very few, although a case can be made out when the interests of a third party or of society itself are involved. For example, this would include detainment and treatment for a mental disorder under mental health legislation or detainment by a magistrate under public health legislation.[99] Non-voluntary treatment is that which is given when the patient is not in a position (or is in a limited position) to have or to express any views as to their management and these will include, first, when the patient is unconscious; second, when the patient's state of mind is such as to render an apparent consent or refusal invalid, both of which can occur when a patient lacks capacity; and, finally, when the patient is a minor: that is, they lack capacity by virtue of their status (for discussion of minors and consent to treatment, see Chapter 9). We now proceed to discuss the legal position of consent to treatment of adults lacking capacity, beginning with the unconscious patient.

8.4.1 THE UNCONSCIOUS PATIENT

In some circumstances, it is possible to visualise non-voluntary treatment as proceeding with consent, although that consent has not been expressed. Thus, when an unconscious patient is admitted to hospital, the treating clinician may argue that their consent could be implied or presumed on the grounds that if they were conscious, then they would

---

[98] *Diamond* (n 93) [34].   [99] For the former, see Chapter 10.

probably consent to their life being saved in this way.[100] This may be true but, while the majority of patients could be expected to endorse the decision to treat in such circumstances, it is something of a fictitious approach to the problem.

An alternative route is to apply the necessity principle. It is widely recognised in both the criminal and civil law that there are times when acting out of necessity legitimates an otherwise wrongful act. The basis of this doctrine is that acting unlawfully is justified if the resulting good effect materially outweighs the consequences of adhering strictly to the law. In the present context, the doctor is justified, and should not be subject to criminal or civil liability, if the value which they seek to protect is of greater weight than the wrongful act they perform—that is, treating without consent—*and* there is no other means by which the end can be achieved.

Thus, necessity will be a viable defence to any proceedings for non-consensual treatment where an unconscious patient is involved *and* there is no known objection to treatment. The treatment undertaken, however, must not be more extensive than is required by the exigencies of the situation. A doctor cannot, therefore, 'take advantage' of the patient being unconscious to perform procedures which are not essential for the patient's immediate survival or well-being. This was established in two well-known Canadian cases where the courts explored the distinction between procedures that are justified by necessity and those which are merely 'convenient', a distinction which is also applied by the UK courts[101] and recognised by professional bodies.[102]

In the first of these, *Marshall* v *Curry*,[103] the plaintiff sought damages for battery against the defendant surgeon who had removed a testicle in the course of an operation for a hernia. The surgeon's case was that the removal was essential to a successful operation and that, had he not done so, the health and life of the patient would have been imperilled because the testis was, itself, diseased. Taking the view that the doctor had acted 'for the protection of the plaintiff's health and possibly his life', the court held that the removal of the testicle was necessary and that it would have been unreasonable to put the procedure off until a later date.

By contrast, in *Murray* v *McMurchy*,[104] the claimant succeeded in an action for battery against a doctor who had sterilised her without her consent. In this case, the doctor had discovered during a Caesarean section that the condition of the plaintiff's uterus would have made it hazardous for her to go through another pregnancy and he tied the fallopian tubes, although there was no pressing need for the procedure to be undertaken. The court took the view that it would not have been unreasonable to postpone the sterilisation until after the claimant's consent had been obtained, and was not justified by the 'convenience' of doing the procedure during the surgery.

The principle that emerges from these two cases is that a doctor is justified by necessity in proceeding without the patient's consent if the treatment is necessary in the sense that it would be, in the circumstances, unreasonable to postpone the operation. Postponement of treatment is, however, to be preferred if it is possible to wait until the patient is in a position to give consent. An English example arose in *Williamson* v *East London and City Health Authority*,[105] in which the plaintiff consented to removal and replacement of a

---

[100] In Scotland, this could be expressed as the doctrine of *negotiorum gestio*.

[101] *Re F* [1990] 2 AC 1 [74]–[77] (Lord Goff).   [102] See GMC (n 27) para 63.

[103] [1933] 3 DLR 260.

[104] [1949] 2 DLR 442. For discussion of these cases, see, in particular, Butler-Sloss LJ in the appeal stage of *F* v *West Berkshire HA* [1989] 2 WLR 1025. *Devi* v *West Midlands Regional Health Authority* [1980] CLY 687 provides an almost exact British parallel.

[105] (1998) 41 BMLR 85. The case reads as a model moral story as to the importance of filing adequate clinical notes.

leaking breast implant. The condition was, however, found at operation to be more serious than had been anticipated and a subcutaneous mastectomy was performed. Although the evidence was conflicting, Butterfield J ruled that consent to such an extensive procedure had not been given. Damages of £20,000 were awarded despite the fact that the court agreed that the operation would have been needed at some time in the future.

The distinction between necessity and convenience is, nevertheless, often delicately balanced—particularly in the light of the sometimes-vague terms of written consent forms. In an unreported Scottish case,[106] the patient signed to the effect: 'I hereby give permission for myself to have a general anaesthetic and any operation the surgeon considers necessary'. The operation proposed was the comparatively simple removal of a supposed branchial cyst but, on exploration, the cyst was in fact found to be a carotid body tumour. Removal of such a mass is a far more difficult procedure and the patient, in fact, sustained paralysis of half his body. The Inner House concluded that permission was not limited by seriousness and that the patient had consented to any operation to the end of removing the swelling, with Lord Robertson stating: 'Consent must be read as covering any operation considered by the surgeon at the time to be in the patient's interest.'[107] Nonetheless, the three judges who had heard the appeal could all foresee different conclusions if the operation lay outside the procedure contemplated by the patient. It is less certain that such a decision would be reached in the England and Wales jurisdiction or, say, in the US, where it has been considered for many years that: 'the so-called authority [of such consent forms] is so ambiguous as to be almost completely worthless'.[108]

8.4.2 CONSENT AND PATIENTS ASSESSED AS LACKING CAPACITY

The provision of treatment for an adult who is assessed as lacking capacity is possible, subject to the terms of the relevant mental health and capacity legislation in various UK jurisdictions.[109] The principle is that treatment may be provided so long as it 'benefits' the patient (as per Scotland) or is in the patient's 'best interests' (as per England and Wales, and Northern Ireland), and we discuss this later in Chapter 10. It is also possible for an adult, when capacitous, to confer lasting powers of attorney on a donee in England and Wales—or on a welfare attorney in Scotland—to take surrogate treatment decisions in the event of them losing the mental capacity to do so. Given that such an appointment has been made, the relevant attorney must be consulted before treatment is given.

In all cases of patients, the conditions underpinning non-consensual treatment will be modified in an emergency—while reasonable steps to satisfy the spirit of the Acts must always be taken, the doctor who deliberately delayed essential treatment in order to comply with the letter would be misinterpreting the law and professional obligation. Furthermore, the Social Action, Responsibility and Heroism (SARAH) Act 2015, which extends to England and Wales, requires courts to have regard to whether a person was

[106] *Craig v Glasgow Victoria and Leverndale Hospitals Board of Management* (22 March 1974, unreported) 1st Division. One has to note that this case is half a century old, and we seriously doubt the open-ended nature of the consent would be acceptable today.

[107] ibid.

[108] *Rogers v Lumbermen's Mutual Cas Co* 119 So 2d 649 (La 1960). Guidance on obtaining consent is provided both by the General Medical Council and the Department of Health, see for example GMC (n 27) paras 54–55; Department of Health and Social Care (n 34).

[109] MCA 2005, s 5; Mental Capacity Act (Northern Ireland) 2016, s 9 (not in force at the time of writing), or Part 5 of the Adults with Incapacity (Scotland) Act 2000.

'acting for the benefit of society or any of its members' when determining the relevant standard of care in negligence cases.[110] The SARAH Act will thus predispose courts to view any mistakes that occur during the provision of emergency assistance in a more forgiving light.[111] Even so, we think it plausible that an emergency doctor's actions would continue to be evaluated against the benchmark of 'good medical practice' and that the guidelines of the General Medical Council would remain relevant.

8.5 REFUSAL OF TREATMENT BY CAPACITOUS ADULTS

As noted earlier in this chapter, there is a strong presumption in law and a core principle of medical ethics that an adult with capacity to consent has a right to determine what shall be done with their own body. This principle is qualified in the case of children and young people, as discussed in Chapter 9, but UK case law over a number of years has confirmed that adults with capacity may exercise autonomy as to what may be done—or not done—to or with their body through consent, and conversely, refusal of treatment.

Re T[112] can be regarded as an early seminal case concerned with refusal of treatment, and was, coincidentally, the first adult Jehovah's Witness case to have come before a UK court. The facts of the case involved a pregnant woman who was involved in a car accident. Following admission to hospital and after speaking with her mother, she signed a form of refusal of blood transfusion. After a Caesarean section and the delivery of a stillborn baby, her condition deteriorated, and a court order was obtained, which authorised the administration of a blood transfusion to her on the grounds that it was manifestly in her best interests. The declaration was upheld by the Court of Appeal. At the heart of the Court's decision was a finding to the effect that an adult patient who suffers from no mental incapacity has an absolute right to consent to medical treatment, to refuse it or to choose an alternative treatment—it exists notwithstanding that the reasons for making the choice are rational, irrational, unknown, or even non-existent.[113] How, then, did the Court reach its decision to support the provision of apparently involuntary treatment?

First, of course, it had to transform involuntary treatment into non-voluntary treatment. This it did by finding that T's mental state had deteriorated to such an extent that she could not make a valid choice as between death and transfusion—and if there was doubt as to how the patient was exercising her right of self-determination, that doubt should be resolved in favour of the preservation of life.[114] An additional factor of great importance to her treating doctors was added when it was stated that the effects of outside influence on a patient's refusal have to be taken into consideration; in short, the question of whether the patient means what they say has to be posed, including whether the decision was reached independently after counselling and persuasion or whether the patient's will was overborne is a matter to be decided by the doctors. At first glance, this looks

---

[110] Social Action, Responsibility and Heroism Act 2015, s 2.

[111] Rachel Mulheron, 'Legislating Dangerously: Bad Samaritans, Good Society, and the Heroism Act 2015' (2017) 8(1) Modern Law Review 88.

[112] *Re T (adult) (refusal of medical treatment)* [1992] 4 All ER 649.

[113] (1992) 9 BMLR 46 [50] (Donaldson J).

[114] For the challenges and disciplinary difficulties of assessing capacity, see Mark Jayes et al., 'How do Health and Social Care Professionals in England and Wales Assess Mental Capacity? A literature review' (2020) 42 Disability and Rehabilitation 2797, and for the relevance of religious belief, see Clayton Ó Néill, *Religion, Medicine and the Law* (Routledge 2018).

suspiciously like opening the door to involuntary treatment—that is, until one comes to Staughton LJ, who stated:

> I cannot find authority that the decision of a doctor as to the existence or refusal of consent is sufficient protection, if the law subsequently decides otherwise. So the medical profession . . . must bear the responsibility unless it is possible to obtain a decision from the courts.[115]

Since this will be possible only rarely in an emergency, *Re T* seems to place a well-nigh intolerable burden on the doctors, not all of whom in the middle of the night will be of consultant status. What, for example, is the young junior doctor to make of Lord Donaldson:

> what the doctors *cannot* do is to conclude that, if the patient still had the necessary capacity in the changed situation [he being now unable to communicate], he would have reversed his decision . . . What they *can* do is to consider whether at the time the decision was made it was intended by the patient to apply in the changed situation.[116]

Even the law is undecided on the definition of undue influence[117] and, again, neither Lord Donaldson[118] nor Butler-Sloss LJ[119] made it any easier by including parents and religious advisers among those who might, as a result of their relationship, lend themselves more readily than others to overbearing the patient's will. Now, however, the Mental Capacity Act 2005 (MCA 2005) Code of Practice recognises this possibility; by the same token, the Code of Practice counsels that these parties should not be cut out of the capacity assessment or decision-making processes simply by virtue of the fact that they might have influence or even conflicting interests. Their personal views and wishes should not, however, influence the assessment itself.[120] To assist in determining the views and wishes of the patient it is now possible, and often desirable, to appoint an Independent Mental Capacity Advocate.[121]

The authority of *Re T* was applied shortly afterwards in the case of *Re C*.[122] Despite being a decision at first instance only, the case is, nevertheless, extremely important in that it was the first in which a test for mental capacity was formulated in UK case law (now reflected in the MCA 2005). The case concerned a 68-year-old patient suffering from paranoid schizophrenia who had developed gangrene in a foot while serving a term of imprisonment in Broadmoor. On removal of the patient to a general hospital, a consultant advised that the patient had only a 15% chance of survival if the gangrenous limb was not amputated below the knee.[123] The patient, however, refused the operation, saying that he preferred to die with two feet than to live with one. The hospital questioned C's capacity

---

[115] (1992) 9 BMLR 46, [68]. For an excellent analysis of undue influence, see *Centre for Reproductive Medicine* v *U* (2002) 65 BMLR 92; supported on appeal: [2002] EWCA Civ 565, and applied in *Evans* v *Amicus Healthcare Ltd and Others* [2005] Fam 1.

[116] [1992] 4 All ER 649, [662].

[117] The discussion in *Re T* is inconclusive; in the context of financial matters, see *Royal Bank of Scotland* v *Etridge* [2002] 2 AC 773. In the context of contraception, see *A Local Authority* v *A and Another (capacity: contraception)* [2011] 3 All ER 706.

[118] [1992] 4 All ER 649 [664].   [119] ibid. [667]–[668].

[120] Department for Constitutional Affairs, 'Mental Capacity Act 2005: Code of Practice' (2013) available at <https://assets.publishing.service.gov.uk/government/uploads/system/uploads/attachment_data/file/921428/Mental-capacity-act-code-of-practice.pdf> accessed 01 September 2022, para 4.49. We note that the Code of Practice is currently undergoing consultation as of the time of writing; it remains unclear the extent to which these provisions may change.

[121] ibid.; see also Chapter 10.   [122] *Re C (adult: refusal of medical treatment)* (1993) 15 BMLR 77.

[123] This was, however, averted by intervention short of amputation: [1994] 1 All ER 819 [821].

to exercise his autonomy in this way; an application for an injunction restraining the hospital from carrying out the operation without his express written consent was lodged with the court on C's behalf.

Thorpe J held that C was entitled to refuse the treatment even if this meant his death. Quoting with approval the dicta of Lord Donaldson in *Re T*, he stated that, prima facie, every adult has the right and capacity to accept or refuse medical treatment. He acknowledged that this might be rebutted by evidence of incapacity, but this onus must be discharged by those seeking to override the patient's choice. When capacity is challenged, as in this case, its sufficiency is to be determined by the answer to the question: has the capacity of the patient been so reduced (by his chronic mental illness) that he did not sufficiently understand the nature, purpose, and effects of the proffered medical treatment? This depends on whether the patient has been able to comprehend and retain information, has believed it, and has weighed it in the balance with other considerations when making his or her choice. As Thorpe J stated:

> Applying that test to my findings on the evidence, I am completely satisfied that the presumption that C has the right to self-determination has not been displaced. Although his general capacity is impaired by schizophrenia, it has not been established that he does not sufficiently understand the nature, purpose and effects of the treatment he refuses. Indeed, I am satisfied that he has understood and retained the relevant treatment information, that in his own way he believes it, and that in the same fashion he has arrived at a clear choice.[124]

A similar situation, but one involving a self-inflicted injury, is found in *Re W (adult: refusal of medical treatment)*.[125] Butler-Sloss P held that a psychopathic prisoner with mental capacity could refuse treatment even though it might lead to his death. In contrast, in *Trust A v H (an adult patient)*, the High Court granted the applicant Trust's declarations to allow them to perform a hysterectomy on a patient who had been detained under section 3 of the Mental Health Act 1983, and who suffered from schizophrenia and had delusional beliefs.[126] Although the Court confirmed that no medical treatment could be given without the consent of an adult patient who was competent to make decisions, it was clear that in this case the patient did not appreciate the seriousness of her condition and the sense of threat to life that it presented if unalleviated.[127]

Several important points arise from *Re T* and *Re C*. First, they reaffirm the commitment of the law to the principle of respect for patient autonomy. There is a prima facie presumption of its existence and value which can only be overridden in established circumstances.[128] Furthermore, the particular facts of the case show that incapacity in one or several areas of one's life does not preclude autonomous behaviour in others, nor does it remove the presumption of competence to refuse. Indeed, the injunction obtained by the claimant extended not only to the particular operation contemplated by the hospital but to *all* future attempts to interfere with his bodily integrity without his express written consent. The significance of this is profound. In effect, it represents the earliest judicial

---

[124] [1994] 1 ALL ER 819 [824].   [125] [2002] EWHC 901.   [126] [2006] EWHC 1230 (Fam).

[127] For another case with similar facts to *Re C*—and the same legal outcome—see *Heart of England NHS Foundation Trust v JB* [2014] EWHC 342 (COP).

[128] For an alternative perspective on the relationship between autonomy and best interests, see Alec Buchanan, 'Mental Capacity, Legal Competence and Consent to Treatment' (2004) 97(9) Journal of the Royal Society of Medicine 415.

recognition of the validity of advance refusals of treatment,[129] which has now been put on a statutory footing under the MCA 2005.[130]

However, the judgment in *Re C* suffers from the wideness of its terms and the opportunities for subjective interpretation that it allows. A patient's competence can be successfully challenged if it can be shown that they do not comprehend or absorb information to the extent that they understand it, if they are thought not to believe the information, or if they cannot balance this information against other considerations when making their choice. In this way, hurdles are placed in the path of those seeking to exercise their autonomy but, at the same time, it remains uncertain how high they must jump in order to clear these hurdles. For example, the requirement that the patient must actually comprehend the information is not easy to assess; it can depend as much on the amount of information which is given to the patient and the manner in which it is provided as on the capacity of the patient to understand. Yet, the test is not '*Can* the patient understand?' but, rather, '*Does* the patient understand?' This imposes an obligation on healthcare professionals to ensure that actual understanding is reached and this, in itself, is paradoxical, given that the treating staff might not want the patient to understand if they disagree with the nature of their decision, as was the case in *Re C*. Many of these weaknesses can also be levelled against the various statutory definitions of capacity in the UK, which virtually reproduce the common law test as set out in *Re C*.

Nor is it exactly clear *what* the patient must understand in light of the *Re C* ruling. The decision talks of the 'nature, purpose, and effects' of the treatment. This is potentially very broad and can encompass elements ranging from the general aim of the procedure to the risks and the consequences of refusal and beyond.

Academic commentators, such as Andrew Grubb, have argued that the category of 'autonomous persons' is reduced to only the most 'comprehending' individuals if excessive amounts of information are required to be disclosed and understood.[131] In order to assist in this regard, reference can be made to Chapter 4 of the MCA 2005 Code of Practice, which explores these issues in much greater depth. It offers carers and doctors examples of what it means for the patient 'to understand'. Anyone assessing capacity must have a reasonable belief that the person in their care lacks capacity to make relevant decisions about their care or treatment. This means that the carer must have taken reasonable steps to establish the presence or otherwise of capacity with respect to the particular decision that is to be taken and that this is assessed at an appropriate time. It goes without saying that it must also be established that the decision is in the person's best interests.[132]

The general trend of the common law was ultimately confirmed in *Re B (adult: refusal of medical treatment)*.[133] Ms B was a 43-year-old patient who was paralysed from the neck down and sustained only by means of a ventilator. Ms B refused this intervention shortly after it was introduced but she was adjudged incompetent to do so by two psychiatrists in April 2001. She was, however, declared competent by an independent clinician in August of that year and, thereafter, the hospital treated her as such. Nevertheless, her attending physicians refused to remove the ventilator, advocating instead that their patient attend

---

[129] Reaffirmed in *Re AK (medical treatment: consent)* [2001] 1 FLR 129.

[130] MCA 2005, s 1(2) (presumption of capacity), and ss 24–26 (advance decisions). This is discussed further in Chapter 17.

[131] See Andrew Grubb, 'Commentary' (1994) 2(1) Medical Law Review 92, 95.

[132] MCA 2005, s 5(1) and Code of Practice, Ch 5.

[133] *Sub nom B* v *NHS Hospital Trust* [2002] 2 All ER 449.

a rehabilitation unit which offered a slim chance of improvement in her condition. Ms B rejected this course of action and repeated her refusal on several occasions. Ultimately, the President of the Family Division attended Ms B's bedside to hear her story. In a poignant ruling, Butler-Sloss P reiterated the fundamental principles that now govern this area, namely, that a competent patient has an absolute right to refuse treatment irrespective of the consequences of her decision, and she issued very clear guidance to doctors as to their responsibilities in such cases. These include keeping the patient as involved in the decision-making process as possible, moving to resolve any dispute as promptly as practicable and finding other clinicians to undertake the course of action if the primary carers feel unable to do so.[134] Perhaps most striking of all, notional damages of £100 were awarded in recognition of the technical assault that the health carers had committed by continuing to treat Ms B against her wishes.[135]

Decisions under the MCA 2005 have followed a similar vein. In *Kings College Hospital NHS Foundation Trust* v *C*,[136] the Trust applied for a declaration under section 15 that a patient lacked capacity to make decisions about her medical treatment. The patient, C, had been refusing life-saving treatment, namely renal dialysis, that her doctors wished to give her following her attempted suicide. MacDonald J affirmed that impairment in decision-making process is not sufficient to overrule a patient's refusal; the patient must lack the mental *capacity* to decide whether or not to accept or refuse treatment as established by failing to satisfy the two-stage capacity test in the Act:

> the question for the court is not whether the person's ability to take the decision is *impaired* by the impairment of, or disturbance in the functioning of, the mind or brain but rather whether the person is rendered *unable* to make the decision by reason thereof.[137]

C was found able to understand the information relevant to the decision, to retain that information, and to communicate her decision. Moreover, the Trust could not prove to the requisite standard that C was *unable* to use and weigh the information relevant to the decision in question. Consequently, MacDonald J ruled that, on balance, C did have capacity to decide whether or not to consent to dialysis, even if this meant ending her life:

> a capacitous individual is entitled to decide whether or not to accept treatment from his or her doctor. The right to refuse treatment extends to declining treatment that would, if administered, save the life of the patient and, accordingly, a capacitous patient may refuse treatment even in circumstances where that refusal will lead to his or her death.[138]

More recent case law illustrates the challenge in determining whether a patient understands relevant information to consent, as well as the importance of upholding a patient's autonomy when they are judged capacitous. In *London NHS Foundation Trust* v *E*,[139] a patient had a long-standing diagnosis of type II diabetes and cardiac failure, but had not been diagnosed with any mental disorder prior to his admission to hospital. He suffered from a severely gangrenous left foot for which the recommended clinical treatment was amputation through the knee. The patient declined the surgery. A capacity hearing was arranged, in which a psychiatrist reported that the patient was unable to process and understand information given to him about the difference between the leg injury, which he had a few years ago, and the current gangrenous leg which developed as a consequence

---

[134] Although note the reservations of Charles J in *NHS Trust* v *T* [2004] EWHC 1279.

[135] For general comment, see Marc Stauch, 'Comment on *Re B (Adult: Refusal of Medical Treatment)* [2002] All England Reports 449' (2002) 28(4) Journal of Medical Ethics 232.

[136] [2015] EWCOP 80.   [137] ibid. [31] (emphasis in original).   [138] ibid. [96].

[139] [2018] EWHC 3367 (Fam).

of his diabetes. The psychiatrist was of the opinion that the patient was unable to under-stand that there was a very high risk of death if the surgery did not take place, but also reported that the patient had said to her that he did not wish to die. The patient suffered from cognitive impairment, the cause of which was thought to be vascular. Accordingly, the psychiatrist concluded that the patient lacked capacity to consent to surgery. That conclusion was supported by an independent expert appointed by the Official Solicitor. Based on this evidence, Francis J concluded that the patient lacked capacity to make deci-sions in respect of his current medical treatment and of the two medical options presented to the court—amputation and conservative management—it was clear that surgery had the prospect of preserving life, whereas conservative treatment would almost inevitably result 'in a most unpleasant death'.[140] Thus, on balance and on the evidence currently available, it was determined that it was in the patient's best interests to proceed with the proposed amputation.

Conversely, in the case of *Lancashire and South Cumbria NHS Foundation Trust v Q*,[141] the Trust sought declarations as to the capacity of the patient (Q) to litigate and take decisions regarding her medical treatment. Q was a 50-year-old woman with a diagnosis of bulimia nervosa, which she struggled, unsuccessfully, to combat for over a decade. Q also had a diagnosis of Emotionally Unstable Personality Disorder (EUPD), recur-rent depression, a background of severe trauma, and symptoms of Post-Traumatic Stress Disorder (PTSD). While she lived independently, she also suffered from episodes of life-threatening metabolic complications, the most significant of these being precariously low potassium level, a condition known as hypokalaemia. The Trust sought declarations, including a whether Q had the capacity to take decisions relating to her treatment for hypokalaemia. There was no dispute, nor could there be, that Q was able to understand the information informing the decision on whether to accept or refuse potassium treat-ment. Neither was there any doubt that she was able to communicate her decision. As Mr Justice Hayden put it:

> Indeed, everybody (and I emphasise without exception), has recognised that Q is a very articulate and reflective woman. Thus, no issue arises in relation to Section 3(1) [MCA 2005] (a), (b), or (d) . . . The sole question which falls for consideration is whether Q is able both to weigh and use information relevant to her potassium treatment for her hypoka-laemia [as required by s 3(1)(c)].[142]

Mr Justice Hayden assessed the evidence from various medical professionals, includ-ing the patient's general practitioner (GP) and a consultant psychiatrist, both of whom believed she had the capacity to take decisions concerning her treatment. A second con-sultant psychiatrist also gave evidence and doubted the patient had such capacity on the basis that he believed she had pervasively low self-esteem and hopelessness, both of which were directly attributable to her mental disorder and fundamentally impaired her abil-ity to weigh matters of life in the balance. The fact that it was a finely balanced decision shifted that balance more closely towards capacitous decision-taking. The assessment of those who knew Q well, most particularly her GP, had to be afforded significant weight. This was not to be confined to the question of best interests, but also went to their evalua-tion of capacity, having regard to the way that the issues at stake have been framed:

> Q does not want to die, but she does not want to live under a medical and mental health regime which she finds oppressive and corrosive of her autonomy. As she puts it, she is sim-ply *'sick of it'*. On paper, that regime may not appear rigorous but for Q, it undoubtedly is.

---

[140] ibid. [14].   [141] [2022] EWCOP 6.   [142] ibid. [31].

I regard her view, if she will forgive me for saying so, to be an unwise one. Whilst I hope that recovering her autonomy may be empowering for her, I consider, on the evidence, not least her own, that it is most likely to hasten her death. I am sure that those who have had regular dealings with her, and her friends will consider that a considerable loss. She is an engaging personality with much to offer. However, whilst her decision may be objectively unwise, it is hers and not mine. I must respect her autonomy.[143]

Straightforward as this may seem, these cases have to be read in conjunction with others in which the autonomy of the patient has been overridden and their right to choose for themselves has been denied. We have already drawn attention to the contradictions within the common law in this respect and there is little doubt that much of the uncertainty is perpetuated in legislation.[144] We now turn to consider this further in the next section.

8.5.1 REFUSAL OF TREATMENT IN LATE PREGNANCY

As previously discussed, the decision of the Court of Appeal in *Re T* was not without its caveats. Lord Donaldson said:

An adult patient who . . . suffers from no mental incapacity has an absolute right to choose whether to consent to medical treatment, to refuse it or to choose one rather than another of the treatments being offered. *The only possible qualification is a case in which the choice may lead to the death of a viable foetus.*[145]

This 'possible qualification' was tested in the subsequent case of *Re S*,[146] in which a health authority applied for a declaration to authorise the surgeons and staff of a hospital to carry out an emergency Caesarean section on a 30-year-old woman who was in labour with her third child. The woman refused to submit to the section on religious grounds. The surgeon in charge, however, was adamant that both patient and baby would die without such intervention and, after six days of Mrs S's being in labour, the health authority sought a judgment from the High Court. The decision of Sir Stephen Brown is approximately one page in length and there is little or no legal argument or analysis in the judgment as to how the declaration was agreed. As the President said:

I [make the declaration] in the knowledge that the fundamental question appears to have been left open by Lord Donaldson MR in *Re T* . . ., and in the knowledge that there is no English authority which is directly in point.

Nevertheless, it was precisely this lack of precedential authority which provoked major criticism of *Re S* insofar as the case, with all its jurisprudential limitations, sought to *provide* that authority. The problems that were generated as a result were considerable. First, the decision was based wholly on the medical evidence. There was no discussion of how the competency of a woman to make such a choice was to be assessed. How would the choice by a woman in S's position be validated? Second, when Lord Donaldson spoke of a 'viable' foetus, he was speaking in relative rather than absolute terms—for viability

---

[143] ibid. [57].

[144] For an assessment of the approach of the 2005 Act to assessing capacity, see Mary Donnelly, 'Capacity Assessment Under the Mental Capacity Act 2005: Delivering on the Functional Approach?' (2009) 29(3) Legal Studies 464.

[145] [1992] 4 All ER 649, [652–3] (emphasis added).

[146] *Re S (adult: refusal of medical treatment)* [1992] 4 All ER 671; (1992) 9 BMLR 69. This case was decided only two and a half months after *Re T*.

results from a combination of gestational age and obstetric expertise. At what stage, therefore, would it be regarded as legally acceptable to enforce the operation? Third, we have to ask what importance a court should place on the danger to the life of the woman herself? Strictly speaking, this should have no influence for, as was said in *Re T* and subsequently confirmed in *Re B*, the right to decide whether to accept treatment persists even if refusal will lead to premature death. Yet we still believe that it is asking a great deal of the healthcare team to stand by and watch their patient die a painful death and it is probable that such considerations were in the mind of the President when he was confronted with an emergency situation. Finally, the decision depended on very doubtful logic in that it was, and is, well-established law that the foetus in utero has no rights of its own and has no distinct human personality.[147]

If, then, we look upon an enforced Caesarean section as a means of resolving a conflict between a woman who is refusing treatment and a foetus who seeks it, there is, in effect 'no contest'. In short, there can be no valid reason behind isolating this particular situation as the one occasion on which the foetus achieves legal dominance over its mother. While we have great sympathy with the President in the particular circumstances of *Re S*, it is hard to see his decision as other than logically and legally untenable.

Nonetheless, it appeared for a time as though *Re S* had indeed set a precedent and, despite fierce criticism of the ruling,[148] the English courts went through a phase in which they were prepared to impose Caesarean sections on unwilling women in the interests of their foetuses—with[149] or without[150] the assistance of the Mental Health Act 1983. It was not until 1997 that the problem was considered in depth in the Court of Appeal. In *Re MB*,[151] the court made clear that a woman carrying a foetus is entitled to the same degree of respect for her wishes as is anyone else. It reiterated the general principle that a person of full age and sound mind cannot be treated against their will without the door being opened to civil and criminal legal consequences. The court stressed that circumstances in which non-voluntary treatment is permissible arise only when the patient cannot give consent and when treatment is in the *patient's* best interests. The court has no jurisdiction to declare medical intervention lawful when a competent pregnant woman decides to refuse treatment, even though this may result in the death or serious disability of the foetus. The question of the woman's own best interests does not arise in such circumstances. On the facts of the particular case, however, the pregnant woman was declared incompetent, because of a fear of needles which had led her to refuse the operation. At the end of the day, she consented, and a healthy child was delivered.

This decision clearly places the autonomy of the woman above any interests of the foetus, including an interest in being born alive. Yet, it is important to bear in mind that all of this is subject to the woman being competent when she makes her refusal. If she is not, she must be treated in her best interests. However, it still remains open to speculation how the patient's best interests should be assessed if there is no clear indication of how the mother feels about the birth. In the final analysis, *Re MB* does little to remove from the medical profession the discretion and power to decide on a patient's capacity

---

[147] The offence of child destruction is not engaged as the Infant Life (Preservation) Act 1929 requires intention to kill the child-to-be.

[148] See e.g. Andrew Grubb, 'Commentary on Re S' (1993) 1 Medical Law Review 92.

[149] *Tameside and Glossop Acute Services Trust* v *CH (a patient)* [1996] 1 FLR 762. For analysis, see Andrew Grubb, 'Commentary' (1996) 4 Medical Law Review 193.

[150] *Norfolk and Norwich Healthcare (NHS) Trust* v *W* [1996] 2 FLR 613. The same judge made a similar decision in *Rochdale Healthcare (NHS) Trust* v *C* [1997] 1 FCR 274.

[151] *Re MB (an adult: medical treatment)* [1997] 8 Med LR 217.

to act autonomously and, ultimately to decide on the patient's best interests in cases of assessment of incapacity.

This discretion has not been removed, although the Court of Appeal's subsequent ruling in *St George's Healthcare NHS Trust v S (Guidelines), R v Collins, ex parte S (No 2)*[152] provided guidance for doctors called upon to decide on the capacity of a patient to consent to or refuse treatment.[153] The case concerned S, a 36-year-old pregnant woman with pre-eclampsia who was advised that she would require to be admitted. Fully cognisant of the risks, and wishing her baby to be born naturally, S refused. As a consequence, she was seen by a social worker and two doctors and admitted to a mental hospital for assessment. On her transfer to another hospital, a declaration was sought and granted to dispense with S's consent and the baby was delivered by Caesarean section. S discharged herself and appealed against the declaration. The Court of Appeal upheld its ruling in *Re MB* to the extent that a capacitous pregnant woman has the absolute right to refuse medical intervention. The actions of the hospital were a trespass and the former declaration was set aside accordingly.[154] Moreover, the Court castigated the use of mental health laws to treat an otherwise healthy woman:

> The Act cannot be deployed to achieve the detention of an individual against her will merely because her thinking process is unusual, even apparently bizarre and irrational, and contrary to the views of the overwhelming majority of the community at large.

The position of the pregnant woman of sound mind was now brought into line with the 'adult of sound mind' referred to in *Re T*. More significantly, the Court of Appeal sought to prevent a repeat of this case and, indeed, others involving the treatment of patients of doubtful capacity. It issued guidelines for future reference extending to ten detailed points, albeit largely concerned with procedure. This was an attempt to provide more certainty for doctors faced with the uncertainties thrown up by the common law. However, it is noteworthy that the courts have consistently shied clear of interfering in clinical matters and were quick to emphasise that the guidelines should not be rigidly adhered to, if to do so put the patient's health or life at risk.

A significant additional feature of *St George's v S* lies in its challenge to the use of mental health legislation as a means of legitimising involuntary treatment. A trend in such a use had, in fact, been emerging in the lead up to this ruling, not only in relation to pregnant women but also in the context of individuals with feeding disorders.[155] The MCA 2005 emerged against this backdrop, but it is notably silent on the challenges thrown up by pregnancy. High policy and politics might, of course, have dictated that the broad principle of respect for autonomy meant that no 'special case' should be made, but as these cases demonstrate, principles and practices can easily diverge; reinforcement of the pregnant woman's absolute right to refuse through the MCA Code of Practice may have been welcomed on a number of fronts. Indeed, as discussed in Chapter 10, it now appears that the MCA 2005 may be a vehicle to make decisions for pregnant women with mental health problems and mental disabilities.

---

[152] [1999] Fam 26.

[153] *St George's Healthcare NHS Trust v S, R v Collins, ex parte S* [1998] 3 All ER 673. In a later case, *Bolton Hospitals NHS Trust v O* [2003] 1 FLR 824, Butler-Sloss followed *Re MB* in re-stating the principles but still finding a woman with post-traumatic stress temporarily incompetent due to panic induced by flashbacks. The case adds little to the established jurisprudence.

[154] The case has since been relied upon as authority that the law is cautious in imposing duties relative to autonomous acts by persons of full capacity. See *Murphy v East Ayrshire Council* [2012] CSIH 47, quoting Lord Hoffmann in *Reeves v Metropolitan Police* [2000] 1 AC 360 [368]–[369].

[155] See the example of *A Local Authority v E* [2012] EWHC 1639 (Fam), discussed further in Chapter 10.

8.6 CONCLUSION

We have stressed throughout this book how fast and far autonomy-based reasoning has come to dominate health and medical law, and consent to treatment is no different. It remains fundamental to the provision of (most) medical treatment, as it provides clinicians with the authority to interfere with a patient's bodily integrity. While there may be some exceptions to the requirement to seek consent, what a clinician may do in such circumstances is limited by the principle of necessity, and the law continues to recognise the right of a capacitous patient to refuse medical intervention. Where the law has developed significantly in recent years surrounds the constituent elements of consent, and in particular, what information needs to be disclosed to a patient to ensure consent is fully informed. The *Montgomery* case, and guidance from professional bodies, has facilitated a shift towards understanding consent as a joint decision-making process between patient and healthcare professional,[156] and away from the *Bolam* ideal of 'doctor knows best'. However, vestiges of *Bolam* still remain, with some 'therapeutic privilege' retained to avoid disclosure of risks in limited situations, and ongoing jurisprudential refinements surrounding disclosure of 'reasonable alternative treatments'. This, coupled with the jurisprudence regarding refusal of treatment in late pregnancy, suggests that deference to medical expertise has not entirely disappeared.

FURTHER READING

1. Emma Cave and Caterina Milo, 'Informing Patients: The *Bolam* Legacy' (2020) 20(2) Medical Law International 103–130.

2. Emma Cave, 'The Ill-Informed: Consent to Medical Treatment and the Therapeutic Exception' (2017) 46(2) Common Law World Review 140–168.

3. Michael Dunn et al., 'Between the Reasonable and the Particular: Deflating Autonomy in the Legal Regulation of Informed Consent to Medical Treatment' (2019) 27(2) Health Care Analysis 110–127.

4. Anne-Maree Farrell and Margaret Brazier, 'Not So New Directions in the Law of Consent? Examining *Montgomery* v *Lanarkshire Health Board*' (2016) 42(2) Journal of Medical Ethics 85–88.

5. Aoife Finnerty, 'The Privilege of Information—An Examination of the Defence of Therapeutic Privilege and its Implications for Pregnant Women' (2021) 29(4) Medical Law Review 639–660.

6. Emily Jackson, 'Challenging the Comparison in Montgomery Between Patients and 'Consumers Exercising Choices'' (2021) 29(4) Medical Law Review 595–612.

7. Bernadette Richards, Mark Taylor, and Susannah Sage Jacobson, 'Consent and Innovation—Embracing the Unknown and Empowering the Patient' in Bernadette Richards, Mark Taylor, and Susannah Sage Jacobson (eds.), *Technology, Innovation and Healthcare: An Evolving Relationship* (Edward Elgar 2022) 45–63.

8. Gemma Turton, 'Informed Consent to Medical Treatment Post-Montgomery: Causation and Coincidence' (2019) 27(1) Medical Law Review 108–134.

---

[156] GMC, (n 27) para 2 (noting the professional duty of a doctor to 'work in partnership with patients' as part of a broader duty of 'communication, partnership and teamwork').

9

CHILDREN AND CONSENT TO MEDICAL TREATMENT

9.1 INTRODUCTION

In this chapter, we examine a range of legal issues involved in the consent to medical treatment in relation to children and young people. Courts act in their best interests with respect to decision-making over their medical treatment, while at the same time seeking to take account of considerations of welfare and autonomy. This approach can be fraught with tension in the context of disputes between treating healthcare professionals (HCPs) and parents who differ over the treatment to be offered to their children. It can also be finely balanced in the case of young people between the ages of 12 and 17 years, particularly where it involves a refusal to consent to what may be life-saving medical treatment.

In relation to the law concerning consent to medical treatment involving children, there is a need to take account of relevant legislation, case law, human rights instruments, the courts' inherent jurisdiction powers, and the role played by key stakeholders. In the first section of the chapter, we provide an introduction to key legislation and the role of the courts in this area so as to provide necessary background context ahead of our examination of case law, starting from the seminal case of *Gillick*. Thereafter, post-*Gillick* case law is explored in select areas, including refusals of medical treatment, objections to treatment due to religious beliefs, other welfare considerations, gender identity, and the care of critically ill young children. The final section briefly reflects on the role of human rights in promoting the autonomy of children and young people in decision-making about their own health care and how this has been approached by the courts. For the purposes of this chapter, we use the term 'child' to refer to a person under the age of 12 years, and 'young person' to refer to someone between the ages of 12 and 17 years, but note that these age groups are often referred to in case law as 'minors' or 'mature minors'. We focus predominantly on the jurisdiction of England and Wales in terms of our review of relevant case law, drawing on case law examples and legislation from other UK jurisdictions where appropriate.

9.2 KEY LEGISLATION AND THE ROLE OF THE COURTS

In England, Wales, and Northern Ireland (NI), a child is defined as a person under the age of 18 years.[1] A competent young person aged 16 or 17 years can consent to 'any surgical, medical or dental treatment'; it will be 'effective consent' and it 'shall not be necessary to

---

[1] Family Law Reform Act 1969 (FLRA 1969), s 1(1); Age of Majority Act (Northern Ireland) 1969 (AMNIA 1969), s 1(1). This is also confirmed in the Children (Northern Ireland) Order 1995, s 2(2).

obtain any consent for it from [their] parent or guardian'.[2] Any such treatment 'includes any procedure undertaken for the purposes of diagnosis, and this section applies to any procedure (including, in particular, the administration of an anaesthetic) which is ancillary to any treatment as it applies to that treatment.'[3]

In particular circumstances, the refusal of a competent young person aged 16–17 years to consent to such treatment may be overridden either by those with parental responsibility for the young person or by a court. It is important to note that this consent applies to the young person's own treatment but does not apply to any proposed intervention that is not likely to be of direct health benefit to them, such as blood donations or non-therapeutic research, for example. However, the young person may be able to consent to such treatments if they are assessed as having *Gillick* competence. We will examine both what constitutes such competence, and how the courts have interpreted 'refusals' by young persons later in this chapter.[4]

Other key legislation that must be taken into account in terms of consent arising in the context of the provision of medical treatment to children and young people are those that establish legal frameworks for the safeguarding and protection of children.[5] While there are differences between the respective pieces of legislation in the UK jurisdictions, they all emphasise the importance of the 'welfare principle': namely, that the welfare of the child is the paramount consideration for anyone with parental responsibility for the child or who otherwise has a duty of care to that child.[6] Courts can make an order authorising (medical) 'treatment' pursuant to relevant legislation or they can rely on their inherent jurisdiction.[7] In England, Wales, and NI, the following issues should be taken into account in terms of determining the 'welfare' of the child or young person:[8]

(a) the ascertainable wishes and feelings of the child concerned, considered in the light of their age and understanding;

(b) their physical, emotional, and educational needs;

(c) the likely effect on them of any change in their circumstances;

(d) their age, sex, background, and any of their characteristics which the court considers relevant;

---

[2] FLRA 1969, s 8(1); AMNIA 1969, s 4(1).   [3] FLRA 1969, s 8(2); AMNIA 1969, s 4(2).

[4] In terms of determining capacity for young people aged 16 and 17 years, the same criteria used for assessing the capacity of adults should be used under the relevant mental health laws in England and Wales, as well as NI (see Chapter 10).

[5] For present purposes relating to medical treatment, the Children Act 1989 (CA 1989) applies in the England and Wales jurisdiction. In NI, the relevant legislation is The Children (Northern Ireland) Order 1995 (NICO). Note that other relevant pieces of Welsh legislation now address issues relating to looked after children and children's social care services. For an overview, see Children's Social Care Law in Wales (2022) available at <https://sites.cardiff.ac.uk/childrens-social-care-law/legislation/primary/> accessed 08 January 2023.

[6] CA 1989, s 1(1); NICO 1995, s 3(1).

[7] Note that the term 'inherent jurisdiction' is an English common law doctrine that holds that a (superior) court has jurisdiction to hear any matter that comes before it unless legislation or other rule circumscribes that authority or otherwise grants exclusive jurisdiction to another court or tribunal. In the case of children, it derives from the right and duty of the Crown acting in line with its *parens patriae* powers to take care of those who are not able to take care of themselves. The application of the inherent jurisdiction in Scotland is discussed in Chapter 17. For a recent UK Supreme Court judgment that examined the nature and scope of the doctrine in a family law case, see *In the Matter of NY (A Child)* [2019] UKSC 49.

[8] CA 1989, s 1(3); NICO 1995, s 3(3).

(e) any harm which they have suffered or are at risk of suffering;

(f) how capable each of their parents, and any other person in relation to whom the court considers the question to be relevant, are of meeting their needs; and

(g) the range of powers available to the court under this Act in the proceedings in question.

If a child lacks capacity to consent, then it can be provided by someone who has parental responsibility for them.[9] In England, Wales, and NI, all mothers have parental responsibility for their children, but not all fathers. In NI, only fathers who are married to the mothers have parental responsibility;[10] in England and Wales, fathers who are married *or* civil partners to the mothers, or who are registered on the child's birth certificate, have parental responsibility.[11] In all three jurisdictions, fathers may enter into parental responsibility agreements with the mothers or apply to the court for parental responsibility orders for the child in question.[12] In England and Wales, 'second female parents' also acquire parental responsibilities for children in a similar way.[13]

If a safeguarding, protection, or other welfare issue involving a child comes before the courts, then it will make an order based on the welfare of the child.[14] In the case of the provision of medical treatment, for example, where parents disagree, or there is a disagreement between parents and treating HCPs, then it may need to be referred to the court for a decision on the matter. While the parents' preferences will be taken into account, the court will ultimately make a decision based on the best interests of the child. The courts can approve or prohibit proposed treatment, but they cannot demand that it be carried out. If there is no consent forthcoming for such treatment on the part of those with parental responsibility for the child, then HCPs responsible for treating the child are nevertheless authorised to provide the treatment under the principle of necessity.[15]

The position in Scotland is somewhat different, with a child being defined as any person under the age of 16 years.[16] From 16 years of age, a person may give consent to any 'transaction' having legal effect.[17] For a person under the age of 16 years, they are considered to have 'legal capacity to consent on [their] own behalf to any surgical, medical or dental procedure or treatment where, in the opinion of a qualified medical practitioner attending [them, they are] capable of understanding the nature and possible consequences of the procedure or treatment.'[18] Scotland also has a legal framework for facilitating the safeguarding and protection of children and young people.[19] Under this framework, it is made clear that the courts should take account of the 'age and maturity of the child concerned'; and 'as far as practicable', give them an opportunity to indicate whether they wish to express their views; and if they do, then to give them an opportunity to do so; and to have regard to such views as they may express. In these circumstances, it can be

---

[9] CA 1989, s 3(1); NICO 1995, s 6(1). Note that term 'parental responsibility' is defined under both pieces of legislation as meaning 'all the rights, duties, powers, responsibilities and authority which by law a parent of a child has in relation to the child and [their] property.'

[10] NICO 1995, s 5(1).   [11] CA 1989, s 2(1).   [12] CA 1989, ss 2(b) and 4; NICO ss 5(2)(b) and 7.

[13] CA 1989, s 4ZA.

[14] In relation to CA 1989, see powers granted to make orders under s 8 of both the CA 1989 and the NICO 1995.

[15] See generally, *F v West Berkshire Health Authority* [1989] 4 BMLR 1. For further details on the applicability of the principle of necessity, see Chapter 8.

[16] Age of Legal Capacity (Scotland) Act 1991, s 1(1).   [17] ibid., s 1(1)(b), 9(d).

[18] ibid., s 2(4).   [19] Children (Scotland) Act 1995, s 16(1).

'presumed' that 'a child [who is] 12 years of age or more will be of a sufficient age and maturity to form a view'.[20] If a child lacks capacity, then it can be provided by someone who has parental responsibilities and rights in relation to such child.[21] All mothers have parental responsibilities and rights in relation to their children. Fathers who are married to, in a civil partnership with, the mothers, or who are registered on the child's birth certificate have parental responsibility.[22] Otherwise, 'natural fathers' or 'second female parents' may enter into an agreement with the mother to acquire parental rights and responsibilities in relation to the child in question.[23] We now turn to consider what is meant by *Gillick* competence and how this has been interpreted by the courts to date, focusing on the England and Wales jurisdiction by way of example.

9.3 *GILLICK* COMPETENCE

Tension between considerations of welfare and autonomy is most acute in the context of young people, particularly between 12 and 16 years of age. While parental authority clearly exists to consent or refuse on behalf of a child acting in their own best interests, uncertainties arise with the growing independence of a child as they become a young person with greater autonomy, maturity, and insight in relation to choices to be made about their health care. In the circumstances, the question becomes at what point should the law recognise these developments have taken place and what consequences should follow from this legal recognition for all the stakeholders concerned. This arose for consideration in the seminal case of *Gillick*, which involved a ruling by the House of Lords in relation to when a child or young person becomes competent to make a decision about their health care.[24] The UK Department of Health and Social Security (as it was then constituted) had issued guidance on the giving of clinical advice, examinations, and treatment on contraception, which was not subject to any limitation with regards to the age of the persons to whom such services could be provided. It stated that it was a matter for the clinician to decide whether to provide contraception advice and treatment and that the confidentiality of a child under the age of 16 years who sought and received such advice should be respected and their parents should not be contacted without their permission.

This guidance was challenged by Mrs Victoria Gillick, a Roman Catholic, who had several daughters under the age of 16 years. She was concerned that none of her daughters should be given contraceptive advice or abortion treatment while they were under 16,

---

[20] ibid., see ss 11(1) and (7) in relation to the Court of Session or Sherriff's Court making orders in relation to parental rights and responsibilities, for example.

[21] ibid., s 1. Note that parental responsibility is defined as involving the safeguarding and promoting of the child's health, development, and welfare, as well as providing in a manner appropriate to the stage or development of the child, direction (under the of 16 years) and guidance (under the age of 18 years). Where the child is not living with the parent, then they shall maintain personal relations and direct contact with the child on a regular basis, and they should act as their child's legal representative but only in so far as compliance with these requirements is practicable and in the interests of the child. Note that the child will be entitled to sue or to defend in any legal proceedings with respect to these responsibilities. This is mirrored in s 2(1) of the Act in relation to recognised parental rights.

[22] ibid., s 3(1).

[23] ibid., s 4(1) (natural fathers); s 4A (second female parent). Pursuant to s 4(2), any such agreement entered into will not have effect unless it is in the prescribed form, and it is registered in the Books of Council and Session.

[24] See *Gillick* v *West Norfolk and Wisbech Area Health Authority* [1986] AC 112.

without her prior knowledge and consent as their parent (although there was no evidence that this was, or would ever be, the case). She subsequently sought court declarations against both the Department and the local health authority that the guidance was unlawful as, among other things, it adversely interfered with her parental rights and duties towards her daughters. Eventually, the case made its way on appeal to the House of Lords, which sought to resolve a number of complex issues it raised. First and foremost, the Lords examined the nature and scope of parental rights to control a young person (or as they stated a 'mature minor') and when they should be able to receive contraceptive advice, or consent to medical treatment, against the wishes or knowledge of their parents. In addition, the Lords also considered when a doctor would (or would not be) guilty of a criminal offence in providing contraception or advice to underage patients in the exercise of their clinical duties to such patients.

The House of Lords dismissed the application made by Mrs Gillick, holding that parental rights, as such, did not exist in relation to the facts of this case, except insofar as necessary to safeguard the best interests of the young person. In some circumstances, such a young person would be able to give consent in their own right, without the knowledge or approval of their parents. In his judgment, Lord Scarman proposed that the test for determining whether a young person has competence to provide such consent, was a question of fact to be determined based on the facts in a given case. This has come to be described as *Gillick* competence.[25] Lord Scarman set out the relevant test for assessing such competence as follows:

> the parental right to determine whether or not their minor child below the age of 16 will have medical treatment terminates if and when the child achieves a sufficient understanding and intelligence to enable him or her to understand fully what is proposed. It will be a question of fact whether a child seeking advice has sufficient understanding of what is involved to give a consent valid in law. Until the child achieves the capacity to consent, the parental right to make the decision continues save only in exceptional circumstances . . .[26]

Lord Scarman went on to state:

> It is not enough that the minor should understand the nature of the advice which is being given; instead, she must also have a sufficient maturity to understand what is involved. There are moral and family questions, especially her relationship with her parents; long-term problems associated with the emotional impact of pregnancy and its termination; and there are the risks to health of sexual intercourse at her age, risks which contraception may diminish but cannot eliminate. It follows that a doctor will have to satisfy himself that she is able to appraise these factors before he can safely proceed upon the basis that she has at law capacity to consent to contraceptive treatment. [27]

In sum, a young person will be assessed as *Gillick* competent if they can show they have sufficient maturity to make the decision in question. If *Gillick* competent, then they can provide legal consent for the medical procedure. In making this assessment, there will be a need to take account of the young person's age, maturity, and mental capacity; their understanding of the issue and what it involves—including advantages, disadvantages, and potential long-term impact; their understanding of the risks, implications, and

---

[25] ibid., (Scarman LJ). Indeed, the term '*Gillick* competent' is a central part of medico-legal lore; see *Re R (a minor) (wardship: medical treatment)* (1992) 7 BMLR 147 [156] (Donaldson LJ).

[26] ibid., [188(H)]–[189(A)] (Scarman LJ).

[27] ibid., [189(C)]–[189(D)] (Scarman LJ).

consequences that may arise from their decision; how well they understand any advice or information they have been given; their understanding of any alternative options, if available; and their ability to explain a rationale around their reasoning and decision making.[28]

In his judgment, Lord Fraser also provided further guidance as to how HCPs should assess whether a young person under the age of 16 years can consent to contraceptive or sexual health advice and treatment.[29] The scope of what have become known as the Fraser guidelines was extended to encompass termination of pregnancy following the later case of *R (Axon)*,[30] where the claimant, a mother of five children, sought a declaration from the court to the effect that a doctor owed no duty of confidentiality to a patient who was a young person in respect of advice and proposed treatment in relation to contraception, sexual health, and termination of pregnancy. The court refused the claimant's application, holding that while the knowledge and agreement of the parents were clearly desirable, an HCP who had made reasonable efforts to encourage their patient to tell their parents—but where the patient refused to do so and proceeded with a termination of pregnancy—would not be subject to sanction in the courts or before their peer registration body (i.e. General Medical Council). The judgment served to underline the importance of recognising the autonomy of young people and preserving their confidentiality in the context of the doctor-patient relationship. In addition, it confirmed that the concept of *Gillick* competence was of wider application in the provision of healthcare advice and treatment by treating HCPs to young people who are their patients.

The current version of the Fraser guidelines provides that advice on contraception, sexual health, and termination of pregnancy can be given to young people by treating HCPs if they take into account the following:

- they have sufficient maturity and intelligence to understand the nature and implications of the proposed treatment;
- they cannot be persuaded to tell their parents or to allow the doctor to tell them;
- they are likely to begin or continue having sexual intercourse with or without contraceptive treatment;
- their physical or mental health is likely to suffer unless they received the advice or treatment, and;
- the advice or treatment is in the young person's best interests.

The only exception to this approach in terms of breaching patient confidentiality is likely to be where the HCP has grounds to believe that the young person may be subject to pressure or coercion to give consent or is otherwise at risk of exploitation.[31] We now turn in the next sections of the chapter to consider select case law examples where courts have sought to grapple with how best to interpret and apply *Gillick* competence across a range of different (and often difficult) circumstances.

---

[28] The concurrence of Scots law on this question has scarcely been disputed and is set out in the Age of Legal Capacity (Scotland) Act 1991, s 2(4).

[29] *Gillick* (n 24), [174(D)]–[174(E)] (Fraser LJ).

[30] *R (Axon)* v *Secretary of State for Health* [2006] EWHC 37 (Admin).

[31] See e.g., NSPCC Learning, 'Fraser Guidelines' (2021) available at <https://learning.nspcc.org.uk/child-protection-system/gillick-competence-fraser-guidelines> accessed 08 January 2023.

9.4 REFUSAL OF LIFE-SAVING MEDICAL TREATMENT

The case of *Re R*[32] was something of a landmark case as it constituted the first time that the relationship between consent to and refusal of treatment by young persons was considered by the UK courts. The case concerned a 15-year-old girl whose increasingly disturbed behaviour required sedative treatment. However, during her lucid phases, in which she appeared rational and capable of making decisions, she refused her medication and the local authority instituted wardship proceedings, the intention being to seek authority to provide anti-psychotic treatment whether she consented or not. R appealed against an order which had been obtained to that effect. In its judgment, the Court of Appeal first made it clear that the powers of the court in wardship were wider than that of parents and the court could override both consent and refusal of treatment by the ward if that was considered to be in their best interests.

The Court then distinguished *Gillick* in that it could not be applied to a child whose mental state fluctuated widely from day to day. However, the most significant aspect of the case lay in its definition of parental powers. Essentially, Lord Donaldson MR considered that the parental right which *Gillick* extinguished was to *determine* the treatment of a young person, including not just a right to consent but also a right to veto. In explanation, he introduced the concept of consent providing the key to the therapeutic door. In the case of a young person, he stated there are two keyholders (themselves and their parents), and therefore consent by either *enabled* treatment to be given lawfully but did not, in any way, *determine* that the young person should be treated.

Academic commentary in the wake of the *Re R* judgment raised several concerns.[33] This was not, primarily, as to the assessment of R's incapacity, which the court considered should be based on the general condition of the patient rather than that at a given moment in time. Rather, academic criticism was directed towards the retention of the parental right to give consent in the face of the child's refusal, an interpretation of the law which was described by one commentator as 'driving a coach and horses through *Gillick*'.[34] But is this, in fact, so? Lord Donaldson's distinction between a parental ability to determine a young person's medical treatment and to consent to such treatment is a legitimate one. Moreover, he was, arguably, doing no more than engaging in statutory interpretation of section 8(1) of the Family Law Reform Act 1969, which provides that a young person aged 16 to 17 years can consent to medical treatment, equivalent to an adult. However, this is subject to the caveat in section 8(3) which states that 'nothing in this section shall be construed as making ineffective any consent which would have been effective if this section had not been enacted'. It has been widely assumed that this section does no more than confirm the common law right of young persons to decide these types of issues for themselves. If this is the correct interpretation, however, then there is a need to question the need for section 8(1) in the first place, a view that is supported by the absence of any such statute in Scotland prior to the Age of Legal Capacity (Scotland) Act 1991, and specifically section 2(4) of the Act (as discussed earlier in this chapter).

---

[32] *Re R (a minor) (wardship: medical treatment)* [1992] Fam 11.

[33] Compare Stephen Gilmore and Jonathan Herring, '"No" is the Hardest Word: Consent and Children's Autonomy' (2011) 23(1) Child and Family Law Quarterly 3; Emma Cave and Julie Wallbank, 'Minors' Capacity to Refuse Treatment: A Reply to Gilmore and Herring' (2012) 20(3) Medical Law Review 423.

[34] Ian Kennedy, 'Consent to Treatment: The Capable Person' in Clare Dyer (ed) *Doctors, Patients and the Law* (Blackwell 1992) ch 3.

It could be argued that the better view is that a parental right to consent on behalf of a child existed before the FLRA 1969 and that section 8(3) simply preserves that right in the case of all those below the age of 18 years. Indeed, this appears to have been the basis of Lord Donaldson's position in his judgment.[35] Nevertheless, academic criticism in the wake of *Re R* demonstrates the difficulties which arise when attempting to apply general philosophical principles to particular cases involving medical treatment. Given R's particular condition, one can well ask what the court's alternative was in any case. This could only have been to accede to her refusal of treatment when capacitous and then to treat her as incapacitous under the principle of necessity, and it is doubtful whether such an approach is ethically sustainable.[36] While it may have been better to confine his judgment to such narrow issues, Lord Donaldson nevertheless consolidated his position on the broader issues at stake, albeit with some reservations, in the following case of *Re W*.[37]

Re W takes us one step further down the road of consent in that it concerned a 16-year-old girl who came within the provisions of section 8(1) of the Family Reform Act 1969. W had been diagnosed with anorexia nervosa and was refusing all treatment, despite a rapid deterioration in her health. The Court of Appeal supported an order that she be treated in a specialist unit for her condition largely on clinical grounds, finding that the disease was capable of destroying her ability to make an informed choice. As such, the wishes of the young woman regarding her refusal of treatment were considered as something which, of themselves, required treatment. In the course of various judgments given by the Court of Appeal, several general issues were either clarified or reinforced. First, it was reiterated that the court had extensive powers in wardship and that these existed irrespective of the provisions of section 8(1) of the Family Law Reform Act 1969. In addition, Lord Donaldson held that the exercise of the court's powers to make a specific issue order did not conflict with those sections of the Children Act 1989 which give a young person the right to refuse psychiatric or medical treatment in defined circumstances.[38] All the judicial opinions emphasised that this position did not conflict with *Gillick*, which was concerned with *parental* powers only. Second, the court disposed in clear terms of the relationship of consent to refusal of treatment, with particular reference to the 1969 Act.[39] In this regard, Lord Donaldson stated: [40]

> No minor of whatever age has power by refusing consent to treatment to override a consent to treatment by someone who has parental responsibility for the minor and a fortiori a consent by the court.

This was also confirmed by Lord Balcombe, who stated: [41]

> I am quite unable to see how, on any normal reading of the words of the section, it can be construed to confer [an absolute right to refuse medical treatment] . . . That the section did not operate to prevent parental consent remaining effective, as well in the case of a child over 16 as in the case of a child under that age, is apparent from the words of sub-s (3).

---

[35] (1992) 7 BMLR 147 [156].

[36] For an argument that the provisions of the Mental Capacity Act 2005 to protect autonomy interests should be applied to young people, see Victoria Chico, 'The Mental Capacity Act 2005 and Mature Minors: A Missed Opportunity?' (2011) 33(2) Journal of Social Welfare and Family Law 157.

[37] *Re W (a minor) (medical treatment)* [1992] 4 All ER 627.

[38] This was clearly restated in *South Glamorgan County Council v W and B* [1993] 1 FCR 626.

[39] For an argument that court powers undermine the concept of 'parental responsibility' see Sarah Woolley, 'The Limits of Parental Responsibility Regarding Medical Treatment Decisions' (2011) 96(11) Archives of Disease in Childhood 1060.

[40] [1992] 4 All ER 627, [639].   [41] ibid., [641].

Of course, this is a legal decision, and it is true, as Lord Balcombe pointed out, that there can be no difference in logical terms between an ability to consent to treatment and an ability to refuse treatment. It is undoubtedly the case that the courts will seek to respect a young person's autonomous wishes in respect of many aspects of their life, including their medical care. For example, in *Torbay Borough Council v News Group Newspapers*,[42] we find Justice Munby upholding the right of a young woman who was almost 17 years of age to decide for herself as to whether to disclose the details of her pregnancy to the media, irrespective of the wishes of her parents.

However, matters are not so clear-cut when the decision relates to medical *treatment* and when a refusal may involve a serious risk of physical or mental harm, or indeed, death. It could be argued, for example, that HCPs know more about the treatment of disease than the average child, and while consent involves acceptance of an experienced professional view, refusal rejects that experience and does so from a position of limited understanding.[43] Prognosis is, admittedly, one of the most difficult exercises in relation to the provision of health care to patients but, by and large, HCPs who are recommending a particular course of treatment will be convinced that the patient's condition can only worsen in its absence. The consequences of refusal are, therefore, likely to be more serious than those of compliance and, on these grounds, refusal of treatment may require greater understanding than does acceptance. In principle, consent and refusal are but reverse expressions of the same autonomous choice; the difference is that the level of understanding at which a choice can be said to be an 'understanding choice' is higher in the latter.

What is clear from both *Re R* and *Re W* is that Lord Donaldson was concerned to protect the HCPs from litigation; his reference in *Re W* to consent providing a flak-jacket for the treating doctors in both cases demonstrates this vividly.[44] It is, therefore, possible to criticise the two decisions as concentrating on this aspect and taking insufficient notice of the developing autonomy of young persons. Nonetheless, the judgments in both cases are at pains to emphasise the importance of respecting their wishes and of giving them greater value in line with increasing maturity. They emphasise that those wishes are not binding; but their tenor is such as to establish the key tenets of *Gillick* competence very firmly in English jurisprudence in terms of addressing these types of cases and to insist that this is breached only in exceptional circumstances.

Having said that, there are always cases that challenge this position. This was illustrated in the case of *Re M (child: refusal of medical treatment)*,[45] in which a young woman aged 15 and a half years, who had acute heart failure, was denied the right to refuse a heart transplant operation. While the High Court emphasised the need to take account of her wishes regarding her medical treatment, it also endorsed the legal view that those wishes are in no way determinative. Justice Johnson was keen that his ruling be very clearly laid out for the young woman to read for herself but, interestingly, he did not seek to ascertain her views before passing judgment. Instead, these were gleaned by a local solicitor and the Official Solicitor who, together, formed the view that the young woman was overwhelmed by her circumstances. She had said that she did not wish to die. By the same token, she had also indicated that she did not want someone else's heart, nor did she relish the thought of taking medication for the rest of her life. In the final analysis, it was held that it was in

---

[42] [2003] EWHC 2927.

[43] For a specific rejection of this view, see Richard Huxtable, 'Case Commentary: Time to Remove the "Flak Jacket"?' (2000) 12 Child and Family Law Quarterly 83.

[44] For discussion see Alasdair Maclean, 'Keyholders and Flak Jackets: The Method in the Madness of Mixed Metaphors' (2008) 3(3) Clinical Ethics 121.

[45] [1999] 2 FLR 1097.

her best interests to receive a new heart and the High Court authorised her treating HCPs to perform the procedure. Whatever one may feel as to its medical merits, this judgment could be said to represent the outermost reaches of acceptable paternalistic practices. While it seems that she finally acquiesced in terms of going ahead with the procedure, it is ethically troubling to consider that the court was prepared to countenance transplantation surgery being forced on the young woman in the event that her resistance to the procedure continued. More broadly, we question if it is ethically correct to earmark a scarce and expensive resource such as a heart for someone who does not want it. In the circumstances, it is no wonder that the judge expressed concern at the gravity of his decision.

The enduring force of the precedent laid down by *Re R* and *Re W* was also demonstrated in *Plymouth Hospitals NHS Trust* v *YZ*.[46] In this case, the High Court granted a declaration that it was in the best interests of a 14-year-old girl to undergo immediate testing and treatment for a suspected paracetamol overdose to avoid the risks of liver damage and death. This was so despite relatively clear opposition from the young woman in question. Indeed, the court lamented the fact that legal proceedings had not been instituted earlier in the dispute between the young woman and her treating HCPs. The key aspects underpinning the court's ruling included: (i) the particular dangers associated with the type of overdose; (ii) the presumption in favour of life; (iii) the time pressure within which effective intervention was possible; (iv) consensus between treating HCPs and the mother of the young woman; and (v) a suggestion that the refusal was merely further evidence of 'oppositional behaviour'.

This last aspect is somewhat troubling and so wide in its potential reach that it has the potential to overwhelm *any* decision by a young person with which a third party might disagree. This seems to be confirmed despite claims to interference with the human rights of a young person arising in the context of a refusal of treatment, even where there is a presumption of capacity over the age of 16 years. This was highlighted in *An NHS Foundation Hospital* v *P*.[47] P was a 17-year-old young woman who had refused life-saving treatment after an overdose. An application was made by the NHS Trust authorising treatment for B's overdose. As treatment could include sedation and restraint, the Trust also sought an order that it would be lawful to take steps amounting to a deprivation of liberty under Article 5 of the European Convention on Human Rights (ECHR), notwithstanding the young woman's rights under Article 8. An on-call consultant psychiatrist had assessed P as having the capacity to make her own decisions. While the court acknowledged that her wishes and feelings were important components of assessing welfare considerations taking account of her rights under Article 8, they were not 'decisive' and did not outweigh courts' obligations to preserve life under Article 2.[48] It was therefore held to be within the court's inherent jurisdiction to overrule the young woman's decision, with her best interests and welfare being the paramount consideration.[49]

In *University Hospitals Plymouth NHS Trust* v *B (A Minor)*,[50] B, a 16-year-old young woman, refused treatment to manage diabetic ketoacidosis, a life-threatening complication of insulin dependent diabetes. Her condition worsened, and an application was made by the treating NHS Trust for an order to administer intravenous fluids and insulin to B. Before the High Court, Justice McDonald undertook a best interests assessment as to whether B's refusal of treatment should be overridden. Although a range of factors were considered, including medical evidence, B's grandfather's statement and B's wishes and feelings. B did not have separate legal representation at the hearing, and the judge did

---

[46] [2017] EWHC 2211 (Fam).   [47] [2014] EWHC 1650 (Fam) (also known as *P (A Child), Re*)).
[48] ibid., [13], [15].   [49] ibid., [12].   [50] [2019] EWHC 1670 (Fam).

not approach her directly to ascertain her wishes and feelings, which were considered separately from the medical evidence presented. Justice McDonald went on to overrule the young woman's refusal, on the grounds that it was in her best interests that she should receive the treatment prescribed by her treating HCPs. The approach taken in this case to dealing with B's wishes and feelings regarding the refusal of treatment is troubling, and stands in contrast to the approach taken in the earlier case of *An NHS Foundation Trust* v *A, M, P, A Local Authority*.[51] In this case, the views and feelings of A, a 15-year-old young woman, were ascertained via email exchange with Justice Hayden as part of a best interests assessment. In the circumstances, it could be argued that it represents a departure from best practice in recognising the autonomy of young people with respect to decision-making involving their health care, which is in line with respect for a children's rights approach.[52]

Legal disputes are, necessarily, concerned with those cases where there is an impasse in terms of medical treatment as between young persons and their parents/treating HCPs. While the refusal of treatment by a young person might be overturned as a matter of strict law, the majority of cases ought to proceed in ways that reflect and respect their wishes in supportive healthcare settings. There can be little doubt that professional obligations should support the promotion of the growing autonomy of young persons as far as this is possible, albeit recognising that at times such an approach must concede to their overall welfare interests.[53] Our review of case law on refusals of treatment nevertheless highlights ongoing judicial discomfort with supporting a children's rights-based approach to such decision-making, an issue to which we shall return later in the chapter.

9.5 RELIGIOUS BELIEFS

Due respect and deference for religious beliefs have become significant factors in our increasingly multicultural society in the UK, meriting further consideration. The welfare of children and young people is not solely determined by their healthcare interests. Indeed, parents will often have strong beliefs and cultural values that they wish to impart to their offspring. An obvious example is religious beliefs. In this section, we consider both parental preferences with respect to treatment involving their children which take account of their religious beliefs, as well as how children and young people themselves have sought to express their own preferences regarding treatment in light of such beliefs.[54] We focus in particular on case law examples involving the refusal of both young people and their parents to agree to blood transfusions as a result of their religious beliefs. This has most often arisen in the case of those who are Jehovah's Witnesses, a Christian sect with strong

---

[51] [2014] EWHC 920 (Fam).

[52] Note that it has been argued that the failure on the part of the court to give sufficient weight to the views and feelings of B 'sets a dangerous precedent' and could be considered contrary to Art 12 of the United Nations Convention on the Rights of the Child (CRC). See Rebecca Limb, 'According Appropriate Weight to Children's Wishes and Feelings: *University Hospitals Plymouth NHS Trust v B (A Minor)* [2019] EWHC 1670 (Fam)' (2021) 29(3) Medical Law Review 524.

[53] On the challenges of this kind of approach, see Emma Cave, 'Maximisation of Minors' Capacity' (2011) 23(4) Child and Fam Law Quarterly 431; Emma Cave, 'Goodbye Gillick? Identifying and Resolving Problems with the Concept of Child Competence' (2013) 34(1) Legal Studies 103.

[54] See Jean McHale, 'Health Law, Health and Health Care Law, Faith(s) and Beliefs: New Perspectives and Dilemmas' (2008) 9(4) Medical Law International 279; Clayton Ó Néill, *Religion, Medicine and the Law* (Routledge 2019).

views about the permissibility of blood transfusions.[55] While we focus on these case law examples, it should be remembered that there are a variety of religious beliefs that may impact on healthcare practice, and the same principles will apply. Equation of this objective assessment with subjective and sincerely held religious beliefs lies at the heart of the court decisions in such cases.

Although there may be little public sympathy for parents who depend upon divine intervention exclusively, or refuse on religious or cultural grounds to consent to blood transfusion for a seriously ill child, it would be a mistake to reject their position out of hand. Ignoring deeply held religious beliefs represents a major change of attitude in a free and diverse society. Such action also entails a significant interference with the principle that parents should have the freedom to choose the religious and social upbringing of their children.[56] On the other hand, the objective assessor may well see a difference between endangering life and expressing lesser social concerns; both the courts and the public may well accept the latter, while seeing the former as unreasonable parenting. It is well-nigh impossible to find a case in the UK and other common law jurisdictions where a court has upheld a parental refusal to recommend life-saving treatment on behalf of their child purely on the basis of their own religious beliefs.

In *Re S (a minor) (medical treatment)*,[57] the court ordered transfusion of a four-year-old child against the wishes of his Jehovah's Witness parents, even though treatment was elective and carried only a 50% chance of success. In handing down his ruling, Thorpe J gave the practical advice that the parents could absolve their consciences in that the decision was now out of their hands. While blood transfusion is, from the technical point of view, a comparatively straightforward form of treatment, causing minimal discomfort to the recipient, the same cannot be said for bone marrow transplants. However, the courts have been prepared in this context to override parental objection on religious grounds when the life of a child is a stake. This is exemplified in the case of *NHS Trust v A (a child)*,[58] where the court granted the Trust's application for a declaration that a bone marrow transplant should be carried out on a seven-month-old child who suffered from a severe genetic defect in her immune system. It was accepted that, without the suggested treatment, the child would die, probably by the age of one. Medical experts had estimated that the transplant had approximately a 50% prospect of effecting a lasting cure and that she would then have a normal life expectancy; they also considered that there was a 10% risk that the child would die as the result of treatment. The parents had not consented to the transplant going ahead, mainly on the grounds that they were convinced the child fell into the latter group; that she would be exposed to undue suffering; and should the treatment prove successful, she would be infertile. Alongside these reasons, they were 'practising Christians' and believed that God could and would effect a miraculous cure.[59] Religious objection to treatment in A's case was, therefore, founded on trust in God rather than on fear of divine retribution which lies at the heart of the Jehovah's Witness' objections. As a result, Justice Holman's approach to declaring a non-consensual transplant to be lawful was, perhaps, made that much easier.[60]

[55] For a comparative view, see Sarah Woolley, 'Children of Jehovah's Witnesses and Adolescent Jehovah's Witnesses: What Are Their Rights?' (2005) 90(7) Archives of Disease in Children 715.

[56] See e.g., Elaine Sutherland, 'A Veiled Threat to Children's Rights? Religious Dress in Schools and the Rights of Young People' (2009) 53(3) Judicial Review 143.

[57] (1993) 1 FLR 377.   [58] (2008) 1 FLR 70.   [59] ibid. [31]–[33].

[60] ibid. [2] where Justice Holman also pointed out that, insofar as A was not hospitalised at the time and no order was given, the parents still retained control of the situation. He drew heavily on his previous judgment in *An NHS Trust v MB* [2006] 2 FLR 319, emphasising the close association between consent, refusal, and medical willingness to treat.

We may also want to consider the less dramatic situation where the general religious dictates of parents demand that life be preserved whenever possible, as in the case of orthodox Judaism or the Islamic faith. In *Re C (a minor) (medical treatment)*,[61] the High Court refused to respect the wishes of parents, on religious grounds, to continue venti- latory treatment for a 16-month-old child who was suffering from the inevitably fatal condition of spinal muscular atrophy. The significance of *Re C* lies in the attitude of the court in determining the extent to which parental power is subjugated to the clinical judgement of HCPs. In reaching its decision, the court assiduously followed existing prec- edents which had eschewed judicial interference with the clinical judgement of HCPs in cases such as this.[62] There was, however, no direct mention in this case of the place for the parents' religious beliefs.

In stark contrast, the decision of Mr Justice Holman in *Central Manchester University Hospitals NHS Foundation Trust v A*[63] is a powerful example of a judge struggling to show sensitivity to the religious beliefs of parents while discharging the legal duty to pronounce in the best interests of the patient. In this case, there were two patients: 14-month-old iden- tical twin boys who were suffering from a progressive and irreversible neuro-degenerative disorder. Long passages of the judgment recount the religious position of the parents, being that it was offensive to their Islamic faith to withdraw life-sustaining support before all brain function had ceased. On the facts, the judge agreed that it could not be said that this state had been reached. However, based on an assessment of cognition, as well as the now- standard balance sheet approach of benefits and burdens, the best interests of the boys were declared to favour the removal of life support.

The foregoing case law examples could be taken as indicating that the law has very little difficulty in discounting religious beliefs when children's welfare is concerned.[64] However, we also need to consider how the courts have taken account of the religious beliefs of young people themselves. In *Re E*,[65] which involved a 15-year-old otherwise competent boy who was refusing blood transfusion as a Jehovah's Witness, Justice Ward held that while 'I respect this boy's profession of faith . . . I cannot discount at least the possibility that he may in later years suffer some diminution in his convictions.'[66] Some would regard this statement as a common-sense direction, whereas others would instead view it as outrageous paternalism. An even more instructive case is the later Jehovah's Witness decision in *Re L (a minor)*,[67] which involved the refusal of blood transfusion by a 14-year-old girl who was described as 'mature for her age'. Sir Stephen Brown P had little hesitation in finding her to be lacking *Gillick* competence on the grounds that her limited experience of life 'necessarily limit[ed] her understanding of matters which are as grave as her own present situation'.[68]

---

[61] [1998] 1 FLR 384.

[62] *Re J (wardship: medical treatment)* [1991] Fam 33; *Re J (a minor) (medical treatment)* [1992] 4 All ER 614; *Re R (a minor) (wardship: medical treatment)* [1992] Fam 11.

[63] [2015] EWHC 2828 (Fam).

[64] See e.g. *In re J (a minor) (prohibited steps order: circumcision)* [2000] 1 FLR 571 in which a ritual cir- cumcision at the age of five was considered not to be in the child's best interests. For academic commentary on the issue, see J Steven Svoboda, 'Circumcision of Male Infants as a Human Rights Violation' (2013) 39(7) Journal of Medical Ethics 469; Joseph Mazor, 'The Child's Best Interests and the Case for the Permissibility of Male Infant Circumcision' (2013) 39 Journal of Medical Ethics 421.

[65] *Re E (a minor)* [1993] 1 FLR 386.   [66] ibid.

[67] *Re L (medical treatment: Gillick competence)* [1998] 2 FLR 810.

[68] ibid. [813]. For commentary on this case, see Caroline Bridge, 'Religious Beliefs and Teenage Refusal of Medical Treatment' (1999) 62(4) Modern Law Review 585.

A recent ruling which highlights the difficulties in reconciling religious beliefs with human rights in the context of refusals of treatment is the case of *Re X (A Child) (No 2): An NHS Trust v X*,[69] which involved a 15-year-old (almost 16-year-old) young woman who had serious sickle cell syndrome. She refused blood transfusions to treat the condition due to her religious beliefs as a Jehovah's Witness. The treating NHS Trust applied for an order that it would be lawful to administer a 'top-up' blood transfusion which was authorised by the court as being in the young woman's best interests. In addition, the Trust also sought a 'rolling order' to enable a blood transfusion to be given as and when necessary to the young woman over a two-year period until she reached 18 years of age. In response, the young woman argued that this type of rolling programme represented a significant interference with her rights under common law, the Mental Capacity Act 2005 (MCA 2005) and Articles 3, 5, 8 and 14 ECHR. She argued that as a young person with capacity, she had the right to make her own decision about her medical care, including the right to refuse consent to blood transfusions.

In giving judgment, Sir James Munby observed that she was 'mature and wise beyond her years' and held that even where a young person is considered to be *Gillick* competent or was otherwise presumed to have capacity under relevant legislation, they should not be considered as 'autonomous' in all circumstances.[70] In the context of a refusal to submit to life-preserving medical treatment, the court was entitled to overrule such a decision sitting in its inherent jurisdiction until the child reached the age of 18 years, if it viewed the decision as not being in the best interests of the child. In seeking to give proper consideration to the young person's *Gillick* capacity and existing ECHR rights, however, he went on to order that a single blood transfusion be administered, but refused to approve a rolling programme of such transfusions over a two-year period. This was on the grounds that it ran the risk of privileging medical paternalism over judicial protection and would diminish the young woman's human dignity.[71] This case continues to highlight ongoing judicial discomfort in respecting *Gillick* competence in the context of a young person's refusal of life-preserving treatment.[72] Interestingly, human rights considerations were only factored into the court's approach with respect to the way in which the treatment was to be administered to the young person, rather than the treatment itself.

The ruling by Sir James Munby may be contrasted with that of Justice Cohen in *Teaching Hospitals NHS Trust v DV (A Child)*,[73] published mere months apart. In this case, DV had been diagnosed with pulmonary osteosarcoma, a form of bone cancer. He urgently required surgery in relation to the spread of the cancer to the lung, which may have necessitated blood transfusions. DV had been baptised as a Jehovah's Witness when he was 14 years of age and did not want to receive blood transfusions. During prior medical treatment, he had been administered a blood transfusion which had caused him huge distress and had subsequently been diagnosed with Post Traumatic Stress Disorder (PTSD). DV's parents were also Jehovah's Witnesses. DV had a good relationship with his treating HCPs, who recognised that if DV did receive blood transfusions it would have a detrimental impact upon him.[74] All parties were in agreement about DV's need for surgery, which could not wait until he was 18 years old. As a result, the treating NHS Trust sought a declaration from the court that not providing blood transfusions in DV's case would not

---

[69] [2021] EWHC 65 (Fam).   [70] ibid. [120].   [71] ibid. [168].

[72] For further commentary on this case, see Emma Cave, 'Confirmation of the High Court's Power to Override a Child's Treatment Decision: *A NHS Trust v X (In the matter of X (A Child) (No 2))* [2021] EWHC 65 (Fam)' (2021) 29(3) Medical Law Review 537.

[73] [2021] EWHC 1037 (Fam).   [74] ibid., [18].

be unlawful. In the High Court, Justice Cohen agreed that DV was *Gillick* competent and set out a list of factors for and against the use of blood transfusions. The factors in favour of not proceeding with blood transfusions in accordance with DV's wishes were that:[75]

- DV's wishes were clear, consent, firmly expressed, and had been held for a considerable period of time;
- DV's age (in eight months he would be 18 years of age);
- DV had deeply held core religious values, which he had thought about carefully and was loyal to the tenets of his faith;
- the risk of psychological harm to DV if blood products were given against his wishes;
- the low risk of haemorrhage to DV;
- it would be counterproductive to proceed against DV's wishes because it might make him reluctant to have future surgery, if needed;
- the sheer practical difficulties of any other course;
- the view of DV's parents who supported his decision and felt strongly that his views should be respected.

The factors in favour of giving blood products to DV were that:[76]

- They might be necessary. The risk was not non-existent to DV, and if blood products were not available during the course of surgery and there was excessive haemorrhaging, then the damage that could be caused to DV could be very serious and potentially fatal.
- DV wanted to survive and he had made it very clear that he wanted to live.

Having weighed up DV's wishes and feelings against the potential adverse consequences of not respecting them, Justice Cohen came to the conclusion that he would respect DV's wishes to refuse the administration of blood products and approved the treatment plan accordingly. The High Court also found that obtaining this order was necessary where treating HCPs considered it to be a 'finely balanced' case,[77] although they were supportive of the wishes of their patients. What proved decisive to the Court was the level of understanding shown on the part of DV and his parents as to the potential risks and consequences at stake. Interestingly, the same legal representatives were involved in representing DV and X (see previously). Justice Cohen stated that they were seeking similar declarations, and that this was clearly an attempt to 're-run the same argument'. He indicated that he did not see 'any uncertainty about the law' and could 'see no benefit in a hearing' on the issue.[78] This reflected the particular circumstances of DV's case, in that he was shortly to turn 18, as well as the fact that the medical issues at stake had been clearly addressed. More broadly, he observed that these types of hearings were very resource-intensive in terms of court and NHS time and monies and concluded that this was not the case to test the relationship between *Gillick* competence, best interests, and human rights.[79]

---

[75] ibid., [21].   [76] ibid. [22].
[77] ibid. [33], drawing on *An NHS Trust and others v Y (by his litigation friend, the Official Solicitor) and another* [2018] UKSC 36, [125] (Black LJ).
[78] ibid. [39].   [79] ibid. [40]–[42].

9.6 OTHER WELFARE CONSIDERATIONS

There is also other case law examples where a range of issues, including the logic of parental decision-making, the severity of the child's condition, and the consequences of the decision, indicate there is no particular judicial approach. Although speculative, it could be argued that this may have been a consequence of socio-cultural and human rights developments over time, whereby there has been a redefinition of the role of the parents in respect of control of their children and that it is no longer possible to regard them as having unfettered power over them. A few examples will suffice. In *Re C (a child) (HIV testing)*,[80] Justice Wilson held that, notwithstanding the opposition of both parents who rejected contemporary medical thinking on the causes and treatment of HIV/AIDS, it was overwhelmingly in the interests of the child that her HIV status be known. Accordingly, he ordered that a blood sample should be taken from the child. In *Re C (a child) (immunisation: parental rights)*,[81] two fathers consented to the immunisation of their daughters against the wishes of their mothers. After a long trial, Justice Sumner held that the girls' best interests must prevail and, accordingly, he ordered that a programme of immunisation should go ahead. The particular interest in this case, however, lies in the fact that the parents disagreed, and the court accepted that if the parents agreed, then they would have a right to choose whether or not to accept medical advice to have their children immunised.

A more recent ruling confirms these principles. In *Re M (children)*,[82] immunisation was held to be in the children's best interests despite parental objection. This involved taking account of factors such as the children's background and physical needs, the risks of harms either way, and the evidence of an independent arbiter. Interestingly, the fact that one parent had a strong view on the matter was a factor that was considered to be of little or no significant weight.'[83] In *Re B (A Child: Immunisation)*[84] the absence of any new peer-reviewed research to cast any further doubt on the MMR vaccine was material in supporting a declaration by the court that it was in a child's best interest to receive the MMR vaccine, despite a dispute between the parents in this regard.

Decisions in favour of parental autonomy are relatively rare, but a case law example of where this was upheld is *Re T (a minor) (wardship: medical treatment)*,[85] where the Court of Appeal held that the parents of a child suffering from biliary atresia, a life-threatening liver defect, could legally refuse a liver transplant on their behalf. This was the case even though there was firmly held medical opinion that a transplant would give the child several years of life beyond their current prognosis. The significance of the court's ruling from the perspective of the law of consent lies in its willingness, indeed, determination, *not* to equate best *medical* interests with the far broader notion of *overall* best interests, which now permeates the entire application of the test. The court may, in fact, take the view that parents who object to life-saving treatment for a child could become bad parents and, as a result, their childhood may be compromised. Alternatively, the child who

---

[80] [2000] Fam 48.

[81] [2003] 2 FLR 1095, also known as *Re B (a child)*. Note that the case was not directly concerned with the MMR (measles, mumps, and rubella) vaccine controversy. Followed in *F v F (MMR Vaccine)* [2013] EWHC 2683 (Fam). For commentary, see: Emma Cave, 'Adolescent Refusal of MMR Inoculation: *F (Mother)* v *F (Father)*' (2014) 77(4) The Modern Law Review 630.

[82] [2016] EWFC 69.

[83] *Cf.* Suchi Agrawal and Stephanie Morain, 'Who Calls the Shots? The Ethics of Adolescent Consent for HPV Vaccination' (2018) 44(8) Journal of Medical Ethics 531.

[84] [2018] EWFC 56.   [85] [1997] 1 All ER 906.

is treated contrary to the parent's religion or other deeply held beliefs might come to be regarded as 'tainted' or 'soiled' by the treatment, leading them to reject the child or treat them adversely. In such cases, the argument could be put that it is in the child's *overall* best interests *not* to receive the said treatment, and this may go some way to explaining the apparently paradoxical decision in *Re T*.

Fraught wardship proceedings culminated in the decision in *Re King (A Child)*,[86] a ruling which saw a degree of leeway granted to parents in determining the child's best interests in unusual circumstances. Parents sought permission to take their child to Prague to undergo proton therapy, which was a form of treatment that was then unavailable in the UK. In the parents' view, this would be a superior treatment for their son following surgery to remove his brain tumour, as it would cause less radiation and tissue damage to other organs than the conventional radiotherapy offered at the treating hospital. Nevertheless, the NHS Trust was not prepared to recommend or fund travel abroad for proton therapy. The parents subsequently removed their child from hospital without permission and travelled to Spain. The local authority became concerned at this course of events, with the result that European arrest warrants were issued for the parents and the child was made a ward of court, requiring him to be presented immediately at the nearest hospital in Spain. The dramatic nature of the case ensured intense media interest.[87] Agreement was eventually reached between the medical teams in the UK, Spain, and the Czech Republic on a treatment plan for proton therapy and evidence of funding was also provided. Justice Baker authorised the proposal on the grounds that proton therapy was a reasonable course of treatment that was compatible with the child's best interests. The case was not one in which the parents were insisting on a manifestly unreasonable course of treatment and ultimately, the outcome and reasoning in this case were consistent with established best interest principles. Nevertheless, it raised broader concerns about how the courts should deal with heightened parental expectations regarding entitlement to a preferred course of treatment, and how the balance should be struck between child welfare, parental autonomy, and resource allocation.

In *An NHS Trust* v *Mr M*,[88] an NHS Trust sought to perform surgery on a ten-year-old boy suffering from cancer of the jaw. His parents objected because they preferred Chinese medicine. The matter was urgent because of the aggressive nature of the cancer, and because of serious medical concern about the extreme suffering that its spread would entail. There was evidence that if prompt action were taken, then the surgery would have a success rate of 55–65%. In holding that the surgery was in the child's best interests, Justice Mostyn stated that:

> The views and opinions of both the doctors and the parents must be carefully considered. Where, as in this case, the parents spend a great deal of time with their child, their views may have particular value because they know the patient and how he reacts so well; although the court needs to be mindful that the views of any parents may, very understandably, be coloured by their own emotion or sentiment. It is important to stress that the reference is to the views and opinions of the parents. Their own wishes, however understandable in human terms, are wholly irrelevant to consideration of the objective best interests of the child save to the extent in any given case that they may illuminate the quality and value to the child of the child/parent relationship.

---

[86] [2014] EWHC 2964 (Fam).

[87] See e.g., BBC News, 'Brain Tumour Boy Ashya King Free of Cancer, Parents Say' (23 March 2015) available at <https://www.bbc.co.uk/news/uk-england-32013634> accessed 09 January 2023.

[88] [2015] EWHC 2832 (Fam).

The previous case demonstrates appreciation on the part of the courts about the relative seriousness of the medical intervention being proposed, and how this might impact on an assessment of best interests. We highlight a number of case law examples in this regard. In *Re C (detention: medical treatment)*,[89] a 16-year-old young woman who had anorexia nervosa was detained using the High Court's inherent protective jurisdiction in order for her to receive 'medical treatment' including, inter alia, force-feeding. This unusual procedure was justified because it was in her best interests to receive 'treatment' for her condition, and therefore it was also a part of those interests that she be detained using reasonable force if necessary, so that the treatment could be carried out. Another interesting point raised by the case was the use by Justice Walls of the three-stage test for competency laid down in *Re C (adult: refusal of medical treatment)*.[90] That case concerned the competency of an adult. As we have seen, the capacity of young persons to agree to or to refuse medical treatment had traditionally relied on the concept of *Gillick* competence, the evaluation of which lies within the discretion of the HCP. This could be said to add judicial weight to the argument that refusal of medical treatment by young people requires a higher standard of competency than does a decision to consent to such treatment.[91]

In the case of *An NHS Trust v A, M and P*,[92] a 16-year-old girl had been detained in hospital for a period of ten months. Although the cause was unclear despite medical investigations, she suffered from persisting vomiting. The vomiting only occurred during daytime, and she was able to sleep through the night. This condition had led to substantial weight loss and at the time the matter came before the court, she only weighed five and a half stone. She was fed intravenously to ensure that she received sufficient nutrition but without this treatment, it was estimated the young girl only had three months to live. Medical opinion had concluded that there appeared to be no gastrointestinal cause for the vomiting, which was disputed by the girl and her mother. Specifically, expert evidence from two psychiatrists considered that the girl lacked capacity and had a disordered relationship with food. The NHS Trust in whose hospital the girl was being treated sought a declaration that it would be lawful to undertake intravenous feeding, and to receive fluids, nutrition and medication, and ongoing psychiatric care. The High Court granted the Trust's application for a declaration to this effect. In giving judgment, Justice Hayden placed considerable weight on the girl's preferences to refuse the proposed course of treatment:[93]

> Accordingly, it is right that I should give thought to A's own wishes and feelings on her treatment . . . All the parties agreed that in the light of A's presentation notwithstanding her age (approaching 16 years), an assessment should be made of her capacity to understand the issues that fall for consideration in this case and in her treatment. I start from the premise that a competent young person under the age of 16 years, who is able to understand all the relevant advice and the consequences of that advice, is to be treated as an autonomous individual and respected as such. That of course would not mean her views would be determinative, but they would be given great weight.

---

[89] [1997] 2 FLR 180.   [90] See Chapter 8.

[91] Note the contrary position adopted by the Scottish courts as highlighted in the case of *Re Houston, Applicant* (1996) 32 BMLR 93, Sheriff McGown interpreted s 2(4) of the Age of Legal Capacity (Scotland) Act 1991 in respect of a 15-year-old boy suffering from mental illness to mean that capacity to consent encompassed a capacity to refuse and, furthermore, it brings to an end the power of a parent to consent on behalf of the young person.

[92] [2014] EWHC 920 (Fam).   [93] ibid. [12] (Hayden J).

However, the Court also recognised that the girl and her mother lacked insight into the reasons for such treatment and ordered that contact between the two be suspended for at least two weeks in order to give the treatment the best chance of success. Due to the level of ongoing conflict between the girl and her treating HCPs, the Court also ordered that she be made a ward of the court. This was done to clarify responsibility for decision-making with respect to provision of health care for the girl.

In *An NHS Trust v ABC & A Local Authority*,[94] a 13-year-old girl attended her GP with her grandmother. Following testing, it was discovered that the girl was 21 weeks pregnant. She was referred on to her local hospital for further care and treatment. The NHS Trust which managed the hospital applied for a declaration with respect to the girl's capacity to consent to either the continuation of, or conversely the termination of, the pregnancy. If she was determined to lack capacity, then a further declaration was sought that it was in her best interests to have the termination. Medical opinion was of the view that the girl had capacity, having assessed that she appeared to have a clear understanding of her position and of available options for further treatment. She was able to explain her wish to have a termination and indicated that if she was forced to continue with the pregnancy then it would cause her considerable distress. She also did not appear to be subject to undue influence from family members and that she had come to this decision on her own. In the High Court, Justice Mostyn granted the NHS Trust's declaration finding that the 13-year-old girl was *Gillick* competent and could decide whether to continue or to terminate her pregnancy. This meant that there was no question of liability being imposed upon the Trust, if she proceeded with the termination. What is striking about Justice Mostyn's judgment is the preparedness to find a young person aged 13 years to be *Gillick* competent, particularly in the context of the highly contested area of abortion. In this regard, it has been argued that the judgment represented a significant departure from earlier post-*Gillick* case law that tended to focus predominantly on best interests.[95]

The case of *Re S (Child as parent: Adoption: Consent)*[96] is of particular interest because it represented the first time that the courts sought to take account of the 'concepts and language' of the MCA 2005 in assessing *Gillick* competence. The facts of the case involved S, a young woman under the age of 16 years, who had developmental delay and learning disabilities. She had a three-month old baby, T, but she did not want to have anything to do with T post-birth and was supportive of him being adopted. The issue was whether she had capacity to consent to T being voluntarily accommodated under section 20 of the Children Act 1989 and thereafter adopted. In considering S's competence to engage in such decision-making, Justice Cobb acknowledged in his judgment that there were fundamental differences between a common law assessment of competence for a young person under the age of 16 years (per *Gillick*) and the assessment of capacity of a person over the age of 16 years under the Act, in particular there being 'no requirement to consider any 'diagnostic' characteristic of a young person under 16 (i.e. impairment of, or a disturbance in the functioning of, the mind or brain) in the assessment of their competence, as there is under section 2(1) of the Act.[97] He also noted that just because S may lack competence in relation to decision-making regarding the placement of T did not mean that she lacked subject matter competence in relation to consent, for example. As would be the approach taken under the MCA 2005, any assessment of competence should be

[94] [2014] EWHC 1445.
[95] See Kirsty Moreton, 'Gillick Reinstated: Judging Mid-Childhood Competence in Healthcare Law: An NHS Trust v ABC & A Local Authority [2014] EWHC 1445 (Fam)' (2015) 23(2) Medical Law Review 303.
[96] [2017] EWHC 2729 (Fam).   [97] ibid. [16].

made on available evidence, and in respect of the current and specific decision at issue. Justice Cobb went on to state:

> For my part, I consider it helpful to test Gillick competence in the way outlined . . . while it is abundantly clear that the Mental Capacity Act 2005 does not apply to those under 16 years of age, there is an advantage in applying relevant MCA 2005 concepts and language to the determination of competence to the under-16s, for this will materially assist in maintaining consistency of judicial approach to the determination of capacity or competence of a parent to give consent to adoption or placement, whether that parent is under or over 16 years of age.[98]

In sum, *Re S* has been viewed as a 'particularly important judgment' in relation to young people under the age of 18 years. It provided more detail on the nature and scope of Gillick competence, bringing greater clarity through referencing the MCA 2005, while also noting fundamental differences as appropriate.[99]

9.7 GENDER IDENTITY

We now turn to consider the *Bell* v *Tavistock* litigation which ignited a good deal of legal, political, and public controversy over the clinical management of gender dysphoria in young people, as well as the extent to which the law should intervene in such management while also seeking to balance questions of autonomy and evolving capacity of young people and parental preferences. At the heart of such litigation, however, was an examination of the nature and scope of *Gillick* competence. There are two key judgments, one at first instance before the High Court,[100] and then in the Court of Appeal.[101] A subsequent leave to appeal by the original claimants to the Supreme Court was refused.[102]

The case involved an application for judicial review in the High Court in the first instance.[103] It was brought by two claimants, Quincy Bell and Mrs A, who sought to challenge the policy and practice of treatment of gender dysphoria at the Gender Identity Development Centre (GIDS), which was run under the auspices of the first defendant, the Tavistock and Portman NHS Foundation Trust. The challenge was brought on a number of grounds: (i) children and young persons under 18 are not competent to give consent to the administration of puberty blocking drugs; (ii) information given to those under 18 years of age by GIDS is misleading and insufficient to ensure such children or young persons are able to give informed consent; and (iii) in the absence of procedural safeguards,

---

[98] ibid. [20].

[99] 39 Essex Chambers, 'Re S (Child as parent: Adoption: Consent)', 39 Essex Chambers Blog (2 November 2017) available at <https://www.39essex.com/information-hub/case/re-s-child-parent-adoption-consent> accessed 09 January 2023.

[100] *Bell & Anor* v *The Tavistock & Portman NHS Foundation Trust & Ors* [2020] EWHC 3274 (Admin).

[101] *Bell & Anor* v *The Tavistock & Portman NHS Foundation Trust & Ors* [2021] EWCA Civ 1363.

[102] The claimants (Quincy Bell and Mrs A) sought leave to appeal to the Supreme Court, but this was refused on 28 April 2022 on the grounds that it did not raise an arguable point of law. See *R (on the application of Bell and another) (Appellants)* v *Tavistock and Portman NHS Foundation Trust (Respondent)* UKSC 2021/0098.

[103] In the *Bell* v *Tavistock* judgments, reference is made to the first instance court being the Divisional Court. This is not a separate division of the High Court but is often used to identify that the matter was heard before several judges. In this case, it was heard before three judges. For present purposes, we use the term High Court.

and the inadequacy of the information provided, there has been an infringement of the rights of such children and young persons under Article 8 ECHR.

In terms of background context, the following accounts were provided by the claimants as part of their judicial challenge. It is important to note that these accounts, particularly regarding medical treatment, were disputed by the defendants. However, a judicial review is focused on the lawfulness of decision-making and actions by a public body rather than resolving factual disputes between the parties involved in the application.[104] Quincy Bell was born female and considered from the age of four or five years that she was gender non-conformist, associating more with male games and clothes. She felt alienated at secondary school and took birth control pills to stop her periods and she did not feel comfortable in her own body. As a result, she suffered from anxiety and depression. From 14 years of age, she began actively to question her gender identity and started watching YouTube videos, as well as undertaking research on the internet, about gender dysphoria and the transition process. At 15 years of age, she was referred to GIDS and was seen for first time when she was 16 years of age. She subsequently had several appointments over a period of just under two years, and after three such appointments, she was prescribed puberty blockers. Prior to being prescribed this medication, she was given advice about the impact on her fertility, but her priority at the time was to be prescribed testosterone. At 16 years of age, she indicated she was not concerned about her fertility and in any event, egg storage was not available on the NHS. At 17 years of age, she commenced on testosterone for a period of three years, which resulted in rapid bodily changes, including to her genitals and voice, in addition to the growth of facial and body hair. At 20 years of age, she underwent a double mastectomy and appreciated that she would need a hysterectomy at a later stage, due to the atrophy of her reproductive organs as a result of taking testosterone. In January 2019, she ceased taking testosterone and began to identify as a woman and wished to change her birth certificate back to her natal sex.[105]

Mrs A, the second claimant, was a mother of a 15-year-old girl with autism spectrum disorder (ASD) and a history of mental ill-health and behavioural problems. According to Mrs A, her daughter was 'desperate to run away from all that made her female' and had been referred to Child and Adolescent Mental Health Services (CAMHS) for further assessment. Mrs A stated that she was very concerned that her daughter would be referred to GIDS and prescribed puberty blockers. At the time of the judicial challenge, her daughter had not been referred to GIDS, but by the time of the Court of Appeal judgment, the referral had taken place. In the circumstances, the High Court noted that Mrs A's interest in the judicial review challenge was 'largely theoretical'.[106]

The application was heard before President Dame Sharp, Lord Justice Lewis, and Justice Lieven; a joint judgment was handed down in December 2020. In the judgment, the documentation and approach to consent processes at GIDS were examined, including standard operating procedures in this regard. In advance of any referral of a young person to an endocrinologist to consider the prescription of puberty blockers, they noted that GIDS clinicians discussed the proposed treatment with the young person. This included checking that the young person's hopes for treatment are realistic, explaining what the treatment can and cannot do, discussing any potential side-effects, discussing fertility

---

[104] For an overview of judicial review, see Courts and Tribunals Judiciary, 'Judicial Review' (2022) available at <https://www.judiciary.uk/how-the-law-works/judicial-review/#:~:text=Judicial%20review%20is%20a%20type,wrongs%20of%20the%20conclusion%20reached> accessed 09 January 2023.

[105] *Bell & Anor* v *The Tavistock & Portman NHS Foundation Trust & Ors* [2020] EWHC 3274 (Admin) [78]–[83].

[106] ibid. [89].

and the potential impact on genital development for birth-registered males. Visual aids are used to support this process.[107] The process of consent was described as 'discursive and iterative', involving multiple discussions and answering any questions the young people or their parents might raise. Where the young person is under 15 years of age, parental support is a prerequisite for the referral for treatment. If the young person had not reached the appropriate stage of physical development, then the referral would be deferred for a period of 6–12 months to better judge their level of emotional cognitive and psychosocial maturity, as well as capacity. GIDS clinicians would only refer a young person if they determined that they were *Gillick* competent with regards to providing the requisite consent for such treatment.

Notwithstanding the consent processes in place at GIDS, the Court expressed concern as to whether young persons were able to provide informed consent even if they were assessed as *Gillick* competent. This was because of the limited scientific evidence available concerning the long-term benefits versus the potential harms of the treatment given that there was uncertainty as to whether a young person would continue to identify as transgender in the future. The Court took the view that the treatment in question, namely the prescribing of puberty blockers, was an 'experimental treatment' and currently of unknown impact. In the circumstances, it went to 'the critical issue of whether a young person can have sufficient understanding of the risks and benefits to be able lawfully to consent to that treatment.'[108] The Court went on to expand upon its concerns in this regard, stating that:

> The combination . . . of lifelong and life changing treatment being given to children, with very limited knowledge of the degree to which it will or will not benefit them, is one that gives significant grounds for concern . . . We do not think that the answer to this case is simply to give the child more, and more detailed, information.[109]

In relation to the question of *Gillick* competence, the Court found that a young person would have to understand not only the implications of taking puberty blockers but also what that was likely to mean in terms of progression towards the use of cross-sex hormones. To have such competence in this context, a young person would have to demonstrate they were able to understand, retain, and weigh up the following:

- the immediate consequences of the treatment in physical and psychological terms;
- that the vast majority of patients taking puberty blockers go on to take cross-sex hormones and therefore they were on a pathway to greater medical interventions;
- the relationship between taking cross-sex hormones and subsequent surgery, with the implications that followed from such surgery;
- the fact that taking cross-sex hormones could adversely impact sexual function and might well lead to infertility;
- the impact that taking this step on the treatment pathway might have on future and life-long relationships;
- the unknown physical consequences of taking puberty blockers, and;
- the fact that the evidence base for this treatment was as yet highly uncertain.[110]

The Court then sought to distinguish competence to consent to the treatment in question as between young persons under the age of 16 years, and those aged 16 and 17 years of age. In relation to young people under the age of 16 years, it held that a young person could

---

[107] ibid., [38].   [108] ibid. [74].   [109] ibid. [143]–[144].   [110] ibid. [138].

only consent to the use of medication intended to suppress puberty where they are competent to understand the nature of the treatment. This included an understanding of the factors outlined in the previous paragraph which it considered would present significant difficulties for a young person under the age of 16 years. The Court was also doubtful that a young person aged 14 or 15 years could understand and weigh the long-term risks and consequences of taking of puberty blockers and considered it highly unlikely that a child aged 13 years and under would be able to do so.[111]

In relation to young people aged 16 and 17 years of age, the Court confirmed that there was a presumption of capacity to consent to treatment under the Family Law Reform Act 1969 and that, absent a dispute with parents, courts usually had no role as long as the young person had capacity and their clinicians considered the treatment to be in their best interests.[112] The Court stated that the potential long term consequences arising from the prescription of puberty blockers were such that clinicians could very well view these types of cases as appropriate to seek authorisation from the court prior to commencing the treatment.[113] Although it recognised that the defendants opposed such an approach viewing the need for such authorisation as an unwarranted intrusion into a young person's autonomy, the Court was adamant that this should be the preferred approach:

> In principle, a young person's autonomy should be protected and supported; however, it is the role of the court to protect children, and particularly a vulnerable child's best interests. Under the inherent jurisdiction concerning medical treatment for those under the age of 18, there is likely to be a conflict between the support of autonomy and the protective role of the court. As we have explained above, we consider this treatment to be one where the protective role of the court is appropriate.[114]

The High Court judgment caused a storm of controversy, with a wide range of concerns expressed about its approach to dealing with, inter alia, the clinical management of gender dysphoria, particularly the claim that puberty blockers are 'experimental treatment';[115] the failure to properly consider the autonomy of competent transgender children in relation to determining their own treatment;[116] and a misunderstanding of the relationship between *Gillick* competence and the level of information provision required for consent to treatment for gender dysphoria,[117] with broader implications for consent processes involving children and young people in health care.[118]

---

[111] ibid. [151].   [112] ibid. [146].   [113] ibid. [152].   [114] ibid. [149].

[115] See e.g. Simona Giordano and Søren Holm, 'Is Puberty Delaying Treatment "Experimental" Treatment?' (2020) 21(2) International Journal of Transgender Health 113. More generally, it has been argued that transgender children should have a legal right to access puberty blockers as the established standard of care, and a lack of access puts them at risk of psychological and physical harm; see Maura Priest, 'Transgender Children and the Right to Transition: Medical Ethics When Parents Mean Well but Cause Harm' (2019) 19(2) American Journal of Bioethics 45.

[116] See Reubs J Walsh, 'A Blow to the Rights of Transgender Children' British Psychological Society Blog (3 December 2020) available at <https://www.bps.org.uk/psychologist/blow-rights-transgender-children> accessed 09 January 2023.

[117] Kirsty Moreton, 'A Backwards-step for Gillick: Trans Children's Inability to Consent to Treatment for Gender Dysphoria—Quincy Bell & Mrs A v The Tavistock and Portman NHS Foundation Trust and Ors [2020] EWHC 3274 (Admin)' (2021) 29(4) Medical Law Review 699.

[118] See e.g. Shannon Fyfe and Elizabeth Lanphier, 'Is a Minor's Decision to Take Puberty-Blockers Exceptional?' (BMJ Blog, 20 January 2021) available at < https://blogs.bmj.com/medical-ethics/2021/01/20/is-a-minors-decision-to-take-puberty-blockers-exceptional/> accessed 09 January 2023; Simona Giordano, Fae Garland, and Søren Holm, 'Gender Dysphoria in Adolescents: Can Adolescents or Parents Give Valid Consent to Puberty Blockers?' (2021) 47 Journal of Medical Ethics 324.

The first instance judgment was subsequently overturned by the Court of Appeal.[119] The grounds for appeal by the defendants were as follows. The High Court had erroneously departed from *Gillick*, which had established that children under 16 years of age could make their own decisions if they were assessed on an individual basis as being competent to do so by their treating clinician. In the circumstances, the High Court had 'intruded into the realm of decisions agreed upon by doctors, patients and their parents, where the court had not previously gone and had erred in deciding between the evidence of competing experts, without that evidence having been properly admitted or tested in cross-examination.'[120]

In its judgment, the Court of Appeal stated that there were two key documents that provided the basis for the judicial review challenge: first, the GIDS service specification, which comprised 61 pages of detailed provisions, including several which addressed with the issue of informed consent; and second, the GIDS standard operating procedure (as at 31 January 2020), which incorporated guidance and documentation in relation to consent for referral to other hospitals for consideration as to whether a patient should be prescribed puberty blockers. In doing, so, the Court of Appeal recognised that the High Court had not had the benefit of the 'focus on these documents that we have had.'[121]

Having reviewed such documentation, the Court of Appeal made clear that it viewed its remit in the context of a judicial review challenge to policy and practice in treating gender dysphoria by GIDS was to 'test their lawfulness' only. In the circumstances, the High Court's position that court authorisation should be sought before puberty blockers are prescribed was incorrect. In line with *Gillick*, [122] this was a matter for a clinician to discuss in consultation with their patient and to then make an assessment with regards to competence to consent to this course of treatment.[123] The Court then went on to find that the High Court had 'placed an improper restriction on the Gillick test of competence':[124]

> the question whether valid consent is given in any case is a question of fact. That depends upon the individual circumstances of any child and the surrounding circumstances of the clinical issues. Both he (Lord Scarman) and Lord Fraser identified at a high level what they could expect a clinician to consider in making a clinical decision. Turning their observations into formal declarations (all the more so if they included immutable facts) would have been inappropriate. It is a matter of clinical judgement, tailored to the patient in question, how to explain matters to ensure that the giving or refusal of consent is properly informed. As Lord Fraser observed . . . medical professionals who do not discharge their responsibilities properly would be liable to disciplinary sanction. The law of informed consent culminating in *Montgomery* also exposes the vulnerability of clinicians to civil action from someone they have treated who shows that they did so without first obtaining informed consent.[125]

The Court of Appeal judgment was warmly received by a range of stakeholders. This included organisations supporting young trans people and their families who were relieved and happy with the judgment, with one seeing it as a 'victory for common sense and young people's bodily autonomy',[126] and another now 'cautiously optimistic that

---

[119] *Bell & Anor* v *The Tavistock & Portman NHS Foundation Trust & Ors* [2021] EWCA Civ 1363.
[120] ibid. [66].   [121] ibid. [14].   [122] ibid. [76].   [123] ibid. [54]–[55].
[124] ibid. [94].   [125] ibid., [81].
[126] Mermaids, 'Mermaids Statement on the Bell v Tavistock Appeal' (17 September 2021) available at <https://mermaidsuk.org.uk/news/mermaids-statement-on-the-bell-v-tavistock-appeal/> accessed 09 January 2023.

things will improve for trans youth and . . . their healthcare needs.'[127] Legal practitioner and academic commentary ranged from positive support for the clarification provided by the Court of Appeal that it is a matter for the treating clinician, and not the courts, to decide whether an individual has the capacity to consent on a case-by-case basis,[128] to welcoming the judgment as a vindication of the 'human rights of trans young people' with the upholding of 'their decisional autonomy'.[129]

The case of *AB v CD & Ors*[130] was decided after the High Court judgment in *Bell v Tavistock* but before the matter came before the Court of Appeal. This was an application by AB, the mother of a child, XY, who was 15 years of age. XY had been born male but came out to her parents as transgender when she was ten years old and had fully transitioned socially in all aspects of her life, including legal paperwork. She changed her name by deed poll in 2016. The mother of XY sought a declaration from the court that she and the child's father could consent to XY taking puberty blockers. Justice Lieven held that unless the parents were overriding the wishes of the young person, then they could consent to puberty blockers on their behalf without the need for a best interests application to the court. This was so notwithstanding the first instance judgment in *Bell v Tavistock*. The judge rejected the suggestion that the prescription of puberty blockers was in a special category of medical intervention which always required the sanction of the court, despite the controversial nature of the treatment.[131] In effect, Justice Lieven resolved the practical difficulties associated with the first instance judgment in *Bell v Tavistock* where the High Court's proposed guidance effectively meant that young people under the age of 16 years could not consent to puberty blockers and that a court order was needed. Instead, she provided that parental consent could be given for the taking of puberty blockers where there was uncertainty over whether their child had the capacity to provide their own consent to the taking of such medication. The judgment was subsequently referred to with approval in the Court of Appeal's judgment in *Bell v Tavistock*.

One of the issues highlighted in the *Bell v Tavistock* litigation was the issue of access to, and the provision of, high-quality gender identity health care. As was noted, there had been a huge growth in referral and waiting times for children and young people seeking consultation and treatment at GIDS, which essentially operated as a single provider for managing gender identity issues, such as gender dysphoria, in England. In this section of the chapter, we provide a brief overview of recent proposals for reform in this area of health care, drawing on England by way of example. In doing so, we recognise that there are different arrangements within the UK's four jurisdictions in relation to the provision of health services in relation to gender identity and gender dysphoria. In Scotland, for example, this is currently provided through several Gender Identity Clinics (GICs) which are part of the National Gender Identity Clinical Network for Scotland, NHS Scotland.[132]

---

[127] Gendered Intelligence, 'Bell v Tavistock Quashed on Appeal' (17 September 2021) available at <https://genderedintelligence.wordpress.com/2021/09/17/bell-v-tavistock-quashed-on-appeal/> accessed 09 January 2023.

[128] Megan Griffiths, 'Appeal Allowed in Bell v Tavistock: The Scope of Declarations in the Judicial Review of Clinical Treatment Decisions' (Clinical Negligence Blog, 12 King's Bench Walk, 4 October 2021) available at <https://clinicalnegligence.blog/2021/10/04/appeal-allowed-in-bell-v-tavistock-the-scope-of-declarations-in-the-judicial-review-of-clinical-treatment-decisions/> accessed 09 January 2023.

[129] Sandra Duffy, 'Bell v Tavistock on Appeal: Court of Appeal Upholds Young Persons' Ability to Consent to Puberty-Blocking Medication' Oxford Human Rights Hub (5 October 2021) available at <https://ohrh.law.ox.ac.uk/bell-v-tavistock-on-appeal-court-of-appeal-upholds-young-persons-ability-to-consent-to-puberty-blocking-medication/> accessed 09 January 2023.

[130] [2021] EWHC 741 (Fam).   [131] ibid. [138].

[132] For further details, see NHS Scotland, 'Gender Identity Clinics' (2022) available at <https://www.ngicns.scot.nhs.uk/gender-identity-clinics/> accessed 09 January 2023.

In Wales, the Welsh Gender Service was established in 2017. It is based in Cardiff, with Local Gender Teams (LGT) based in each Health Board.[133] In Northern Ireland, there are separate NHS services for children and adults. For children, Knowing Our Identity is a service which supports trans and gender variant children and adolescents, up to the age of 18 years. For adults, the Regional Gender Identity & Psychosexual Service (Brackenburn Clinic) provides adults with assessment, psychological support, and onward referral, where appropriate, for hormone replacement therapy and surgery.[134]

In 2020, the Care Quality Commission (CQC) conducted an inspection of GIDS due to concerns reported by HCPs and the Children's Commissioner for England related to clinical practice, safeguarding procedures, and assessments of capacity to consent to treatment. In January 2021, it published a highly critical report of the service, which it rated as overall 'inadequate', with evidence of poor leadership, poor record-keeping, and overwhelming caseloads.[135] As a result, it found that GIDS was leaving 'thousands of vulnerable young people at risk of self-harm as they wait years for their first appointment'.[136] In the wake of the findings from the report, the CQC took immediate enforcement action against the Tavistock and Portman NHS Foundation Trust, demanding improvements including monthly updates on plans to reduce current waiting lists.[137]

In light of the increasing difficulties with young people being able to access gender identity health care through GIDS, NHS England commissioned an independent review into the management of gender identity services for children and young people.[138] Known as the Cass Review, named after its Chair Dr Hilary Cass, a consultant paediatrician and former President of the Royal College of Paediatrics and Child Health,[139] the Review published an interim report on its work in early 2022.[140] The key findings are summarised in the section on Key Points from Cass Review Interim Report 2022 (see below). The report confirmed the ongoing problems experienced at GIDS, which operated as a single specialist service providing gender identity services for children and young people in England. The Review found that a single national provider for gender identity services

[133] For further details, NHS Wales, 'Welsh Gender Service' (2022) available at <https://cavuhb.nhs.wales/our-services/welsh-gender-service/> accessed 09 January 2023.

[134] Transgender NI, 'Healthcare for Transpeople' (2022) available at <https://transgenderni.org.uk/healthcare/> accessed 09 January 2023.

[135] Care Quality Commission, 'Tavistock and Portman NHS Foundation Trust, Gender Identity Services' (20 January 2021) available at <https://www.cqc.org.uk/provider/RNK/inspection-summary#genderis> accessed 09 January 2023.

[136] See Libby Brooks, 'Gender Identity Development Service for Children Rated Inadequate' *The Guardian* (20 January 2021) available at <https://www.theguardian.com/society/2021/jan/20/gender-identity-development-service-for-children-rated-inadequate> accessed 09 January 2023.

[137] Care Quality Commission, 'Care Quality Commission Demands Improved Waiting Times at Tavistock and Portman NHS Foundation Trust' (20 January 2021) available at <https://www.cqc.org.uk/news/releases/care-quality-commission-demands-improved-waiting-times-tavistock-portman-nhs> accessed 09 January 2023.

[138] NHS England, 'Independent Review into Gender Identity Services for Children and Young People' (2022) available at <https://www.england.nhs.uk/commissioning/spec-services/npc-crg/gender-dysphoria-clinical-programme/gender-dysphoria/independent-review-into-gender-identity-services-for-children-and-young-people/> accessed 09 January 2023.

[139] The Cass Review, 'Independent Review of Gender Identity Services for Children and Young People' (2022) available at <https://cass.independent-review.uk/> accessed 09 January 2023.

[140] The Cass Review, 'Independent Review of Gender Identity Services for Children and Young People: Interim Report' (2022) available at <https://cass.independent-review.uk/publications/interim-report/> accessed 09 January 2023. For commentary on the findings and impact of the report, see Editorial, 'The Observer View on Gender Identity Services for Children' *The Guardian* (20 March 2022) available at <https://www.theguardian.com/commentisfree/2022/mar/20/observer-view-cass-review-gender-identity-services-young-people> accessed 09 January 2023.

(such as GIDS), was not a sustainable model in the longer term, and that further research was needed about why referrals to GIDS were taking place. The Review noted the lack of consensus and open discussion about the nature of gender dysphoria and about the appropriate clinical response. It also recognised that the clinical approach and overall service design of GIDS had not been subjected to normal quality controls that are typically applied when new or innovative treatments are introduced.[141]

Key Points from Cass Review Interim Report 2022[142]

1. Children and young people with gender incongruence or dysphoria must receive the same standards of clinical care, assessment and treatment as every other child or young person accessing health services.

2. There needs to be agreement and guidance about the appropriate clinical assessment process that should take place at primary, secondary and tertiary level, underpinned by better data and evidence.

3. Addressing the challenges will require service transformation, with support offered at different levels of the health service. A fundamentally different service model is needed which is more in line with other paediatric provision, to provide timely and appropriate care for children and young people needing support around their gender identity. This must include support for any other clinical presentations that they may have. It is essential that these children and young people can access the same level of psychological and social support as any other child or young person in distress, from their first encounter with the NHS and at every level within the service. The Review team will work with NHS England, providers and the broader stakeholder community to further define the service model and workforce implications.

4. The Review's research programme will not just build the evidence base in the UK but will also contribute to the global evidence base, meaning that young people, their families, carers and the clinicians supporting them can make more informed decisions about the right path for them. At this stage the Review is not able to provide advice on the use of hormone treatments due to gaps in the evidence base. Recommendations will be developed as our research programme progresses.

On 19 July 2022, Dr Cass wrote to NHS England setting out a more detailed proposal for a regionalised model of care for the management of gender identity and gender dysphoria involving children and young people.[143] Essential components of the new model would include the following:

- A comprehensive patient and family centred service and package of care is needed to ensure children and young people who are questioning their gender identity or experiencing gender dysphoria get on the right pathway for them as an individual.

---

[141] The Cass Review, 'Interim Report' (2022) available at <https://cass.independent-review.uk/publications/interim-report/> accessed 09 January 2023.

[142] ibid.

[143] The Cass Review, 'Letter from Dr Hilary Cass to Mr John Stewart, National Director Specialised Commissioning NHS England' (19 July 2022) available at <https://cass.independent-review.uk/publications/> accessed 09 January 2023.

- Regional centres should be commissioned as specialist centres to manage the case-load of children requiring support around their gender identity. The regional centres should be experienced providers of tertiary paediatric care to ensure a focus on child health and development, with strong links to mental health services. They should have established academic and education functions to ensure that ongoing research and training is embedded within the service delivery model.

- Regional centres will need to work collaboratively with local services within their geography, including designated local specialist services drawing on a number of designated specialist services within Child and Adolescent Mental Health Services (CAMHS) and paediatrics.

- Regional centres should be responsible for overseeing the shared care model, working through an operational delivery network (ODN) or similar mechanism.

- Consideration should be given to intake procedures that ensure that children and young people referred to these services are able to access the most appropriate package of support at the earliest feasible point in their journey.

- A formal national provider collaborative with an integral research network should be established, bringing together clinical and academic representatives from the regional centres. There should be independent oversight of data collection, audit and quality improvement (for example, through a Healthcare Quality Improvement Partnership-commissioned approach) to ensure the highest possible standards of data management and utilisation.

- There should be a rapid establishment of research infrastructure to address the gaps in the evidence base regarding all aspects of gender care for children and young people, from epidemiology through to assessment, diagnosis, support, counselling, and treatment.

On this last point, Dr Cass suggested young people being considered for hormone treatment should be asked to enrol in a prospective study with adequate follow up into adulthood, with a more immediate focus on the questions regarding puberty blockers. As she pointed out:

> Without an established research strategy and infrastructure, the outstanding questions will remain unanswered and the evidence gap will continue to be filled with polarised opinion and conjecture, which does little to help the children and young people, and their families and carers, who need support and information on which to make decisions. [144]

In July 2022, it was announced that GIDS would close in spring 2023 as part of the shift towards a more regionalised model for providing gender identity services in England, as recommended by the Cass Review. In the short term, this will involve the establishment of two new centres in London and the North West of England, which will be situated within specialist children's hospitals, such as Great Ormond Street and Alder Hey.[145] Between October and December 2022, NHS England held a consultation on an interim service specification for services for children and young people with gender

---

[144] ibid.
[145] Jasmine Andersson and Andre Rhoden-Paul, 'NHS To Close Tavistock Child Gender Identity Clinic' (BBC News, 28 July 2022) available at <https://www.bbc.co.uk/news/uk-62335665?at_medium=RSS&at_campaign=KARANGA> accessed 09 January 2023.

dysphoria. At the time of writing, NHS England is analysing responses and a report summarising feedback received will be published in 2023, alongside the final interim service specification.[146]

The shift towards creating a new model for the provision of healthcare services in relation to gender identity issues has been welcomed by a range of stakeholders, given the growing recognition that waiting times to access GIDS had become 'unacceptable'.[147] However, the provision of such services forms part of wider public debates about transgender rights, as well as how best to support children and young people who are either questioning or wishing to change their gender identity.[148] It is also important that we examine the role of law and the courts in such debates. In *AB v CD*, Justice Lieven suggested that courts should be wary of 'becoming too involved in highly complex moral and ethical issues on a generalised, rather than case specific basis'; instead, these types of matters 'were best assessed in a regulatory and academic setting and not through litigation'.[149] In the circumstances, critical engagement with the law, as well as what is or should constitute an ethically principled approach to gender identity health care, is vital.[150]

9.8 CRITICALLY ILL YOUNG CHILDREN

As highlighted previously, any decision by the courts must be based on the best interests of the child.[151] The courts rely on their inherent jurisdiction in doing so,[152] as well as taking into account (where appropriate) relevant legislation which recognises the paramountcy of the welfare principle and human rights instruments.[153] By way of example, we now turn to consider several high-profile cases in recent times involving disputes between treating HCPs and parents in relation to the care of their critically ill young children.

The first case we consider is that of Charlie Gard who was born in August 2016 and suffered from infantile onset mitochondrial DNA depletion syndrome (MDDS). This involved the significant drop of mitochondria in his tissues, resulting from genetic

---

[146] NHS England, 'Interim Service Specification for Specialist Gender Dysphoria Services for Children and Young People – Public Consultation' (04 December 2022) available at <https://www.engage.england.nhs.uk/specialised-commissioning/gender-dysphoria-services/> accessed 09 January 2022.

[147] Andersson and Rhoden-Paul (n 145).

[148] See e.g. Sally Hines and Ana Cristina Santos, 'Trans* Policy, Politics and Research: The UK and Portugal' (2018) 38(1) Critical Social Policy 35; Anna Carlile, 'The Experiences of Transgender and Non-Binary Children and Young People and Their Parents in Healthcare Settings in England, UK: Interviews with Members of a Family Support Group' (2020) 21(1) International Journal of Transgender Health 16; Luke Tryl, 'Forget Toxic Twitter Debates: The UK Isn't As Divided on Trans Rights as You Think' *The Guardian* (16 June 2022) available at <https://www.theguardian.com/commentisfree/2022/jun/16/twitter-trans-rights-gender-identity-report> accessed 09 January 2023.

[149] *AB v CD & Ors* (n 133) [121]–[122] (Lieven J).

[150] See e.g. Karl Gerrtise et al., 'Decision-Making Approaches in Transgender Healthcare: Conceptual Analysis and Ethical Implications' (2021) 24(4) Medicine Health Care and Philosophy 687; Robert Rowland, 'Integrity and Rights to Gender-Affirming Healthcare; (2022) 48(11) Journal of Medical Ethics 832.

[151] See e.g. *An NHS Trust v MB* [2006] EWHC 507 (Fam), [16] (Holman J).

[152] See *Kings College Hospital NHS Foundation Trust v Takesha Thomas, Lanre Haastrup, Isaiah Haastrup* [2018] EWHC 127 (Fam).

[153] See e.g., the case of *F (mother) and F (father)* [2013] EWHC 2683 (Fam) where the parents of two children aged 11 and 15 years of age, were in dispute over whether their children should receive the measles-mumps-rubella (MMR) vaccine. When the matter came before the court, it noted the young people's views as being both against having the vaccines, but the court ultimately held that their views were not 'balanced', and they should therefore receive the vaccine based on the welfare principle.

mutations within his DNA. It is a condition that leads to progressive muscle weakness, including those which control breathing, contributing to respiratory failure. In some cases, the brain may be affected, causing seizures, stroke-like episodes, movement disorders or developmental delay. Other parts of the body commonly affected also include the liver, kidney and gastrointestinal tract and hearing loss. Over time, Charlie's condition deteriorated, he became seriously ill with MDDS symptoms, and was treated at Great Ormond Street Hospital in London. Charlie's parents wanted to take him to the United States so he could receive nucleoside therapy, considered an experimental treatment for his condition. The cost of taking Charlie for treatment was sourced through a successful crowd funding campaign run by his parents. In relation to the proposed experimental treatment in the United States, the doctor who offered the treatment had not yet examined Charlie and, in addition, there had not been any clinical trials showing any benefit to children such as Charlie.

Social media campaigns supporting Charlie's parents depicted the state as interfering with parents' rights to make decisions about their children. His treating doctors, who were based at Great Ormond Street Hospital, were also criticised in such campaigns, particularly as they considered it would not be in Charlie's best interests to undergo experimental treatment in the United States which they argued had no chance of succeeding. An application was subsequently brought by the hospital Trust seeking a court declaration that the removal of Charlie who was then aged eight months to the United States for experimental treatment was not in his best interests.

In *Great Ormond Street Hospital for Children NHS Foundation Trust* v *Yates and others*,[154] Justice Francis in the High Court provided a detailed overview in his judgment of the medical treatment provided to Charlie, as well as the advantages and disadvantages of pursuing experimental treatment in the United States. While he had enormous sympathy for Charlie and this parents, Justice Francis agreed with the hospital's position that it would not be in Charlie's best interests to pursue treatment in the United States. The parents subsequently appealed the High Court decision. In *Yates* v *Great Ormond Street Hospital for Children NHS Foundation Trust*,[155] counsel for Charlie's parents argued that there was a need to distinguish between two types of disputes between parents and doctors treating their children. In category 1 cases, the parents were not proposing a viable alternative form of treatment. In category 2 cases, such as Charlie's, his parents were proposing a viable alternative treatment and, in such cases, the courts should not interfere with parental choice unless it would be likely to cause significant harm.[156] The Court of Appeal held that receiving the experimental treatment in the United States had zero prospect of success and would only prolong Charlie's life, which all agreed could no longer be justified in his best interests. As such, Justice Francis was entitled at first instance to conclude on the facts before him that this treatment was not a viable option for Charlie.[157] The Court of Appeal disagreed with the parents' submission that there was a threshold of significant harm that should determine whether a court should interfere with parental choice about decision-making regarding viable alternative treatment for their children.[158] While the court agreed that for the most part parental preferences will be respected and

---

[154] [2017] EWHC 972 (Fam).   [155] [2017] EWCA Civ 410.
[156] ibid., [58] (McFarlane LJ). For academic commentary on the threshold criterion of 'significant harm', see Douglas Diekema, 'Parental Refusals of Medical Treatment: The Harm Principle as Threshold for State Intervention' (2004) 25(4) Theoretical Medicine and Bioethics 243; Imogen Goold and Cressida Auckland, 'Parental Rights, Best Interests and Significant Harms' (2019) 78(2) Cambridge Law Journal 287.
[157] ibid. [97] (McFarlane LJ).   [158] ibid. [105] (McFarlane LJ).

indeed be determinative, however, when there is a dispute between treating clinicians and parents, the best interests test must prevail.[159] Following the Court of Appeal judgment, Charlie's parents attempted to appeal without success to the Supreme Court, and the European Court of Human Rights declined to formally intervene in the case. Following withdrawal of treatment and the provision of palliative care, Charlie passed away on 28 July 2017.[160]

Shortly after the Gard case, the case of Alfie Evans also attracted a good deal of media attention, which included high-profile social media campaigns conducted by his parents. Alfie was born in 2016 and had a serious neurodegenerative condition that had destroyed almost all of his brain. His treating doctors at Alder Hey hospital in Liverpool were of the view that any further treatment was both futile and inhumane. Alfie's parents disagreed and instead wished to take him to Italy to receive treatment to prolong his life. The hospital Trust brought an application to the court that continued ventilatory support was not in Alfie's best interests and, in the circumstances, it was not lawful for such treatment to continue. Alfie's parents objected to the application and despite mediation, no agreement had been reached by the parties to the application as to a way forward.[161] Justice Hayden held that it would be in Alfie's best interests for treatment to be withdrawn, finding that Alfie deserved peace, quiet and privacy and good palliative care which would keep him as comfortable as possible in the final stages of his life.[162] Taking him to Italy would involve removing him from the intensive care unit at the hospital and would likely make him more vulnerable to infection. His need for constant medication would likely be compromised as a result of travelling to Italy and there were concerns that he might die in transit.[163] The judge suggested that the position might have been different if the parents had been able to demonstrate that the proposed treatment was likely to offer a clear benefit to Alfie, but no such evidence was available. In the circumstances, the removal of Alfie to Italy for such treatment was not in his best interests.[164]

The judgment of Justice Hayden was subsequently confirmed on appeal. Alfie's parents then brought separate legal proceedings based on a habeas corpus writ in which it was alleged that Alfie had been unlawfully detained at his treating hospital. This was dismissed at first instance and on appeal.[165] In the Supreme Court, it has held that his parents did not have unfettered rights to make choices and exercise rights on behalf of Alfie. The rights of the child will prevail where they are inconsistent with that of the parents.[166]

While disputes between treating doctors and parents over the treatment of their children ending in the courts have been a feature of this area of law, what marked the cases of Charlie Gard and Alfie Evans as unusual was the parents' preparedness to engage in high-profile mainstream and social media campaigns, as well as a range of legal proceedings, in support of parental choice with regards to treatment preferences involving their children. This was combined with advocacy on the part of their legal representatives in support of a threshold of significant harm as a key determinant in promoting such choice. As has been highlighted, the courts in both cases rejected the parents' claim that the test

---

[159] ibid. [112] (McFarlane LJ).

[160] For an overview of the Gard litigation, see Natasha Hammond-Browning, 'When Doctors and Parents Don't Agree: The Story of Charlie Gard' (2017) 14(4) Journal of Bioethical Enquiry 461.

[161] *Alder Hey Children's NHS Foundation Trust* v *Evans* [2018] EWHC 308 (Fam) [1]–[2].

[162] ibid. [62].   [163] ibid. [63].   [164] ibid. [66].

[165] For an overview of these various proceedings, see *Evans & Anor* v *Alder Hey Children's NHS Foundation Trust & Anor* [2018] EWCA Civ 805.

[166] *In the matter of Alfie Evans (No 2)*, U SC, 20 April 2018 [9] (Hale, Kerr, and Wilson LJJ).

for interference with parental autonomy should be constituted by considering whether parents' decision-making places their child at risk of significant harm. Nevertheless, they tested the boundaries of how we should understand the relationship between parental choice, best interests and the welfare of the child in decision-making involving the treatment of critically ill young children.[167]

We also highlight the case of Tafida Raqeeb, which differs from Gard and Evans cases in several respects. This case involved a five-year-old girl who suffered a brain bleed, which was caused by a ruptured arteriovenous malformation (AVM). This is a rare condition and was undetected and asymptomatic in her case. Tragically, the ruptured AVM caused extensive and irreversible damage to her brain. Tafida's treating doctors considered that further life-sustaining treatment was not in her best interests. However, her parents wished for her to be transferred to an Italian hospital which was prepared to offer her palliative care. The consensus of the medical opinion was that Tafida was ventilator dependent, although the Italian doctors were open to considering whether she could be weaned off a ventilator following a tracheostomy. If she was aware, then she was minimally so, and her everyday life did not appear to cause her pain. In respect of the options for her treatment and care, it was agreed that she would not make a substantial recovery and continued medical intervention would be aimed at sustaining her life as close as possible to current condition. If she was maintained on mechanical ventilation, then medical opinion was also of the view that she would likely live for a substantial period of time. Unlike in the earlier cases examined in this section, it was agreed that any transfer to the hospital in Italy could take place with a minimum of risk to Tafida.

There were two sets of proceedings involving Tafida: the first was a judicial review application where the parents argued that the decision of the hospital Trust to refuse Tafida's transfer to Italy was unlawful and should be quashed; and the second involved an application by the hospital Trust for an order under section 8 of the Children Act 1989 and declarations under the court's inherent jurisdiction that it was in Tafida's best interests to go to Italy for treatment.[168]

On behalf of the parents, it was submitted that Tafida's death was not imminent, provided that she continued to receive life-sustaining treatment, which meant that she could potentially live for a further number of years. There was no evidence that she was in pain, and ongoing treatment would not be overly burdensome to her. It was unlikely she would suffer any pain or discomfort as a result of her transfer to Italy for treatment. In terms of her wishes and feelings, Tafida understood her religion before she suffered her catastrophic injury; she had expressed a wish to live in accordance with her Islamic faith, and her death would not be in accordance with her religious beliefs. Although the continuation of Tafida's life might be considered medically futile, life-sustaining treatments uphold the sanctity of life and that was also important to the religious beliefs of Tafida and her family. In the circumstances, it was argued, her right to life under Article 2 ECHR should be protected.

In contrast, the Trust submitted that it was not in Tafida's best interests to receive life-sustaining treatment due her medical condition which involved minimal change of

---

[167] There is a wealth of legal and ethical commentary on the Gard and Evans cases, see e.g., Jo Bridgeman, 'Gard and Yates v GOSH, the Guardian and the United Kingdom: Reflections on the Legal Process and the Legal Principles' (2017) 17(4) Medical Law International 285; Emma Cave and Emma Nottingham, 'Who Knows Best (Interests)? The Case of Charlie Gard' (2018) 26(3) Medical Law Review 1; Dominic Wilkinson and Julian Savulescu, 'Alfie Evans and Charlie Gard—Should the Law Change?' (2018) 361 British Medical Journal k1891; David Benbow, 'An Analysis of Charlie's Law and Alfie's Law' (2020) 28(2) Medical Law Review 223.

[168] *Barts Health NHS Trust v Raqeeb* [2019] EWHC 2530 (Fam); *Raqeeb and Barts Health NHS Trust* [2019] EWHC 2531 (Admin).

recovery and there was no benefit to her continuing treatment. The religious beliefs of her parents were not relevant to considering Tafida's best interests. There had also been no breach of her human rights; specifically, her Article 9 ECHR rights to freedom of thought, conscience, or religion given the nature of her current condition and limited brain activity; and her right to life under Article 2 as she derived no benefit from life and therefore any concerns about upholding the sanctity of life were outweighed by other considerations.

When the matter came before the court, Justice McDonald considered the respective submissions of the parties and undertook a 'careful and balanced evaluation' of the factors impacting a best interests assessment involving Tafida. Having undertaken that assessment, he came to the following conclusion:

> In circumstances where, whilst minimally aware, moribund and totally reliant on others, Tafida is not in pain and medically stable; where the burden of the treatment required to keep her in a minimally conscious state is low; where there is a responsible body of medical opinion that considers that she can and should be maintained on life support with a view to placing her in a position where she can be cared for at home on ventilation by a loving and dedicated family in the same manner in which a number of children in a similar situation to Tafida are treated in this jurisdiction; where there is a fully detailed and funded care plan to this end; where Tafida can be safely transported to Italy with little or no impact on her welfare; where in this context the continuation of life-sustaining treatment is consistent with the religious and cultural tenets by which Tafida was being raised; where, in the foregoing context, transfer for treatment to Italy is the choice of her parents in the exercise of their parental responsibility and having regard to the sanctity of Tafida's life being of the highest importance, I am satisfied, on a fine balance, that it is in Tafida's best interests for life sustaining treatment to continue.[169]

Justice McDonald recognised that this was a difficult case in which to undertake a best interests assessment where the child in question was not in pain or aware of their situation. In such circumstances:

> The answer to the objective best interests tests must be looked for in subjective or highly value laden ethical, moral or religious factors extrinsic to the child, such as futility (in its non-technical sense), dignity, the meaning of life and the principle of the sanctity of life, which factors mean different things to different people in a diverse, multicultural, multifaith society. Nevertheless, the gold standard against which cases of this nature are measured and determined remains that of the child's best interests and as the march of medical innovation continues to bring cases of this nature before the courts the courts will be required to apply this standard to the best of their ability. That is what I have endeavoured to do in this very sad case.[170]

Having reached this conclusion, Justice McDonald declined to grant relief in relation to the judicial review application brought on Tafida's behalf, in addition to dismissing the applications made by the Trust for an order under section 8 of the Children Act 1989 and declarations under the court's inherent jurisdiction. Tafida's parents were free to organise her transfer to Italy for life-sustaining treatment.[171]

---

[169] ibid. [187].   [170] ibid. [191].

[171] For academic commentary on the case, with particular reference to the implications of Justice McDonald's interpretation of 'best interests', see Emma Cave, Joe Brierley, and David Archard, 'Making Decisions for Children – Accommodating Parental Choice in Best Interests Determinations: Barts Health NHS Trust v Raqeeb [2019] EWHC 2530 (Fam); Raqeeb and Barts Health NHS Trust [2019] EWHC 2531 (Admin)' (2020) 28(1) Medical Law Review 183.

Our final example involves the recent *Battersbee* litigation, where the courts considered what constitutes best interests in relation to the provision of life-sustaining treatment involving a critically ill young child. Note that the litigation also examined the circumstances in which a declaration of legal death can be made on the basis of brain stem testing, which is examined in more detail in Chapter 13. The facts of the case involved Archie Battersbee, who was 12 years of age when he suffered traumatic brain injuries in April 2022 and subsequently fell into a coma. A dispute arose between his parents and treating doctors over whether life-sustaining treatment should be continued in his case. His treating doctors viewed Archie's brain damage as so extensive that they considered him to be brain stem dead; however, this could not be confirmed on testing. When the matter came before the High Court, Justice Arbuthnot held that Archie was 'probably' dead and had died on the day that he had undergone an MRI scan (i.e. 31 May 2022) and his life support treatment should now cease.[172] It was further held that in the event that the court had not been prepared to make a declaration of death in Archie's case, then it would have been in his best interests for mechanical ventilation to be withdrawn.[173] The parents appealed the ruling to the Court of Appeal.[174] In giving judgment, the court criticised the ruling by Justice Arbuthnot on a number of grounds, including the way in which the best interests assessment had been undertaken in relation to the withdrawal of treatment in Archie's case.[175] In the circumstances, the court remitted the case to the High Court in order for a best interests assessment to be undertaken with regards to withdrawal of life-sustaining treatment.

The assessment was subsequently undertaken by Justice Hayden who emphasised in his ruling that the investigation into where best interests lie 'requires unswerving focus on Archie',[176] and needs to extend beyond the medical issues at stake:

> [In] determining where Archie's best interests lie ... It is important that I place him, his personality, his wishes, at the centre of this process. Respect for Archie, as a person, involves a clear recognition that as a human being, he is more than the raft of medical complexity that I have set out above. He is not, in my judgment, simply who he is now, but he is also who he has been throughout his short life.[177]

In taking account of both medical and non-medical factors, Justice Hayden went on to find that it would not be in Archie's best interests to continue with ventilation. In the circumstances, the court could no longer continue to authorise such treatment as 'it compromises Archie's dignity, deprives him of his autonomy, and becomes wholly inimical to his welfare. It serves only to protract his death, whilst being unable to prolong his life.'[178] Archie's parents then sought leave to appeal from Justice Hayden's judgment. In refusing leave to appeal,[179] the Court of Appeal made the following observations in relation to the best interests assessment:

> Standing back, against the judge's findings on the medical evidence, in circumstances where Archie is unable to experience anything that occurs to him or around him (either painful or pleasurable), the judge was entitled to hold, as he did, that the medical regime 'serves only

---

[172] *Barts Health NHS Trust v Dance & Battersbee* [2022] EWHC 1435 (Fam) [180]–[181].
[173] ibid. [183]–[195].   [174] *Barts Health NHS Trust v Dance & Battersbee* [2022] EWHC 1435 (Fam).
[175] ibid. [37].
[176] *Barts Health NHS Trust v Dance & Ors (Re Archie Battersbee)* [2022] EWFC 80 [2].
[177] ibid. [25].   [178] ibid. [46].
[179] *Dance & Anor v Barts Health NHS Trust* [2022] EWCA Civ 1055.

to protract his death, whilst being unable to prolong his life'. In those circumstances his findings as to dignity and autonomy, futility and burden were fully open to him and entirely justified. Specifically, the judge was entitled to find that the treatment carried a burden for Archie, even though he has no capacity to experience pain and no conscious awareness . . .[180]

Whilst it is, most sadly, correct that it was the medical evidence that ultimately determined the outcome of the judge's best interest determination, he had clearly taken full account of the countervailing factors. Those factors, and in particular Archie's individual feelings and religious beliefs, were insufficient to avoid a finding that the continuation of life-sustaining treatment was no longer in the best interests of this moribund child, who is weeks away from a death which will otherwise occur from a gradual further deterioration and then failure of his organs followed by the failure of his heart. Consent can only be given to medical treatment where it is in the patient's best interests and the consequence of the judge's assessment is that continued life-sustaining treatment for Archie will not be lawful, even for a period of days or weeks.[181]

As has been highlighted in the select case law examples we have examined in this section, the courts have been prepared to override parental decision-making regarding the issue of consent to, or conversely the refusal of, medical treatment involving their critically ill young children. In what has been described as their role as the 'judicial reasonable parent',[182] the courts have made clear that the key consideration remains what is ultimately in the child's best interests.

9.9 CHILDREN, YOUNG PEOPLE, AND HUMAN RIGHTS

As has been highlighted in this chapter, human rights considerations have come to play an increasingly important role in applications to the courts regarding decision-making and consent processes involving the treatment of children and young people. In this section of the chapter, the aim is to highlight human rights instruments of relevance in this regard, as well as to briefly reflect on the judicial approach to incorporating human rights in this area of health and medical law. First and foremost, the Human Rights Act 1998 (HRA), as well as how it has been interpreted in case law jurisprudence, form part of the human rights-based framework applicable in this area in the UK. ECHR rights which are relevant in the context of decision-making and consent processes involving medical treatment of children and young people include Article 3 (prohibition of torture, inhuman or degrading treatment or punishment), Article 5 (right to liberty and security), Article 8 (right to respect for family and private life), and Article 14 (right not to have ECHR rights secured in a discriminatory way).

Other relevant human rights instruments include the United Nations Convention on the Rights of People with Disabilities (UNCRPD), which is applicable to children with disabilities (Article 7).[183] Specifically, Article 7(2) notes that in all actions concerning children with disabilities, the best interests of the child shall be a primary consideration.

---

[180] ibid. [38].   [181] ibid. [71].
[182] *X (A Child) (No. 2), Re* [2021] EWHC 65 (Fam) [21] (Sir James Munby).
[183] United Nations Convention on the Rights of People with Disabilities, adopted 13 December 2006, UN General Assembly, Sixty-First Session, A/RES/61/106, available at <https://www.un.org/development/desa/disabilities/convention-on-the-rights-of-persons-with-disabilities.html> accessed 09 January 2023, discussed in more detail in Chapter 10.

Under Article 7(3), the state must ensure that such children have the right to express their views freely on all matters affecting them, their views being given due weight in accordance with their age and maturity, on an equal basis with other children. The UK ratified the Convention in 2009 but has not incorporated it into domestic law to date.

Of particular importance is the United Nations Convention of the Rights of the Child (CRC), which came into force in 1990.[184] Key CRC rights which are relevant to questions of consent or conversely refusal to consent to treatment involving children and young people, include Article 3 (best interests of the child shall be a primary consideration), Article 5 (parents/guardians should act in a child's best interests while also recognising their evolving capacity), Article 12 (respect for children's views in all matters which impact their lives; this requires the child to be provided the opportunity to be heard in legal and administrative proceedings), and Article 24 (child's right to the highest standard of health). Although the CRC was ratified by the UK in 1991, it has not yet been incorporated into domestic law to date. However, Scotland recently sought to incorporate key aspects of the CRC into Scots law.[185]

The aim of the UNCRC Bill is to 'deliver a proactive culture of everyday accountability for children's rights across public services in Scotland', in all Scottish public authorities would be required 'to take proactive steps to ensure the protection of children's rights in their decision-making and service delivery and make it unlawful for public authorities, including the Scottish Government, to act incompatibly with the UNCRC requirements as set out in the Bill.'[186] In 2021, a Supreme Court challenge was brought by the UK Government in relation to the Bill on the grounds that it was outside the powers of the Scottish Parliament pursuant to the Scotland Act 1998. This was upheld in part by the Supreme Court and the Bill was subsequently referred back to the Scottish Parliament for further consideration in light of the judgment.[187] At the time of writing, the Scottish Government remains committed to incorporating the UNCRC into Scots law to the 'maximum extent possible'.[188] Stakeholder consultations have been undertaken in relation to the necessary amendments to be made to the Bill in order to address the Supreme Court judgment and a revised Bill will be presented for consideration by the Scottish Parliament in 2023.[189]

With a range of human rights instruments available in terms of either being directly legally enforceable (i.e. ECHR through the HRA) or otherwise able to be used as a reference point (i.e. UNCRPD or UNCRC), the question is how the UK courts have sought to take human rights considerations into account in the context of decision-making and

---

[184] United Nations Convention on the Rights of the Child, adopted 20 November 1989, UN General Assembly Resolution 44/25, available at <https://www.ohchr.org/en/instruments-mechanisms/instruments/convention-rights-child> accessed 09 January 2023.

[185] For an overview, see Scottish Parliament, 'United Nations Convention on the Rights of the Child (UNCRC) (Incorporation) Scotland Bill 2021' (2022) available at <https://www.parliament.scot/bills-and-laws/bills/united-nations-convention-on-the-rights-of-the-child-incorporation-scotland-bill> accessed 09 January 2023.

[186] Scottish Government, 'Children's Rights' (2022) available at <https://www.gov.scot/policies/human-rights/childrens-rights/#:~:text=The%20UNCRC%20is%20the%20most,the%20right%20to%20be%20heard> accessed 09 January 2023.

[187] Reference by the Attorney General and the Advocate General for Scotland—United Nations Convention on the Rights of the Child (Incorporation) (Scotland) Bill, Case ID: 2021/0079, 6 October 2021.

[188] Scottish Government, 'Pledge on Children's Rights' (6 October 2021) available at <https://www.gov.scot/news/pledge-on-childrens-rights> accessed 09 January 2023.

[189] Scottish Government, Children's Rights (n 186).

consent processes involving medical treatment of children and young people. For one commentator, the approach has been 'extraordinarily haphazard'.[190] As our examination of case law in this chapter has highlighted, it would be safe to say that the approach taken by the courts has been grounded in addressing the particular facts of a given case, rather than pursuing a coherent strategy in relation to the application of a human rights framework to healthcare decision-making involving children and young people.

In *Gillick*, Lord Scarman recognised that children were 'right-holders', finding that where they are considered of 'sufficient intelligence and understanding', the 'parental right yields to the child's right to make [their] own decisions'.[191] Where reference is made to human rights instruments in case law, however, they are viewed as evidencing support for the recognition of young people's evolving autonomy but not as determinative.[192] With some notable exceptions, judicial support for viewing young people as rights-bearers seem to be subordinate, if not disappear, in cases where there is a refusal of life-saving treatment. In such cases, even where a young person may be *Gillick* competent, when this is balanced against medical opinion and/or parental preferences, the courts invariably revert to a protective role, employing a best interests assessment in line with their inherent jurisdiction powers.[193]

Part of the problem for the courts in assessing questions of evolving capacity may reflect not only the gravity of adverse healthcare consequences that may result for the young person but also the evidence they hear from treating HCPs which highlight the difficulties in assessing capacity in their young patients.[194] Accessing and according 'due weight' to young people's ability to make decisions, as well as how best to take account of their wishes and feelings, can be difficult to conceptualise and define in the medico-legal context. In practice, courts may find themselves on safer ground in shifting their focus to best interests rather than rights-based considerations. However, the end result of this shift is troubling for young people who are *Gillick* competent and find their wishes and feelings circumscribed with respect to autonomous decision-making about their own healthcare.

9.10 CONCLUSION

In this chapter, we examined key case law, legislation, and human rights instruments relevant to consent to medical treatment involving children and young people. Our examination highlighted that this area of health and medical law is fraught with a range of tensions arising from seeking to balance considerations of welfare and autonomy in healthcare decision-making. While *Gillick* competence has the potential to assist in this regard, it is clear the courts continue to struggle with the concept in the context of the evolving capacity of young people. This was highlighted in the context of refusal of life-saving

---

[190] See Jane Fortin, 'Accommodating Children's Rights in a Post Human Rights Act Era' (2006) 69(3) Modern Law Review 299, 300.

[191] *Gillick* (n 27) [186] (Scarman LJ).

[192] *Mabon v Mabon and others* (2005) Fam 366 [32].

[193] We note with interest the comments by Lady Hale in the UK Supreme Court judgment, *In the Matter of D (A Child)* [2019] UKSC 42 at [50], where she observed that a human rights-based approach would not necessarily draw a distinction between those over and under 16 years of age as is the case under the common law (albeit she was specifically referencing Art 5 ECHR on the deprivation of liberty).

[194] It has been argued that while assessment of children's capacity may be grounded in intuition and experience for HCPs, it should nevertheless be done 'via a process which is rights-based'; see Aoife Daly, 'Assessing Children's Capacity' (2020) 28(3) International Journal of Children's Rights 471.

medical treatment by young people, particularly those with deeply held religious beliefs. In cases involving critically ill young children, questions of parental choice in deciding whether, and if so, what sort of medical treatment they wish their offspring to receive, can clash with courts' assessment of their best interests, which must take precedence over their wishes. A human rights-based approach may offer a way forward in managing the tensions between welfare and autonomy, but the courts appear reluctant to fully embrace such an approach, tending to find safer ground in their reliance on best interests.

FURTHER READING

1. Priscilla Anderson et al., 'Living Bioethics, Theories and Children's Consent to Heart Surgery' (2022) 17(3) Clinical Ethics 272.

2. Imogen Goold, Jonathan Herring, and Cressida Auckland (eds), *Parental Rights, Best Interests and Significant Harms: Medical Decision-making on Behalf of Children Post-Great Ormond Street Hospital v Gard* (Hart 2019).

3. Imogen Goold and Cressida Auckland, 'Resolving Disagreement: A Multi-Jurisdictional Comparative Analysis of Disputes about Children's Medical Care' (2020) 28(4) Medical Law Review 643.

4. Julian März, 'What Does the Best Interests Principle of the Convention on the Rights of the Child Mean for Paediatric Healthcare?' (2022) 181 European Journal of Paediatrics 3805.

5. Michelle Taylor-Sands and Georgina Dimopoulos, 'Judicial Discomfort over "Innovative" Treatment for Adolescents with Gender Dysphoria' (2022) 30(3) Medical Law Review 479.

10

MENTAL HEALTH LAW

10.1 INTRODUCTION

Mental health law, and the practices of psychiatry that accompany it, have long been a controversial aspect of health and medical law, as well as ethics. Yet poor mental health is not uncommon; approximately 1 in 4 people in the UK experience some form of mental health problem in their lifetime, with 1 in 6 having a mental health problem at any one time,[1] and over 1.5 million people in the UK have a learning disability.[2] In spite of this prevalence, the regime for providing care and treatment for adults with poor mental health or mental disabilities remains distinct from physical health. While law and ethics considers the consent of a patient as (almost always) essential when giving treatment, under mental health law it is permissible and legal to treat a patient without their consent, and at times, when they are actively objecting to it. This may require some form of compulsion and detention in an acute mental healthcare facility, with restrictions placed on individual liberty and autonomy, in order to provide treatment for the patient, or to mitigate the risk they pose to others.

But mental health law is not only focused on offering treatment for acute 'mental disorder'; individuals with long-term conditions or mental disabilities also fall within its remit. They may be viewed as requiring protection, and it may be necessary to detain them in an acute setting to provide this. Alternatively, they may be held to lack capacity to make decisions about daily aspects of their lives, with others making decisions on their behalf. This raises questions about the extent of lawful interference in the lives of individuals with disabilities and the appropriateness of a separate legal framework for decision making where they are concerned.

And, as the modern system for health and social care is not confined to hospital settings, mental health law reaches into the community and even at times into individuals' homes. This creates the potential for significant intrusion into their lives. From this context, two key challenges emerge: 1) how mental health law can balance its stated need to treat and protect vulnerable individuals with the degree of compulsion and control required to achieve this aim, and 2) what safeguards or opportunities ought to be available to resist or challenge compulsion. In this chapter, we discuss how each of the UK jurisdictions has responded to these challenges.

As this book is primarily concerned with health and medical law, the focus of this chapter is on the civil aspects of mental health law; that is to say, aspects which permit

---

[1] Public Health Scotland, 'Mental Health and Wellbeing' (24 December 2021) available at <http://www.healthscotland.scot/health-topics/mental-health-and-wellbeing/overview-of-mental-health-and-wellbeing> (accessed 10 August 2022).

[2] Mencap, 'How Common is Learning Disability?' (2022) available at <https://www.mencap.org.uk/learning-disability-explained/research-and-statistics/how-common-learning-disability> accessed 04 September 2022.

decision making on behalf of individuals and treatment without consent. The management of forensic matters and the interface between mental health law and the criminal
justice system are not discussed. This chapter also focuses on the situation with adults; the
position regarding children is discussed in Chapter 9. We first provide a brief overview of
the legislative frameworks within the UK and the system it creates, before considering the
key concepts and justifications engaged through it. We then examine in detail legislation
across the UK, focusing first on compulsory treatment regimes and then on questions of
capacity. The chapter concludes by considering human rights issues engaged in mental
health law, and the potential for reform in the area.

10.2 THE UK LEGISLATIVE FRAMEWORK: A LANDSCAPE SKETCH

In the majority of the UK jurisdictions, mental health law consists of two linked statutory
frameworks, one which concerns the treatment of a patient's 'mental disorder', on a compulsory basis if necessary (often referred to as 'detention'), and the other which focuses
on decision-making (including but not limited to medical treatment) for adults whose
capacity to decide for themselves is impaired. The exception is Northern Ireland, where
a 'fusion approach' has been adopted, with one piece of legislation covering both areas of
law (but yet to be fully implemented).

10.2.1 TREATING MENTAL HEALTH PROBLEMS

In England and Wales, the Mental Health Act 1983 (MHA 1983)[3] governs the process for
admission to and treatment in acute mental health facilities. The Mental Health Care and
Treatment (Scotland) Act 2003 (MHCTA 2003)[4] provides a comparable framework. The
provisions of these statutes are discussed in more detail below, but both provide (among
other areas):

- the legal basis for admission and detention in hospital on a compulsory basis for the
  purpose of treating 'mental disorder';

- the process for authorising specific procedures, including those which require a second opinion from a medical practitioner;

- mechanisms for compulsory outpatient care;

- details of specific statutory roles to support patients, such as the Nearest Relative or
  Named Person role, and advocacy roles; and

- procedures for ending compulsory treatment and detention, including via appeal to
  the relevant Tribunal.

The legal (and ethical) basis for compulsory treatment under both Acts is a 'mental
disorder plus risk' paradigm, meaning the risk (to the patient or to others) posed by the
level of 'disorder' cannot be mitigated without requiring the patient to receive treatment.

Clinical expertise is crucial in determining that this threshold is met. Indeed, the
medical profession has always been involved in making decisions regarding compulsory

---

[3] As amended by the Mental Health Act 2007, hereafter referred to in its amended form as the MHA 1983.
[4] As amended by the Mental Health (Scotland) Act 2017.

treatment and detention, with admission to an institution based on the assessment of two medical practitioners since the nineteenth century.[5]

In spite of the importance of medical (and in particular, psychiatric) experience, clinical roles in the mental health system have diversified. Treatment is provided through a multi-disciplinary team in hospital and community settings, with other important professions such as nurses, and allied healthcare professionals such as clinical psychologists and social workers, providing input from their distinct professional viewpoint.

Broadly, statutory clinical roles include those who take responsibility for a patient's care, those who support a patient throughout their admission to hospital, and those who may be called on to provide a second opinion, should a serious treatment be considered (the procedure for this is discussed in more detail). **Table 10.1** provides an overview of some of the key roles contained in the MHA 1983 and MHCTA 2003.

Professionals who carry out these statutory roles are required to adhere to the relevant codes of practice. Under the MHA 1983, the purpose of the Code of Practice is to provide guidance to professionals and include a statement of principles to inform decision-making under the Act.[6] The principles currently contained within the English Code of Practice are:

- **Least restrictive option and maximising independence** (patients should be treated without detention, their independence should be encouraged and recovery supported wherever possible).
- **Empowerment and involvement** (patients should be fully involved in decisions about their care and treatment, with the views of families and carers taken into account).
- **Respect and dignity** (patients, families and carers should be listened to and treated with respect and dignity).
- **Purpose and effectiveness** (care and treatment decisions should be tailored to the patient with clear aims to promote recovery, based on current evidence, guidance, and best practice).
- **Efficiency and equity** (service providers and other organisations should work together to ensure high quality services for mental health, as an equal priority to physical health, and facilitate safe discharge).[7]

The Welsh Code of Practice largely mirrors these principles, except it contains an additional principle—'keeping people safe'—and replaces 'purpose and effectiveness' with 'effectiveness and efficiency', and efficiency and equity with 'fairness equity and equality'.[8] While these codes are highly persuasive in assessing whether the conduct of professionals and services has met appropriate standards, they are considered guidance and not instruction. As such, departure from their standards is possible, but only where the professional or service has a good, cogent reason to do so.[9]

---

[5] The Lunatics Act 1845.

[6] MHA 1983, s 118.

[7] Department of Health and Social Care, 'Mental Health Act 1983: Code of Practice' (2017) available at <https://www.gov.uk/government/publications/code-of-practice-mental-health-act-1983> accessed 04 September 2022.

[8] Welsh Government, 'Mental Health Act 1983: the Code of Practice for Wales' (2016) available at <https://gov.wales/mental-health-act-1983-code-practice> accessed 04 September 2022.

[9] R (Munjaz) v Ashworth Hospital Authority [2005] UKHL 58.

Table 10.1 Key statutory roles involved in compulsory care and treatment

Title	Legislation	Profession	Responsibilities
Coordination and oversight of compulsory care			
Responsible Clinician (RC)[10] (*England and Wales*)	s 34 MHA 1983.	An Approved Clinician (AC) who is a medical practitioner, psychologist, nurse, occupational therapist, or social worker (with appropriate qualifications)—the majority are psychiatrists.	Responsible for assessing the patient and overseeing compulsory treatment, both in inpatient and community setting. Can grant leave of absence, recall the patient to hospital and make decisions around discharge. Must keep necessity of detention under review.
Responsible Medical Officer (RMO) (*Scotland*)	s 230 MHCTA 2003.	Medical practitioner, usually one who is an Approved Medical Practitioner (AMP).	Coordinate care. Where long-term detention is required, must sign the application to request detention, and prepare a care plan (s 76). AMP may also grant/revoke a certificate to allow detention on a short-term basis.
Providing support for the patient			
Approved Mental Health Professional (AMHP) (*England and Wales*)	ss 13, 114-115 MHA 1983.	Social worker, nurse, occupational therapist, or psychologist who meets the criteria and has completed relevant training. Approved and appointed by social services authorities.	Coordinating and participating in admission process, identifying and contacting a patient's Nearest Relative, and involved in community treatment. Must ensure patients' rights are respected, wishes are taken into account, and non-discrimination.
Mental Health Officer (MHO) (*Scotland*)	ss 32, 45, 57-62, 85, 89, 138, 147, 151, 155, 181, 205, 229, 231, 255 MHCTA 2003.	Social worker appointed by the local authority.	Provide patients with information about their rights (including right of appeal), involvement in short term detention, responsible for making application for long-term detention and liaising with patient's Named Person.
Providing a second opinion			
Second Opinion Appointed Doctor (SOAD) (*England and Wales*)	Part IV MHA 1983	Medical practitioner appointed by the Care Quality Commission.	Section 57 treatments—must confirm patient is able to consent *and* provide second opinion that treatment is appropriate. Section 58 treatments—confirm patient is able to consent *or* provide second opinion that treatment is appropriate.
Designated Medical Practitioner (DMP) (*Scotland*)	Part 16 MHCTA 2003, s 233.	Medical practitioner appointed by the Mental Welfare Commission for Scotland.	Can interview and examine the patient and review records, must confirm whether patient is capable or incapable or consent and whether they are objecting to treatment or not, confirm proceeding with treatment is in the patient's best interests.

[10] For a detailed discussion, see Nicola Glover-Thomas and Judith Laing, 'Mental Health Professionals' in Lawrence Gostin et al. (eds.) *Principles of Mental Health Law and Policy* (OUP 2010).

In Scotland, the principles are provided in MHCTA 2003 itself (with the accompanying Code of Practice providing guidance to persons who discharge functions under the Act),[11] and as such they have the force of law. The principles require professionals discharging functions under the Act to consider:

(a) the relevant 'present and past wishes and feelings of the patient';

(b) the views of individuals close to the patient, such as their named person or carer;

(c) 'the importance of the patient participating as fully as possible';

(d) 'the importance of providing information and support' to enable their participation;

(e) 'the range of options available';

(f) 'the importance of providing the maximum benefit to the patient';

(g) 'the need to ensure that, unless it can be shown that it is justified in the circumstances, the patient is not treated in a way that is less favourable than the way in which a person who is not a patient might be treated in a comparable situation'; and

(h) 'the patient's abilities, background and characteristics, including, without prejudice to that generality, the patient's age, sex, sexual orientation, religious persuasion, racial origin, cultural and linguistic background and membership of any ethnic group.'[12]

10.2.2 DECISION MAKING FOR ADULTS WHO LACK CAPACITY

In England and Wales, the Mental Capacity Act 2005 (MCA 2005)[13] provides the legal basis for taking decisions for adults deemed to lack capacity to decide for themselves. The foundations and ethos of the MCA 2005 differ considerably from the MHA 1983. The Act emphasises allowing the individual (referred to as 'P') to participate in decision-making even when they are unable to decide from themselves, placing them at the heart of decisions, and providing protection where they cannot decide for themselves,[14] a far cry from the risk-based approach of the MHA 1983.

The MCA 2005 is underpinned by a series of statutory principles (having taken inspiration from its Scottish counterpart), which require that all individuals are presumed to have capacity to make decisions, even if those decisions are considered unwise.[15] Where an individual is found to lack capacity to make a particular decision, any course of action taken must be in their best interests,[16] with regard to whether the purpose could be achieved in a less restrictive manner, by reference to the person's rights and freedoms.[17] The MCA 2005 also contains provisions to authorise P's care and treatment arrangements where these result in a deprivation of their liberty which is not covered by the MHA 1983 (under the 'Deprivation of Liberty Safeguards' or 'DoLS' scheme).[18] Whether the Act has lived up to its stated aim is debateable; post-legislative scrutiny by the House of Lords

---

[11] MHCTA 2003, s 274; Scottish Government, 'Mental Health (Care and Treatment) (Scotland) Act 2003: Code of Practice' (2005) available at <https://www.gov.scot/publications/mental-health-care-treatment-scotland-act-2003-code-practice-volume-3-compulsory-powers-relation-mentally-disordered-offenders/> accessed 04 September 2022.

[12] MHCTA 2003, s 1(3).   [13] As amended by the Mental Health Act 2007.

[14] Office of the Public Guardian, 'Mental Capacity Act Code of Practice' (2013) available at <https://www.gov.uk/government/publications/mental-capacity-act-code-of-practice> accessed 04 September 2022.

[15] MCA 2005, ss 1(2)-(4).   [16] ibid., s 1(5).   [17] ibid., s 1(6).

[18] MCA 2005, Sch A1, as will be discussed in detail.

suggests there are significant gaps in practice, a lack of awareness and understanding, and prevailing cultures of risk-aversion and paternalism that mean the rights conferred by the MCA 2005 have not been realised.[19]

In Scotland, the Adults with Incapacity (Scotland) Act 2000 (AWIA 2000) provides the framework for treating individuals incapable of providing consent. Although it is similar to the MCA 2005, it focuses on intervention in the affairs of an adult, who is defined as a person over 16 years old, rather than basing its *raison d'être* in empowerment and protection. In Chapter 10, we focus solely on the provisions relating to capacity and medical treatment.

The AWIA 2000 contains five statutory principles,[20] which are as follows:

1. The intervention must **benefit** the person and be the only reasonable way to achieve that benefit.

2. The intervention must be the **least restrictive option**, taking account of its purpose.

3. In taking the decision, the **person's wishes and feelings** must be taken into account, with assistance provided to allow these to be communicated.

4. The decision maker must take account of the **views of others with an interest**, for example the named person, close family, an attorney or guardian.

5. Anyone exercising a function under the Act **must encourage the adult to make their own decisions and develop the necessary skills** to do so, where required.

Adherence to the principles provides decision makers with a general defence against allegations of breach of duty. In this way, they are fundamental to the operation of the Act.

In the health and social care context, the majority of decisions taken under the MCA 2005 and AWIA 2000 are taken by health and social care workers (in absence of appointed deputies or attorneys). However, in some instances, intervention from a court is required.

Both the MCA 2005 and AWIA 2000 are supported by their own Codes of Practice, which provide detailed guidance to those involved in their decision-making processes.[21] Under the MCA 2005, where an aspect of the Code—or a failure to comply with it— becomes apparent in legal proceedings, courts or tribunals must take this failure this into account when making a determination on the matter in question.[22] But it bears remembering that, per the previous discussion, the Codes of Practice are binding on professionals and local authorities.

The interface between the capacity-based Acts and the involuntary treatment Acts remains complex. It remains possible that an adult detained under the MHA 1983 or MHCTA 2003 may lack capacity under the MCA 2005 or AWIA 2000. When it comes to the MCA 2005's DoLS in particular, the interface with the MHA 1983 is highly complex, given the potential for overlap (both can, in theory, be used in the same hospital setting).[23] Which Act is utilised may rely on whether the patient expresses an objection or not, but the practice of identifying if this is the case may not be straightforward.[24]

---

[19] UK Parliament, 'Select Committee on the Mental Capacity Act 2005 – Report' (2005) available at <https://publications.parliament.uk/pa/ld201314/ldselect/ldmentalcap/139/13902.htm> accessed 04 September 2022.

[20] AWIA 2000, s 1.

[21] Office of the Public Guardian (n 14). The AWIA 2000 is supported by six Codes of Practice for different actors. See Scottish Government, 'Adults with incapacity: forms and guidance' (2022) available at <https://www.gov.scot/collections/adults-with-incapacity-forms-and-guidance/> accessed 04 September 2022.

[22] MCA 2005, s 42(5).

[23] For a discussion, see Neil Allen, 'The (Not So) Great Confinement' (2015) 5(1) Elder Law Journal 45.

[24] ibid.; for general rules on which Act to apply in Scotland, see Jill Stavert and Henry Patrick, *Mental Health, Incapacity and the Law in Scotland* (2nd edn, Bloomsbury 2016) 405.

10.2.3 A FUSION APPROACH

Prior to 2016, mental health law in Northern Ireland largely reflected the approach taken in the other UK nations. The Mental Health Order 1986 (MHO 1986) largely mirrored the MHA 1983 and the traditional approach to mental health legislation (i.e. an involuntary treatment framework). However, with the passage of the Mental Capacity Act (Northern Ireland) in 2016 (MCANI 2016), Northern Ireland has begun to move in a separate direction. The MCANI 2016 aims to bring together or 'fuse' mental health and capacity legislation, providing treatment under a single legal basis: impairment of decision-making capacity and best interests. First proposed by Dawson and Szmukler, a fusion approach intends to avoid the discriminatory elements of mental health legislation by applying a single capacity-based model for medical decision making, rather than a separate legal framework for mental health.[25] It therefore moves away from the 'mental disorder plus risk' paradigm to justify intervention in the lives of adults. Through this, it seeks to enhance patient autonomy, promote patient rights, and reduce the stigmatisation of mental disorder.[26]

The MCANI 2016 is underpinned by a series of principles, which reflect those in the MCA 2005. These include:

- the presumption of capacity;
- lack of capacity should not be established based on assumptions about any conditions or characteristics of the person or because a decision appears unwise; and
- lack of capacity should not be established 'unless all practicable help and support to enable the person to make a decision about the matter have been given without success'.[27]

Like the MCA 2005, the MCANI 2016 also requires that where a person lacks capacity, the act or decision made must be in their best interests,[28] and has provisions relating to authorising a deprivation of liberty to provide care.[29]

The MCANI 2016 is undergoing a phased implementation and once this is complete, the MHO 1986 will be repealed.[30] The lack of full implementation means it is not possible to evaluate whether a fusion approach will meet its stated aims of enhancing patient autonomy and protecting rights. It is reliant on the idealist reading of capacity law as empowering individuals and placing them at the heart of decision-making. As discussed, in practice this has not necessarily been realised under the MCA 2005. Complete implementation may take ten to fifteen years and has been further delayed by the Covid-19 pandemic. To be successful in its aim, a significant shift away from a risk-based culture would be required. The system will also require appropriate financial resourcing to ensure its success. It seems likely that the other UK nations will continue to watch NI's process when considering whether such a model is appropriate to adopt in the future.

---

[25] John Dawson and George Szmukler, 'Fusion of Mental Health and Incapacity Legislation' (2006) 188(6) British Journal of Psychiatry 504.

[26] ibid.   [27] MCANI 2016, ss 1(2)–1(5).   [28] ibid., s 2(2).   [29] ibid., ss 24–27, Sch 2.

[30] Department of Health (Northern Ireland), 'Mental Capacity Act Background' (2022) available at <https://www.health-ni.gov.uk/mental-capacity-act-background#:~:text=The%20Act%20provides%20 a%20statutory,future%20when%20they%20lack%20capacity.> accessed 04 September 2022.

10.2.4 REGULATORY OVERSIGHT

The existence of a government-sponsored oversight body for facilitating compliance and enforcement with regulatory standards in mental health care has been an important part of the mental health law system since the eighteenth century. In particular, it has been seen as a vital check on ensuring that those who are wielding compulsory powers under such laws do so appropriately. In England and Wales, the Madhouses Act 1774 created the first regulatory body. Through the enhanced powers granted by the Lunatics Act 1845, this body became the Lunacy Commission. Arguments supporting a regulatory authority arose out of concern over the poor conditions and practices in eighteenth century institutions and a need to bring 'private madhouses' within the control of law. With the advent of the NHS, the regulatory functions were absorbed into what then became known as the Health Advisory Service (the precursor of the UK Department of Health).

In England and Wales, the Care Quality Commission (CQC) now regulates acute mental health services and those provided within social care, although it does not have powers in relation to supported living arrangements, so its reach into community settings is more limited. As part of its statutory role, it is required to promote and protect the rights of service users, in particular individuals detained under the MHA 1983 or deprived of their liberty under the MCA 2005.[31] The CQC is responsible for licensing mental health providers, ensuring that such services meet its standards, and monitoring use of the MHA 1983's compulsory mechanisms and MCA 2005's DoLS scheme. It has powers to inspect mental health services and to investigate complaints. It produces annual reports in relation to this monitoring work.[32] As noted, the CQC is also responsible for the appointment of SOADs and will monitor how often the SOAD procedures are used. While the CQC aims to utilise a rights-based approach,[33] its regulatory approach been widely criticised, not least for its failures to detect and prevent instances of abuse in private hospitals for adults with learning disabilities and autism, for example in Winterbourne View in 2011,[34] and again at Whorlton Hall in 2019.[35]

In Northern Ireland, the Regulation and Quality Improvement Authority (RQIA) fulfils an analogous regulatory role to the CQC and produces reports regarding its inspection of facilities, as well as scrutinising detentions to ensure they remain appropriate (with powers to terminate 'improper detention').[36]

The position differs slightly in Scotland; although the Mental Welfare Commission for Scotland (MWCS) has a statutory function to monitor the Scottish Acts in a similar way, it is not a formal regulatory authority. The MWCS instead states that its function is 'to protect and promote the human rights of people with mental health problems,

[31] Health and Social Care Act 2008, s 4(1)(d).

[32] Care Quality Commission, 'Monitoring the Mental Health Act in 2020/21' (2022) available at <https://www.cqc.org.uk/publications/major-report/monitoring-mental-health-act> accessed 04 September 2022.

[33] Judy Laing, 'Protecting the Rights of Patients in Psychiatric Settings: A Comparison of the Work of the Mental Health Act Commission with the Care Quality Commission' (2014) 36(2) Journal of Social Welfare and Family Law 149.

[34] BBC, 'Timeline: Winterbourne View Abuse Scandal' (20 December 2012) available at <https://www.bbc.co.uk/news/uk-england-bristol-20078999> accessed 04 September 2022.

[35] Glynis Murphy, 'CQC Inspections and Regulation of Whorlton Hall 2015–2019: an Independent Review' (March 2020) available at <https://www.cqc.org.uk/sites/default/files/20020218_glynis-murphy-review.pdf> accessed 04 September 2022.

[36] The Regulation and Quality Improvement Authority, 'What We Do: Mental Health and Learning Disability' (2022) available at <https://www.rqia.org.uk/what-we-do/mental-health-learning-disability/> accessed 04 September 2022.

learning disabilities, dementia and associated conditions.'[37] Through its monitoring function, it produces annual reports on the use of the MHCTA 2003 and AWIA 2000 and 'themed visit reports' on specific areas of legislation to identify trends and issues in how the law is used.[38] It also uses its position to influence and challenge mental health law and policy in Scotland, and provides patients and families with advice and information. Like the CQC, the MWCS appoints DMPs and monitors the regulatory that DMP second opinions are required.[39]

10.3 KEY CONCEPTS AND PRINCIPLES

Having outlined key aspects of the UK legal frameworks in mental health, we now turn to consider in more detail some of the key concepts that have underpinned the development of such frameworks, including whether they are justified by reference to promoting individual autonomy and empowerment.

10.3.1 PROTECTION, RISK, AND DANGEROUSNESS

A key justification offered for the existence of compulsory treatment powers is that they are necessary to protect the patient. They might pose a danger to themselves, and even if they are refusing treatment, it will restore their health or save their life. Protection might also be warranted because the individual's mental health condition makes them incapable of making decisions for themselves (i.e. they lack capacity), yet decisions are needed about care, living arrangements, or other aspects of their life. The law allows decisions to be taken on their behalf by their healthcare practitioners or a court in order to protect them, including when they disagree. In this context, protection appears to be a form of justifiable paternalism because the act is done with the intention of protecting the individual from harm.

To focus only on protection at this personal level would be to neglect its second facet, where the individual may not pose a risk to themselves but is considered a risk to others. Detaining them and providing treatment may be necessary to provide public protection and control the risk posed to members of society. This so-called 'dangerousness' of mental health patients has played an important role in conceptualising mental health law and, fuelled in part by the mainstream (and now social) media depictions of individuals with mental health problems perpetrating violence, has driven narratives around policy reform in recent decades.[40]

A consequence of the predominance of this narrative is that a risk-based model remains firmly embedded in medical decision-making throughout the process of detention, treatment, and discharge. However, it may well be that the prediction of dangerousness is a pragmatic and imprecise—and, perhaps, fruitless—exercise.[41] Many attempts have been made to determine an objective concept of dangerousness, but none have

[37] Mental Welfare Commission for Scotland, 'Who We Are and What We Do' (2022) <https://www.mwcscot.org.uk/about-us/who-we-are-and-what-we-do> accessed 22 July 2022.

[38] Mental Welfare Commission for Scotland, 'Monitoring the Acts' (2022) available at <https://www.mwcscot.org.uk/law-rights/monitoring-acts> accessed 04 September 2022.

[39] MHCTA 2003, s 233.

[40] Peter Bartlett and Ralph Sandland, *Mental Health Law: Policy and Practice* (OUP 2007) 239–243.

[41] See e.g. Eileen Munro and Judith Rumgay, 'Role of Risk Assessments in Reducing Homicides by People with Mental Illnesses' (2000) 176(2) British Journal of Psychiatry 116.

succeeded in allaying doubts as to the strong element of subjectivity that is inherent in such judgments.[42]

When it comes to decisions under the MCA 2005, questions of risk and public protection also feature, for example in decisions regarding deprivation of liberty, and the recent UK Supreme Court judgment in *A Local Authority* v *JB*,[43] which is examined in more detail later in this chapter.

10.3.2 AUTONOMY, EMPOWERMENT, AND LIBERTY

Given the potential for 'protection' to interfere with broad aspects of individuals' lives, it is little wonder that questions about autonomy arise, with two portrayed as a fundamental tension in mental health law—it must balance a patient's right to autonomy with the need to protect them, or the public, when they are unwell. Against a background where facilitating patient autonomy is recognised as important in the context of providing treatment in healthcare settings (as discussed in Chapter 8), calls continue to be made for patient autonomy to be afforded a greater role in the mental health system, and for patients to be given more choice over what treatment they are given (see discussion on reform). Of course, what facilitating patient autonomy looks like will turn on what interpretation is adopted and what dimension we are interested in (as discussed in Chapter 2), and is potentially challenging in the context of a compulsory treatment environment where opportunities for choice may be restricted. Indeed, choice and empowerment are considered central to capacity-based legislation; its stated aim is to encourage and support individuals to choose for themselves, or, as a minimum, take their wishes and views into account in the decision-making process.[44] However, as various commentators have noted, empowerment as a concept can itself be stigmatising, portraying the individual as in need of 'fixing' to obtain a particular standard of normality. It can even lead to compulsory treatment on the basis that such treatment will allow the individual to obtain greater independence.[45] This demonstrates the potential paradoxical outcomes that 'empowerment' and the autonomy we consider we are fostering might bring.

Closely linked to autonomy and empowerment is the concept of liberty. With detention or care and treatment plans entailing control of an individual's daily life,[46] questions arise as to the extent to which interference with liberty is justifiable in the interests of protection. Again, much will turn on what 'liberty' itself looks like, engaging with questions of well-being and the ability to live life in accordance with one's own wishes. We will discuss this in detail in the human rights context, but what constitutes liberty in mental capacity law is not tied to a particular location or context, and may instead be viewed as being a question of the extent to which an individual who lacks capacity is subject to control and supervision over daily life.[47]

---

[42] See, in general, John K Mason, 'The Legal Aspects and Implications of Risk Assessment' (2000) 8(1) Medical Law Review 69; and, more specifically, James McMillan, 'Dangerousness, Mental Disorder and Responsibility' (2003) 29(4) Journal of Medical Ethics 232.

[43] [2021] UKSC 52.

[44] Mental Capacity Act 2005, ss 1–45; AWIA 2000, s 1; MCANI 2016, Part 1.

[45] Beverley Clough, *The Spaces of Mental Capacity Law: Moving Beyond Binaries* (Routledge 2022); Lucy Series, *Deprivation of Liberty in the Shadows of the Institution* (Bristol University Press 2022) 23.

[46] *Guzzardi* v *Italy* [1980] ECHR 5.

[47] *Cheshire West and Chester Council* v *P and another* [2014] UKSC 19.

10.3.3 VULNERABILITY

In the mental health context, vulnerability is generally understood to mean that individuals with mental health problems are at increased risk of harm because of their condition. It follows that a liberal society has an obligation to protect its most vulnerable, and mental health law thus provides a framework to tackle this vulnerability. This account has been criticised because of its connotations of weakness and helplessness, which it is argued have been used to justify paternalism.[48] Indeed, the label vulnerable is ascribed in this context to certain individuals to justify a range of paternalistic action, including where the perceived vulnerability is not necessarily linked to the mental health problem itself.[49] On this basis, some disability scholars reject the term.[50] As discussed in Chapter 2, other theorists argue that responses to vulnerability ought to foster (instead of undermine) autonomy and the two concepts should not be viewed as oppositional.[51] This is not the approach currently adopted by the mental health systems in the UK; as noted, policy and legal responses to the protection of the vulnerable and enhancing autonomy are presented as being in tension in both ethical and legal terms.[52]

As we now turn to consider specific elements of each legislative framework in greater detail, it remains important to keep in mind how these concepts are deployed to shape the legislation, its application by judges, and calls for its reform.

10.4 COMPULSORY TREATMENT

10.4.1 WHAT IS A MENTAL DISORDER?

As discussed, the diagnosis of a mental disorder is crucial to the operation of compulsory treatment powers. Who is within the scope of these powers therefore turns on the definition given to 'mental disorder'.

In England and Wales, the MHA 1983 currently operates under a single broad definition, defining 'mental disorder' as 'any disorder or disability of the mind'.[53] Only two exclusions exist, learning disability and autism, which are not considered a mental disorder for the purposes of certain provisions of the Act unless 'associated with abnormally aggressive or seriously irresponsible misconduct'[54] and dependence on alcohol and drugs.[55]

The breadth of the definition and limited exclusions potentially permit a finding of disorder based on a lack of compliance with predominant social norms (impacting mainly on minoritised groups); for example, gender dysphoria is in principle included. The

---

[48] Beverley Clough, 'Disability and Vulnerability: Challenging the Capacity/Incapacity Binary' (2017) 16(3) Social Policy and Society 469.

[49] Michael Dunn, Isabel Clare, and Anthony Holland, 'To Empower or Protect? Constructing the Vulnerable Adult in English Law and Public Policy' (2008) 28(2) Legal Studies 234.

[50] Andrea Hollomotz, 'Beyond "Vulnerability": an Ecological Model Approach to Conceptualizing Risk of Sexual Violence Against People with Learning Difficulties' (2008) 39(1) British Journal of Social Work 99.

[51] Catriona Mackenzie, Wendy Rogers, and Susan Dodds, *Vulnerability: New Essays in Ethics and Feminist Philosophy* (OUP 2013).

[52] Simon Wessely et al., 'Modernising the Mental Health Act: Increasing choice, reducing compulsion' (GOV.UK, 2018) available at <https://assets.publishing.service.gov.uk/government/uploads/system/uploads/attachment_data/file/778897/Modernising_the_Mental_Health_Act_-_increasing_choice__reducing_compulsion.pdf> accessed 04 September 2022, 166–167.

[53] MHA 1983, s 1(2).   [54] ibid., s 1(2A).   [55] ibid., s 1(3).

original MHA 1983 had a more granular definition of mental disorder with specific categories of disorder. It also contained exclusions relating to promiscuity or other immoral conduct and sexual deviancy, but this was removed in 2007 to ensure paedophiles could be detained. The breath of the definition also ensured that personality disorder could be managed under the Act.[56] The potential inclusion of learning disability and autism, even in limited circumstances, has also been criticised as discriminatory on disability grounds[57] because it treats individuals who are not ill as if they are (a criticism in theory also applicable to personality disorder).

In Scotland, the MHCTA 2003 has a similarly wide definition, defining 'mental disorder' as any mental illness, personality disorder, or learning disability[58] (and as such, criticisms relating to including learning disability are equally applicable). A key point of difference is found in the MHCTA 2003's exclusions: individuals cannot be considered mentally disordered on the basis of sexual orientation, sexual deviancy, transsexualism, transvestism, dependence on or use of drugs or alcohol, alarming or distressful behaviour, or imprudent activity.[59] However, if the conduct is evidence of an underlying disorder (for example, severe distress related to a psychotic episode), then the Act would continue to apply.

10.4.2 ADMISSION FOR ASSESSMENT AND TREATMENT

Having established the existence of 'mental disorder', a patient must meet the legal criteria to be admitted to an acute setting, and the required formalities must be met. This, and the process to be followed, differs based on the duration and purpose of the admission.

In England and Wales, the MHA 1983 contains two key types of admission.[60] A patient may be admitted for assessment under section 2 for up to 28 days. Should they require treatment, admission is under section 3 for up to six months in the first instance. An application under both sections is made to the hospital by the AMHP or a patient's Nearest Relative and must be supported by the recommendations of two medical practitioners. The practitioners must have examined the patient and be an 'approved practitioner' in line with section 12.

To be admitted for *assessment*, the individual must be 'suffering from mental disorder of a nature or degree' warranting detention for assessment, and they 'ought to be so detained in the interests of [their] own health or safety or with a view to the protection of other persons'.[61] The degree of discretion this affords those applying for and supporting admission is considerable. They need not be correct as to existence of the disorder; as long as they used their 'best judgement', this is sufficient.[62] Even if the degree of the disorder is not enough to justify admission, the nature of the condition may be. This broadness means that regardless of the current state of the patient's health, they could in theory be detained if they are felt to meet the risk criteria. The admission is therefore largely reliant

---

[56] For discussion, see Phillip Fennell, 'The Statutory Definition of Mental Disorder and the Availability of Appropriate Treatment' in Lawrence Gostin et al. (eds.), *Principles of Mental Health Law and Policy* (OUP 2010).

[57] Sheila Hollins, Keri-Michèle Lodge, and Paul Lomax, 'The Case for Removing Intellectual Disability and Autism from the Mental Health Act' (2019) 215(5) British Journal of Psychiatry 633.

[58] MHCTA 2003, s 328(1).   [59] ibid., s 328(2).

[60] There are various other ways patients can come to be admitted, including in emergency situations or through the police. See Peter Bartlett, 'Civil Confinement' in Lawrence Gostin et al. (eds.), *Principles of Mental Health Law and Policy* (OUP 2010).

[61] MHA 1983, s 2(2).   [62] *St George's Healthcare NHS Trust v S* [1998] 3 WLR 936 (CA) [961].

on psychiatric assessment of risk, which may be influenced by fear of getting the assessment wrong and causing harm.[63] A section 2 admission cannot be renewed on the 28-day expiry but can be converted into a section 3 detention, should the criteria be met.

The requirements for admission and detention for *treatment* under section 3 are more stringent. The mental disorder must be of a nature or degree such that it is appropriate for treatment to be given in hospital, and it must be necessary on the basis of risk to self or others that treatment should be given, and it cannot be provided without a section 3 detention.[64] In addition to this, appropriate medical treatment must be available to the patient.[65] As such, detention must be for the purpose of medical treatment for the disorder, and treatment must *in fact* (not in principle) be available. There is currently no statutory requirement that the treatment will benefit the patient. Although the Code of Practice indicates the purpose of treatment should be to alleviate the condition or prevent it worsening, academic commentators such as Bartlett have argued there is no need to ensure the efficiency of treatment in doing so.[66] Detention must also be the only means to provide the treatment, meaning the individual cannot be admitted voluntarily or treated in the community. The Responsible Clinician (RC, discussed previously) can renew a section 3 detention in the final two months, provided the conditions continue to be met.[67]

In Scotland, there are similarly two main forms of civil detention (for non-forensic patients) available under the MHCTA 2003,[68] but the process to utilise them is markedly different. The usual route to admission is under a short-term detention certificate.[69] Granted by an AMP in consultation with the patient's MHO, the certificate requires the patient's transfer to hospital within 72 hours, and the patient may be kept in hospital for up to 28 days. During this time, a RMO must be appointed, and medical treatment can be given in the patient's best interests without consent. If the patient's condition worsens or they require long-term care in hospital, the MHO must make an application to the Mental Health Tribunal for Scotland (MHTS) for a Compulsory Treatment Order (CTO), which permits detention for up to six months (extendable by a further six months).[70] As such, rather than long-term detention turning on medical discretion, the matter is determined by a panel of three members: one judicial, one medical, and one layperson.[71]

For both types of detention, the grounds to be met differ compared to the MHA 1983.[72] There are a number of similarities—there must be a mental disorder, with medical treatment available which will either prevent the disorder worsening or alleviate its symptoms or effects. Also, without treatment, there must be a significant risk to the patient's health, safety, or welfare, or the safety of another person (reflecting the risk plus disorder paradigm). When it comes to the question of risk, the Act does not contain guidance as to the extent of the risk and again, judgement as to the level of the risk will fall to the MHTS or RMO making the order.

The MHCTA 2003 also requires that for an order to be given, the patient's ability to make decisions about the treatment must be significantly impaired because of the mental disorder. Significantly impaired decision-making ability (known as SIDMA) is a unique concept to Scots law. No definition is given for the term in the MHCTA 2003, meaning

---

[63] Simon Wessely et al. (n 52).   [64] MHA 1983, s 3(2).   [65] ibid.

[66] Peter Bartlett (2010) (n 60).   [67] MHA 1983, s 20.

[68] Patients may also be detained in an emergency for up to 72 hours, under an emergency detention certificate; see MHCTA 2003, s 36.

[69] ibid., s 44.

[70] For a detailed explanation of each of these, see Stavert and Patrick (n 24), 173–184.

[71] For more details on membership, see MHCTA 2003, Sch 2, Part 1.

[72] See for example MHCTA (2003), ss 44(4) or 64(5).

it is for the MHO and/or RMO supporting the application to form a view based on (the evidence) as to whether the person's decision-making ability is significantly impaired. Although the impairment must be caused by the condition, the lack of definition gives wide discretion to those caring for the patients. Subsequent published empirical research on the issue has pointed to some challenges in implementation and poor practice, as well as reliance on insight as a reason for SIDMA.[73] SIDMA is similar to capacity but is intended to be more flexible and adopts a lower threshold; therefore, it may be possible that a person would have capacity but their ability to take decisions in relation to the treatment is nevertheless impaired by their condition (and compulsion might therefore be appropriate). This to ensure that someone who has capacity, but whose viewpoint is distorted by their condition, can still benefit from treatment.

Finally, the Order itself must also be necessary to make. This requires consideration of less restrictive measures (such as informal admission or treatment under the AWIA 2000).

10.4.3 WHAT TREATMENT CAN BE GIVEN?

Having discussed how patients come to be compulsorily admitted and detained in acute units, we now turn to consider what treatment they may be given for their 'mental disorder'. Decisions will usually involve a patient's RC or RMO, but at times, a second opinion may be required to authorise it. As mentioned, in both England and Wales and in Scotland, 'treatment' must be available to the patient for them to be admitted, but what this consists of is construed broadly.

General Treatment in Detention

In Scotland, 'medical treatment' includes nursing, care, psychological intervention, habilitation (education and training in work, social and independent living skills), and rehabilitation.[74] In deciding whether to grant a CTO, the MHTS must be satisfied that medical treatment is available to the patient and, in accordance with the principles of the Act, will be of benefit to them. In granting the order, MHTS will also agree what treatment can be given and the RMO in then authorised to carry this out. The treatment to be given will be detailed in the patient's care plan, drawn up by the RMO.[75]

For the first two months of an order, the patient may be given medication without consent if treatment is in their best interests. After this timeframe, the RMO is required to seek a second opinion from a Designated Medical Practitioner (DMP, discussed previously) as to whether the treatment should continue. When making a decision, the DMP must take account of the MHCTA 2003's statutory principles and any advance statement of the patient.[76]

In England and Wales, the majority of treatments do not require the patient's consent,[77] affording the RC a broad discretion as to what interventions are required to treat the disorder (the most common being medication). The key is that treatment must be *for* the mental disorder, either to alleviate its severity or to prevent further deterioration. Physical illnesses or conditions may only be treated under the MHA 1983 insofar

---

[73] Wayne Martin et al., 'SIDMA as a Criterion for Psychiatric Compulsion: An Analysis of Compulsory Treatment Orders in Scotland' (2021) 78 International Journal of Law and Psychiatry 101736.

[74] MHCTA 2003, s 329.   [75] ibid., s 76.

[76] The advance statement can be overridden, but if the DMP does so, they must write to the patient and explain the reasons and send a copy to their named person and the MWCS.

[77] MHA 1983, s 63.

as the illness is ancillary to the mental disorder (for example, treating self-harm wounds caused by a depressive illness).[78] However, this has been construed widely; in *Tameside and Glossop Acute Services Trust v CH*,[79] the court held that a Caesarean section could be given under section 63 because the success of the patient's pregnancy and delivery of a living child was a necessary part of treating her paranoid schizophrenia.

Where treatment is given for more than three months, a patient must either consent (and be certified as having competence to consent), or, in absence of consent or competence, the treatment must be certified by a Second Opinion Appointed Doctor (SOAD, discussed previously) as appropriate to continue.[80]

Safeguarded Treatments

For certain treatments to be given (those considered particularly invasive) in any UK jurisdiction, further safeguards are required, which include the patient's consent, a second medical opinion, or both together. A patient with capacity who has consented may withdraw consent at any time during the course of these treatments.

The first type of safeguarded procedures concern very serious treatments. In England and Wales, the only treatments currently in this category are surgical operations which impact on brain tissue or function, such as neurosurgery.[81] In Scotland, surgical treatments including neurosurgery for mental disorder and deep brain stimulation are included.[82] The necessary conditions for providing such treatment apply to *any* patient, whether they are subject to compulsory treatment or not:[83]

- the patient must consent; *and*
- a SOAD or DMP and two other appointed persons, not being medical practitioners, have certified as to the patient's capacity to consent; *and*
- the SOAD has certified that it is appropriate that the treatment be given (or in Scotland, a DMP has certified that treatment is in their best interests).

Under the MHA 1983, the SOAD must have consulted two other persons who have been professionally concerned with the patient's treatment: a nurse and someone who is neither a nurse nor a medical practitioner. In Scotland, if the patient is incapable of consenting, then very serious treatments can only be authorised by the Court of Session, who must be satisfied (on evidence from the DMP, RMO, and two laypersons) that the treatment would be in the patient's best interests and they are not objecting to it.[84]

Specific safeguards also apply in England and Wales for Electro-Convulsive Therapy (ECT),[85] and in Scotland, for ECT, vagus nerve stimulation, and transcranial magnetic stimulation.[86] In both cases, treatment cannot be given to a patient who has capacity and refuses the treatment.[87]

Where a patient lacks capacity, treatment can be given in Scotland if supported by a DMP or second opinion *and* the patient does not object. In the face of an objection, treatment may only be given on an urgent basis (discussed further below).[88] In England and Wales, ECT can be given to a patient who lacks capacity if a SOAD agrees that it is

---

[78] *B v Croydon Health Authority* [1995] 1 All ER 819.   [79] [1996] 1 WLUK 90.

[80] MHA 1983, s 58.   [81] ibid., s 57.

[82] MHCTA 2003 s 234(2); The Mental Health (Medical treatments subject to safeguards) (Section 234) (Scotland) Regulations 2005 (SI 2005/291).

[83] MHA 1983, s 56(1); MHCTA 2003 s 234(1).   [84] MHCTA 2003, s 236.

[85] MHA 1983, s 58A.   [86] MHCTA 2003, s 237.

[87] MHA 1983, s 58A(2); MHCTA 2003 s237(2).   [88] MHCTA 2003, ss 243(3) and (5).

appropriate, and confirms it does not conflict with a valid and applicable advance decision, or with a decision made by a donee or by the Court of Protection (the latter is discussed further).[89]

In Scotland, the MHCTA 2003 also requires that medication aimed to reduce sex drive or artificial nutrition without consent must be supported by a second opinion, under the same conditions as giving the patient medication on a long-term basis.[90]

The ability to seek a second opinion for serious treatments is intended as a safeguard and means to ensure treatment is truly clinically appropriate. However, the second opinion may not offer a significantly different viewpoint. According to the CQC, 76% of treatments were approved by SOADs in England and Wales in 2020/21, with variations to treatment plans most commonly concerning changes in dosage or medication.[91] It is also unclear as to whether the view of the SOAD or RC should be given more weight.[92]

Moreover, it remains possible for serious treatments to administered to a patient on an urgent basis without using the second opinion procedures. In England and Wales, when treatment is immediately necessary to save the patient's life, or if reversible, immediately necessary to prevent serious deterioration, alleviate serious suffering, or prevent violent or dangerous behaviour, it can be given without reference to a SOAD.[93] The use of such powers more than doubled during the Covid-19 pandemic, with the CQC raising concern about whether they were genuinely required.[94] In Scotland, urgent medical treatment may be given to save the patient's life, prevent a serious deterioration or alleviate serious suffering, or prevent them from behaving violently or being a danger to themselves or others.[95] However, this can only be done if the treatment is 'not likely to entail significant physical hazard to the patient'.[96] It is also important to note that not all restrictive and invasive practices are covered by the second opinion processes—for example, use of seclusion and restraint, or in England and Wales, where nasogastric feeding without consent can be done without additional safeguards.

10.4.4 COMPULSORY COMMUNITY TREATMENT

A key change introduced by the Mental Health Act 2007 to the MHA 1983 was provisions for Supervised Community Treatment (SCT). This aimed to allow patients discharged from hospital to be subject to compulsory management in community settings (under a 'Community Treatment Order'), ensuring compliance with treatment plans after discharge, assisting recovery and avoiding the need for hospitalisation (but preserving the potential for recall to hospital if necessary). The number of patients under SCT has consistently risen since the 2007 Act was implemented, with far more patients subject to them today than was originally envisaged. Despite their proliferation, they remain a controversial tool. SCT is not necessarily efficient at reducing readmission rates,[97] and essentially allows the MHA 1983 to reach out of the hospital setting and exert control over patients in community settings, raising questions as to the appropriateness of interferences with

---

[89] MHA 1983, s 58A(5).   [90] MHCTA 2003, ss 240(2)-(3).
[91] Care Quality Commission (n 32), 86.
[92] See *R (Wilkinson)* v *Responsible Medical Officer Broadmoor Hospital and another* [2001] EWCA Civ 1545, as discussed in Neil Munro, 'Treatment in Hospital' in Lawrence Gostin et al. (eds.), *Principles of Mental Health Law and Policy* (OUP 2010).
[93] MHA 1983, s 62.   [94] Care Quality Commission (n 32), 87–88.
[95] MHCTA 2003, s 243(3).   [96] ibid., s 243(4)(a).
[97] See Tom Burns et al., 'Community Treatment Orders for Patients with Psychosis (OCTET): a Randomised Controlled Trial' (2013) 381(9879) The Lancet 1627.

their liberty. The ability to invoke a Community Treatment Order rests with the patient's RC (with agreement of their AMHP) at the point of discharge; as such, their use can be variable, dependent on availability of services in the community, the RC's views about the likelihood of compliance with the treatment plan, and their perceptions of risk.[98] There is also significant variation of use in relation to age, gender, and ethnicity, with Black or Black British patients over 11 times more likely to be placed under SCT than their White counterparts.[99]

A Community Treatment Order may be made (for six months in the first instance) where:

(a) the patient is suffering from mental disorder to a nature or degree that it is appropriate for them to receive treatment (and appropriate treatment is available);

(b) treatment is necessary for their health and safety or protection of others;

(c) the patient is subject to recall powers, treatment can be provided without the patient's detention in hospital; and

(d) it is necessary that the RC can recall the patient to hospital.[100]

The RC is also required to consider the patient's history, risk of deterioration in the community, and other relevant factors.[101] The RC may also place conditions on the Order,[102] with failure to comply resulting in the potential for recall the patient to hospital.[103] Patients under SCT with capacity cannot be given treatment without their consent, including in emergencies.[104] For safeguarded treatments, the SOAD procedures continue to apply.

In Scotland, there are no separate orders for community treatment. Instead, the MHTS has powers to grant a Community Compulsory Treatment Order (CCTO) under the MHCTA 2003. These are authorised using the same criteria as for orders authorising hospital treatment.[105] When making a CCTO, the MHTS may impose certain conditions on the patient, such as a requirement to attend at a set time and location for treatment. If the patient fails to comply, the RMO may have them taken into custody and removed to the location for treatment, or to any other hospital.[106] The patient may also be recalled to hospital if the RMO concludes it is likely the patient's non-compliance will result in a deterioration in their health.[107] This may lead to seeking an order for detention in hospital.

Like SCT, an increasing proportion of compulsory orders under the MHCTA 2003 are CCTOs, and similar concerns about their impact on minoritised groups and their effectiveness arise.[108] In commenting on them, the MWCS noted with optimism the decrease in hospitalisation, but raised concern about a trend in compulsion overall, as the increase in CCTOs suggested increasing levels of compulsion as a practice.[109]

---

[98] Ritz De Ridder et al., 'Community Treatment Orders in the UK 5 Years On' (2016) 40(3) Psychological Bulletin Journal 119.

[99] NHS Digital, 'Mental Health Act Statistics, Annual Figures, England 2021-2022' (2022) available at <https://digital.nhs.uk/data-and-information/publications/statistical/mental-health-act-statistics-annual-figures/2021-22-annual-figures> accessed 31 October 2022.

[100] MHA 1983, s 17A(5).   [101] ibid., s 17A(6).   [102] ibid., s 17B.   [103] ibid., s 17E.

[104] ibid., Part 4A.   [105] MHCTA 2003, s 63.   [106] ibid., s 112.   [107] ibid., s 113.

[108] Mental Welfare Commission for Scotland, 'Characteristics of Compulsory Treatment Orders in Scotland: An Analysis to Inform Future Law Reform' (2022) available at <https://www.mwcscot.org.uk/sites/default/files/2022-06/CharacteristicsOfCTOs_June2022.pdf> accessed 04 September 2022, 8.

[109] ibid., 28.

10.4.5 SUPPORT DURING DETENTION

Family and Friends

As those often closest to the individual and at times acting as their carers, family members and close friends may well be in a position to offer support to a loved one subject to compulsion, or provide those caring for them with an understanding of what they would want. However, families in mental health law occupy an uneasy position. At times they are depicted as the individual's advocate, able to defend their rights against law's encroachments. Conversely, they may also be seen as overbearing, difficult, and exerting their own views rather than prioritising those of the individual, and presenting barriers to their empowerment and independence.[110] Within capacity-related legal frameworks, decision-makers are required to take account of the views of those close to the individual and this often involves seeking views of family members. These views are not necessarily determinative and, at times, the COP actively rejects the family's view, or even P's, for example, if they conclude the views of P cannot be separated from an overbearing parent.[111] This paradox is reflected in the statutory roles frequently fulfilled by family members, which we now turn to discuss.

In England and Wales, a patient's Nearest Relative (NR) has certain rights and responsibilities arising from detention, guardianship, or SCT under the MHA 1983. These comprise of rights to:

- apply for the individual to be detained or placed under guardianship;
- object to an application for detention or guardianship, or challenge whether less restrictive options have been considered;
- discharge the patient from detention, or apply to the tribunal if this is refused by the RC;
- ask for an independent advocate to be appointed; and
- be consulted and given information regarding treatment in detention.

The role is seen as an important safeguard of the patients' rights, yet from this list, we can distil a mixture of custodian and advocacy-based rights, with NRs both able to seek compulsory treatment on the patient and challenge it. The ability of the NR to act on their powers is also limited in that NRs deemed to be unreasonably objecting or failing to act in the interests of the patient can be 'displaced' (and therefore removed from their role) through an application to a County Court by the patient, their AMHP, or other relatives.[112] The apparent willingness of the courts to displace a NR, as well as the priority that is afforded to medical knowledge in these matters, had led commentators to view the NR as an ineffective safeguard.[113]

A further concern is whether the appropriate person fulfils the role. Section 26 MHA 1983 provides a hierarchical list of family members who may act as NR, based on proximity of their relationships to the patient; whoever is highest on the list will act as the NR. This has been criticised for prioritising blood relatives over the quality of other relationships,

---

[110] Lucy Series (2022) (n 45), 80–82.

[111] See *A Local Authority* v *M* [2014] EWCOP 33; *A Primary Care Trust* v *H* [2008] EWHC 1403 (Fam).

[112] MHA 1983, s 29.

[113] Kirsty Keywood, 'Nearest Relatives and Independent Mental Health Advocates: Advocating for Mental Health' in Lawrence Gostin et al. (eds.), *Principles of Mental Health Law and Policy* (OUP 2010), 328–336.

failing to recognise non-cohabiting families, and leading to unsuitable individuals inappropriately receiving information about the patient's treatment.[114] Although as stated, the patient can apply to displace their NR, the default will be the next person down on the list. Whether they do so will also depend on their ability to begin proceedings for displacement, a process which is far from straightforward.[115]

In Scotland, patients can choose to nominate a Named Person (NP) to be involved with their care. Further to amendments to the MHCTA 2003 by the Mental Health (Scotland) Act 2015, a NP cannot be appointed by default in absence of an express choice.[116] The NP has rights to be consulted and have their views taken into account regarding the patient's care and treatment. They can also apply and appeal to the MHTS. Although the nomination process deals with some of the concerns about the NR, the NP can still be displaced by the MHTS if they view the choice of person as unsuitable or feel the person is not acting to safeguard the patient's interests.[117] This can be viewed as a positive, as it ensures the NP represent *the patient* and not their own views, but points to a similar ease with which this safeguard may be disregarded in favour of medical expertise. The role's effectiveness may also be limited by a lack of uptake, understanding, and awareness.[118]

In Northern Ireland, the MHO 1986 has similar NR provisions to the MHA 1983. This will be replaced by s 69 MCANI when it comes into force, when individuals will be able to appoint a Nominated Person or if they do not, a default is appointed for them (based on the NR hierarchical list).[119] They may not make decisions on behalf of P when they lack capacity, but can make sure the individual's views are considered as part of best interests assessments or when authorisation for a deprivation of liberty is being considered. Once implemented, the MCANI 2016 contains a duty to consult the Nominated Person in relation to particular interventions.[120]

Advocacy

Advocacy in mental health aims to provide information, representation, and support, seeking to allow the patient's voice to be heard.[121] Advocacy is considered necessary to redress power imbalances between a patient subject to compulsion and the services with which they engage.[122] Statutory independent advocacy services exist in all the UK jurisdictions.

When it comes to compulsory treatment, both the MHA 1983 and MHCTA 2003 provide a statutory right to independent advocacy. Scottish health boards and local authorities must collaborate to ensure independent advocacy services are available to individuals with mental disorder. These services are defined as ones 'of support and representation', which aim to enable the person 'to have as much control of, or capacity to influence' their care.[123] Similarly, in England and Wales social services authorities and health boards are required to make Independent Mental Health Advocates (IMHAs)

---

[114] Judy Laing et al., 'The Nearest Relative in the Mental Health Act 2007: Still an Illusionary and Inconsistent Safeguard?' (2018) 40(1) Journal of Social Welfare and Family Law 37; *JT v United Kingdom* [2000] ECHR 133.
[115] ibid.   [116] MHCTA 2003, s 250.   [117] MHCTA 2003, s 257.
[118] Kathryn Berzins and Jacqueline Atkinson, 'Service Users' and Carers' Views of the Named Person Provisions of the Mental Health (Care and Treatment) (Scotland) Act 2003' (2009) 18(3) Journal of Mental Health 207.
[119] MCANI 2016, ss 73–76.   [120] MCANI 2016, s 15.
[121] Karen Newbigging et al., 'Characteristics of Compulsory Treatment Orders in Scotland: An Analysis to Inform Future Law Reform (Independent Mental Welfare Commission for Scotland 2022)' available at <https://www.mwcscot.org.uk/sites/default/files/2022-06/CharacteristicsOfCTOs_June2022.pdf> accessed 04 September 2022, 8.
[122] ibid., 26–27.   [123] MHCTA 2003, s 259.

available for 'qualifying patients'.[124] IMHAs help patients understand the Act, what restrictions have been imposed on them, what treatment is proposed for their care, and what their rights are. IMHAs are also able to provide support to patients at tribunal. Patients qualify for an IMHA if they are detained, subject to a Community Treatment Order or to guardianship, or are on conditional discharge.

The implementation of IMHA services remains a mixed picture. Understanding of the role is variable across England and Wales, with differences in local commissioning processes meaning the nature of available services differs dependent on location.[125] Some academic commentators have also argued that because the advocacy services have been professionalised, they may lack independence from the viewpoint of services.[126] Because of this, existing services may not provide culturally appropriate advocacy, to the detriment of patients from minoritised populations.[127]

10.4.6 ENDING COMPULSORY CARE

Discharge from compulsory care can come about in several ways. Under the MHA 1983, patients may be discharged through an order (in writing) by their RC if they conclude the criteria for ongoing treatment are no longer met.[128] Similarly, in Scotland, a patient's RMO may revoke a CTO (and therefore discharge the patient) if, in the course of their required regular review of detention, they believe the required grounds are no longer met.[129] A patient will also be discharged if the detention is not renewed at the end of the relevant timeframe. Ending compulsion does not necessarily mean discharge from hospital; for example, a patient may be discharged from their section 3 detention/CTO but remain in hospital as an informal patient and treated with their consent.

Where a patient is discharged from hospital, they have a right to aftercare,[130] and the MHA 1983 Code of Practice states that planning for aftercare should start 'as soon as the patient is admitted' with particular reference to how the patient's needs will be met after discharge.[131] As noted, under the Act, a patient's NR can also discharge a patient by giving 72 hours' notice to the hospital, although the RC can prevent discharge if they consider the patient would, if discharged, 'likely act in a manner dangerous to other persons or himself'.[132] Should this happen, the NR is unable to discharge the patient for a period of six months.[133]

Patients also have the opportunity to contest their continued detention and bring about their discharge. The main vehicle to do so is via appeal to the relevant tribunal (although it is also possible to request a review by the hospital manager under the MHA 1983).[134] The function of tribunals is to ensure detention and any compulsory treatment is lawful and in compliance with patients' rights. Tribunals consist of three members—one judicial, one medical, and one lay member—who have experience and knowledge in mental health. At tribunal hearings, there is usually attendance by the patient and their nominated representative, their treating clinician, nurse, and social worker.

---

[124] MHA 1983, ss 130A (England) and 130E (Wales).   [125] Karen Newbigging et al. (n 121), 50.
[126] Kirsty Keywood (n 113).   [127] Simon Wessely et al. (n 52).   [128] MHA 1983, s 23.
[129] MHCTA 2003, s 80.   [130] ibid., s 117.
[131] Department of Health and Social Care (2017) (n 8), 33.13–33.15. The Code advocates for a 'care programme approach', which aims to ensure services are coordinated.
[132] ibid., s 25.   [133] ibid., s 25(1)(b).   [134] MHA 1983, s 23.

In England and Wales, the Mental Health Review Tribunal for Wales and the Mental Health Tribunal (MHT) in England[135] hear applications from any patient (including offender patients) or their Nearest Relative who has been admitted under section 2 or section 3, or is subject to guardianship or SCT under the MHA 1983. There is a limit on the number of applications possible; in most cases, one application may be made in the first six months of detention, and once thereafter in periods of renewal.[136] Hospital managers are under a duty to refer patients to a tribunal who have not applied themselves within six months.[137] The tribunal has various powers, including to order the patient's discharge (with conditions where required) if they consider the criteria for the relevant order is not (or no longer) met.[138] If it does not order discharge, the tribunal may also make recommendations to a patient's RC regarding a leave of absence, or transfer to a hospital or into guardianship.

In Northern Ireland, the MCANI 2016 establishes a right to apply to the 'Review Tribunal' by the patient or their Nominated Person against authorisations of deprivation of liberty (discussed further).[139] The tribunal presently also considers applications against detention or guardianship under the MHO 1986 in a similar manner to the MHA, although once it has been repealed, such applications will cease.

The role of the Mental Health Tribunal for Scotland (MHTS) differs significantly in that, as discussed previously, its primary function is to make, grant, and approve CTOs. As well as granting orders, the MHTS hears appeals against detention (from the patient or their Named Person), meaning at times it will hear appeals against decisions that it has made. The Sheriff Court hears subsequent appeals against MHTS decisions in the first instance for civil cases (restricted patient cases proceed directly to the Court of Session), though grounds of appeal are similarly limited.[140]

It is important to note that the vast majority of tribunals do not conclude with the discharge of the patient.[141] Equally, access to tribunals will depend on patients knowing about their right to apply, and then taking the steps to do so. Tribunals are often criticised for the dominance of medical considerations, their focus on legal technicalities, and a lack of meaningful patient involvement.[142] Although tribunal decisions may be subject to further review, this is only possible in very limited circumstances.[143] As a result, the ability to uphold the rights of patients and provide an avenue for them to seek justice remains limited by the discretion the respective UK Acts afford to treating healthcare professionals.

10.5 MENTAL HEALTH AND CAPACITY

Having discussed the legal framework for compulsory treatment, we now turn to consider legislation focused on capacity.

---

[135] See Part V Mental Health Act 1983. Section 65 establishes Wales' MHRT, and England's MHT is part of the First-tier Tribunal established by s 3 of the Tribunals Courts and Enforcement Act 2007, with appeal to the Upper Tribunal.

[136] MHA 1983, ss 66 and 69.   [137] ibid., s 68.   [138] ibid., ss 72–75.

[139] MCANI 2016, s 45.   [140] MHCTA 2003, s 324.

[141] In 2020/21, about 10% of cases resulted in discharge; see Care Quality Commission (n 32).

[142] Aisha Macgregor, Michael Brown, and Jill Stavert, 'Are Mental Health Tribunals Operating in Accordance with International Human Rights Standards? A Systematic Review of the International Literature' (2019) 27(4) Health & Social Care in the Community e494.

[143] See *R v Upper Tribunal, ex parte Cart* [2011] UKSC 28. For a detailed summary of relevant cases across all stages of the tribunal process, see Peter Bartlett and Ralph Sandland (2007) (n 40), 508–563.

10.5.1 WHAT IS CAPACITY?

In England and Wales, lack of capacity can only be established where P is 'unable to make a decision' (the 'functional test') in relation to the matter at the material time because of 'an impairment of, or a disturbance in the functioning of, the mind or brain' (the 'diagnostic test').[144] The starting point is the functional test; P must be unable to make a decision if they are unable to understand, retain, use, or weigh the information relevant to the decision, or communicate the decision.[145] This inability to make a decision must be caused by the person's impairment – a 'causative nexus' must be established between the functional and diagnostic elements. It is not necessary, however, to demonstrate a precise pathology make this out, as Hayden J held in *Pennine Acute Hospitals NHS Trust* v *TM*:

> It is a misunderstanding of section 3 MCA 2005 to read it as requiring the identification of a precise causal link when there are various, entirely viable causes. Insistence on identifying the precise pathology as necessary to establish the causal link is misconceived. Such an approach strikes me as inconsistent with the philosophy of the MCA 2005. What is clear, on the evidence, is that the Trust has established an impairment of mind or brain and that has, in light of the consequences I have identified, rebutted the presumption of capacity.[146]

Those assessing capacity need only be satisfied that, on the balance of probabilities, there exists an impairment which causes the person to be unable to make a decision; multiple possible diagnoses which could cause the inability to decide, an uncertain diagnosis, or the absence of a formal diagnosis are no impediment to satisfying the causative nexus.

What information is considered relevant to a decision for the purposes of the functional test will turn on the specific circumstances of 'the matter', as we discuss further below. Crucially, an individual can only be seen as unable to take a decision if all practical steps have been taken to assist them without success.[147]

In Scotland, the AWIA 2000 defines 'incapacity' as being incapable of acting, or making, communicating, understanding, or retaining the memory of decisions, by reason of mental disorder (as defined in the MHCTA 2003).[148] A finding of incapacity may not be made if the adult can be assisted 'by human or mechanical aid' to communicate their decision.[149] The definition is broadly similar to the MCA 2005 and many requirements also bear similarity. For example, all steps must be taken to allow person to take own decisions.[150] The principles emphasise a need to ensure the adult's capacity is maximised and their decision-making is supported wherever possible. The adult concerned or anyone else claiming an interest in the matter may contest a finding of incapacity in the Sheriff Court.[151] The Court of Session hears Appeals against Sheriff Courts' decisions.

In Northern Ireland, the definition of lack of capacity largely mirrors the MCA 2005, with assessment based on a diagnostic and functional test, specific to the decision in question at the time it is made.[152] An individual is to be treated as unable to make a decision where they are unable to understand, retain, use, or weigh information, or unable to communicate the decision.[153] The standard of proof in a court setting is the balance of probabilities, but as long as reasonable steps have been taken to establish a reasonable belief of lack of capacity, in compliance with the principles, this is sufficient.[154] The MCANI 2016 requires in addition that three steps are taken to support the individual to take their own decision, namely the provision of relevant information (in an accessible manner), that the matter is raised at a time and place which will assist them to make the decision, and involving others who will likely assist as well.[155]

---

[144] MCA 2005, s 2(1).   [145] ibid., s 3(1).

[146] [2021] EWCOP 8, [37]. See also *Newcastle Upon Tyne NHS Foundation Trust v MB* [2022] EWCOP 43.

[147] MCA 2005, s 1(3).   [148] AWIA 2000, s 1(6).   [149] ibid.   [150] ibid., s 1(5).   [151] ibid., s 14.

[152] MCANI 2016, s 3(1).   [153] ibid., s 4.   [154] ibid., s 6.   [155] ibid., s 5(2).

Although in each case capacity is to be assessed in relation to a specific decision (and not on a universal basis), it remains a binary threshold. Either the individual has capacity, and are capable of deciding for themselves, or they do not, and decisions are made on their behalf. All individuals with mental health conditions are potentially in the scope if their diagnosis renders them unable to make a decision. The assessment of capacity may be significantly challenging in the case of a mental health condition, where an individual's state of mind may fluctuate in a short space of time.

10.5.2 HOW ARE DECISIONS MADE?

In England and Wales, if P is found to lack capacity in relation to a matter, decisions are based on an assessment of their best interests.[156] This requires consideration of all the relevant circumstances, including P's wishes, feelings, beliefs, and values which might influence their decision, the views of others close to them, and any potential for them to regain capacity.[157] Best interests does not reflect medical best interests, but rather takes a broader approach in consideration of P as an individual and their social circumstances. The factors do not accord to any hierarchy, and the weight afforded to each will depend on the factual scenario at hand. Notably, although P's views are important, they are not necessarily determinative; the decision may go against P's express wishes if the circumstances dictate. This position is somewhat unsatisfactory as it allows P's preferences to be readily discounted. Indeed, the Law Commission of England and Wales recommended in 2017 that the MCA 2005 should be amended to ensure *particular* weight is afforded to P's views in the best interests assessment.[158] However, this amendment did not feature in the subsequent reform of the legislation which took place via the Mental Capacity Amendment Act 2019 (discussed further going forward). Consequently, determining best interests remains a complex balancing act of the relevant factors.

In Scotland, a different approach is taken through the prism of 'benefit', as reflected in the AWIA 2000's principles.[159] This arose from an explicit rejection of best interests, with the Scottish Law Commission viewing it as too vague, failing to give due consideration to the wishes of the person, and inappropriate for the adult context due to its genesis in child law.[160] Conversely, in drafting the MCA 2005, the UK Parliament concluded that the notion of 'benefit' was overly prescriptive and the best interests standard would allow a more holistic approach.[161] The difference between the two in practice is perhaps narrower, with the Sherriff Courts using the terms interchangeably.[162]

The MCANI 2016 also adopts the best interests approach, with requirements to take account of all the relevant circumstances, encouraging P's involvement and in consultation with those around P.[163] When it comes to P's wishes, the MCANI 2016 requires that 'special regard' is given to P's wishes, beliefs, values, and factors they would likely consider if they could.[164] Again, a reasonable belief that the action is in the individuals' best interests will suffice.[165]

---

[156] MCA 2005, s 1(5).   [157] ibid., s 4.

[158] Law Commission, 'Mental Capacity and Deprivation of Liberty' (GOV.UK, 2017) available at <https://www.lawcom.gov.uk/project/mental-capacity-and-deprivation-of-liberty/> accessed 04 September 2022.

[159] AWIA 2000, s 1(2).

[160] Scottish Law Commission, 'Report on Incapable Adults' (1995) available at <https://www.scotlawcom.gov.uk/files/5013/2758/0994/rep151_1.pdf> accessed 04 September 2022.

[161] Joint Committee on the Draft Mental Incapacity Bill, 'Draft Mental Incapacity Bill, Session 2002-03, Volume I' (2003) available at <https://publications.parliament.uk/pa/jt200203/jtselect/jtdmi/189/189.pdf> accessed 04 September 2022.

[162] Alex Ruck Keene and Adrian Ward, 'With and Without "Best Interests": the Mental Capacity Act 2005, the Adults With Incapacity (Scotland) Act 2000 and Constructing Decisions' (2016) 22 International Journal of Mental Health and Capacity Law 1.

[163] MCANI 2016, s 7.   [164] ibid., s 7(6).   [165] ibid., s 8.

Medical Treatment

The AWIA 2000 contains specific rules for administering medical treatment to adults who lack capacity to consent. It defines medical treatment as 'any procedure or treatment designed to safeguard or promote physical or mental health'.[166] If a healthcare professional believes a patient lacks capacity to consent to medical treatment (and some form of treatment is being considered), they should issue a 'section 47 certificate of incapacity' using the prescribed form. The certificate provides a general authority to the healthcare professional to give the requisite treatment, in accordance with the AWIA 2000's principles. A new certificate is not required for each type of treatment; the certificate instead will specify a single treatment or an overall treatment plan. The certificate lasts for one year, or up to three years in case there is a severe or profound learning disability, dementia, or severe neurological disorder where the condition is unlikely to improve.[167] The expectation is that treating healthcare professionals would review the patient's capacity on a regular basis.[168] The adult or anyone claiming an interest in their welfare may appeal a treatment decision to the Sheriff's Court, or with their leave, the Court of Session.[169]

There are certain decisions excluded from the general authority to treat under the Act. If the adult has a welfare attorney or guardian with competence to make medical decisions on their behalf, that person should be approached to provide consent to the treatment in the first instance.[170] If the medical decision-maker disagrees with the proposed treatment, the treating professional requires a supportive second opinion from a DMP to administer it.[171] Where a medical decision-maker is involved, any appeal must be heard by the Court of Session.[172] The general authority to treat does not allow the use of force or detention 'unless it is immediately necessary', admission to a psychiatric hospital or treatment subject to the MHCTA, or treatment where there it would be inconsistent with a court ruling.[173] Should there be an ongoing court case regarding treatment, only life-saving treatment or treatment to prevent a serious deterioration in the medical condition may be given.[174]

Mirroring the MHCTA 2003, certain treatment may not be given under the general authority to treat because they require specific safeguards. These are generally treatments considered irreversible or hazardous.[175] Only the Court of Session can approve treatments involving neurosurgery, non-therapeutic sterilisation, or surgical implantation of hormones to reduce sex drive.[176] A second opinion from a DMP is required for drugs seeking to reduce sex drive, ECT, abortion, or medical treatment which is likely to lead to sterilisation 'as an unavoidable result'.[177] In accordance with the principles, this treatment can only be given where it is the least-restrictive alternative and it will confer a benefit.

---

[166] AWIA 2000, s 47(4).
[167] Adults with Incapacity (Conditions and Circumstances Applicable to Three Year Medical Treatment Certificates) (Scotland) Regulations 2007.
[168] Scottish Government, 'Adults With Incapacity: Code of Practice for Medical Practitioners' (20 October 2020), available at <https://www.gov.scot/publications/adults-incapacity-scotland-act-2000-code-practice-third-edition-practitioners-authorised-carry-out-medical-treatment-research-under-part-5-act/> accessed 10 August 2022.
[169] AWIA 2000, s 52.   [170] ibid., s 50(2)(c).   [171] ibid., s 50(4).
[172] ibid., ss 50(3), 50(6)–(7).   [173] ibid., s 47(7).   [174] ibid., s 47(9).
[175] ibid., s 48(2).
[176] The Adults with Incapacity (Specified Medical Treatments) (Scotland) Regulations 2002 (SI 2002/275), reg 3 and Sch 1.
[177] ibid., reg 4 and Sch 2.

Once its provisions relating to medical treatment are implemented, the MCANI 2016 will require additional safeguards for treatments with 'serious consequences', especially where P or their Nominated Person objects.[178] Such treatments include: those that cause serious pain, serious distress, or serious side-effects; major surgery; those that affect seriously the options that will be available to that person in the future, or have a serious impact on their day-to-day life; and those that in any other way have serious consequences for that person, whether physical or non-physical.[179] Such treatment must be authorised under Schedule 1 by a Trust panel. These panels within the relevant Health and Social Care (HSC) Trust, and consist of healthcare workers from various backgrounds who have undertaken specific training. The treatment must also satisfy the 'prevention of serious harm' condition, defined as a risk of serious harm to P or others, and the treatment is proportionate to the likelihood and seriousness of the harm.[180] Section 35 of MCANI 2016 also requires Independent Mental Capacity Advocates to be made available for patients when best interests decisions are made for 'relevant' acts under section 36 (which are similar to those in the MHA 1983).

In England and Wales, the MCA 2005 does not contain an equivalent framework for particular kinds of medical treatment; however, guidance is provided regarding when cases concerning 'serious medical treatment' should be brought before a court for determination.[181]

10.5.3 COURT PROCEEDINGS UNDER THE MCA 2005

When matters relating to the MCA 2005 in England and Wales require court involvement, decisions are taken in the specialist Court of Protection (COP).[182] No such equivalent exists in Scotland; as discussed, the Sheriff Court adjudicates on matters relating to the AWIA 2000. The COP has specific powers to make declarations in relation to whether P lacks capacity to make a decision on a particular matter and if they do, whether a proposed course of action or treatment would be in their best interests.[183] The COP is also able to authorise deprivations of liberty under the Act, or vary or terminate DoLS authorisations where it considers the criteria are not (or are no longer) met.[184] The COP has various other powers in relation to financial and welfare matters that are outwith the scope of this chapter.

In the COP, a judge[185] will hear representations and take evidence from various parties. Involved parties often include the protected party at the centre of the case (P), representatives of the relevant hospital or local authority, treating healthcare professionals, and P's family or others close to them. Although decisions concern P, they may not always be a party to the proceedings. Where P is party to proceedings but lacks capacity to conduct the proceedings, they will be appointed a litigation friend,[186] most often via the Official Solicitor. Litigation friends do not represent the individual and advance a case based on their interests, but rather take an independent position on best interests for the court to consider. They may also consent to certain applications on P's behalf. The approach

---

[178] MCANI 2016, ss 19–23.   [179] ibid., s 21.   [180] ibid., s 22.

[181] Applications relating to medical treatment: guidance authorised by the honourable Mr Justice Hayden, the Vice President of the Court of Protection [2020] EWCOP 2.

[182] MCA 2005, s 45.   [183] ibid., s 15.   [184] ibid., s 21A.

[185] For details on who can be a judge in the COP, see MCA 2005, s 46.

[186] Court of Protection Rules 2017, r 1.2(4)(a).

may at times mean the Official Solicitor takes a position which is directly contrary to P's express wishes, something that has attracted criticism as failing to give P proper representation in COP proceedings.[187]

Once said to be 'Britain's most secret court',[188] the COP has made recent endeavours to increase the transparency of its decisions, and in 2016 the 'Court of Protection Transparency Project' was launched allowing observers to attend hearings.[189] The pilot was subsequently adopted into COP procedures, with many hearings open to observers. The Open Justice Court of Protection (OJCOP) project in particular attends and blogs on many hearings to promote transparency in the COP.[190] Despite this, some concerns continue to be voiced about 'closed' proceedings in the COP. The case of *Re A (Covert Medication: Closed Proceedings)*[191] serves as a recent example. In 2020, A, a young woman with Primary Ovarian Failure (POF), mild learning disability, and autism spectrum disorder had been removed from her mother (B)'s care against the wishes of them both (based on concerns about undue influence of B over A) and into a placement. This placement was for the purposes of treating the OF using medication. B commenced proceedings in the COP, asking for her daughter to be returned to her on the understanding that no treatment had been given over the course of two years, and a hearing to consider this took place in April 2022. It subsequently emerged in a further hearing in September 2022 that the medication had been administered to A on a covert basis and that this had been concealed from B and B's legal team. The covert medication had been approved in parallel closed proceedings which the mother had not been notified of (by order of the court) at the time of the hearing in April 2022. This information was then revealed to the mother in the hearing in September.

The concealment of this significant fact from B and the public proceedings raises concern about the commitment to transparency in the COP. While this may have been done with the best of intentions to protect A, the obscuring of the covert medication meant that B's arguments proceeded on a false basis. It is perhaps telling that B subsequently withdrew her application. The wider public were also misled in this case; the OJCOP attended the hearing in April 2022 and blogged based on the information available (that no medication had been given), unaware of the parallel closed proceedings. Their reflection on the case was as follows:

> It makes a mockery of transparency if members of the public are admitted to hearings in which information is deliberately withheld from us such that we then publish information that is not accurate or true . . . As a supporter and proponent of the judicial commitment to transparency and open justice, I am very disappointed that the decision of the court to conduct the proceedings in this manner has put the Open Justice Court of Protection Project in such an invidious position.[192]

While there may be compelling reasons for hearings to be held in private (for example, if the case is particularly sensitive or there are concerns about medical confidentiality), the existence of parallel proceeding which undermine those taking place in public is

---

[187] Alex Ruck Keene, Peter Bartlett, and Neil Allen, 'Litigation Friends or Foes? Representation of "P" before the Court of Protection' (2016) 24(3) Medical Law Review 333.

[188] Christopher Booker, 'The Terrifying Tale of How Britain's Most Secret Court Imprisoned a Grandmother' (*The Telegraph*, 2016) available at <https://www.telegraph.co.uk/news/2016/10/16/the-terrifying-tale-of-how-britains-most-secret-court-imprisoned/> accessed 24 October 2022.

[189] Open Justice, 'Promoting Open Justice in the Court of Protection' (2021) available at <https://openjusticecourtofprotection.org/about/> accessed 24 October 2022.

[190] ibid.   [191] [2022] EWCOP 44.   [192] Open Justice (n 189).

a cause for concern and might benefit from further practice directions to clarify their use and scope.

In the next section, we explore some specific cases that arise regularly in the COP and the challenges these bring.

Life-threatening Situations

As discussed in Chapter 8, the law recognises the right of a capacitous adult to refuse any form of medical treatment, regardless of whether the refusal would result in death. But where P lacks capacity, the COP may determine that life-saving treatment is required in the face of active objection as long as it is held to be in their best interests. Common examples of such cases are the amputation of a gangrenous body part,[193] decisions regarding force-feeding for patients with eating disorders,[194] or cancer treatment.[195] In determining the question of capacity, as in all cases, judges will consider whether P's mental health condition prevents them being able to understand, retain, weigh, or use information. In amputation cases (which usually centre on Ps with schizophrenia or schizoaffective disorders), a lack of capacity often turns on whether hallucinations or delusional beliefs affect their ability to *weigh* the information about the severity of their condition appropriately. While the individual understands the information imparted by healthcare providers, a lack of capacity might be established due to a lack of trust in what they are being told, or a belief that the leg will be healed by a god (which is judged indicative of an inability to weigh information).[196]

Although the existence of a mental health condition is insufficient to demonstrate lack of capacity, where it comes to a patient with anorexia, a refusal to eat will often be determinative. As Jackson J held in *A Local Authority* v *E*:

> E's obsessive fear of weight gain makes her incapable of weighing the advantages and disadvantages of eating in any meaningful way. For E, the compulsion to prevent calories entering her system has become the card that trumps all others. The need not to gain weight overpowers all other thoughts.[197]

Jackson J noted that this leaves people like E in a 'catch-22' situation, in that 'by deciding not to eat, she proves that she lacks capacity to decide at all.'[198] Assessing capacity is evidently challenging where the decision is intimately linked to the symptoms of P's mental health condition. It may be unclear what represents the authentic desires of the individual or whether their ability to understand, weigh, and retain information has been impacted by their condition.

Having established a lack of capacity (which may be accepted by the parties prior to the case coming to court), the COP will consider whether there is an applicable advance decision to refuse treatment[199] and if there is not, what course of action is in P's best interests. The starting point is a strong presumption that it will be in the person's best interests to stay alive.[200] Whether this will win out in the balancing act will then depend on medical opinion, the views of family and those close to them, and, vitally, the weight afforded to P's wishes. This can be highly variable dependent on the facts of the individual case.

---

[193] *An NHS Foundation Trust* v *ZA* [2021] EWCOP 39.
[194] *A Mental Health NHS Trust* v *BG* [2022] EWCOP 26.
[195] *The Newcastle upon Tyne Hospitals NHS Foundation Trust* v *RB* [2021] EWCOP 11.
[196] *Wye Valley NHS Trust* v *B* [2015] EWCOP 60; *East Lancashire Hospitals NHS Trust* v *PW* [2019] EWCOP 10.
[197] [2012] EWHC 1639 (COP) [49].   [198] ibid. [52].
[199] MCA 2005, ss 24–26 (discussed in Chapter 17).
[200] *Aintree Hospitals NHS Foundation Trust* v *James* [2013] UKSC 67.

For example, in *Wye Valley NHS Trust v B*[201] and *An NHS Foundation Trust v ZA*,[202] amputation was judged not to be in either individual's best interests. Both had consistently expressed their opposition to the amputation, and the judges in each case emphasised the importance of the individual's quality of life for the time they had left. As Jackson J stated in *B*:

> I am quite sure that it would not be in Mr B's best interests to take away his little remaining independence and dignity in order to replace it with a future for which he understandably has no appetite and which could only be achieved after a traumatic and uncertain struggle that he and no one else would have to endure. There is a difference between fighting on someone's behalf and just fighting them. Enforcing treatment in this case would surely be the latter.[203]

In contrast, in *East Lancashire Hospitals NHS Trust v PW*,[204] amputation was found to be in PW's best interests. Lieven J pointed to the fact that PW did not want to die and is 'labouring under a delusion that there is an alternative' where there was not.[205] Alongside the better prospects of recovery when compared to B, this led to the determination the operation should proceed.

Similarly, in *A Local Authority v E*, despite E's opposition to force-feeding and her parents' view that her wishes should be respected, Jackson J nonetheless concluded that it was in her best interests to proceed with the treatment. He held the presumption in favour of life was not displaced and although treatment was burdensome, it was not futile and represented a final chance of helping E, a vulnerable young woman, recover.[206] This is in contrast to *A Mental Health NHS Trust v BG*, where Sir Johnathan Cohen concluded that force-feeding was not in BG's best interests because nothing more could be done to help her, and as such, continued treatment would be futile.[207] In these instances, differing medical evidence on the futility of treatment appeared to have a greater bearing on the outcome than the wishes of the person at the centre of the case.

Reproductive Decisions

The COP is often asked to make declarations in relation to capacity and best interests for reproductive matters, be they relating to the provision of contraception (from medication to intrauterine devices), an abortion, or occasionally non-therapeutic sterilisation (as discussed in Chapter 15). Whether an individual has capacity to make a decision will depend on what information is considered relevant. For capacity to consent to contraception, 'information relevant to the decision' consists of the medical facets, i.e. the reason for using it, likelihood of pregnancy, advantages and disadvantages of the type of contraception, and side effects.[208] It does not include the ability to care for a child or wider social consequences. In contrast, in *S v Birmingham Women's and Children's NHS Trust*, which concerned capacity to consent to termination of a pregnancy, Hilder J found that relevant information (for this case specifically) included what the termination process is, the effect of the procedure and its finality, the risks to physical or mental health of undergoing it, and the possibility of 'safeguarding measures in the event of a live birth' (i.e. that the baby may be taken into care).[209] This perhaps reflects the different nature of each decision, but also demonstrates how the construction of the relevant matter can have an impact on whether the individual is considered to have capacity to make the decision and the breadth of issues they must be able to understand.

---

[201] [2015] EWCOP 60.   [202] [2021] EWCOP 39.   [203] [2015] EWCOP 60 [45].
[204] [2019] EWCOP 10.   [205] ibid. [32].   [206] [2012] EWHC 1639 (COP) [137]–[140].
[207] [2022] EWCOP 26 [48]–[50].
[208] *Re A (Capacity: Refusal of Contraception)* [2010] EWHC 1549 (Fam).
[209] [2022] EWCOP 10 [52].

In recent years, the COP has made various anticipatory declarations[210] relating to pregnant women with mental health conditions (frequently schizophrenia or schizoaffective disorder) who disagree with their healthcare providers' views on the preferable mode of delivery for their child. In such cases, the woman is considered to have capacity to make decisions regarding her obstetric care at the time of the hearing. However, the treating healthcare professionals, expressing concern that they might lose capacity during labour, request declarations from the COP that should capacity be lost, it would be in her best interests to administer a Caesarean section (against her expressed view).[211] Although an anticipatory declaration may seem at odds with the requirement that capacity is established in relation to a decision made at the relevant time, in *United Lincolnshire NHS Hospitals Trust v CD*,[212] Francis J relied on the wording of section 15(1)(c), which allows the COP to determine the lawfulness of an act 'yet to be done' in relation to P. He considered this provision permitted anticipatory declarations of lawfulness in exceptional circumstances (such as where the life of CD and her baby is at risk).[213]

The assessment of best interests in these cases is heavily reliant on medical evidence as to why a Caesarean is preferable. Following the approach in *CD,* the case of *Guys and St Thomas' NHS Foundation Trust v R*[214] concerned a woman who was 39 weeks pregnant. R was reported as having told healthcare staff that a Caesarean section would be 'the last thing she would want'. However, medical evidence was that there would be a 'real risk' that it would be necessary to ensure safe delivery.[215] As such, the COP made declarations allowing a Caesarean section to take place, should R be assessed as lacking capacity. The declarations provided for R's 'transfer and treatment' and authorised a deprivation of liberty if required (given that transfer potentially involved taking her against her will from the psychiatric unit for obstetric care). In the end, R went on to give birth to a healthy child without the need for a Caesarean section.

Assessment of best interests cannot technically take into account the interests of the foetus, not only because it has no legal personality but also because best interests focuses on P's interests and not those of others. However, these cases indicate some concern about the impact refusing a Caesarean section would have on the foetus, and judges will often infer the woman's preference will be in favour of a safe delivery. For example, in the case of *Miss K*, Lieven J stated: 'I have no reason to believe her wishes would be anything other than to have the safest birth possible.'[216] In *R,* Hayden J equally noted that: 'The case law has emphasised the right of a capacitous woman, in these circumstances, to behave in a way which many might regard as unreasonable or "morally repugnant"', including the right to jeopardise the life and welfare of her foetus, but '[w]hen the Court has the responsibility for taking the decision, I do not consider it has the same latitude. It should not sanction that which it objectively considers to be contrary to P's best interests.'[217] He went to reason that:

> The statute prohibits this by its specific insistence on 'reasonable belief' as to where P's best interests truly lie. It is important that respect for P's autonomy remains in focus but it will rarely be the case, in my judgement, that P's best interests will be promoted by permitting the death of, or brain injury to, an otherwise viable and healthy foetus.

[210] MCA 2005, s 15.

[211] *Guys and St Thomas' NHS Foundation Trust (GSTT) and South London and Maudsley NHS Foundation Trust (SLAM) v R* [2020] EWCOP 4.

[212] [2019] EWCOP 24.   [213] ibid. [16].   [214] [2020] EWCOP 4.   [215] ibid. [4].

[216] *University Hospitals Dorset NHS Foundation Trust and Another v Miss K* [2021] EWCOP 40, [18].

[217] *GSTT and SLAM v R* (n 211), [63].

In this case it may be that R's instincts and intuitive understanding of her own body (which it must be emphasised were entirely correct) led to her strenuous insistence on a natural birth. Notwithstanding the paucity of information available, I note that there is nothing at all to suggest that R was motivated by anything other than an honest belief that this was best for both her and her baby. It is to be distinguished, for example, from those circumstances where intervention is resisted on religious or ethical grounds. In the circumstances therefore, it seems reasonable to conclude that R would wish for a safe birth and a healthy baby.[218]

What we are left with, then, is a fine jurisprudential line between respecting a capacitous pregnant women's right to exercise her autonomy and refuse medical treatment above any interests of the foetus, and—in the case of a pregnant woman with a mental health problem—over what it considers objectively to be her best interests in protecting a viable and healthy foetus. Across this line, however, the stated goal is promotion of autonomy and ability to exercise her own choices, as Mr Justice Hayden was keen to emphasise in *R*:

> The inviolability of a woman's body is a facet of her fundamental freedom but so too is her right to take decisions relating to her unborn child based on access, at all stages, to the complete range of options available to her. Loss of capacity in the process of labour may crucially inhibit a woman's entitlement to make choices. At this stage the Court is required to step in to protect her, recognising that this will always require a complex, delicate and sensitive evaluation of a range of her competing rights and interests. The outcome will always depend on the particular circumstances of the individual case.

As Neal has observed, and with which we agree, recent jurisprudence would indicate that:

> the foetus of a pregnant person who lacks capacity might be said to enjoy a *kind* of legal status, not as anything of value in its own right, but insofar as it is known, or presumed, to matter to P. As a valued child-to-be, it wins a place in the consideration of P's own best interests, despite lacking any *legal* interests of its own.[219]

Sexual Relations

Not only does the COP consider the reproductive consequences of sexual activity; it also makes determinations regarding capacity in relation to having sexual relations. The MCA 2005 states that no person can consent to sexual relations on behalf of another,[220] therefore if someone lacks capacity in this regard, any sexual activity with them is considered a sexual offence. A starting point in understanding the development of jurisprudence in relation to the question of capacity to consent to sexual relations is *X City Council v MB, NB and MAB*.[221] Although the case concerned capacity in relation to marriage, Munby J found that capacity to marry would include capacity to consent to sexual relations, with the information relevant to the decision including the sexual nature of the act, reasonably foreseeable consequences (such as pregnancy), and the capacity to decide whether to give or withhold consent to sexual intercourse.

---

[218] ibid.
[219] Mary Neal, '"Not Nothing"? The Late Term Foetus in the Court of Protection' (Open Justice, 2021) available at <https://www.strath.ac.uk/humanities/lawschool/blog/notnothingthelatetermfoetusinthecourtofprotection/> accessed 21 July 2022.
[220] MCA 2005, s 27.   [221] [2006] EWHC 168 (Fam).

Following the implementation of the MCA 2005, jurisprudence in the COP has continued to consider P's capacity to consent to sexual relations. Unlike many decisions under the MCA 2005, 'the matter' in this context is assessed in a broad way, in relation to the *act* of sexual relations rather than the *identity* of a particular sexual partner (i.e. capacity is act-specific, not person-specific). As Baker J reasoned in *A Local Authority v TZ*, if the COP was required to step in whenever sexual relations are contemplated, this would be a significant intrusion into P's private life,[222] as well as highly impractical, especially where P's sexual activities are unknown.[223]

Cases before the COP in this area often focus on individuals considered vulnerable to sexual abuse or exploitation, and therefore reflect an underlying motivation to protect P from risk of harm.[224] However, the UK Supreme Court was faced with an unusual fact situation in this regard in the recent case of *A Local Authority v JB*.[225] JB was a 38-year-old man with autistic spectrum disorder and various other problems related to cognitive function. He demonstrated a 'strong desire' to have sexual relations with women, and this had led to at times aggressive sexual behaviour towards women and in particular, vulnerable women. His treating clinical psychologist concluded he posed a 'moderate risk of sexual offending to women',[226] as he appeared unable to weigh his desire for sexual intercourse with the need to secure their consent. The local authority commenced proceedings in the COP, seeking a declaration that JB lacked capacity to consent to sexual relations. The parties agreed in advance of the hearing (the official solicitor acting as JB's litigation friend) that he lacked capacity to make decisions about who he could have contact with, where he lived, his care, access to social media, and to conduct legal proceedings.

At first instance, Roberts J found that he had capacity to consent to sexual relations, as the information relevant to the decision did not include understanding the other person had to give ongoing consent. The Court of Appeal overturned the decision, and recast 'the matter' as capacity to *engage in* (rather than consent to) sexual relations. They held that information relevant to the decision may include:

(1) the sexual nature and character of the act of sexual intercourse, including the mechanics of the act;

(2) the fact that the other person must have the capacity to consent to the sexual activity and must in fact consent before and throughout the sexual activity;

(3) the fact that P can say yes or no to having sexual relations and is able to decide whether to give or withhold consent;

(4) that a reasonably foreseeable consequence of sexual intercourse between a man and woman is that the woman will become pregnant; and

(5) that there are health risks involved, particularly the acquisition of sexually transmitted and transmissible infections, and that the risk of sexually transmitted infection can be reduced by the taking of precautions such as the use of a condom.[227]

This formulation was upheld by the UK Supreme Court. In its judgment, the Court rejected counsel for the Official Solicitor's argument that the MCA 2005 was solely confined to the protection of P, considering that the Act can afford practical protection

---

[222] [2013] EWHC 2322 (COP), [23].
[223] *IM v LM and others* [2014] EWCA Civ 37.
[224] *A Local Authority v P and others* [2021] EWCIO 48.   [225] [2021] UKSC 52.
[226] ibid. [37].   [227] [2020] EWCA Civ 735 [100].

to the public by including the other person's ability to consent in 'information relevant to the decision'.[228] The Court refined the Court of Appeal's test further, stating that whether the assessment of capacity to engage in sexual relations was act-specific or person-specific would depend on the circumstances. For example, it could be person-specific where it involved a couple in a long-standing relationship. In such circumstances, the information relevant to the decision might be different and would not necessarily include all the factors listed.[229]

To date there have only been limited cases reported from the COP which consider P's capacity to engage in sexual relations, so the implications of the ruling by the UK Supreme Court have yet to be fully understood. It does appear that the ability to vary between act-specific and person-specific determinations of capacity may allow for a more nuanced suggestion in a case where concerns of abuse are raised in relation to a particular sexual partner.[230] Yet this also raises concerns as to how the test could (potentially) be manipulated to provide what a particular judge considers is the 'right' outcome in a given case. Questions may also be posed as to how capacity to engage in sex can properly be separated from capacity to decide to have contact with individuals (another issue which is frequently considered in the COP). As Poole J stated in *Hull City Council v KF*:

> It is difficult to see how a person who lacks capacity to decide to have contact with a specific person could have capacity to decide to engage in sexual relations with that person. Sexual intimacy is a form of contact with another or others.[231]

Should an individual be found to lack capacity to engage in sexual relations on an act-specific basis, the ruling has profound implications for them, as was noted by Roberts J in *JB* at first instance:

> The outcome for P in this context is binary. If judged incapacitous because he or she has no comprehension that his or her consent is required before engaging in acts of a sexual nature, he or she is potentially consigned to celibate abstention unless capacity is established at some point in the future.[232]

This discussion demonstrates the fluidity of best interests decision making and capacity assessments, which take place in often stark contexts and have life-altering implications for the individuals at the centre of such discussion. In face of the MCA 2005's focus on empowerment, many of these COP decisions reflect an ethos of protection, of the individual, of those at risk from them, and perhaps at times, of an unborn child.

10.6 MENTAL HEALTH LAW AND HUMAN RIGHTS

Human rights form an essential element of mental health law in the UK. Any legislative framework or judicial interpretation of such law has to take full account of the implications of the rights detailed in the European Convention on Human Rights (ECHR), which has substantive force in UK law. When considering which rights are engaged, numerous ECHR Articles come to mind. Mental health law affects broad aspects of an individuals' private and family life (Article 8), and as discussed, touches on many intimate decisions. Restraint and seclusion measures could be considered inhuman or degrading treatment

---

[228] [2021] UKSC 52 [92].   [229] ibid. [71]–[72].
[230] See e.g. *Hull City Council v KF* [2022] EWCOP 33.
[231] ibid. [24].   [232] [2019] EWCOP 39 [78].

(Article 3), yet measures must be taken to protect patient's lives, such as prevent a suicidal patient in hospital from taking their own life (Article 2). Patients require access to an independent body to challenge detention (Article 6). Arguably, the most important of these is Article 5, which sets out the right to liberty.

Beyond the ECHR, a 'new paradigm' model for disabled person's rights now exists through the UN Convention on the Rights of Persons with Disabilities (CRPD). Ratified by the UK in 2009, the CRPD requires that such persons enjoy rights on an equal basis with all others. We reflect on the profound challenge this poses to mental health legislation in the next section.

10.6.1 DEPRIVATION OF LIBERTY AND ARTICLE 5

Article 5 ECHR requires that no one shall be deprived of their liberty, save for in the circumstances prescribed for by law *and* in six specific cases, one of which is the detention of persons of unsound mind.[233] The European Court of Human Rights (ECtHR) jurisprudence has not defined 'unsound mind', but the Court has nevertheless required that expert medical evidence 'reliably show' that the person is of unsound mind, that their condition is of a kind warranting compulsory detention, that detention is necessary in the circumstances, and that the condition persists during detention.[234] The rationale for this provision follows the same contours as that of compulsory mental health law; individuals of unsound mind (or the 'socially maladjusted') may be dangerous to the public, and might require therapeutic intervention in their own interests.[235] To be compliant with Article 5, individuals must be able to challenge the lawfulness of the detention,[236] and they have a right to compensation should it be found to be unlawful.[237]

What Does it Mean to be Deprived of Liberty?

Whether Article 5 is engaged in any given situation will turn on whether an individual's circumstances amount to a deprivation of liberty. From relevant ECtHR jurisprudence, three elements must be present:

- the person must be confined 'in a restricted space for a not negligible length of time' (the objective element);[238]
- they have not provided valid consent (the subjective element); and
- the state is responsible for their confinement.

The ECtHR has been clear that the context of the measures is critical, starting from the person's concrete situation and taking account of duration of the measure, its type, effects, and its implementation. Considering these elements, measures taken to protect the individual or taken in their interests may still amount to a deprivation of liberty.[239]

Informal Treatment

It appears obvious that detention in a mental health unit is a deprivation of the patient's liberty. Indeed, the procedures and safeguards around admission, and ability to challenge it at tribunal, bear great similarity to the ECtHR's criteria for lawful interference with Article 5. But the answer becomes less obvious if the patient is not subject to compulsory

---

[233] ECHR, Art 5(1)(e).   [234] *Wintwerp v Netherlands* (1979) 2 EHRR 387.
[235] *Guzzardi v Italy* (1980) 3 EHR 333.   [236] ECHR, Art 5(4).   [237] ibid., Art 5(5).
[238] *Storck v Germany* [2005] ECHR 406.   [239] *Guzzardi v Italy* (1980) 3 EHR 333.

powers. As alluded to in the previous section, not all patients treated in acute units in the UK are formally detained or there against their will. In England and Wales, the Mental Treatment Act 1930 first introduced 'voluntary admission' to allow patients to be admitted for treatment without the stigma of a formal detention, either with their agreement or where they did not object.[240] The possibility of non-compulsory admission was retained by the MHA 1983, which allows for the admission of 'informal patients'.[241]

Initially, the distinction between formal (detained) and informal patients came down to whether the patient resisted or objected to their placement in hospital, rather than their capacity to consent to an informal admission.[242] However, a patient admitted informally who does not appear to object may not in fact be able to leave hospital (because they would be detained if they tried). Informal patients are also unable to challenge their placement in hospital before a tribunal. As such, questions arise as to whether the situation amounts to a deprivation of liberty, and if it does, whether the legal safeguards are sufficient for Article 5 compliance.

This scenario was considered in the case of *R v Bournewood Community and Mental Health NHS Trust, ex parte L*,[243] which related to an autistic man who was an informal patient under the MHA 1983 but lacked capacity to consent to his placement in hospital. The House of Lords, overturning the Court of Appeal, held that he was not deprived of his liberty. The Lords (with Lord Steyn dissenting) based their findings on L's lack of objection and the fact he had not been restrained (although had he tried to leave, he would have been prevented from doing so). The finding in part reflected a desire to encourage informal admission where possible, and the potential implications for thousands of other patients like L not just in hospital, but in nursing homes, who lacked capacity to consent, and may need to be detained for treatment to continue.[244]

L's family appealed to the ECtHR, which in *HL v UK*[245] overturned the House of Lords decision, holding that the situation amounted to a deprivation of liberty even if he was not objecting or attempting to leave. The Court pointed to the lack of procedural safeguards available to L when compared to patients admitted formally under the MHA 1983, and that this gap essentially allowed healthcare professionals complete discretion when it came to treating him and incapacitous adults in analogous positions. In response to the ruling, and to remedy what became known as the 'Bournewood gap', the UK Government developed a system of safeguards to lawfully deprive individuals of their liberty in cases where they are not detained under the MHA 1983. This resulted in the creation of the Deprivation of Liberty Safeguards (DoLS) scheme, which was introduced to the MCA 2005 through the MHA 2007. These apply only to England and Wales and are discussed further going forward.

It bears remembering that the MHA 2007 did not do away with informal admission. Instead, in England and Wales it is now explicitly reserved for patients who have capacity to consent to the admission.[246] But the extent to which such admissions are truly consensual remains questionable. Recalling that deprivation of liberty is a matter of 'degree and intensity' rather than 'nature of substance',[247] informal detention occupies a position on the edge of compliance. Patients admitted informally who attempt to leave may well be formally detained, and may also be coerced to consent to admission through a 'choice' of informal admission or detention.[248] In England and Wales, patients

---

[240] Mental Treatment Act 1930, s 1.   [241] MHA 1983, s 131.   [242] Lucy Series (2022) (n 45), 146.
[243] [1999] 1 AC 458.   [244] Lucy Series (2022) (n 45), 152.   [245] [2005] 40 EHRR 32.
[246] Office of the Public Guardian (n 14), para 14.14.
[247] *Guzzardi* v *Italy* (1980) 3 EHR 333, 93.
[248] Rachel Bingham, 'The Gap Between Voluntary Admission and Detention in Mental Health Units' (2012) 38(5) Journal of Medical Ethics 281.

informally admitted continue to lack procedural safeguards afforded to formally detained patients; they cannot challenge their detention in a tribunal, and in England, they do not have access to an IMHA unless certain invasive treatments are considered (although this is not the case in Wales).[249] In Scotland, informal patients have a right to apply to the MHTS if they consider they have been unlawfully detained.[250] The MWCS also provides guidance as to the specific rights of detained patients in terms of ability to leave and to refuse treatment.[251]

The Deprivation of Liberty Safeguards (DoLS) Scheme under the MCA 2005

The DoLS scheme applies to individuals in hospitals and care homes in England and Wales who are deprived of their liberty for the purposes of treatment.[252] The care provider must apply to a 'supervisory body' (usually the local authority) for authorisation. To make such an authorisation, a Best Interests Assessor (BIA), who may be a social worker, psychologist, nurse, or occupational therapist, and a Mental Health Assessor (a medical professional) must carry out a DoLS assessment. These professionals are appointed by the local authority and must have had no previous involvement in the individual's care. The assessment must confirm the six qualifying requirements are met:

(1) Age: P is over 18.

(2) Mental health: P must be suffering from a mental disorder (in line with the MHA but including learning disability).

(3) Mental capacity: P lacks capacity to decide regarding their accommodation in hospital or the care home for treatment.

(4) Best interests: the detention must be in P's best interests, must be necessary, and proportionate to the likelihood and seriousness of harm occurring.

(5) Eligibility: P is not detained under the MHA and does not meet the criteria for detention.

(6) No refusals: no relevant advance decision exists to refuse treatment.[253]

BIAs are key to the DoLS scheme. Their focus is on whether the arrangements are truly in the patient's best interests, and they must determine also whether the situation amounts to a deprivation of liberty. BIAs have significant authority to delineate the extent of the deprivation of liberty; they can challenge the necessity of the arrangements, may suggest conditions on the authorisation to reduce the impact of the deprivation of liberty on the person, or the need for an ongoing authorisation.[254]

DoLS authorisations should be for the shortest time possible and can last for up to a year, with renewal possible for a further year at each asking. If authorisation is granted, a representative must be appointed to support P, and both must be informed of the possibility of appeal.[255] In practice, very few DoLS authorisations are subject to appeal.[256]

Independent Mental Capacity Advocates (IMCAs) must be made available to individuals where (1) decisions are made about changes in accommodation, serious treatment,

---

[249] MHA 983, s 130G.   [250] MHCTA 2003, s 291.

[251] Mental Welfare Commission for Scotland, 'Good Practice Guide: Human Rights in Mental Health Services' (2017) available at <https://www.mwcscot.org.uk/sites/default/files/2019-06/human_rights_in_mental_health_services.pdf> accessed 04 September 2022.

[252] MCA 2005, Sch. A1.   [253] ibid., Part 3.

[254] For a full discussion of this role, see Lucy Series (2022) (n 45).

[255] MCA 2005, Sch. A1, s 59. Appeals are heard in the COP under s 21A.

[256] Lucy Series (2022) (n 45) 154.

or a potential deprivation of liberty, (2) they lack capacity, and (3) there is no one else independent of the services providing accommodation or treatment who could be consulted.[257] IMCAs provide support to the individual to enable decision-making, ascertain their wishes and feelings and any alternatives, and may obtain information relevant to the decision in order to discuss what should happen with the decision-maker.

Cheshire West and the 'Acid Test'

The aim of the DoLS was to ensure compliance with the Article 5 rights of those who lack capacity. Their operation again turns on the precise definition of deprivation of liberty; this determines who is in scope for a DoLS authorisation, but also the resource implications of the scheme, as higher numbers require more applications to local authorities, which in turn means more authorisations, more assessments, and more BIAs. The question of definition returned to the UK Supreme Court in the Cheshire West case,[258] which concerned care arrangements for three individuals: P, MIG, and MEG. None of them were cared for in hospitals or care homes: P lived in a supported residential facility, MEG was in an NHS residential home, and MIG lived with her foster carer. All were able to leave their facilities and homes on certain days but required help and support with aspects of their life, and at times P and MEG were subject to restraint or intervention. MIG and MEG were both under age 18 at the time proceedings commenced. The Court of Appeal held that none of the individuals had been deprived of their liberty, pointing to the 'relative normality' of their lives as compared to someone of their age and characteristics.[259] The UK Supreme Court, however, held that the purpose of a placement, its normalcy, and whether the person objects to it, are not relevant in determining whether there was a deprivation of liberty. Giving the leading judgment, Lady Hale, reflecting on ECtHR case law, identified what she described as an 'acid test' for deprivation of liberty, which meant that the individual is under continuous supervision and control, and is not free to leave.[260] In rejecting the 'relative normality' requirement, she underlined that the threshold should not be different for those with disabilities compared to those without, and the entire point of human rights is that they apply equally to everyone.[261]

Crucially, the acid test in Cheshire West established that deprivation of liberty does not turn on a specific location. As long as the state is responsible for care arrangements, it does not matter if these are provided in a domestic setting; an individual may still be deprived of their liberty in a place they consider to be home. The Court concluded that P, MIG, and MEG had all been deprived of their liberty because they were under continuous supervision and control, and unable to leave.

The Implications of Cheshire West

Cheshire West had repercussions across the UK jurisdictions. In England and Wales, criticisms of the unwieldly nature of the DoLS system and its complexity pre-dated the case, but the decision brought its shortcomings into sharper focus. In the aftermath, the number of DoLS applications rose dramatically, placing considerable strain on supervisory bodies, who were unable to keep up with demand and faced spiralling costs.[262] Subsequent cases brought some refinement; for example, Ferriera clarified

[257] MCA 2005, s 35.   [258] Cheshire West (n 47).
[259] Surrey County Council v P and others [2011] EWCA Civ 190; Cheshire West and Chester Council v P [2011] EWCA Civ 1257.
[260] Cheshire West (n 47) [49].   [261] ibid. [38].
[262] Law Commission of England and Wales, 'Mental Capacity and Deprivation of Liberty' (2017) Law Com No 372, para 2.22.

that a patient who died in the intensive care unit was not in 'state detention' and deprived of their liberty, because it was their illness, and not the actions of the hospital, which caused their loss of liberty.[263]

DoLS themselves also contain limitations; they are not applicable to anyone under the age of 18 years, nor do they deal with questions of liberty outside of hospital or care home settings. Yet the acid test made clear that DoLS do not cover all deprivations of liberty that take place in this context. Any deprivations of liberty which fell outwith the DoLS scheme would need to be authorised by the COP, and as such the lack of a complete scheme raised the prospect of either a significant volume of court applications for authorisations, or, if these were not given in a timely manner, numerous instances of unlawful interference with individuals' Article 5 rights.

The House of Lords' post-legislative scrutiny of the MCA 2005 (arriving mere months before *Cheshire West*) had already recommended starting again with DoLS, considering that their focus on risk did not sit well with the MCA 2005's ethos of empowerment.[264] In light of these developments, the UK Government asked the Law Commission of England and Wales to provide recommendations for a system to replace DoLS, with the final report delivered in March 2017.[265] In response to the proposals, the UK Government brought forward the Mental Capacity (Amendment) Act 2019, which contains the framework for the new Liberty Protection Safeguards (LPS) scheme.[266] The 2019 Act remains a contentious piece of legislation, with the final version differing significantly from the Commission's original proposals.[267] At the time of writing, the LPS scheme has not been implemented and when and if it will be remains an open question. The scheme would authorise 'arrangements' for the care of patients over the age of 16 years which amount to a deprivation of liberty and is not limited to hospitals and care homes. Instead, it would in any setting, including a patient's own home. Authorisation would be given by a responsible body (this may now be the hospital providing treatment, to help streamline the process) under three conditions: P must lack capacity, have a mental disorder, and the arrangements must be necessary to prevent harm to P, and be proportionate to the likelihood and seriousness of harm.[268]

Authorisation would be granted through a pre-authorisation review of the necessary documentation. It is unclear who would be responsible for undertaking the review or the required assessments. The role of BIA does not feature; instead, an Approved Mental Capacity Professional (AMCP) would review the arrangements in specific circumstances, such as where it appears the person may object to the arrangements, or if the deprivation of liberty will be in an independent hospital.[269] AMCPs would have expanded powers to take action and block authorisation (rather than make recommendations), but only in cases referred to them.[270] Authorisation under the LPS would be for a maximum of one year, subject to renewal.[271]

In spite of its untethering from a specific location, and attempts to capture wider populations who may be deprived of their liberty, the LPS rely on a very similar model to the DoLS, i.e. they aim to ensure deprivations of liberty are lawful and in line with established

[263] *R (Ferreira)* v *HM Senior Coroner* [2017] EWCA Civ 31.
[264] House of Lords, 'Mental Capacity Act 2005: Post-Legislative Scrutiny' (2014) available at <https://publications.parliament.uk/pa/ld201314/ldselect/ldmentalcap/139/139.pdf> accessed 04 September 2022.
[265] Law Commission of England and Wales (n 262).   [266] MCA 2005, Sch AA1.
[267] For a detailed discussion and key criticisms, see Lucy Series, 'On Detaining 300,000 people: The Liberty Protection Safeguards' (2019) 25 International Journal of Mental Health and Capacity Law 79.
[268] MCA 2005, Sch AA1, s 13.   [269] ibid., Sch AA1, s 24(2).
[270] ibid., Sch AA1, ss 24 and 38.   [271] ibid., Sch AA1, ss 29, 32–36.

norms. As such, while it aims to ensure Article 5 ECHR compliance, it does not offer a radically altered alternative.

The other UK jurisdictions also took stock of *Cheshire West* and its implications for their legislation. When the ruling was handed down, the Scottish Law Commission was already considering how the AWIA 2000 should be amended in light of *HL v UK*. In October 2014, cognisant of the findings in *Cheshire West,* the Commission recommended introducing a legal procedure to authorise measures preventing an adult from going out of a hospital. The recommendations included a heightened legal process to consider 'significant restrictions of liberty', rejecting the term 'deprivation of liberty' as unhelpful.[272] The Scottish Government consulted on the report in 2016 and in 2018 made proposals for reform. These maintained the Commission's distinction between decisions as to where a person lives, and *how* a person lives, and adopted a 'graded guardianship' regime for significant restrictions on liberty, reflective of an adult's lack of consent and the existence of any objection.[273] Under the proposals, a significant restriction on liberty may be established where the acid test in *Cheshire West* is satisfied, where there are barriers which limit the adult's access to certain areas of their residence, and where force, restraint, medication, or surveillance is used to control their actions.[274] The proposals further state that measures applying to all adults in a given location (e.g. CCTV) which do not disadvantage them 'excessively or unreasonably' will not in or of themselves create a significant restriction on liberty.[275] These proposals have yet to progress to a Bill in the Scottish Parliament, and appear likely to be superseded by the recommendations of the Scottish Mental Health Law Review (discussed in detail going forward).

In Northern Ireland, the partial implementation of the MCANI 2016 has focused primarily on an equivalent DoLS scheme. This was implemented in December 2019, in part because it was necessary in the wake of *Cheshire West* to ensure Article 5 ECHR compliance. An individual who lacks capacity within the meaning of the MCANI 2016 and is in hospital must have their deprivation of liberty authorised through a 'short term detention authorisation' which lasts for 14 days (renewable for a further 14) and is authorised by two healthcare professionals.[276] In other health and social care settings or private homes, applications for authorisation are made to a Trust panel (discussed previously).[277] The DoLS Code of Practice provides detailed guidance as to the scheme's operation, which reflects MCANI's statutory principles and definitions.[278] To make an application, the Code of Practice requires that:

1. the individual has been deprived of their liberty in line with the acid test;[279]
2. they lack capacity;[280]

---

[272] Scottish Law Commission, 'Report on Adults with Incapacity, Report No 240' (2014) available at <http://www.scotlawcom.gov.uk/files/6414/1215/2710/Report_on_Adults_with_Incapacity_-_SLC_240.pdf> accessed 04 September 2022.
[273] Scottish Government, 'Adults with Incapacity (Scotland) Act 2000: Proposals for Reform' (2018) available at <https://www.gov.scot/publications/adults-incapacity-scotland-act-2000-proposals-reform/> accessed 04 September 2022.
[274] ibid.   [275] ibid.   [276] MCANI 2016, Sch 2.   [277] ibid., Sch 1 s2(2)(b).
[278] Department of Health, 'Deprivation of liberty safeguards code of practice' (November 2019) available at <https://www.health-ni.gov.uk/publications/mcani-2016-deprivation-liberty-safeguards-code-practice-november-2019> accessed 04 September 2022.
[279] ibid., para 2.6.   [280] ibid., para 2.11.

3. the deprivation of liberty is necessary to prevent serious harm, proportionate to the likelihood and seriousness of harm;[281] and

4. the deprivation of liberty is in their best interests.[282]

Currently, a DoLS authorisation may not be given if the treatment may be administered under the MHO 1986, although this will change once the MCANI 2016 is fully implemented. As mentioned, DoLS authorisations can be challenged in the Review Tribunal.[283] It is still unclear whether the NI DoLS scheme will be effective or will avoid the criticisms levied at its English and Welsh counterpart. The scheme was also amended by Covid-19 emergency legislation, meaning it has had little opportunity to function as initially intended to date.[284]

Regardless of the prevailing legal framework, the UK jurisdictions continue to grapple with the implications of Article 5 ECHR for mental health law. For example, in England and Wales, the issue continues to be contested in the COP. In spite of this, it remains important to remember that Article 5 does not make deprivation of liberty unlawful when it comes to managing mental health or disability. Rather, it provides protection against arbitrary detention, seeking to ensure that any deprivations of liberty track legally and socially acceptable paths, and are accompanied by sufficient legal safeguards to limit any discretionary action. It is reflective of the traditional ethos of mental health law, and the necessity of detention for certain elements of the population. We now turn to consider the CRPD's alternative vision.

10.6.2 UN CONVENTION ON THE RIGHTS OF PERSONS WITH DISABILITIES

The CRPD focuses on the rights of persons with disabilities, which is defined as '[t]hose who have long-term physical, mental, intellectual or sensory impairments which in interaction with various barriers may hinder their full and effective participation in society on an equal basis with others.'[285]

The CRPD is founded on a commitment to the full and equal enjoyment of human rights by persons with disabilities and requires states to take measures to promote and protect this. Anti-discrimination and reasonable accommodation is fundamental, and as such all exclusions or restrictions of rights and freedoms on the basis of disability should, under the terms of the Convention, be eliminated.[286] Substantive rights include the right to life,[287] access to justice,[288] freedom from exploitation, violence and abuse,[289] protecting the integrity of the person,[290] and the right to health[291] and an adequate standard of living.[292] Through these articles, the CRPD embodies a social model of disability, with the rights listed previously focused on enabling social responses to allow persons with disabilities the full enjoyment of all rights.[293] As such, it aims to tackle inadequate social responses to disabled persons' needs, and advocates

[281] ibid., paras 7.6–7.11.   [282] ibid., chapter 6.   [283] MCANI 2016, s 45.

[284] Anne-Maree Farrell and Patrick Hann, 'Mental Health and Capacity Laws in Northern Ireland and the COVID-19 Pandemic: Examining Powers, Procedures and Protections Under Emergency Legislation' (2020) 71 International Journal of Law and Psychiatry 101602.

[285] UNCRPD, Art 1.   [286] ibid., Art 5.   [287] ibid., Art 10.   [288] ibid., Art 13.

[289] ibid., Art 16.   [290] ibid., Art 17.   [291] ibid., Art 25.   [292] ibid., Art 28.

[293] United Nations, 'Convention on the Rights of Persons with Disabilities' (CRPD), (6 May 2022), available at <https://www.un.org/development/desa/disabilities/convention-on-the-rights-of-persons-with-disabilities.html> accessed 10 August 2022.

for their full inclusion in society, ability to take decisions for themselves, and respect for their dignity, autonomy, and independence.[294]

The CRPD also established the Committee on the Rights of Persons with Disabilities. The Committee provides commentaries on interpreting the CRPD's articles, and signatories are required to submit reports on how implementation is progressing. For countries that have signed the Optional Protocol, individuals may also complain to the Committee where they consider their rights have been breached, with the Committee arbitrating on such disputes. The UK is a signatory to the CRPD and optional protocol. As such, the Convention is in force as international law, and the UK is required to submit reports on its progress.[295] In spite of this, judicial interpretation in the UK of the CRPD is sparse. Although Lady Hale drew on the CRPD to support the 'universal nature' of human rights in her judgment in *Cheshire West,* the courts have noted that because the CRPD has not been incorporated into national law, they cannot examine purported violations of it,[296] nor are they required to take notice of requests for interim measures made by the Committee.[297]

The CRPD presents a substantial challenge to UK mental health and capacity laws, in the main because of its outright rejection of differential treatment or legal frameworks where thresholds for intervention are based on disability.[298] Article 12(2) CRPD requires that states recognise the enjoyment of legal capacity for persons with disabilities on an equal basis, suggesting at least a degree of incompatibility with frameworks which assess capacity based on a diagnostic threshold (like the MCA 2005 and AWIA 2000). Article 12(3) further requires that states respect the wills and preferences of individuals. The Committee's interpretation of this Article engenders the abolition of substitute decision-making regimes (like best interests) and replacement with a supported decision-making paradigm, based on the individual's wills and preferences.[299] The Committee's interpretation of Article 12 remains controversial. Criticisms include lack of guidance regarding how the standard would apply to individuals unable to express a 'will or preference', such as those in prolonged disorders of consciousness; that an individual's views might be perversely influenced by manipulation of those close to them; and how this might be implemented while priority continues to be afforded to risk.[300]

The response of the UK jurisdictions to the Committee's interpretation has been mixed. The Wessely Review rejected it because it would not allow intervention where someone is refusing help.[301] Conversely, the MWCS has produced guidance as to how approaches based on supported decision-making could be adopted through the existing

---

[294] CRPD, Art 3.

[295] For the UK Government's response to the Committee's latest inquiry see Disability Unit and Department for Work and Pensions, 'Disabled People's rights: UK 2021 Follow-Up Report to UNCRPD 2016 Inquiry' (Gov.UK, 14 December 2021) available at <https://www.gov.uk/government/publications/disabled-peoples-rights-the-uks-2021-report-on-select-recommendations-from-the-uncrpd-periodic-review> accessed 10 August 2022.

[296] *A Local Authority* v *JB* [2021] UKSC 52 [120].

[297] *Holly Dance and Paul Battersbee* v *Barts Health NHS Trust and Archie Battersbee,* [2022] EWCA Civ 1106.

[298] For detailed analysis, see Peter Bartlett, 'The United Nations Convention on the Rights of Persons with Disabilities and Mental Health Law' (2012) 75(5) Modern Law Review 752.

[299] UN Committee on the Rights of Persons with Disabilities, 'General Comment No 1 Article 12: Equal recognition before the law CRPD/C/GC1' (2014) available at <https://digitallibrary.un.org/record/779679?ln=en> accessed 04 September 2022.

[300] These challenges (and counterarguments) are discussed in Piers Gooding, 'Navigating the Flashing Amber Lights of the Right to Legal Capacity in the United Nations Convention on the Rights of Persons with Disabilities: Responding to Major Concerns' (2015) 15 Human Rights Law Review 45.

[301] Simon Wessely et al. (n 52) 64.

framework, suggesting a more open perspective to CRPD thinking in Scotland,[302] which is further reflected in recent reform proposals.

Aside from Article 12, a second challenge comes through Article 14, which requires the right to liberty on equal basis and no deprivation of liberty based on disability. As such, all measures permitting detention, either in an acute hospital setting under the MHA 1983 and MHCTA 2003, or through DoLS, do not appear compliant.[303] The CRPD's stance explicitly diverges from Article 5(1)(e) ECHR, which allows detention on the basis of mental impairment. The ECtHR acknowledged this in *Rooman* v *Belgium*, but reinforced their view that, even if impermissible under the CRPD, derogations from Article 5 for 'persons of unsound mind' were acceptable:

> it is necessary to acknowledge expressly, in addition to the function of social protection, the therapeutic aspect of the aim referred to in Article 5 § 1 (e), and thus to recognise explicitly that there exists an obligation on the authorities to ensure appropriate and indi- vidualised therapy, based on the specific features of the compulsory confinement, such as the conditions of the detention regime, the treatment proposed or the duration of the detention. On the other hand, the Court considers that Article 5, as currently interpreted, does not contain a prohibition on detention on the basis of impairment, in contrast to what is proposed by the UN Committee on the Rights of Persons with Disabilities.[304]

Article 14 CRPD also challenges the ethical basis of the MHA 1983 (risk plus mental dis- order), refusing to recognise the validity of any form of detention based on the presence of mental disorder. The UK Government does not appear to accept this incompatibility, considering that the safeguards contained in the MHA 1983 and MCA 2005 ensure that deprivations of liberty are compliant with law.[305]

Notably, although arguments for fusion legislation are, like the CRPD, rooted in non- discrimination, it is not immune to CRPD-based critique. The MCANI 2016 still relies on a diagnostic threshold for capacity and continues to permit deprivations of liberty on the basis of lack of capacity. As such, while some commentators argue that this approach would be compliant with the CRPD,[306] full compliance remains doubtful.[307]

10.7 REFORM

As may be evident from the discussion in the previous section, mental health law in the UK appears subject to constant amendments, refinements, and programmes of reform, which are often fraught and drawn-out affairs.[308] Programmes of reform are ongoing in each of the UK jurisdictions (not least, the implementation of the MCANI 2016).

---

[302] Mental Welfare Commission for Scotland, 'Supported Decision Making: Good Practice Guide' (2020) available at <https://www.mwcscot.org.uk/sites/default/files/2021-02/Supported%20Decision%20 Making%202021.pdf> accessed 04 September 2022.

[303] Peter Bartlett (n 298), 772–775; see also Lucy Series (2022) (n 45), 102–106.

[304] [2019] ECHR 105, [205].

[305] Office for Disability Issues, 'UK Initial Report on the UN Convention of the Rights of Persons with Disabilities' (2011) available at <https://www.gov.uk/government/publications/un-convention-on-the-rights- of-persons-with-disabilities-initial-report-on-how-the-uk-is-implementing-it> accessed 04 September 2022.

[306] George Szmukler, Rowena Daw, and Felicity Callard, 'Mental Health Law and the UN Convention on the Rights of Persons with Disabilities' (2014) 37(7) International Journal of Law and Psychiatry 245.

[307] Eilionóir Flynn, 'Mental (in)capacity or Legal Capacity? A Human Rights Analysis of the Proposed Fusion of Mental Health and Mental Capacity Law in Northern Ireland' (2020) 64(4) Northern Ireland Legal Quarterly 485.

[308] See e.g. Patrick Brown, 'Risk Versus Need in Revising the 1983 Mental Health Act: Conflicting Claims, Muddled Policy' (2006) 8(4) Health & Risk Society 343.

In 2017, motivated by rising rates of detention under the MHA 1983 and concern for its disproportionate impact on minoritised groups, the UK Government commissioned an Independent Review of the MHA 1983, led by Sir Simon Wessely.[309] The review's final report was published in December 2018, and made 154 recommendations for reform.[310]

On 27 June 2022, the Government announced a draft Mental Health Bill (the Bill)[311] to reform the MHA based on some of the Wessely Review's recommendations. Not all have been adopted. For example, while the draft Bill is reflective of the Review's principles of choice and autonomy, least restrictions, therapeutic benefit, and the person as individual,[312] they are not statutory principles, as was recommended. Key clauses in the draft Bill which relate to the topics discussed in this chapter are highlighted going forward.

First, the Bill amends the definition of learning disability, by providing definitions of what constitutes 'autism', 'leaning disability', and 'psychiatric disorder' for the purpose of the Act.[313] It provides that individuals may only be admitted for treatment if they are suffering from psychiatric disorder. This means individuals with autism or a learning disability may only be admitted for *assessment,* unless they have a co-occurring mental health condition which requires treatment.[314] This clause aims to prevent an individual being detained solely on grounds of learning disability or autism, but it has attracted concern that such individuals could simply be detained under DoLS or the LPS instead.[315]

The Bill also makes changes to the admission process. It contains a definition for 'appropriate medical treatment', which will mean that which '(i) has a reasonable prospect of alleviating, or preventing the worsening of, the disorder or one or more of its symptoms or manifestations, and (ii) is appropriate in the person's case'.[316] Under the Bill, admission under section 2 or 3 MHA 1983 will only be available where 'serious harm may be caused' to self or others, and section 3 admissions will be shortened to three months in the first instance (renewable for six months, then a year).[317] This aims to ensure detention is only justified where it will assist the patient and the magnitude of risk is greater.

[309] Department for Health and Social Care, 'Independent Review of the Mental Health Act' (2019) available at <https://www.gov.uk/government/groups/independent-review-of-the-mental-health-act> accessed 10 August 2022.

[310] Simon Wessely et al. (n 52).

[311] Department of Health and Social Care and Ministry of Justice, 'Draft Mental Health Bill 2022' (2022) available at <https://www.gov.uk/government/publications/draft-mental-health-bill-2022> accessed 04 September 2022. For a detailed discussion see Judy Laing, 'Reforming the Mental Health Act: Will More Rights Lead to Fewer Wrongs?' (2022) 30(1) Medical Law Review 158.

[312] Department of Health and Social Care and Ministry of Justice, 'Draft Mental Health Bill, Explanatory Notes' (2022) available at <https://assets.publishing.service.gov.uk/government/uploads/system/uploads/attachment_data/file/1085872/draft-mental-health-bill-explanatory-notes.pdf> accessed 04 September 2022.

[313] Department of Health and Social Care and Ministry of Justice, 'Draft Mental Health Bill 2022' (2022) (n 311), cl 1.

[314] ibid., cl 3.

[315] See e.g. Rosie Harding, 'Initial Thoughts on the Draft Mental Health Bill: Autism and Learning Disability Provisions' (29 June 2022) available at <https://legalcapacity.org.uk/crpd/initial-thoughts-on-the-draft-mental-health-bill-autism-and-learning-disability-provisions/> accessed 26 July 2022.

[316] Department of Health and Social Care and Ministry of Justice, 'Draft Mental Health Bill 2022' (2022) (n 311), cl 6.

[317] ibid., cl 3.

The Bill proposes a number of changes to treatment under the Act, chiefly introducing statutory care and treatment plans which set out the patient's views and how these are taken into account when decisions about treatment are made.[318] The Bill would require healthcare professionals, in making decisions about medical treatment, to take into account the patient's wishes and feelings, and take steps to allow them to participate in the decision-making process (similar to the MCA 2005 best interests requirements).[319] The proposals also contain a substantial overhaul of Part IV. A patient with capacity who objects to medical treatment, or who has an advance decision objecting to said treatment, cannot be given it unless it is supported by a SOAD, and there is a 'compelling reason' to do so.[320] Any treatment given beyond two months (not three) will required SOAD approval,[321] and patients who have capacity and are refusing urgent treatment cannot have it administered the basis of serious suffering (capacitous patients will have a 'right to choose to suffer').[322]

The Bill makes several changes to CTOs, chiefly requiring the involvement and agreement of the supervising community clinician in decisions relating to the use and operation of the CTO. Where the patient is recalled to hospital, the community clinician must be consulted wherever possible. The Bill also seeks to amend the conditions placed on a patient to ensure that only those that are necessary can be used.[323]

The Bill also makes changes to patient support, and would replace the role of NR with a 'Nominated Person', aligning with the Scottish and Northern Irish models.[324] It would also extend IMHA support to informal patients in England, imposing duties on hospitals to notify services about patients who qualify for support and ensuring those services seek to interview such patients to identify if they wish to access an IMHA.[325] Finally, the Bill would see the powers of mental health tribunals expanded, with patients able to apply more quickly and more regularly to tribunals.[326]

The reform process is equally active in Scotland, for both the AWIA 2000 (as discussed) and the MHCTA 2003. Concerning the latter, the Scottish Mental Health Law Review (SMHLR) concluded in May 2022.[327] The SMHLR's final report, published in September 2022, makes proposals for wide changes to both Acts. In particular, the SMHLR recommended the Scottish Government adopt an approach to mental health law which reflects human rights and the CRPD.[328] This includes the adoption of a framework for 'human rights enablement, supported decision making and autonomous decision making'.[329] This means enabling human rights to be actively respected in line with a CRPD vision and seeking to ensure patients' wills and preferences are given 'special regard'. To reflect this, the SMHLR recommended that the purpose of the new legislation should be 'to ensure that all the human rights of people with mental and intellectual disability . . . are respected, protected and fulfilled',[330] and suggested the legal frameworks should move away from diagnosis as the threshold for support and intervention. The SMHLR also proposed that and the 'ultimate long term goal' should be fused or unified legislation, but, recognising

---

[318] ibid., cl 18.   [319] ibid., cl 9.   [320] ibid., cl 11.   [321] ibid., cl 12.   [322] ibid., cl 15.
[323] ibid., cll 4, 19, and 20.   [324] ibid., cll 21–25, Sch 1.   [325] ibid., cl 34, Sch 3.
[326] ibid., cll 5, 27–29.
[327] Scottish Mental Health Law Review, 'Consultation: March 2022' (2022) available at <https://consult.gov.scot/mental-health-law-secretariat/scottish-mental-health-law-review/> accessed 04 September 2022.
[328] Scottish Mental Health Law Review, 'Final Report' (2022) available at <https://cms.mentalhealthlaw-review.scot/wp-content/uploads/2022/09/SMHLR-FINAL-Report-.pdf> accessed 12 October 2022.
[329] ibid., Chapter 8.
[330] ibid., p 87.

this would take many years to develop and embed, in the interim, a unified set of principles for each Act should be developed to ensure greater alignment and parity.[331] The Report made intermediate recommendations for urgent changes to the AWIA 2000, including the development of a scheme to authorise deprivations of liberty.[332]

On comparison of these two approaches, it seems likely that mental health law in England and Wales and Scotland will diverge further in the future. The recommendations of the SMHLR reflect a rights-based approach to law which embraces the social model of disability and goes further than the current proposals for reform in England and Wales, which fundamentally overhaul the compulsory framework, and further than the MCANI 2016 with its human rights focus. While Scotland advocates for a unified or fusion approach, England and Wales instead have opted to bring the MHA 1983 and MCA 2005 'up to date' and await the outcome of the NI experience.[333] Of course, we will need to await the completion of each jurisdiction's reform process, and the final form of any legislation passed by the respective Parliaments, before seeing the impact any divergence would have on the experience of patients within the system.

10.8 CONCLUSION

As should be clear, mental health law remains a dynamic area and continues to be, for many, deeply unsatisfactory. While traditional legal frameworks based on the 'risk plus disorder' paradigm persist in the UK, wide concerns continue to be raised about the disproportionate impact of the law on minoritised groups and the wide discretion it continues to afford to those making decisions, rather than prioritising the views of the patients subject to it. This deep tension between patient rights and autonomy on the one side, and risk and protection on the other, appears to contribute to the near-constant state of flux that characterises the law in this area. Although legislation based on capacity (including fusion legislation) relies on the separate paradigm of empowerment, they are not immune from the draw of protection, at times supporting courses of action that conflict directly with an individual's expressed wishes, and indeed, the decisions taken under their auspices appear at least as restrictive as traditional mental health law.

Human rights discourse in this area is equally dynamic, with the exigences of the right to liberty driving significant reform in capacity legislation and posing searching questions as to what 'freedom' ought to mean for persons with mental disabilities. While the ECHR continues to reflect the risk paradigm, the CRPD, in contrast, provides a different and arguably radical vision of what mental health law should be, even if this is yet to be embraced by UK legislatures and courts. Further changes in the law seem certain, and as the UK jurisdictions move forward with their increasingly distinct approaches to tackling poor mental health, it appears likely that many of the challenges highlighted in this chapter will persist.

---

[331] ibid., p 111.   [332] ibid., Chapter 13.   [333] Simon Wessely et al. (n 52), 222–223.

FURTHER READING

1. Gordon R Ashton, His Honour Judge Marc Marin, and the Rt Hon Lord Justice Baker, *Mental Capacity: Law and Practice* (4th edn, 2018).

2. Peter Bartlett and Ralph Sandland, *Mental Health Law: Policy and Practice* (OUP 2007).

3. Beverley Clough, *The Spaces of Mental Capacity Law: Moving Beyond Binaries* (Routledge 2022).

4. Lawrence Gostin, Peter Bartlett, Phil Fennell, Jean McHale, and Ronnie MacKay (eds.) *Principles of Mental Health Law and Policy* (OUP 2010).

5. Lucy Series, *Deprivation of Liberty in the Shadows of the Institution* (Bristol University Press 2022).

6. Jill Stavert and Henry Patrick, *Mental Health, Incapacity and the Law in Scotland* (2nd edn, Bloomsbury 2016).

11

MEDICAL CONFIDENTIALITY AND DATA PROTECTION

11.1 INTRODUCTION

This chapter deals with the protection of patient privacy and the associated potential tensions that arise from the prospect that additional—alternative—value can be produced from use of patient data beyond the confines of the doctor–patient relationship. The starting principle is clear: a general common law duty is imposed on doctors to respect the confidences of their patients. The nature of this obligation—which applies to all confidential information and not only to medical material[1]—was discussed by the House of Lords in *A-G v Guardian Newspapers Ltd (No 2)*,[2] in which it was affirmed that there is a public interest in the protection of confidences received under notice of confidentiality or in circumstances where the reasonable person ought to know that the information was confidential. In *Hunter v Mann*, the court stated that 'the doctor is under a duty not to [voluntarily] disclose, without the consent of the patient, information which he, the doctor, has gained in his professional capacity'.[3]

In the very significant case of *W v Egdell*,[4] which we discuss in greater detail later, the court accepted the existence of an obligation of confidentiality between a psychiatrist and his patient, an obligation which counsel submitted was based not only on equitable grounds but also on implied contract. The House of Lords then confirmed in *Campbell v Mirror Group Newspapers Ltd*[5] that details of one's medical circumstances are 'obviously private' and deserving of the full protection of the law of confidence, albeit now subject to the slant afforded to the law by the Human Rights Act 1998, which we also consider further later.

Added to this, by statute, the processing of 'personal data' is governed by the principles embodied in the Data Protection Act 2018, which, in turn, implements and supplements the terms of the UK General Data Protection Regulation (hereafter, the GDPR). This system is overseen by the UK-wide Information Commissioner's Office, and there is a plethora of professional organisations and persons part of whose remit is to respect and monitor the confidentiality of patients' information. These include the General Medical

---

[1] The duty to respect confidences is to be distinguished from the (broader) notion of respecting individual privacy, although the two are obviously related. Although the House of Lords confirmed that there is general tort of invasion of privacy in English law, as per *Wainwright v Home Office* [2003] UKHL 53, this is not at all the same as saying that privacy interests are not protected. Moreover, Scotland has now recognised a right of privacy in the common law as per *C v Chief Constable of the Police Service of Scotland* [2019] CSOH 48 and, as discussed going forward, UK courts now recognise a stand-alone tort of misuse of private information.

[2] [1990] AC 109.   [3] [1974] QB 767 [772] (Boreham J).   [4] [1990] Ch 359.
[5] [2004] 2 AC 457.

Council (GMC), the British Medical Association (BMA), individuals known as Caldicott Guardians within NHS organisations and local authorities which provide social services, and the Confidentiality Advisory Group, which operates in England and Wales under the auspices of the Health Research Authority to offer advice on whether an application to process identifiable patient information without consent for medical purposes should or should not be approved.[6] This field is, in fact, in a state of considerable current flux and concern surrounding the legitimate and lawful uses of medical data—and this has only accelerated following the purported beneficial uses of patient data for combatting the Covid-19 pandemic.[7]

In what follows, this chapter will provide an overview of data protection law, with a focus on the medical and scientific research context, before turning to the common law duty of confidentiality and the circumstances in which confidential information may be lawfully disclosed. Brief coverage also will be provided on the emerging tort of misuse of private information. The chapter will conclude with a discussion of access to patient medical records, remedies that individuals may seek when their private or confidential information is misused, and the use of medical information upon one's death.

11.2 THE CONTOURS OF THE LANDSCAPE

The protection of medical confidentiality is complicated because it is a terrain consisting of, and influenced by, three overlapping spheres of interest: the professions, law, and ethics. We can, therefore, look not only at what the patient feels is their legal entitlement but also at the ethical requirements of the medical profession itself. Here there are a number of sources from which the doctor can seek guidance. The Hippocratic Oath makes several demands which can scarcely be regarded as binding on the modern doctor; nonetheless, its stipulations as to professional confidentiality are still firmly endorsed. The relevant modern translation runs: 'Whatever things seen or heard in the course of medical practice ought not to be spoken of, I will not, save for weighty reasons, divulge.' The Declaration of Geneva (last amended in 2017) imposes much the same obligation on the doctor, requiring them to 'respect the secrets that are confided in me, even after the patient has died'.[8]

There can be no doubt that confidentiality is taken seriously by lawyers and ethicists alike. Most critics, however, see the concept as being something of a pretence in that bureaucracy, fuelled by modern administrative technology, is increasingly invasive of the principle; never-ending advances in information technology merely facilitate wider and faster dissemination of patient information, heighten concerns about the risk of unauthorised disclosure, and generally exacerbate the problem. Certainly, patients' records must circulate fairly widely—and among professionals who might be less deeply indoctrinated as to confidentiality than their medical colleagues. But early suggestions that institutions should take over custodianship of confidences and impose an overall standard of

---

[6] See Confidentiality Advisory Group, 'About Us' (2022) available at <https://www.hra.nhs.uk/about-us/committees-and-services/confidentiality-advisory-group/> accessed 08 November 2022.

[7] Department of Health and Social Care, 'Data Saves Lives: Reshaping Health and Social Care With Data' (June 2022) available at <https://www.gov.uk/government/publications/data-saves-lives-reshaping-health-and-social-care-with-data/data-saves-lives-reshaping-health-and-social-care-with-data> accessed 08 November 2022.

[8] World Medical Association, 'WMA Declaration of Geneva' (2017) available at <https://www.wma.net/policies-post/wma-declaration-of-geneva/> accessed 08 November 2022.

duty on all who work in healthcare institutions have now come to represent the position, both at common law[9] and by statute.[10] Indeed, sensitivity towards patient confidentiality and data protection has probably never been greater, with NHS organisations holding training sessions for staff at regular intervals.

Even so, the special position of the doctor is unlikely to change in the foreseeable future and they are currently bound by the authority of, and are subject to the discipline of, the GMC. Subject to certain exceptions, which we discuss further later, the GMC imposes a strict duty on registered medical practitioners to refrain from disclosing voluntarily to any third-party information about a patient which they have learnt directly or indirectly in their professional capacity. A breach of this duty will be a serious matter, exposing the doctor to a wide range of potential professional penalties.[11] We now turn to look at these regimes, starting with data protection law.

11.3 OPERATION OF DATA PROTECTION LAW

Medical information is further protected under the Data Protection Act (DPA) 2018,[12] which supplements the UK GDPR.[13] It is not necessary for the purposes of this chapter to examine the provisions of the Act or GDPR in any great depth. In any event, the UK Government recently introduced the Data Protection and Digital Information Bill to Parliament in the 2022–23 session,[14] which aims to update and simplify the UK's data protection framework, specifically the GDPR, and pivot towards a pro-innovation, post-Brexit regulatory environment. In the scientific and medical context, proposed changes are relatively straightforward. For example, the Bill proposes to insert a definition of what constitutes processing personal data for scientific research under the UK GDPR, and to

---

[9] *A-G v Guardian Newspapers Ltd (No 2)*. There is a duty placed on all those who receive confidential information in circumstances which objectively (and reasonably) import a duty of confidence. Communications in a hospital are a paradigm example of this: see *W, X, Y and Z v Secretary of State for Health et al.* [2015] EWCA Civ 1034.

[10] Data Protection Act 2018 and the Health and Social Care Act 2012.

[11] GMC, 'Confidentiality: Good Practice in Handling Patient Information' (2018). This guidance and related documentation and toolkits are available at <https://www.gmc-uk.org/ethical-guidance/ethical-guidance-for-doctors/confidentiality> accessed 08 November 2022. See also BMA, 'Confidentiality Toolkit: A Toolkit for Doctors' (2021) available at <https://www.bma.org.uk/media/4283/bma-confidentiality-and-health-records-toolkit-july-2021.pdf> accessed 08 November 2022.

[12] The Data Protection Act 2018 came into force on 25 May 2018, in line with the EU's General Data Protection Regulation.

[13] The DPA 2018 originally supplemented EU Regulation (EU) 2016/679 (the EU General Data Protection Regulation); in post-Brexit UK, the GDPR itself now has become domesticated and reformulated as the 'UK GDPR'. Separate from the EU, there is a general and strong European interest in the subject which is reflected elsewhere in the Council of Europe's Recommendation No R (97) 5 on the Protection of Medical Data (1997). This recommendation not only includes general principles that should guide national laws on the confidentiality of medical information but also embraces specific recommendations relating to such matters as storage of data, their transmission across borders, and the use of data in medical research. See also Council of Europe, Recommendation CM/Rec(2019)2 (2019) on Protection of health-related data (2019), which aims to facilitate the full application of the principles of the Council of Europe's Convention for the Protection of Individuals with regard to Automatic Processing of Personal Data ('Convention 108') as well as to take into account the principles developed in the modernised Convention (known as 'Convention 108+') and to apply them to a modern environment in which health-related data are exchanged and shared.

[14] UK Parliament, 'Data Protection and Digital Information Bill' (2022) available at <https://bills.parliament.uk/bills/3322> accessed 08 November 2022.

clarify that research into public health only falls under the definition of scientific research if it is in the public interest. The Bill also proposes to amend the UK GDPR by clarifying a way for data controllers processing for scientific research purposes to obtain consent to an area of scientific research where it is not possible to identify fully the purposes for which the personal data is to be processed at the time of collection. It would clarify when consent in such cases will meet the existing definition under the UK GDPR. As of the time of writing, it remains to be seen what final shape the UK's data protection framework will take; indeed, a slightly revised version of the Bill, known as the Data Protection and Digital Information (No. 2) Bill, was proposed in early 2023. This said, the material that follows in this section is expected to retain broad application.

It is sufficient simply to note certain key features of the legal regime.[15] Data protection law operates closely with the law of confidentiality, but the two regimes operate separately if not in parallel. Data protection law protects the rights of individuals in respect of the processing of their personal data. This means that personal data revealed in a medical context that has not been recorded in any way (for example, some of the confidential personal details of a patient explained to a doctor but not written down in medical notes) will be covered by the law of confidentiality, but not data protection law.[16] To lawfully process personal data, one must have a 'legal basis', of which six exist under the GDPR.[17] Additionally, a specific exception (or exemption) is needed to process special category personal data, of which ten exist under the GDPR.[18]

'Personal data' is defined as 'any information relating to an identified or identifiable natural person; an identifiable natural person is one who can be identified, directly or indirectly, in particular by reference to an identifier such as a name, an identification number, location data, an online identifier or to one or more factors specific to the physical, physiological, genetic, mental, economic, cultural or social identity of that natural person'.[19] The law regulates the processing of such data by reference to a set of principles that ensure, inter alia, that data are only processed when it is fair and lawful to do so, that data are processed and kept only so far as is necessary for the purposes for which they were obtained, that the data are accurate and kept up to date, and that they should be processed in a secure manner. A logical first step in determining whether the GDPR (and DPA 2018) applies at all—beyond determining whether data are 'personal data'—is to establish whether data are being 'processed'. The GDPR envisages an incredibly wide scope for this term including:

> any operation or set of operations which is performed on personal data or on sets of personal data, whether or not by automated means, such as collection, recording, organisation, structuring, storage, adaptation or alteration, retrieval, consultation, use, disclosure by transmission, dissemination or otherwise making available, alignment or combination, restriction, erasure or destruction.[20]

One might think there is little that could be done with data which would not fall within such a definition! Nonetheless, in *Johnson* v *Medical Defence Union Ltd*,[21] the Court of Appeal held that it was not 'processing' (as defined similarly in the previous EU Data

---

[15] For a guide to the GDPR, see Information Commissioner's Office (ICO), 'Guide to the UK General Data Protection Regulation (UK GDPR)' (2022) available at <https://ico.org.uk/for-organisations/guide-to-data-protection/guide-to-the-general-data-protection-regulation-gdpr/> accessed 08 November 2022.

[16] UK GDPR Art 2(5) states that the GDPR only applies to the processing of personal data 'wholly or partly by automated means' or by other means where they form 'part of a filing system or are intended to form part of a filing system'.

[17] UK GDPR, Art 6(1).   [18] UK GDPR, Art 9(2).   [19] UK GDPR, Art 4(1).

[20] UK GDPR, Art 4(2).   [21] [2007] 3 CMLR 9.

Protection Directive) for an employee of the Union to carry out a risk assessment of a member based purely on complaints against him (irrespective of whether any complaint was well founded), even when this led to the termination of his membership. There is an important distinction to draw between 'fair processing' and 'fair' decisions. The former is a technical requirement of law that is linked to dealing with information in a 'relevant filing system' and it is to be distinguished from decisions taken by human beings with which one might disagree. Damages were awarded in *Grinyer* v *Plymouth Hospitals NHS Trust* (2011, unreported) for unlawful access to medical records—a sum of £12,500 (exacerbation of pre-existing injury) and £4,800 (loss of earnings). Unlawful processing of personal data can lead to recovery for 'moral damages' for affront to privacy even when there is no pecuniary loss.[22]

Data protection law attempts to categorise information into three distinct groupings. These are (i) regular categories of personal data; (ii) special categories of personal data (i.e. sensitive personal data); and (iii) anonymised or anonymous data. All are of relevance in the healthcare setting. Data which are 'pseudonymised' are still considered personal data and thus subject to data protection law. The GDPR defines pseudonymisation as:

> the processing of personal data in such a manner that the personal data can no longer be attributed to a specific data subject without the use of additional information, provided that such additional information is kept separately and is subject to technical and organisational measures to ensure that the personal data are not attributed to an identified or identifiable natural person.[23]

Data which are anonymised are not covered by the provisions of the GDPR and DPA 2018.[24] It has been a matter of considerable contemporary debate since the days of the EU Data Protective Directive and Data Protection Act 1998, however, as to what constitutes 'anonymised' data. In *Common Services Agency* v *Scottish Information Commissioner*,[25] the House of Lords had to rule on a dispute regarding the disclosure of rare incidences of childhood leukaemia in the Dumfries and Galloway postal areas. A request had been made under freedom of information legislation, but this would not need to be complied with if the data were 'personal data', which would clearly have been the case if names, ages, and addresses were released. The Commissioner had ruled, however, that the applicant could and should have been provided with data subjected to a process known as 'barnardisation' which can be applied to tables of data involving very small numbers in order to protect individual privacy.[26] Was this sufficient to anonymise the data? The question was unresolved by their Lordships and considered to be a question of fact to be remitted to the Commissioner himself.[27] In legal terms, the position remains unsatisfactory: against which legal standard must an Information Commissioner or any other party determine whether a sufficient level of anonymity is reached? It is well recognised as a matter of practice that a 'spectrum of identifiability'[28] exists with respect to fragments of information about individuals which can be pieced together by a variety of means, and

---

[22] *Vidal-Hall* v *Google Inc.* [2015] EWCA Civ 311.   [23] UK GDPR, Art 4(5).

[24] Advice to organisations on many matters of data protection is available, however, from the Information Commissioner's Office.

[25] [2008] UKHL 47.

[26] This technique randomly adds 0, +1, or –1 to all values between 2 and 4 in cells of data, and adds 0 or +1 to entries where the value is 1. A cell containing 0 remains unchanged. In this way, it is argued, the data are 'perturbed' and anonymity is protected.

[27] For comment see Graeme Laurie and Renate Gertz, 'The Worst of all Worlds? *Common Services Agency* v *Scottish Information Commissioner*' (2009) 13 Edinburgh Law Review 330.

[28] For discussion, see William Lowrance, *Privacy, Confidentiality and Health Research* (CUP 2012).

that *absolute* anonymity is elusive if not illusory.[29] Anonymisation is often referred to as a craft. Anonymity and identifiability are, instead, *relative* concepts:

> To determine whether a natural person is identifiable, account should be taken of all the means reasonably likely to be used … either by the controller or by another person to identify the natural person directly or indirectly. To ascertain whether means are reasonably likely to be used to identify the natural person, account should be taken of all objective factors, such as the costs of and the amount of time required for identification, taking into consideration the available technology at the time of the processing and technological developments.[30]

Note, too, circumstances can change over time—so the status of whether anonymised data remains as such must be kept under regular review.

In contrast, 'special categories of personal data' are defined as data revealing racial or ethnic origin, political opinions, religious or philosophical beliefs, or trade union membership; the processing of genetic data, biometric data for the purpose of uniquely identifying a natural person; data concerning health; and data concerning a natural person's sex life or sexual orientation.[31] Additional protection is afforded to such data and, as we have seen elsewhere in this book, the primary point of reference is the concept of consent. In principle, one might expect then that 'explicit consent' would be the most common and obvious factor to legitimate processing of sensitive personal data.[32] However, a wide range of alternative justifications for processing accompanies this protection. Indeed, in the biomedical context, the legal basis to process personal data is more commonly a task performed in the public interest (namely the carrying on of health services in the NHS),[33] and the exemption to permit processing of special category personal data such as health data is one of the following:

- Where the processing is necessary for scientific research purposes, is carried out in accordance with Article 89(1) of the GDPR (as supplemented by section 19 of the Data Protection Act 2018) and is in the public interest.[34]

- Where the processing is necessary to protect the vital interests of the data subject or of another person where the data subject is physically or legally incapable of giving his consent.[35]

- Where the processing is necessary for medical purposes where the processing is undertaken by a health professional or someone else who owes an equivalent duty of confidentiality.[36]

- Where the processing is necessary for reasons of public interest in the area of public health.[37]

The GDPR also enables the UK Government to create exemptions on the basis of 'substantial public interest'.[38] According to the DPA 2018, special provisions in the UK are made for, among others, preventing fraud, the investigation and prosecution of crime, and legitimate journalistic activities.[39]

---

[29] Harald Schmidt and Shawneequa Callier, 'How Anonymous is "Anonymous"? Some Suggestions Towards a Coherent Universal Coding System for Genetic Samples' (2012) 38(5) Journal of Medical Ethics 304.
[30] UK GDPR, Recital 26.   [31] UK GDPR, Art 9(1).   [32] UK GDPR, Art 9(2)(a).
[33] UK GDPR, Art 6(1)(e).   [34] Data Protection Act 2018, s 4 of Part 1 of Sche 1.
[35] UK GDPR, Art 9(2)(c).   [36] UK GDPR, Art 9(2)(h).   [37] UK GDPR, Art 9(2)(i).
[38] UK GDPR, Art 9(2)(g).   [39] See Part 2 of Sch 1 of the Data Protection Act 2018.

Regarding the scientific research exemption, the law creates a number of important protections for researchers using personal data obtained from data subjects. Specifically, the DPA 2018 provides for derogations from the rights of information access, data rectification, restrictions on processing, and objection to data processing.[40]

The GDPR and DPA 2018 provisions are all-encompassing of identifiable personal data. Consent has a role to play but, as we have seen, it certainly does not emerge as a trump card. Indeed, some might argue that the broad and indistinct categories of justifications for processing personal data without consent potentially weaken the protection that is afforded to informational privacy interests. The model, however, is, as always, a search for a balance and few could deny that absolute protection of one's medical information may sometimes bow to public interests. We observed this most pronouncedly in the Covid-19 pandemic. It bears emphasising that the essential purpose of the GDPR is to legitimate the free flow of information, not to prevent it, and in times of public health emergencies, data flows are especially important to protect the health of the population. The devil is in the detail, though, of determining which interests should be weighed in the balance and how far privacy should be compromised in any given case, and the extent to which individually identifying data must be disclosed. The example of scientific research is particularly apt. The UK has mechanisms for allowing research using identifiable patient data without consent, subject to rigorous review, and we discuss these later.

We now turn to discuss the common law duty of confidentiality, otherwise known as the duty of confidence. As will be discussed, the common law and statutory provisions must be read together and these two legal regimes of data protection and confidentiality do not offer entirely the same levels of protection, nor do they serve the same objectives.

11.4 THE DUTY OF CONFIDENCE AND ITS EXCEPTIONS

All the classic codes of practice imply some qualification of an absolute duty of professional secrecy. Thus, the Hippocratic Oath has it: 'All that may come to my knowledge . . . which ought not to be spread abroad, I will keep secret', which clearly indicates that there are some things which may be published. The Declaration of Geneva modifies this prohibition to: 'I will respect the secrets that are confided in me', and the word 'respect' is open to interpretation. The GMC, while always emphasising its strong views as to the rule dictating professional secrecy, lists five general headings under which confidential patient information may or must be disclosed.[41] In this section, we focus on three key exceptions: disclosure required by law, disclosure by way of patient consent, and disclosure on the grounds of public interest. In the following section, we focus on another increasingly important but ethically fraught exception: where disclosure is permitted or has been approved under a statutory process that sets aside the common law duty of confidentiality.

---

[40] Data Protection Act 2018, s 15(2)(f) and Part 6 of Sch 2.

[41] GMC, 'Confidentiality' (n 11) para 9. The guidance states that personal information can be disclosed under the following scenarios: 1) the patient consents, whether implicitly or explicitly, for the sake of their own care or for local clinical audit; 2) the patient has given their explicit consent to disclosure for other purposes; 3) the disclosure is of overall benefit to a patient who lacks the capacity to consent; 4) the disclosure is required by law or the disclosure is permitted or has been approved under a statutory process that sets aside the common law duty of confidentiality; and 5) the disclosure can be justified in the public interest.

11.4.1 DISCLOSURE REQUIRED OR RESTRICTED BY LAW

Various statutes may require doctors to disclose confidential patient information to identified authorities. For example, the Abortion Act 1967 and relevant regulations[42] require any practitioner terminating a pregnancy to provide specified information to the Chief Medical Officer, namely the reference number and the date of birth or age and postcode of the woman concerned. In England and Wales, there is a statutory duty to notify the police when it is identified that an under-18-year-old has had female genital cutting.[43] The Public Health (Control of Disease) Act 1984 and Health Protection (Notification) Regulations 2010 and Health Protection (Notification) (Wales) Regulations 2010—and equivalents in Scotland[44] and Northern Ireland[45]—require a doctor to notify actual or suspected cases of patients suffering various forms of infectious disease to the proper officer of the local authority. Similarly, under section 172 of the Road Traffic Act 1988, any person may be required to give information which may lead to the identification of a driver alleged to be guilty of certain offences. Finally, under the Terrorism Act 2000, any person must inform police as soon as possible of any information that may help to prevent an act of terrorism, or help in apprehending or prosecuting a terrorist.[46]

Conversely, there are also statutes that impose heightened restrictions on disclosing information about patients. For example, under section 22 of the Gender Recognition Act 2004, it is an offence to disclose 'protected information' when that information is acquired in an official capacity. 'Protected information' is defined as information about a person's application for gender recognition and a person's gender history after that person has changed gender under the Act. Section 22 also sets out a series of exceptions where disclosure is considered to be justified.[47] Similarly, section 33A(1) of the Human Fertilisation and Embryology Act 1990, as amended, protects the information kept by clinics and the Human Fertilisation and Embryology Authority, subject to certain exceptions.[48] Finally, another example are regulations that prohibit disclosure of information capable of identifying an individual who is examined or treated for any sexually transmitted disease, to anyone other than to a medical practitioner in connection with the treatment of the individual in relation to that disease or for the prevention of the spread of the disease.[49]

11.4.2 CONSENT

Perhaps the most easily recognisable exception to the duty of confidentiality is when the patient, or their legal proxy, consents to the disclosure of information. The situation is simple when viewed from the positive angle. A positive consent to release of information elides any obligation to secrecy owed by the person receiving that consent; equally, an explicit request that information should not be disclosed is binding on the doctor save in the most exceptional circumstances—a matter which is of major concern in relation to

---

[42] Abortion Regulations 1991 (England and Wales) (and amendments); Abortion (Scotland) Regulations 1991; Abortion (Northern Ireland) (No 2) Regulations 2020.

[43] Female Genital Mutilation Act 2003 (as amended by the Serious Crime Act 2015).

[44] Public Health etc. (Scotland) Act 2008.   [45] Public Health Act (Northern Ireland) 1967.

[46] Terrorism Act 2000, s 19.

[47] See also The Gender Recognition (Disclosure of Information) (England, Wales and Northern Ireland) Order 2005 (SI 2005/916) and The Gender Recognition (Disclosure of Information) (Scotland) Order 2005 (SSI 2005/15).

[48] Human Fertilisation and Embryology Act 1990, s 33A(2).

[49] NHS Trusts and Primary Care Trusts (Sexually Transmitted Diseases) Directions 2000; National Health Service (Venereal Diseases) Regulations 1974 (SI 1974/29).

communicable disease. Note, however, that, even granted the consent of a patient, a doctor is not absolved of fair processing requirements under data protection law.

The position is not so clear when looked at from the negative aspect—that is, when the patient has neither consented to nor dissented from disclosure—and it may, indeed, be frankly unsatisfactory. How many patients know whether the person standing with the consultant at the hospital bedside is another doctor, a social worker, or just an interested spectator? Would they have consented to their presence if they had been informed? The consultant may be responsible if, as a result, there is a breach of confidence—but this is small consolation to the patient who feels that their rights have been infringed. What patient at a teaching hospital outpatient department is likely to refuse when the consultant asks, 'You don't mind these young doctors being present, do you?'—the pressures are virtually irresistible and truly autonomous consent is well-nigh impossible, yet the confidential doctor–patient relationship which began with their general practitioner has, effectively, been broken.

It is obvious that such technical breaches must be, and generally are, accepted in practice—a modern hospital cannot function except as a team effort and new doctors have to be trained, the return for a technical loss of privacy being access to the best diagnostic and therapeutic aids available.[50] The GMC recognises this in permitting the sharing of information with other practitioners who assume responsibility for clinical management of the patient and, to the extent that the doctor deems it necessary for the performance of their particular duties, with other healthcare professionals who are collaborating with the doctor in their patients' management.[51]

An implication cannot, however, be taken for granted—especially as to the particular need for the information to be imparted. In *Cornelius v De Taranto*,[52] for example, the question of whether consent had been given to the referral of a patient to a consultant was disputed; what was clear, however, was that there was no justification for including information in the referral note that had no therapeutic relevance. It was confirmed, moreover, that it is the doctor's responsibility to ensure that those entitled to information appreciate that it is being imparted in strict professional confidence.[53] The doctor's duty is thereby restricted in a reasonable way; it is difficult to see how they can be expected to carry the onus for any subsequent actions by their associates. Once again, common law, UK GDPR, and the DPA 2018 must be read together. The guidance from the Information Commissioner's Office in respect of using and disclosing health data takes a pragmatic approach in stating that:

> Healthcare providers generally operate on the basis of implied consent to share patient data for the purposes of direct care, without breaching confidentiality. Implied consent for direct care is industry practice in that context. But this 'implied consent' to share confidential patient records is not the same as consent to process personal data in the context of a lawful basis under the UK GDPR. In the healthcare context consent is often not the appropriate lawful basis under the GPDR. This type of assumed implied consent would

---

[50] See e.g. NHS England, 'Confidentiality Policy' (2016) available at <https://www.england.nhs.uk/wp-content/uploads/2019/10/confidentiality-policy-v5.1.pdf> accessed 08 November 2022, which lays down principles that must be observed by all who work within NHS England (including contractors) and have access to person-identifiable information or confidential information.

[51] GMC, 'Confidentiality' (n 11) paras 8 and 26–29, although the guidance emphasises the importance of informing patients of the fact that information will be shared for both care and other reasons, such as service planning or medical research.

[52] (2001) 68 BMLR 62, CA.   [53] ibid.

not meet the standard of a clear affirmative act – or qualify as explicit consent for special category data, which includes health data. Instead, healthcare providers should identify another lawful basis (such as vital interests, public task or legitimate interests). For the stricter rules on special category data, Article 9(2)(h) specifically legitimises processing for health or social care purposes. Even if you are required to get a patient's consent to the medical treatment itself, this is entirely separate from your data protection obligations. It does not mean that you have to rely on consent for your processing of the patient's personal data.[54]

Thus, there is a distinction in law between implied consent to use patient data for the purposes of direct care, without breaching confidentiality, and consent to process personal data in the context of a lawful basis under the GDPR. As the ICO notes, any requirement to obtain consent to the medical treatment itself does not mean that there is a requirement to get 'GDPR consent' to undertake processing of personal data; other lawful bases are likely to be more appropriate in the healthcare context.[55]

A related issue arises in the context of consent, confidentiality, public interest, and the family: how is the doctor to treat medical information that has significant health implications for family members, and the patient refuses consent to have that information be disclosed to such members? The case of *ABC* v *St George's Healthcare NHS Foundation Trust*[56] involved a disclosure dilemma involving a high penetrant and predictive genetic condition: Huntington's disease. The central legal question was the existence of a healthcare professional's duty of care to the daughter of a man suffering from Huntington's disease, which is a dominant genetic disorder where the risks to children are 50:50 for each child. In tragic family circumstances, the father had shot and killed the claimant's mother and was being held under the Mental Health Act 1983. The father refused to allow medical staff to tell the daughter of his condition, despite the fact that she attended family therapy sessions with him, and irrespective of the fact that she was pregnant. In the event, the daughter was subsequently diagnosed with the condition; because of the ethical practices of not testing children for late onset disorders, it was not known whether the condition had also been passed to her newborn. Notwithstanding, it was the argument of the daughter in this case that—had she been informed at a suitable time—she would have taken a test and terminated the pregnancy on the positive diagnosis. Accordingly, she brought an action claiming (a) negligence on the part of the healthcare professionals responsible for her father's care, and (b) violation of her human rights under Article 8 of the European Convention on Human Rights (ECHR).

Mrs Justice Yip of the High Court held that the daughter was indeed owed a duty of care by one of the NHS Trusts (specifically, the family therapy team) to 'balance her interest in being alerted the genetic risk against the interest of [the father] and the public interest in confidentiality'.[57] However, on the facts, there was no breach of that duty. This suggests that courts may *allow* lawful disclosure of confidential information on the grounds of

---

[54] Information Commissioner's Office, 'When is Consent Appropriate?' (2022) available at <https://ico.org.uk/for-organisations/guide-to-data-protection/guide-to-the-general-data-protection-regulation-gdpr/consent/when-is-consent-appropriate/> accessed 08 November 2022.

[55] ibid.   [56] [2020] EWHC 455 (QB).

[57] ibid. [166]. The case thus instantiates in law what had already been in place in professional guidance for some time: a doctor may owe a third person who is in a close proximal relationship with the patient a duty of care to balance their interest in being informed of their genetic risk against the patient's interest and the public interest in maintaining confidentiality. The scope of that duty extends to conducting a balancing exercise between the interests of the patient and the at-risk third person, and to acting in accordance with its outcome.

public interest when a patient refuses to consent to such disclosure, where there are exceptional circumstances of danger or harm to others, but in general, they remain reluctant to *require* it. We now proceed to elaborate on the public interest exception to the duty of confidentiality.

11.4.3 PUBLIC INTEREST

It is ethical to break confidentiality without a patient's consent when it is in their own interests to do so and when it is undesirable on medical grounds or seriously impracticable to seek such consent. The recipient of the information may be another healthcare professional, or a close relative or, as in a case where the doctor suspects that the patient is a victim of neglect or physical or sexual abuse, an unrelated third party[58]—but it remains the doctor's duty to make every reasonable effort to persuade the patient to allow the information to be given, and to make clear to the third party that the information is given in confidence. When these situations occur, decisions rest, by definition, on clinical judgement. A properly considered clinical decision cannot be unethical whether it proves legally right or wrong and, in the event of action being taken on the basis of breach of confidence, the fact that it was a justifiable breach would offer a complete defence both in the civil courts and before disciplinary proceedings of the GMC. The GMC does, however, stress the need for caution when the patient has insufficient understanding, by reason of immaturity, of what the treatment or advice being sought involves.

Insofar as it rests on subjective definitions, the doctor's overriding duty to society represents what is arguably the most controversial permissible exception to the rule of confidentiality. Society is not homogeneous, but consists of groups amenable to almost infinite classification—regional, political, socio-economic, by age, and so on. It follows that what one person regards as a duty to society may be anathema to another. Individual doctors are bound to weigh the scales differently in any particular instance while, in general, all relative weighting must change from case to case—there is, for example, a great deal of difference in respect of confidentiality between being stung by a bee and suffering from venereal disease. While it is clear that no hard rules can be laid down, some aspects of this societal conflict are sufficiently important to merit individual consideration.

The most dramatic dilemma is posed by the possibility of violent crime. What is the doctor to do if they know their patient has just committed sexual assault—particularly if there is evidence that this is but one of a series of attacks? Perhaps even more disconcertingly, what if it becomes apparent that their patient is *about* to commit such an offence? Statute law is helpful here only in a number of negative senses—the DPA 2018 permits the processing of personal data to assist in the detection and prosecution of crime,[59] and legislation establishing professional bodies provides likewise.[60] If the police lack a court

---

[58] For an interesting discussion of possible liability for failure to report suspected abuse, see *C v Cairns* [2003] Lloyd's Rep Med 90, QB. Note too, the GMC Guidance states that: 'If you consider that failure to disclose the information would leave individuals or society exposed to a risk so serious that it outweighs the patient's and the public interest in maintaining confidentiality, you should disclose relevant information promptly to an appropriate person or authority . . . You should not ask for consent if you have already decided to disclose information in the public interest but you should tell the patient about your intention to disclose personal information, unless it is not safe or practicable to do so. If the patient objects to the disclosure you should consider any reasons they give for objecting.' See GMC, 'Confidentiality' (n 11) paras 67–68.

[59] Data Protection Act 2018, Part 3.

[60] See *General Dental Council v Savery* [2011] EWHC 3011 (Admin) and Dentists Act 1984, s 27.

order or warrant, they may ask for a patient's health records to be disclosed voluntarily under the DPA 2018.[61] However, health professionals have no obligation under this law to disclose the records to the police in the absence of a court order or summons, or in the absence of the patient's consent or overriding public interest.

Common law may appear less clear-cut. There is case law to the effect that the doctor need not even assist the police by answering their questions concerning their patients, although they must not give false or misleading information.[62] The obligation on the prosecution to disclose to the defence all unused material which might have some bearing on the offences charged has also caused some difficulty for forensic physicians. Generally speaking, an accused gives consent to disclosure of specific information only. Other information may, however, come to light during an examination; once this is in their notes, the police may feel it their duty to include it in their 'disclosure', despite the fact that there is no consent to their so doing. The forensic physician may, therefore, feel it their ethical imperative to conceal their knowledge—but the decision must, at times, be difficult to make.

Broadly, the justification for disclosure in such cases rests with the doctrine of the public interest as applied to medicine. This crystallised in the case of *W v Egdell*.[63] Here, a prisoner in a secure hospital sought a review of his case with a view to transfer to a regional secure unit. His legal representatives secured a report from an independent consultant psychiatrist that was, in the event, unfavourable to W; as a result, the application for transfer was aborted. W was, however, due for routine review of his detention and the psychiatrist, becoming aware that his report would not be included in the patient's notes, feared that decisions would be taken on inadequate information with consequent danger to the public. He therefore sent a copy of his report to the medical director of the hospital and a further copy reached the Home Office; W brought an action in contract and in equity alleging breach of a duty of confidence. The trial judge, Scott J, considered that, in the circumstances:

> The question in the present case is not whether Dr Egdell was under a duty of confidence; he plainly was. The question is as to the breadth of that duty.[64]

Attention was drawn to the advice of the GMC as to the circumstances in which exception to the rule of confidentiality is permitted. The GMC's guidelines which applied at the time were contained in the so-called 'Blue Book'. Paragraph 79 stated:

> Rarely, cases may arise in which disclosure in the public interest may be justified, for example, a situation in which the failure to disclose appropriate information would expose the patient, or someone else, to a risk of death or serious harm.

Scott J based his conclusions on broad considerations—that a doctor in similar circumstances has a duty not only to the patient but also to the public and that the latter would require them to disclose the results of their examination to the proper authorities if, in their opinion, the public interest so required; this would be independent of the patient's instructions on the point.

---

[61] Data Protection Act 2018, Sch 2, paras 2, 5.

[62] *Rice v Connolly* [1966] 2 QB 414 and more recently *A Health Authority v X and Others* [2001] 2 FLR 673. The European Court of Human Rights (ECtHR) has confirmed that it is not a breach of the right to respect for private life for national law to require doctors to disclose records to police authorities provided that each person in receipt of the information is under a duty to continue to respect the individual's privacy: *Z v Finland* (1997) 25 EHRR 371.

[63] [1990] Ch 359; [1990] 1 All ER 835.   [64] [1990] Ch 359, [389]; [1989] 1 All ER 1089 [1102].

The Court of Appeal unanimously confirmed the trial judge's decision to dismiss the action but did so with rather more reservation—particularly as expressed in the judgment of Bingham LJ. The concept of a private interest competing with a public interest was rejected in favour of there being a *public* interest in maintaining professional duties of confidence; the 'balancing' of interests thus fell to be carried out in circumstances of unusual difficulty. Doubts, which we share, were cast on the applicability of paragraph 78(b) of the Blue Book to a doctor acting in the role of an independent consultant; disclosure would have to be justified under paragraph 78(g) and, here, it was for the court, not the doctor, to decide whether such a disclosure was or was not a breach of contract. Moreover, there was no doubt that section 76 of the Mental Health Act 1983 showed a clear parliamentary intention that a restricted patient should be free to seek advice and evidence for specific purposes which was to be accepted as confidential. Only the most compelling circumstances could justify a doctor acting contrary to the patient's perceived interests in the absence of consent. Nevertheless, in the instant case, the fear of a real risk to public safety entitled a doctor to take reasonable steps to communicate the grounds of their concern to the appropriate authorities.

Looked at superficially, it is easy to view *Egdell* as a serious intrusion into the relationship of confidential trust between doctor and patient; it is equally possible to perceive the principle as emerging relatively unscathed. W's case was clearly regarded as extreme and, although we cannot exclude some concern, there is no evidence in the judgment that the courts would condone a breach of confidence on less urgent grounds. The danger, then, is that what is acceptable medical activity—or what are regarded as extreme circumstances—can only be delineated retrospectively. In *R v Crozier*,[65] a psychiatrist called by the accused, concerned that his opinion should be available to the court, apparently handed his report to counsel for the Crown; the now sentenced accused appealed on the grounds that the breach of confidentiality between doctor and patient had denied him the opportunity of deciding whether medical evidence would be tendered on his behalf. The Court of Appeal again thought that there was a stronger public interest in the disclosure of the psychiatrist's views than in the confidence he owed to the appellant; the psychiatrist was found to have acted responsibly and reasonably in a very difficult situation. But what if a doctor acts unreasonably in such circumstances? The damage to the patient is done and they will get little satisfaction from the fact that the doctor is censured; it is surely a thoroughly paternalistic practice that should be carefully restrained.

Still to date, however, the common law public interest exception to the duty of confidence remains frustratingly ill-defined. *Egdell* confirms that a threat of physical harm to third parties clearly justifies a breach, as will reasonable assessments by doctors that such a threat may be founded on a person's state of health—an obvious example is the need to report a sick patient to the Driver and Vehicle Licensing Authority (DVLA) regarding their fitness to drive. Even this, however, may not be straightforward, as is shown by an example reported from New Zealand. There, a bus driver underwent a triple coronary bypass operation and was subsequently certified as fit to drive by his surgeon. His general practitioner, however, asked that his licence to drive be withdrawn and, furthermore, warned his passengers of their supposed danger. The practitioner's activities resulted in a report to the Medical Practitioners' Disciplinary Committee and a finding that he was 'guilty of professional misconduct in that he breached professional confidence in informing lay people of his patient's personal medical history'. Dr Duncan sought judicial review of this decision. The High Court accepted the propriety of breaching medical

[65] (1990) 8 BMLR 128.

confidentiality in cases of clear public interest, but refused the application on grounds which can be summed up: 'I think a doctor who has decided to communicate should discriminate and ensure the recipient is a responsible authority.'[66] Seldom can there have been a case which demonstrates the 'need to know' principle so forcibly.

Access to patient records in order to carry out internal and external investigations regarding the proper discharge of healthcare responsibilities can also be justified on this basis[67] and, beyond these specific examples, a few general parameters can be laid down. We recall the classic dictum of Lord Wilberforce in *British Steel Corporation v Granada Ltd*[68] in which he drew the crucial distinction between what is *in the public interest* and that which the *public is interested in*—journalists take note! Furthermore, a disclosure should only occur where it is *necessary* to achieve the public interest in question, when there is a *reasonable likelihood* that it can do so, and when the disclosure is to those persons or agencies who can further that interest. The onus of justification is placed firmly on the shoulders of the doctor.[69] Within the framework of human rights, the House of Lords confirmed that the correct approach if an individual's human rights are engaged by conduct involving disclosure of confidential information is to ask (i) whether the disclosure pursues a legitimate aim, such as the protection of the rights and interests of others or freedom of expression, and (ii) whether the benefits achieved by disclosure are proportionate to the harm which might be done by the interference with an individual's privacy rights. If the answers are affirmative, then the disclosure will be lawful.[70]

In *W v M (An Adult Patient)*,[71] the Court of Protection gave guidance on the kinds of factors that should be taken into consideration when determining how far details of medical cases involving vulnerable patients can be reported. The instant case involved the lawfulness of withholding artificial feeding and hydration from a patient in a minimally conscious state, a matter of clear public interest and whose substance we discuss later. For present purposes, the question was how much of the circumstances could be reported. The resultant guidance highlights the following factors: (i) the general rule is that hearings should take place in private unless there is good reason to deviate; (ii) the balance of consideration is as between the right to respect for private life and the right to freedom of expression; and (iii) this could include wider considerations such as whether other Convention rights are engaged (e.g. fair trial), the rights and interests of family members, the nature and strength of evidence of harm, and the fact that the public interest is most often likely only to extend to the general medical issues and not the private circumstances of the patient; equally, there is a public interest in the workings of the Court of Protection being more widely understood. On such a balance, the prohibition against disclosure in the instant case was upheld.[72]

---

[66] *Duncan v Medical Practitioners' Disciplinary Committee* [1986] 1 NZLR 513 [521] (Jeffries J).

[67] *A Health Authority v X and Others* [2001] 2 FLR 673. Statutory obligations of disclosure are, by definition, more clear-cut, as we discuss later. See, too, *Re General Dental Council's Application* [2011] EWHC 3011 (Admin), in which it was confirmed that the Council was lawfully entitled to pass on patient records, even without consent, to its Practice Committee and investigatory body when exploring instances of insurance fraud with respect to its members and patient treatment.

[68] [1981] AC 1096 [1168].

[69] Biomedical research is generally (but certainly not always) considered a matter of public benefit.

[70] *Re Attorney General's Reference (No 3 of 1999)* [2009] UKHL 34; [2009] 2 WLR 142.

[71] [2012] 1 WLR 287.

[72] See also Chapter 10 for discussion on transparency in Court of Protection proceedings. *Cf. A Healthcare NHS Trust v P* [2015] EWCOP 15; ordering disclosure to the press of the identity of an incapacitated individual when a reporting restriction order was applied for, and in the interests of transparency. Note, however, any further disclosure by the press would be a contempt of court if the order were granted.

11.5 TORT OF MISUSE OF PRIVATE INFORMATION

The House of Lords considered the state of the breach of confidence action post-Human Rights Act 1998 in *Campbell* v *Mirror Group Newspapers Ltd*.[73] Although great play was made in the House of Lords that it was the complainer's medical status that was particularly in issue, *Campbell* is not strictly within the common scenario of 'medical confidentiality' insofar as no medical practitioner was involved in its disclosure. However, the case demonstrates a number of important points which would clearly influence the courts' approach to such a breach; therefore, it merits consideration in depth. The circumstances were that an internationally renowned supermodel accepted that she had previously lied publicly about her being addicted to drugs, and did not seek to prevent publication of the fact. She did, however, bring an action in breach of confidence for the publication of additional details of her therapy and of photographs taken of her, covertly, in the street as she left her clinic; it was claimed that these acts interfered with her right to respect for private life (Article 8 ECHR). The defendant, in turn, argued the case for freedom of expression (Article 10 ECHR) and for the public interest in publishing the materials in order to correct the claimant's earlier untrue statements.[74] But how were these rights and freedoms to be balanced in the shadow of the Human Rights Act 1998? Lord Hope remarked that the language of the breach of confidence action had now changed from a balance of public interests to a balance of ECHR rights—but he still doubted whether 'the centre of gravity has shifted'. Furthermore, he considered that the balancing exercise is essentially the same but that it is, now, 'more carefully focused and penetrating'.[75]

Yet case law subsequent to *Campbell* has clarified that while analysis to determine a breach of confidence must take account of Human Rights Act 1998 and in particular Article 8 ECHR, the core elements of the test have been retained, namely: (1) only where the relevant information is confidential will the law restrain its disclosure (i.e. the information must have the necessary quality of confidence about it); (2) the information must be imparted in particular circumstances (e.g. a doctor–patient relationship); and (3) the confidential information must have been misused or is threatened to be misused.

What is new, however, is a *separate* cause of action, known as the tort of misuse of private information. In *OBG Ltd* v *Allan and Douglas* v *Hello!* Lord Nicholls clarified that:

> As the law has developed breach of confidence, or misuse of confidential information, now covers two distinct causes of action, protecting two different interests: privacy, and secret ('confidential') information. It is important to keep these two distinct. In some instances information may qualify for protection both on grounds of privacy and confidentiality. In other instances information may be in the public domain, and not qualify for protection as confidential, and yet qualify for protection on the grounds of privacy. Privacy can be invaded by further publication of information or photographs already disclosed to the public. Conversely, and obviously, a trade secret may be protected as confidential information even though no question of personal privacy is involved.[76]

In assessing a claim for misuse of private information, courts generally adopt a two-stage process addressing two broad issues: (1) whether the claimant objectively had a *reasonable expectation of privacy* in respect of the relevant information; (2) if this is shown,

---

[73] [2004] 2 AC 457.
[74] Campbell also claimed compensation for violation of the provisions of the Data Protection Act 1998, s 13, to which the defendant claimed the public interest exception under s 32.
[75] *Campbell* (n 5) [86] (Lord Hope).   [76] [2007] UKHL 21, [255].

then the issue to consider is whether that reasonable expectation of privacy is outweighed by other relevant considerations and countervailing interests of the defendant, such as the defendant's own rights, the rights of others, and/or the public interest. This would suggest that, linking to Article 8 ECHR's protection of one's right to privacy, if there is a reasonable expectation of privacy in relation to the information, then the fact that the information has been made public by a third party will not relieve the doctor of any duty of confidence that they owe in relation to it.[77]

With respect to private information, i.e. the focus on information rather than the person (or relationship) that gives rise to an obligation of confidence (or secrecy), the focus is now notably on the underlying values that support respect for private life—values based on privacy and personal autonomy.[78] Also, the focus of such a claim, and the test to be applied as to whether a sound cause of action arises, lies not within the conscience of the receiver of the information but, rather, on the reasonable expectation of privacy that the subject of the information might have.[79] Moreover, we now have a clearer idea of how the process of considering competing claims to control confidential information should be managed. The entire House agreed with Lord Hope that the court must, first, ask if Article 8 is engaged. If it is, then a balance of considerations, applying a proportionality test, is to be undertaken as between the respective claims under Articles 8 and 10 (or other rights or considerations to be included in the balance).

11.6 PRIVACY AND CONFIDENTIALITY IN MEDICAL RESEARCH

Medical research is a matter of significant public interest. Patient-participant consent to the use of their information in research should be obtained, but this is not always possible or practicable. Identifiable patient information may be disclosed if necessary for the purposes of a medical research project if there is a legal basis for the disclosure and the project has been approved by a recognised ethics committee or other authorising body. The matter is included in the general discussion of medical research in Chapter 6. Here, we must note the fragility of these approaches and their susceptibility to political change and public disquiet.

The delicate nature of the balance of interests has long been appreciated by governmental and regulatory bodies. The guidelines on medical confidentiality from the GMC emphasise the important public interests in epidemiology, research, and public health surveillance that can be gained from further uses of patient data (i.e. uses of information other than those for which they were initially gathered).[80] While stressing that the consent of the patient to such uses should normally be sought, the GMC accepts that consent is not always possible or practicable and that it is possible (and justifiable) for doctors to disclose identifiable information to further such a public interest so long as certain safeguards are respected. The advice of a Caldicott Guardian or similar expert

---

[77] See also *Bloomberg LP v ZXC* [2022] UKSC 5, in which Lord Hamblen and Lord Stephens endorsed this two-stage test. For the first stage, it is confirmed that whether there is a reasonable expectation of privacy is an objective question. The expectation is that of a reasonable person of ordinary sensibilities placed in the same position as the claimant and faced with the same publicity. The question whether there is a reasonable expectation of privacy is a broad one, which takes account of all the circumstances of the case.

[78] See *A-G v Guardian Newspapers Ltd (No 2)* [1990] AC 109.

[79] On this, see *Murray v Express Newspapers plc* [2008] 3 WLR 1360.

[80] GMC, 'Confidentiality' (n 11) para 77.

adviser (e.g. data protection officer) should be sought, and, if existing statutory routes for disclosure can be used then these should be preferred.[81]

In England and Wales, the Health Service (Control of Patient Information) Regulations 2002 (known colloquially as the COPI Regs) were passed in June 2002 and currently sit under section 251 of the NHS Act 2006.[82] They support processing of patient information for medical purposes, including the purposes of medical research, the operations of cancer registries, and processing to protect public health with respect to communicable diseases and other similar risks. The COPI Regs set aside the common law duty of confidence:

> Anything done by a person that is necessary for the purpose of processing patient information in accordance with these Regulations shall be taken to be lawfully done despite any obligation of confidence owed by that person in respect of it.[83]

Subject to the restrictions contained within regulation 7, regulation 5 grants the Secretary of State the power to authorise the processing of 'confidential patient information' for 'medical purposes' in circumstances set out in the Schedule of the Regulations. As discussed in the next section, the Health Research Authority (HRA) is responsible for appointing a committee for the purposes of giving advice to the Secretary of State and the HRA on the application of the COPI Regs and the disclosure of confidential patient information, for both research and non-research medical purposes, without patient consent. The committee that has been appointed by the HRA for this purpose is known as the Confidentiality Advisory Group (CAG).

The Health and Social Care Act 2012, which largely applies only to England, makes it a clear duty of the Secretary of State to promote research on matters relevant to the health service.[84] The same Act established the Health and Social Care Information Centre (subsequently called NHS Digital, and which in 2023 was merged with NHS England), which, inter alia, has duties to maintain standards, promote the core function of health services, and to develop a confidentiality code of practice accordingly.[85] All of this builds on statutory provision established by section 251 of the NHS Act 2006 that allows the Secretary of State to make provisions for the processing of patient medical data for medical purposes where (i) neither consent nor anonymisation are possible nor practicable, and (ii) when otherwise it would be a breach of confidence to use those data.[86] The HRA has responsibility to administer these powers since 2013. Applications and proposals for research uses, together with providing advice on draft regulations, are delegated to CAG, which advises decision makers—the HRA or the Secretary of State—whether applications to process confidential patient information without consent should be approved or not.[87] Under Schedule 7 to the Care Act 2014, CAG also advises NHS Digital (subsequently NHS England) on aspects relating to its dissemination function of identifiable information or information that may become identifiable.

---

[81] ibid., paras 103, 108.

[82] Section 251 contemplates two types of regulations: (i) those requiring disclosure of specified information to patients or others on their behalf; and (ii) those requiring or authorising disclosure or other processing of specified information between specified individuals subject to certain conditions. The COPI Regs pertain to the latter type.

[83] Health Service (Control of Patient Information) Regulations 2002 (SI 2002/1438), reg 4.

[84] Section 6 of the 2012 Act, inserting s 1E into the National Health Service Act 2006.

[85] Jamie Grace and Mark Taylor, 'Disclosure of Confidential Patient Information and the Duty to Consult: The Role of the Health and Social Care Information Centre' (2013) 21(3) Medical Law Review 415.

[86] These provisions only apply in England and Wales.

[87] See Confidentiality Advisory Group (n 6).

ML

A similar function to CAG has historically been performed in Scotland by the Privacy Advisory Committee (PAC), which was an independent ad hoc body, established in the early 1990s, to advise on these sensitive issues. It was replaced in 2015 by a more widely constituted Public Benefit and Privacy Panel (PBPP) for Health and Social Care, but with much the same remit. The PBPP and the CAG both act in an advisory capacity with respect to the activities outlined earlier. Ultimately, responsibility rests with the Secretary of State in England and Wales and NHS National Services Scotland. A similar committee operates in Northern Ireland, known as the Privacy Advisory Committee. It advises on some considerations about using patient information, but it lacks statutory powers and thus cannot give lawful authority to disclosures of identifiable information without consent.

Regulation 3 of the COPI Regs came to play an important role during the Covid-19 pandemic. Regulation 3 both *permits* the processing of confidential patient information and allows the Secretary of State to *mandate* processing for a range of public health purposes. With respect to the power to mandate processing, COPI regulation 3(4) empowers the Secretary of State to require processing for these purposes by issuing a 'notice' to require a body or person specified in regulation 3(3) to process that information for the purpose and time period specified in the notice. These are known as 'COPI Notices'. In March 2020, the Secretary of State for Health and Care issued four COPI Notices, requiring, among other things, that NHS England, GPs, local authorities, combined authorities, and arm's-length bodies of the Department of Health and Social Care process confidential patient information to support the Secretary of State's response to Covid-19 (known as a 'Covid-19 purpose').[88] These Notices were renewed repeatedly over the course of the pandemic and most eventually expired in 2022, although at least one was extended to carry on through 2023. This meant that researchers and others relying on a COPI Notice and who needed to process confidential patient information for Covid-19 purposes after it expired required an alternative legal basis for processing of confidential patient information thereafter, which could include obtaining patient consent, regulation 3 support, or applying to the CAG to transition to regulation 5 support.

All this indicates that the COPI Regs and the Health and Social Care Act 2012 have given a legal basis for the widespread collection of identifiable patient-level data from healthcare providers. This may lead to concerns about trust and uses of one's patient information that are not in accordance with one's reasonable expectation of privacy. Indeed, previous attempts in England to collect such data without patient consent has led to significant problems. A decade ago, the *care.data* initiative was launched, whereby data would be extracted from GP surgeries into a central database through the General Practice Extraction Service (GPES). It was stated that the data would be used in an anonymised form, including—potentially—wider uses by third parties. Where anonymised use was not possible, approval was to be sought from the CAG to authorise identifiable, non-consented uses 'in the public interest'. Leaflets were sent to 26.5 million households, albeit not addressed to individuals. Moreover, this information contained no direct mention of *care.data*. Concerns were also raised that the data were not in fact anonymised, but only pseudonymised. This led to suspension of the programme within weeks of its launch in early 2014 after strong professional and patient objections and concerns about potential commercial access. The programme

[88] See e.g. Department of Health and Social Care, 'Coronavirus (COVID-19): notification to organisations to share information' (2022) available at <https://www.gov.uk/government/publications/coronavirus-covid-19-notification-of-data-controllers-to-share-information> accessed 08 November 2022.

was abandoned in 2016 following a review (known as 'Caldicott 3') by the National Data Guardian for Health and Care, in which a new consent/opt-out model was recommended to give people a clear choice about how their personal confidential data is used for purposes beyond their direct care: specifically, that people should be able to opt out from personal confidential data being used beyond their own direct care.[89] The associated lessons from *care.data* are salutary ones: no administration should believe when it comes to patient privacy that mere legal authority can necessarily command social legitimacy. Moreover, there is a real and present danger in attempting to borrow 'social licence' from the trust people have in public professionals such as GPs to undertake wider social benefit programmes without serious forethought and robust consultation.[90]

Following the public reaction and political fallout from *care.data,* and in line with the recommendations of the National Data Guardian in her 'Review of Data Security, Consent and Opt-Outs',[91] in 2018, NHS Digital announced a new 'national data opt-out programme' (NDOO) for England, which allows patients to opt out of their confidential patient information being used for research and planning.[92] Use of confidential patient data for purposes beyond individual care remains subject to data protection legislation and common law duty of confidentiality considerations. Unless patients opt out, access to confidential patient information will be given to research bodies and organisations, such as universities, hospitals, and pharmaceutical companies researching new treatments. Access will not be given to bodies and organisations for marketing purposes and insurance purposes, unless patients specifically request this. Patients can change their mind and update their NDOO choice at any time, and can choose to opt out but still agree to take part in a specific research project or clinical trial. A patient's opt-out will not apply where: 1) the data are legally required to be shared, 2) there is an overriding public interest to share the data, 3) the data are required to be shared for the monitoring and control of communicable disease and other risks to public health; or 4) the patient has given explicit consent to the use of their data for a specific purpose.[93] People can access NHS England's Data Uses Registers to find out how their data has been used by for purposes beyond their individual care.[94]

By mid-2022, NHS Digital required all health and care organisations to have applied patient preferences in all research and planning situations in which confidential patient information is used. NHS Digital has encouraged health and care staff to download leaflets, posters, and other resources to use when informing patients about the NDOO, and in turn over the past few years has been pushing a website where patients can find out more

---

[89] National Data Guardian for Health and Care, 'Review of Data Security, Consent and Opt-Outs' (2016) available at <https://www.gov.uk/government/publications/review-of-data-security-consent-and-opt-outs> accessed 08 November 2022.

[90] Pam Carter, Graeme Laurie, and Mary Dixon-Woods, 'The Social Licence for Research: Why *Care. Data* Ran Into Trouble' (2015) 41(5) Journal of Medical Ethics 404.

[91] National Data Guardian, (n 89).

[92] NHS Digital, 'National Data Opt-Out Programme' (2022) available at <https://digital.nhs.uk/services/national-data-opt-out/compliance-with-the-national-data-opt-out> accessed 08 November 2022. The national data opt-out will apply when 1) confidential patient information is used for purposes beyond an individual's care and treatment, and 2) the legal basis to use the data is approval under reg 2 or 5 of the Control of Patient Information Regulations 2002, s 251 of the NHS Act 2006.

[93] NHS Digital, 'National Data Opt-out Operational Policy Guidance Document' (2020) available at <https://digital.nhs.uk/services/national-data-opt-out/operational-policy-guidance-document> accessed 08 November 2022.

[94] NHS Digital, 'Register of Approved Data Releases' (2022) available at <https://digital.nhs.uk/services/data-access-request-service-dars/data-uses-register> accessed 30 May 2023.

about the programme and set their opt-out choice. Time will tell whether the NDOO programme adequately ensures people can make informed choices about how their data are used, and whether people feel that their confidential patient data are kept secure and only used in line with their reasonable expectations.

Indeed, there is some concern that the lessons from *care.data* and other schemes still do not appear to have been learnt, as seen in a more recent scheme launched in England in 2021. That year, NHS Digital announced that a new General Practice Data for Planning and Research (GPDPR) scheme would be launched to replace GPES. The scheme planned to use data to support the planning and commissioning of health and care services, the development of health and care policy, public health monitoring and interventions (including Covid-19), and enable different areas of research. The data included diagnoses, symptoms, observations, test results, medications, allergies, immunisations, referrals, recalls and appointments, all of which contain information about physical, mental, or sexual health. Names and addresses, written notes, images, letters, and documents would not be collected, however. Again, significant concerns were raised by general practitioners and members of the public regarding lack of transparency in the processes of the extraction, the extent of the data extraction, and the extent of robust security and privacy safeguards.[95] Similar to *care.data*, the GPDPR launch date was first postponed by a few months and then eventually frozen for an indefinite period so that a 'listening exercise' and consultation process could take place before launching a public information campaign and a possible relaunch at a later date.[96] As of the time of writing, it is unclear whether in fact the GPDPR scheme will be relaunched.

11.7 PATIENT ACCESS TO MEDICAL RECORDS

Only in recent times have patients had a right to see their medical records. An important early development came with the Access to Medical Reports Act 1988, as amended.[97] The reports to which the Act refers are limited to those prepared by a medical practitioner who is or has been responsible for the clinical care of the individual and which are intended for direct supply to the patient's employer, prospective employer, or to an insurance company.[98] Reports by health professionals who have had only a casual, non-caring professional association with the patient are excluded. Such reports as are included have always been subject to the patient's consent but the applicant must now positively seek such consent and must inform them of their rights of access.[99] The patient can see the report before it is sent and, unless they have done so, issue of the report must be delayed for three weeks.[100] They have the right to ask the doctor to alter anything that they feel is inaccurate and they may add a dissenting statement should the doctor refuse to do so.[101] Access may be withheld if disclosure would cause serious harm to the patient's physical

[95] Talha Burki, 'Concerns Over England's New System for Collecting General Practitioner Data' (2021) 3(8) The Lancet Digital Health E469.

[96] See NHS Digital, 'General Practice Data for Planning and Research (GPDPR)' (2022) available at <https://digital.nhs.uk/data-and-information/data-collections-and-data-sets/data-collections/general-practice-data-for-planning-and-research> accessed 08 November 2022.

[97] See also the Access to Personal Files and Medical Reports (Northern Ireland) Order 1991.

[98] Access to Medical Reports Act 1988, s 2.   [99] ibid., s 3.   [100] ibid., s 4.   [101] ibid., s 5.

or mental health—or to that of any other person—but, in those circumstances, the patient may withdraw their consent to its promulgation.[102]

The power of control of medical data provided to the individual by the 1988 Act is clearly limited and is confined to a very specific aspect of the doctor–patient relationship. The individual is likely to be far more concerned over dissemination of personal details that are gathered as a result of their status as a *patient*. Statutory protection as to the confidentiality of information such as that contained in hospital notes was, for a short time, provided by the Access to Health Records Act 1990. That Act was, however, repealed to a very large extent by, and its contents were assimilated into, the Data Protection Act 1998, and subsequently the Data Protection Act 2018, which is now the main determinant of what may and may not be done with a patient's records.[103] Under the 2018 Act, the 'data subject' has a right to information as to the purposes for which data about them are being processed and the persons who will have access to the data.[104] The protection of those about whom information is stored lies in preventing the holding of inaccurate information or of concealing the fact that information is stored at all. As a consequence, a patient has the right to be told by the 'data controller'—which could be any healthcare body holding records—whether any such information is held and, if it is, to be supplied with a copy of that information. Initial access must be provided free of charge (including postage costs) unless the request is 'manifestly unfounded' or 'excessive'—in which case a 'reasonable' fee can be charged.[105]

Under Part 2 of Schedule 3 to the Data Protection Act 2018, data concerning health may be withheld from a patient if in the opinion of the relevant health professional, it is likely to cause serious physical or mental harm to the patient or another person.[106] The BMA notes that the circumstances in which information may be withheld on the grounds of serious harm are extremely rare, and this exemption does not justify withholding comments in the records because patients may find them upsetting.[107] The BMA guidance gives support to doctors who are faced with subject access requests (SARs).[108]

---

[102] See also BMA, 'Access To Medical Reports: Guidance From The BMA Medical Ethics Department' (2019) available at <https://www.bma.org.uk/media/1788/bma-access-to-medical-reports-oct-19.pdf> accessed 08 November 2022.

[103] The only significant remnant of the 1990 Act relates to the records of a deceased person (s 3(1)(f)). See also Access to Health Records (Northern Ireland) Order 1993. It also worth noting that under The National Health Service (General Medical Services Contracts) Regulations 2015 (SI 2015/1862), as amended by The National Health Service (General Medical Services Contracts and Personal Medical Services Agreements) (Amendment) Regulations 2020 (SI 2020/226), NHS England introduced an obligation for practices to give patients access to their *prospective* (future) medical record online, including free text and documents. In late 2022, NHS England had planned to switch on automatic access, via the NHS App, to prospective GP record patients at practices using TPP and EMIS systems. This does not change the status of GPs as a data controller or alter existing obligations to promote and offer access to historic information. See NHS Digital, 'Offering Patients Access To Their Future Health Information' (2022) available at < https://digital.nhs.uk/services/nhs-app/nhs-app-guidance-for-gp-practices/guidance-on-nhs-app-features/accelerating-patient-access-to-their-record/offering-patients-access-to-their-future-health-information> accessed 08 November 2022. However, following talks with the BMA, NHS England paused automatic access (at least temporarily) for any practices that requested more time; see Elisabeth Mahase, 'NHS England Halts Mass Rollout of Automatic Patient Access to GP Records' (2022) 379 BMJ o2902.

[104] There are, of course, some exceptions to this, such as medical research uses that do not affect the patient directly and the results do not identify them.

[105] UK GDPR, art 12(5).

[106] Additional grounds for when medical records and health data may not be disclosed to patients are found in BMA, 'Access to Health Records: Updated to Reflect The General Data Protection Regulation and Data Protection Act 2018' (2019) available at <https://www.bma.org.uk/advice-and-support/ethics/confidentiality-and-health-records/access-to-health-records> accessed 08 November 2022, p 6.

[107] ibid.   [108] BMA, 'Access to Health Records', (n 106).

This helpfully covers requests for access to both the records of living and deceased persons as well as requests from a variety of people, including parents, children, individuals authorised to make proxy decisions on behalf of adults lacking capacity, next of kin, police, and lawyers. Where access is to be denied, there is clear instruction about the basis upon which this should be justified. We have noted earlier concern by the BMA about insurers using access provisions to secure disclosure of patients' entire medical record, most likely in contravention of the UK GDPR and Data Protection Act 2018. This has led to further specific guidance to doctors on how to manage such cases.[109] The BMA advises that insurance companies should use the provisions of the Access to Medical Reports Act 1988 to seek a GP report.

The European Court of Human Rights (ECtHR) has confirmed that access to records containing personal information is, prima facie, a matter of entitlement under Article 8 ECHR and is part of the state's obligation to respect the private and family lives of its citizens.[110] It is not, however, an absolute right and other interests may be in play. For example, in *MG v United Kingdom*,[111] the applicant sought access to social service records to confirm his suspicions of childhood abuse at the hands of his father. It was recognised by the ECtHR that the authorities had legitimate concerns about the privacy of third parties in such a case (such as the siblings), and that this might be a legitimate reason to deny full access. Notwithstanding this, the absence of an appeal body to challenge a refusal of access constituted a breach of the applicant's human rights. This has now been remedied in the UK whereby the Information Commissioner's Office can hear appeals against denial of access to personal records.[112] In contrast, in *KH and Others v Slovakia*,[113] the ECtHR held that the right to respect for one's private and family life must be practical and effective and that there is a positive obligation on the part of states to make available to patients copies of their medical records: '[T]he Court does not consider that data subjects should be obliged to specifically justify a request to be provided with a copy of their personal data files. It is rather for the authorities to show that there are compelling reasons for refusing this facility.'[114]

The right of access to information about oneself is, then, unassailable. But to what extent is it meaningful to talk about 'my record' or 'my medical notes'? This is common parlance but it has no legal basis. The ownership of the intellectual property contained in a record—that is, the copyright—is held by the person who has created the notes or their employer, and not by the subject of those notes. Moreover, the physical notes themselves are owned by the GP practice and health service organisation. The patient is therefore unlikely ever to have a successful property claim over their records.[115]

---

[109] BMA, 'Requests for Medical Information From Insurers' (2021) available at <https://www.bma.org.uk/advice-and-support/ethics/confidentiality-and-health-records/requests-for-medical-information-from-insurers> accessed 08 November 2022.

[110] *MG v United Kingdom* (App no 39393/98) [2002] 3 FCR 413.   [111] ibid.

[112] For the human rights dimension more broadly see *MS v Sweden* (1999) 28 EHRR 313.

[113] *KH and Others v Slovakia* (2009) 49 EHRR 34.

[114] ibid. [48.] In *RR v Poland* (2011) 53 EHRR 31, [188] it was confirmed that '[c]ompliance with the state's positive obligation to secure to their citizens their right to effective respect for their physical and psychological integrity may necessitate, in turn, the adoption of regulations concerning access to information about an individual's health'.

[115] In *R v Mid Glamorgan Family Health Services, ex parte Martin* [1995] 1 All ER 356, the court accepted that medical records were owned by the health authority, and a similar view was taken by the High Court of Australia in *Breen v Williams* (1996) 138 ALR 259. See also *Phipps v Boardman* [1966] UKHL 2, in which the House of Lords ruled that confidential information itself is not to be regarded by the law as property. The weight of jurisprudential authority continues to support this view.

11.8 THE REMEDIES

A patient can recover damages for improper disclosure of information about their health—be it under breach of confidence or a tort of misuse of private information claim—even if they have suffered no financial loss as a result. The damages might, of course, be only nominal; on the other hand, they might be considerable were it possible to show loss of society, severe injury to feelings, mental distress, job loss, interference with prospects of promotion, or the like. In *Cornelius* v *de Taranto*, for example, the High Court awarded damages for distress caused by a doctor breaching confidence through wrongly disclosing a medical report on the patient to other medical staff.[116] As Morland J wrote:

> In my judgment it would be a hollow protection of that right [to privacy under Article 8 ECHR] if in a particular case in breach of confidence without consent details of the confider's private and family life were disclosed by the confidant to others and the only remedy that the law of England allowed was nominal damages.
>
> . . .
>
> In the present case in my judgment recovery of damages for mental distress caused by breach of confidence, when no other substantial remedy is available, would not be inimical to "considerations of policy" but indeed to refuse such recovery would illustrate that something was wrong with the law.[117]

Often, however, damage has already been done because information has already been made public and, even if it is achieved, victory in a damages action can be pyrrhic: Ms Campbell, for example, received only £3,500 in compensation.[118] Damages are also payable for contravention of the provisions of the Data Protection Act 2018 where a data subject suffers damage or distress. Any such payments have, however, at least under the previous Data Protection Act 1998, been consistently paltry. In *AB* v *Ministry of Justice*,[119] compensation of £2,250 was for distress arising from a breach of the Data Protection Act 1998 concerning processing of information about the claimant's deceased wife. Interestingly, this was awarded even though there was no 'damage' in the sense of a further loss. Moreover, the compensation was separate from the damage from the technical breach, which was awarded only in the sum of £1. This said, the enforcement powers of the Information Commissioner's Office (ICO) have been radically increased. Under the Data Protection Act 1998, the ICO could levy fines up to £500,000. Now, under the UK GDPR, fines can be up to £17.5 million, or in the case of an undertaking, up to 4% of the total worldwide annual turnover of the preceding financial year, whichever is higher.[120] Heavy fines have been imposed on NHS bodies for breaches of the law.[121]

Injunctive relief (interdict) is another common remedy in this area of law. This includes both a final injunction to prevent continuation of the wrongful conduct and a *quia timet* (precautionary) injunction to prevent threatened breach of confidentiality. Given that the real fear at the core of a breach of confidence action is public disclosure of

---

[116] [2001] EMLR 12.   [117] ibid. [66], [69].   [118] *Campbell* (n 5).
[119] [2014] EWHC 1847 (QB).   [120] Data Protection Act 2018, s 157.
[121] See, for example, Tavistock & Portman NHS Foundation Trust, which was fined £78,400 in June 2022 for using Outlook to send bulk emails to 1,781 Gender Identity Clinic service users and failing to comply with Chapter II GDPR, specifically arts 5(1)(f), and 32(1) and (2). See ICO, 'The Tavistock & Portman NHS Foundation Trust' (2022) available at <https://ico.org.uk/action-weve-taken/enforcement/the-tavistock-portman-nhs-foundation-trust/> accessed 08 November 2022.

private facts, the 'gagging order' will, in many cases, be more desirable to the claimant than damages—and the utility of this remedy endures, as cases such as *X* v *Y* and *H* v *Associated Newspapers* demonstrate.[122]

11.9 CONFIDENTIALITY AND DEATH

Final reflection might, appositely, be concerned with death. The Declaration of Geneva says: 'I will respect the secrets that are confided in me, even after the patient has died.' This view is also endorsed by the GMC in its guidance to doctors:

> Your duty of confidentiality continues after a patient has died . . . There are circumstances in which you must disclose relevant information about a patient who has died . . . In other circumstances, whether and what personal information may be disclosed after a patient's death will depend on the facts of the case.[123]

Likewise, the BMA states that:

> the obligation to respect a patient's confidentiality extends beyond death. However, this duty needs to be balanced with other considerations, such as the interests of justice and of people close to the deceased person. There may be some circumstances where it is obvious that there may be some sensitivity about information in health records. In these limited circumstances healthcare professionals may wish to consider speaking to their patients about the possibility of disclosure after death with a view to soliciting their views about disclosure.[124]

In professional ethical terms, there can be no doubt that a post-mortem report merits the same degree of confidentiality as does the report of the clinical examination; insurance companies and the like have an obvious interest in its content but their right to disclosure is the same as the right to discovery of hospital records—in the absence of a court order, consent to disclosure from the next of kin of the deceased is essential. The personal representative of a deceased patient or someone who might have a claim arising from their death can request access to the patient's records under the only remaining live provision of the Access to Health Records Act 1990.[125]

But has the public at large any rights to details of the medical history of the dead? While the principle remains irrespective of personalities, this is essentially a problem of public figures—and it is remarkable how rapidly professional ethics can be dissipated, say, in describing to the media the wounds of US President John F Kennedy or the psychiatric history of the principals in any *cause célèbre*. The former physician to President François Mitterrand of France faced professional disbarment, a fine, and up to one year's imprisonment for publishing his book, *Le Grand Secret*, immediately after the President's death in January 1996. The book detailed Mitterrand's long battle with cancer throughout his presidency, which had been hidden from the French public. The affair caused a storm of controversy over the appropriate balance between the public's 'right to know' and the

---

[122] See *X* v *Y* [1988] 2 All ER 648 (in which a newspaper sought, and obtained, an injunction to prevent the publication of the names of two doctors being treated in hospital for AIDS) and *H (a healthcare worker)* v *Associated Newspapers* [2002] EWCA Civ 195 (in which the court upheld an injunction naming an HIV-positive dentist and the health authority for which he worked).

[123] GMC, 'Confidentiality' (n 11) paras 134–136, which offer examples of whether disclosure might or might not be justifiable.

[124] BMA, 'Confidentiality Toolkit' (n 11) p 9.   [125] 1990 Act, s 3(1)(f).

individual's 'right to privacy':[126] in the end the French courts followed up an interim injunction on sales with a permanent injunction on publication, the publishers received a hefty fine, and the author was given a four-month suspended sentence.

The ECtHR, however, declared France to be in breach of human rights over its reaction to the book, holding that, while the state could defend its laws imposing civil and criminal liability for breach of confidence as 'necessary in a democratic society', the continued ban on distribution of the book no longer met a 'pressing social need' and was disproportionate to the aim pursued; it was, in effect, a breach of the right to freedom of expression.[127] It is easy to say, 'History will out, let it be sooner than later', but it is less easy to decide at what point revelations become history. The ECtHR, however, felt confident that the imposition of a permanent publication ban nine-and-a-half months after the death of the French President was inappropriate.[128]

Returning to the British perspective, as we saw earlier, the GMC has stated that a duty of confidence persists after the patient's death; whether or not disclosure after death will be improper depends, inter alia, on whether there was any specific requests to keep information confidential, whether disclosure may cause distress to, or be of benefit to, or reveal the identity of the patient's partner or family, and whether the information is already public knowledge or can be anonymised. The GMC does not specify any time limit; a practitioner must be prepared to justify and explain every disclosure. Moreover, a bark in this context carries a bite—no less a person than a former editor of the BMJ has been taken to task for reporting information concerning the health of a well-known, albeit controversial, general after his death.[129] Arguments can be made from an ethical perspective that the dead retain interests that are primarily based on reputation and dignity, and that these justify a continued duty of confidence, albeit eventually reduced and limited with the passage of time.[130]

And so, finally, what of the law? The legal position has long been unclear although it has been argued that, since confidence is, prima facie, a personal matter, the legal duty ends with the death of the patient; contrariwise, it has been suggested that, 'Equity may impose a duty of confidentiality towards another after the death of the original confider. The question is not one of property (whether a cause of action owned by the deceased has been assigned) but of conscience.'[131] Statute sends equally mixed messages. The provisions of the UK GDPR and Data Protection Act 2018 do not apply to information relating to deceased persons, but we have seen that the Access to Health Records Act 1990 continues to apply to the dead and that access is limited to the dead person's personal representative and those with a claim on the estate. The courts, for their part, may apply the principles of medical confidentiality by insisting that an order imposing anonymity in judicial proceedings should remain in force after the subject's death in cases of major sensitivity—such as those involving declarations as to the withdrawal of treatment from the incompetent.[132] Not only does this appear logical but post-mortem publicity may,

---

[126] Alexander Dorozynski, 'Mitterrand Book Provokes Storm in France' (1996) 312 BMJ 201.

[127] *Plon (Société) v France* (2006) 42 EHRR 36, [50].   [128] ibid. [53].

[129] Stephen Lock, 'A Question of Confidence' (1984) 288 BMJ 123, 125.

[130] Daniel Sperling, *Posthumous Interests: Legal and Ethical Perspectives* (CUP 2008), esp ch 5.

[131] Charles Phipps, William Harman and Simon Teasdale, *Toulson & Phipps on Confidentiality* (4th edn, Sweet & Maxwell 2020), para 10-060.

[132] *Re C (adult patient: publicity)* [1996] 2 FLR 251—though this may not hold if the public interest dictates otherwise. For the balance of private and public interests and the imposition of anonymity in general, see *Re G (adult patient: publicity)* [1995] 2 FLR 528. See, too, *Practice Direction* [2002] 1 WLR 325 and *A v East Kent Hospitals University NHS Foundation Trust* [2015] EWHC 1038 (QB). *Cf.*, the House of Lords has ruled that the anonymity of a dead child and the mother accused of its murder should not be restrained merely to protect the privacy of the surviving child who was not directly involved in the trial: *Re S (a child) (identification: restriction on publication)* [2005] 1 AC 593.

in turn, raise questions as to the ethics of previous non-disclosure. The law in fact seems to be moving in this direction. The Information Commissioner has taken the view that the common law duty of confidentiality applies after death and this has been supported by the Information Tribunal.[133]

11.10 CONCLUSION

Confidentiality remains the undeniable stalwart of the doctor–patient relationship. While its iconic status might be overshadowed at times by the seemingly never-ending development of the role of consent, confidentiality remains the constant that binds patient and doctor together, even when they are in dispute. It marks the contours of the relationship and provides the foundation upon which trust in medical professionals is built. Its importance—and fragility—cannot be overstated, nor should it ever be overlooked. However, this is an area of medicine that is becoming increasingly complex, with ever increasing amount of regulation governing access to and use of patient information, be it from the legal regimes of confidentiality, data protection, or privacy, and an area that is currently under significant reform with UK Government efforts to make better use of patient data for direct care as well as for research and innovation.

FURTHER READING

1. Vicky Chico and Mark Taylor, 'Using and Disclosing Confidential Patient Information and the English Common Law: What Are the Information Requirements of a Valid Consent?' (2018) 26(1) Medical Law Review 51–72.

2. Edward Dove and Mark Taylor, 'Signalling Standards for Progress: Bridging the Divide Between a Valid Consent to Use Patient Data Under Data Protection Law and the Common Law Duty of Confidentiality' (2021) 29(3) Medical Law Review 411–445.

3. Angus Ferguson, *Should a Doctor Tell? The Evolution of Medical Confidentiality in Britain* (Ashgate 2013).

4. Charles Phipps, William Harman, and Simon Teasdale, *Toulson & Phipps on Confidentiality* (4th edn, Sweet & Maxwell 2020) Ch 10.

5. Mark Taylor and Tess Whitton, 'Public Interest, Health Research and Data Protection Law: Establishing a Legitimate Trade-Off between Individual Control and Research Access to Health Data' (2020) 9(1) Laws 6, 1–23.

6. Paul Wragg, 'Recognising a Privacy-invasion Tort: The Conceptual Unity of Informational and Intrusion Claims' (2019) 78(2) Cambridge Law Journal 409–437.

---

[133] See *Bluck v The Information Commissioner and Epsom & St Helier University NHS Trust* (2007) 98 BMLR 1. In *Lewis v Secretary of State for Health* [2008] EWHC 2196, the court ordered the release of deceased persons to the Redfern Inquiry on nuclear facilities and effects on human tissue. For comment see, Kartina Choong and Jeanne Mifsud Bonnici, 'Posthumous Medical Confidentiality: The Public Interest Conundrum' (2014) 1(2) European Journal of Comparative Law and Governance 106.

12

CLINICAL NEGLIGENCE

12.1 INTRODUCTION

In this chapter, we consider key elements of bringing a claim in clinical negligence, where a patient alleges that they have suffered harm in a healthcare setting. To bring a successful common law action in the tort of negligence, it is necessary to establish several key elements, including duty of care and breach of the duty of care, factual and legal causation, and that there was a legally recognised harm. We also highlight by way of example how existing case law has approached various types of clinical negligence, including treatment, diagnosis, and protecting patients from themselves. Having looked at wrongful conception, birth, and life claims, we then turn to consider some specific cases, such as the problem of the novice, the use of innovative techniques, complementary medicine, and the doctrine of *res ipsa loquitur*. Thereafter, an overview is provided of key aspects of criminal negligence, before moving on to examine alternatives to clinical negligence litigation, including recent proposals for reform, such as the creation of no-fault schemes for medical injury.

While we recognise that there may be varied approaches in differing UK jurisdictions about the conduct of clinical negligence claims, we focus predominantly on England, with examples drawn from other UK jurisdictions where appropriate. Regarding terminology, our preference is to use the term 'clinical negligence', but we recognise other terms such as 'medical negligence' and 'medical malpractice' are also in use in other parts of the UK, as well as in other countries. We also note that the main parties to clinical negligence claims are referred to different ways, depending on the UK jurisdiction. In the England and Wales jurisdiction, the preferred terms are 'claimant' and 'defendant'; in Northern Ireland, 'plaintiff' and 'defendant'; and in Scotland, 'pursuer' and 'defender'. For the purposes of this chapter, we use the terms 'claimant' and 'defendant'.

12.2 THE BASIS OF LIABILITY FOR CLINICAL NEGLIGENCE

Most claims in respect of clinical negligence are brought in tort; that is, based on a non-contractual civil wrong. The reason for this is that patients within the NHS are not in a contractual relationship with the doctor treating them. By contrast, there will be a contractual relationship in the private sector where it is, therefore, possible to bring an action for damages in contract.[1] In practice, there is very little difference between the two remedies,[2] although the law of contract may provide a remedy for an express or implied

---

[1] *Pfizer Corporation v Ministry of Health* [1965] AC 512; *Reynolds v Health First Medical Group* [2000] Lloyd's Rep Med 240; *Reynolds v Health First Medical Group* [2014] SLT 495.

[2] For a useful discussion of the distinction between contractual and tortious remedies in this context, see Michael Jones, *Clinical Negligence* (5th edn, Sweet & Maxwell 2018); and Judith Laing and Jean McHale (eds.), *Principles of Medical Law* (4th edn, OUP 2016).

warranty given by a doctor.[3] In a Canadian case, *La Fleur* v *Cornelis*,[4] the court held that a plastic surgeon was bound to an express contractual warranty that he had made to the patient. This warranty arose when he was unwise enough to say: 'There will be no problem. You will be very happy.' However, this type of case will be comparatively unusual.

For all practical purposes, any discussion of clinical negligence can confine itself to liability under the law of tort, in which the first question to be asked is, 'Whom do we sue?' An injury to a claimant may have been caused by any one or more of the healthcare professionals (HCPs) who have treated them. Locating negligence may be simple in some cases, but in others, the patient may have to identify the responsible party from a large group, such as a general practitioner (GP), or any HCP within the hospital treating team. Locating the specific act of alleged negligence which caused the injury may also involve a considerable degree of disentanglement.

The claimant may proceed directly against the doctor in question if an allegation is made of negligence on the part of a GP. The GP in the UK is solely responsible for the treatment of their patients; all partners in a practice may, however, be liable for the actions of one of their number and they must have approved indemnity cover.[5] This was because GPs were not covered by the Crown indemnity which continues to apply to hospital doctors working within the NHS. In England, this situation has now changed, which we examine in more detail later in this chapter.[6]

The position is different if the alleged negligence occurs after the GP has referred the patient for further treatment within the NHS. If the negligent act is committed by an NHS employee in the course of their NHS duties, then usually the patient will make a claim against the legal entity which employs them (e.g. the NHS Trust or Health Board). In this case, liability may be based on either of two grounds: (i) the direct duty of a hospital to care for patients; or (ii) the vicarious liability of the Trust for the negligence of its employees. There has been some doubt as to whether a hospital owes a non-delegable duty to use skill and care in treating its patients.[7] In both *A (a child)* v *Ministry of Defence*[8] and *Farraj* v *Kings Healthcare NHS Trust*,[9] the courts declined to hold that there was a non-delegable duty, but these can be explicable in that (i) it was the NHS, not the Ministry of Defence, that was responsible for providing health care, and (ii) *Farraj* involved no material discussion one way or the other about the validity of a non-delegable duty, and was later overturned on the ground that there was no good reason for extending the general limits of a hospital's duty of care beyond the ambit of medical treatment. In *S* v *Lothian Health Board*,[10] the court considered the scope of this duty, on the premise that what is

---

[3] An issue which arose in *Thake* v *Maurice* [1984] 2 All ER 513; reversed [1986] QB 644.

[4] (1979) 28 NBR (2d) 569, NBSC.   [5] Medical Act 1983 (as amended), s 44C.

[6] From 1 April 2019, a new state indemnity scheme for general practice was introduced in England which is known as the Clinical Negligence Scheme for General Practice (CNSGP). The scheme covers clinical negligence liabilities arising in general practice in relation to incidents that occurred on or after this date. See later in this chapter but also generally, NHS Resolution, 'Clinical Negligence Scheme for General Practice (CNSGP)' (2022) available at <https://resolution.nhs.uk/services/claims-management/clinical-schemes/general-practice-indemnity/clinical-negligence-scheme-for-general-practice> accessed 07 December 2022.

[7] For discussion, Christine Beuermann, 'Do Hospitals Owe a So-Called "Non-Delegable" Duty of Care to Their Patients?' (2018) 26(1) Medical Law Review 1.

[8] [2004] 3 WLR 469.

[9] [2008] EWHC 2468 (QB). The Court of Appeal rejected the trial conclusion that a hospital's non-delegable duty to a patient, if there was one, extended to supervising the quality of tests contracted out to an independent laboratory: [2009] EWCA 1203. For a distinction between contracted-out treatment and investigation, see *M* v *Calderdale and Kirklees HA* [1998] Lloyd's Rep Med 157.

[10] 2009 SLT 689.

relevant is whether the hospital assumes responsibility for contracted-out services that lead to negligent harm, not whether it had a degree of control over the work done. This was confirmed by the Supreme Court in *Woodland* v *Swimming Teachers Association and Others*:

> The true test reflects the factors which suggest that control is important, but has more nuance. I would express it thus. A school or hospital owes a non-delegable duty to see that care is taken for the safety of a child or patient who (a) is generally in its care, and (b) is receiving a service which is part of the institution's mainstream function of education or tending to the sick.[11]

The question, then, depends very much on the precise nature of the delegation but it is still of some importance, particularly in respect of staff whose group or personal cover may be less comprehensive than is that of the professions.[12] If claiming, however, that a safe and proper system has not been provided, it should be argued clearly which elements or features of the said system are thought to be lacking.[13] In this regard, the UK Supreme Court has drawn attention to the kinds of factors that should be considered in identifying when liability may be at issue: (i) because of the practical connection between the tortfeasor and the defendant, notably that activities were undertaken by the former for the latter; (ii) vicarious liability can arise even in the absence of a contract of employment; and (iii) the activity in question was integral to the business activities of the defendant. Here 'business' is not to be understood necessarily as a commercial concern.[14]

It should be borne in mind that the employer may still be held vicariously liable even if the employee acts in direct contradiction of their employer's instructions or prohibitions. The vicarious liability of hospitals throughout their hierarchy has been clearly established for half a century[15] and requires no further discussion.[16] If anything, it may be expanding. In *Godden* v *Kent and Medway Strategic Health Authority*,[17] it was held to be an arguable ground of action that a health authority could be held vicariously liable for the acts of a GP who had indecently assaulted and possibly negligently treated his patients. In a further extension of the principle, it was held in *Barclays Bank Plc* v *Various Claimants*[18] that the bank was vicariously liable for the sexual assaults of a doctor who it had nominated to carry out medical assessments on its staff. This was so, even given the status of the doctor as an independent contractor because 'the medical examinations were sufficiently closely connected with the relationship between the doctor and the bank; they were the purpose of that relationship'.

---

[11] [2013] UKSC 66.

[12] The issue does, in fact, seem to have been effectively decided in the ratio of *Re R (a minor) (No 2)* (1997) 33 BMLR 178, [197] (Brooke LJ), a case including inadequate hospital communications (sub nom *Robertson* v *Nottingham Health Authority* [1987] 8 Med LR 1).

[13] See *Campbell* v *Borders Health Board* [2011] CSOH 73.

[14] *Cox* v *Ministry of Justice* [2016] UKSC 10, affirmed in *Armes* v *Nottinghamshire CC* [2017] UKSC 60.

[15] *Roe* v *Minister of Health*; *Woolley* v *Ministry of Health* [1954] 2 QB 66; *Hayward* v *Board of Management of the Royal Infirmary of Edinburgh* and *Macdonald* v *Glasgow Western Hospitals Board of Management* [1954] SC 453.

[16] It is also possible to sue the Secretary of State for policy-based operational failures in the delivery of health care: see *Re HIV Haemophiliac Litigation* (1998) 41 BMLR 171.

[17] [2004] EWHC 1629 (QB).   [18] [2018] EWCA Civ 1670.

12.3 BRINGING A CLAIM IN CLINICAL NEGLIGENCE

The key elements that the claimant must establish in bringing a clinical negligence claim are that:

(i)   the defendant owed a duty of care to the claimant;

(ii) there was a breach of the duty of care, which amounts to a requirement to demonstrate that the standard of the treatment given by the defendant fell below the standard expected of them by the law, and;

(iii) as a result the defendant's acts or omissions which gave rise to this sub-standard treatment, the claimant suffered a legally recognised harm (e.g., physical injury or psychiatric illness).[19] This is otherwise known as causation, which must be established in fact and in law.

If successful in proving all these key elements, the claimant is entitled to financial compensation which is designed to restore them as far as is possible to the position they would have been in, if the negligence had not occurred. In realising this entitlement to financial compensation in a clinical negligence claim, however, it is important to recognise that harm may be both financial and non-financial; therefore, the compensation paid can only approximate the total of loss and harm suffered by the claimant.

The concept of clinical negligence has experienced a schism in recent decades. On the one hand, we have the standard line of cases in which there has been a technical failure or misadventure—in other words, cases associated with medical treatment in one form or another. On the other, there has been a rapid growth in claims of negligence arising before treatment has started. These have become known as information disclosure cases, based on the rights of the patient to make an informed choice as to their treatment, which may be described as a 'consent-based negligence' action, and we discuss this in more detail in Chapter 8. We therefore confine discussion in this chapter to the established field of medical misadventure, most often involving alleged negligence arising in relation to diagnosis and treatment in healthcare settings. In the next section, we turn to consider in more detail each of the key elements which must be established to succeed in a clinical negligence claim.

12.3.1 DUTY OF CARE

How does an individual know if a doctor owes them a duty of care? The answer, in most cases, is disarmingly simple: because they are your doctor. That is, an automatic legal duty of care arises if a doctor has agreed to treat the individual, or they have successfully registered at a GP practice in the UK. A duty will also arise in the case of a private patient by virtue of their contractual relationship with their doctor (or the hospital) and, within a public national health system, the duty arises when the patient presents for treatment

---

[19] Cf. *Fairlie* v *Perth and Kinross Healthcare NHS Trust* 2004 SLT 1200 (OH) in which 'distress'—in the absence of an identifiable psychiatric or psychological condition or illness—was not considered a legally relevant harm. But see also *D* v *East Berkshire Community Health NHS Trust; K* v *Dewsbury Healthcare NHS Trust, K* v *Oldham NHS Trust* [2005] UKHL 23, in which the House of Lords dismissed appeals by three sets of parents who had been falsely accused of child abuse, holding that the parents were not owed a duty of care by the defendant HCPs for psychiatric harm caused by the false allegations, even though they had suffered a recognised form of psychiatric injury.

and is admitted. It does not follow, of course, that the individual patient is entitled to everything they demand. This is a question of the standard of care that can be expected, and
we return to this later in the chapter.

Duties in law can be assumed or imposed. The paradigm example of an assumed obligation (of care) is that of contract, where parties voluntarily agree to be bound to each
other. As we have noted, however, this is not the legal basis for the operation of the NHS;
rather, tort law dictates if and/or when a duty of care arises. In the seminal case of *Caparo*
v *Dickman*, the House of Lords stated that a three-stage test should be used to determine whether such a duty arises.[20] First, the relationship between the claimant and the
defendant must be sufficiently 'proximate'; second, that harm following the defendant's
actions/omissions was 'reasonably foreseeable'; and finally, it would be fair, just, and reasonable to impose such a duty in the given circumstances.[21] This, in essence, is a question of how directly a claimant might be affected by the behaviour of another. The more
direct the likelihood of harm, the more likely it will be that a duty of care will be imposed.
In the later case of *Robinson* v *Chief Constable of West Yorkshire Police*,[22] the Supreme
Court took the opportunity to revisit *Caparo*. Lord Reed (with whom Lady Hale and Lord
Hodge agreed) made clear that any suggestion that the tripartite test applies generally in
the tort of negligence, and in consequence the 'court will only impose a duty of care where
it considers it fair, just and reasonable to do so on the particular facts is mistaken'.[23] The
court then went on to highlight a range of cases where it would be appropriate not to do
so before identifying that it is likely to be only in a 'novel type of case,' where courts may
need to move beyond established principles in line with *Caparo*:

> The courts . . . have to exercise judgement when deciding whether a duty of care should be
> recognised in a novel type of case. It is the exercise of judgement in those circumstances
> that involves consideration of what is 'fair, just and reasonable'.[24]

One thing that is unquestionable is that a public health service owes a duty of care to the
patients it accepts for treatment, which on any analysis is a fair and reasonable legal position. However, is it possible for personnel not to accept patients and so to reject this duty?
What of the over-tired junior doctor who is fed up dealing with the drunks who stagger
into the Accident and Emergency (A&E) on a Saturday night after a fight? Can they be
turned away? Quite simply, no, they cannot, the reason being that the hospital is holding
itself out as offering emergency services, which, self-evidently, is a public statement that
it will respond to the public need, however unpleasant that may be.[25] Moreover, as confirmed by the Supreme Court *in Darnley* v *Croydon Health Services NHS Trust*,[26] patients
who present at A&E are owed a duty that includes the timely receipt of accurate information, for example, about how long they might expect to wait to be seen by a doctor. Where
the A&E Department operates a triage system, it is part of the duty of care to require the
presenting patients to be given this kind of information, either orally by a receptionist

[20] See, principally, *Caparo Industries plc* v *Dickman* [1990] 2 AC 605; also see, e.g., *Kent* v *Griffiths (No 3)*
[2001] QB 36, and now *Darnley* v *Croydon Health Services NHS Trust* [2018] UKSC 50.
[21] ibid.; see also *Goodwill* v *British Pregnancy Advisory Service* [1996] 2 All ER 161; *Vowles* v *Evans* [2003]
1 WLR 1607, CA.
[22] [2018] UKSC 4.   [23] ibid. [21].   [24] ibid. [27].
[25] The same applies to the ambulance service where there is a legal duty to respond to a call for help:
Kent v *Griffiths* [2000] 2 WLR 1158. For a discussion see: Kevin Williams, 'Litigation Against English NHS
Ambulance Services and the Rule in *Kent* v *Griffiths*' (2007) 15(2) Medical Law Review 153. In Scotland,
a private law action was confirmed as justiciable in *Aitken* v *Scottish Ambulance Service* [2011] CSOH 49.
[26] [2018] UKSC 50.

or in a prominent notice. On the facts of this case, a patient presented with a head injury and was told that the wait to be seen by a doctor would be between four and five hours; however, the policy was that such patients would be seen within 30 minutes. In the event, the patient left after 19 minutes only to collapse later, and the delay was proven to have been causal in permanent brain damage. The claim was successful both on duty of care and causation (see later in this chapter).

By the same token, it does not follow that any public healthcare establishment must accept whosoever presents. It is arguably fair and reasonable for a hospital not to offer emergency services and to direct patients elsewhere. The same applies to the individual doctor.[27] Whatever one might think of moral obligations, it is no part of the general law in the UK that a doctor must respond to someone in medical need when that person is not already their patient. The doctor need not then raise their hand in response to a request for medical assistance for the airline passenger who has collapsed on an airline flight.[28] However, a duty of care will clearly arise should they do so and begin to examine the patient and what is then required of them becomes determined by the relevant standard of care. Let us turn, then, to consider the second element of the negligence action, namely, the standard of care, where we examine what the content of any duty entails.

12.3.2 BREACH OF THE DUTY OF CARE

The case of *Barnett v Chelsea and Kensington Hospital Management Committee*[29] establishes several of the key elements needed to succeed in a clinical negligence claim, including breach of the duty of care. The case concerned three workmen who suffered serious illness after drinking tea. They presented to the local hospital, but the doctor was ill himself. The nurse phoned the doctor with the symptoms and he advised that the men go home and see their own doctors. In the event, one of the men died from arsenic poisoning and the action was brought by his widow. The court held that the doctor not only owed a duty of care to those who presented to his casualty unit but that, in these circumstances, he should have ensured that the patients were properly examined. Ultimately, however, as we shall see, Barnett's widow did not recover, despite there being a duty of care and despite the ruling that the requisite standard had not been met. In this case, the standard was about examining emergency patients, but how are we to know what that standard is across the whole spectrum of medical care? There have been many judicial pronouncements by the courts on the subject. As early as 1838 we find Tindall CJ ruling that:

> Every person who enters into a learned profession undertakes to bring to the exercise of it a reasonable degree of care and skill. He does not undertake, if he is an attorney, that at all events you shall gain your case, nor does a surgeon undertake that he will perform a cure; nor does he undertake to use the highest possible degree of skill.[30]

---

[27] But see National Health Service (General Medical Services Contracts) Regulations 2015 (SI 2015/1862). Part 5 Contracts: required terms, reg 17 with respect to general practitioners who are obliged to provide immediate care after accident or emergency in their practice area in core hours.

[28] Note the professional perspective on such inaction: 'You must offer help if emergencies arise in clinical settings or in the community, taking account of your own safety, your competence and the availability of other options for care', which could be said to leave some leeway for subjective decision-making, General Medical Council (GMC), 'Good Medical Practice' (2019) available at <https://www.gmc-uk.org/ethical-guidance/ethical-guidance-for-doctors/good-medical-practice> accessed 07 December 2022.

[29] [1968] 2 WLR 422.   [30] *Lanphier v Phipos* (1838) 8 C & P 475 [478].

An echo of this is to be found in *R* v *Bateman*,[31] where the court explained that:

> If a person holds himself out as possessing special skill and knowledge, by and on behalf of
> a patient, he owes a duty to the patient to use due caution in undertaking the treatment . . .
> The jury should not exact the highest, or very high standard, nor should they be content
> with a very low standard.

If the doctor is not expected to be a miracle worker guaranteeing a cure for their patient, then what standard are they expected to meet? During the course of addressing the jury in the case, McNair J provided the classic answer to this question in *Bolam* v *Friern Hospital Management Committee*:[32]

> The test is the standard of the ordinary skilled man exercising and professing to have that
> special skill. A man need not possess the highest expert skill at the risk of being found
> negligent. It is a well-established law that it is sufficient if he exercises the ordinary skill of
> an ordinary man exercising that particular art.

Nevertheless, the doctor is professing a particular skill and, in the further immortal words of McNair J, the test of that skill 'is not the test of the man on the top of the Clapham omnibus because [that man] has not got this special skill'.[33]

The doctor having that degree of competence expected of the ordinary skilful doctor sets the standard. They are the practitioner who follows the standard practice of their profession or, at least, follows practices that would not be disapproved of by responsible opinion within the profession; they have a reasonably sound grasp of medical techniques and are as informed of new medical developments as the average competent doctor would expect to be. The circumstances in which a doctor treats their patient will also be considered. A doctor working in an emergency, with inadequate facilities and under great pressure, will not be expected by the courts to achieve the same results as a doctor who is working in ideal conditions.[34] This was alluded to by Mustill J in *Wilsher* v *Essex Area Health Authority*[35], where he said that, if a person was forced by an emergency to do too many things at once, then the fact that they do one of them incorrectly 'should not lightly be taken as negligence'.[36]

The reasonably skilful doctor has a duty to keep themselves informed of major developments in practice, but this duty obviously cannot extend to the requirement that they should know all there is to be known in a particular area of medicine. In *Crawford* v *Board of Governors of Charing Cross Hospital*,[37] the claimant had developed brachial palsy because of his arm being kept in a certain position during an operation. Six months prior to the operation an article had appeared in *The Lancet* pointing out just this danger, but the anaesthetist against whom negligence was being alleged had not read the article in question. The Court of Appeal eventually found in favour of the anaesthetist, Lord Denning stating that:

> It would, I think, be putting too high a burden on a medical man to say that he has to read
> every article appearing in the current medical press; and it would be quite wrong to sug-
> gest that a medical man is negligent because he does not at once put into operation the

---

[31] (1925) 94 LJKB 791 [794].   [32] [1957] 2 All ER 118 [121].

[33] A test approved by the Privy Council: *Chin Keow* v *Government of Malaysia* [1967] 1 WLR 813.

[34] This is in accordance with the general principle in the law of torts that errors of judgement are more excusable in an emergency: *The Metagama* 1928 SC (HL) 21; the strength of this precedent was confirmed in the non-medical personal injury case of *Morris* v *Richards* [2003] EWCA Civ 232.

[35] [1987] QB 730, [777].   [36] ibid. [749].   [37] (1953) *The Times*, 8 December, CA.

suggestions which some contributor or other might make in a medical journal. The time may come in a particular case when a new recommendation may be so well proved and so well known, and so well accepted that it should be adopted, but that was not so in this case.[38]

Failure to read a single article, it was said, may be excusable, while disregard of a series of warnings in the medical press could well be evidence of negligence. In view of the rapid progress currently being made in many areas of health and medicine, and in view of the amount of information confronting the average doctor, it is unreasonable to expect a doctor to be aware of every development in their field. At the same time, they must be reasonably up to date and must know of major developments. The practice of medicine has, however, become increasingly based on principles of scientific elucidation and report, which has been referred to as 'evidence-based medicine'. As a result of such developments, the pressure on doctors to keep abreast of current developments is now considerable, rather than just relying on long clinical experience.[39]

The 'custom test'—the test whereby a defendant's conduct is tested against the normal usage of their profession or calling—is one that is applied in all areas of the law of negligence. The courts have given expression to this test in the medical context in several decisions. In the important Scottish case of *Hunter v Hanley*, for example, there was a clear endorsement of the custom test in Lord Clyde's dictum:

> To establish liability by a doctor where deviation from normal practice is alleged, three facts require to be established. First of all it must be proved that there is a usual and normal practice; secondly it must be proved that the defender has not adopted that practice; and thirdly (and this is of crucial importance) it must be established that the course the doctor adopted is one which no professional man of ordinary skill would have taken if he had been acting with ordinary care.[40]

This attractively simple exposition of the law, however, conceals a hurdle at the outset. It may, in many cases, be possible to prove that there is a 'usual and normal practice'—this is particularly so if there are guidelines covering a procedure.[41] On the other hand, there will obviously be disagreement as to what is the appropriate course to follow in several medical scenarios. In some circumstances, the existence of two schools of thought may result in more than one option being open to a practitioner. If this is so, then what are the liability implications of choosing a course of action which a responsible body of opinion within the profession may well reject? Precisely this question arose in *Bolam*,[42] where the claimant had suffered fractures because of the administration of electro-convulsive therapy without an anaesthetic. At the time, there were two schools of thought about anaesthesia in such treatment, one holding the view that relaxant drugs should be used,

---

[38] ibid.

[39] For an example of the evidence-based approach which seeks to produce systematic reviews of primary research in human health care and policy, see Cochrane, 'The Cochrane Library' (2022) available at <https://www.cochrane.org/> accessed 07 December 2022.

[40] 1955 SC 200 [206]. The rigid simplicity of Lord Clyde's definition was defended in an anonymous article 'Clinical Negligence: *Hunter v Hanley* 35 years on' 1990 SLT 325. *Hunter* was specifically approved by Lord Scarman in *Maynard v West Midlands Regional Health Authority* [1985] 1 All ER 635 and would seem to be the relevant test in Ireland: *Dunne (infant) v National Maternity Hospital* [1989] IR 91 per Finlay CJ.

[41] See Ash Samanta, Jo Samanta, and Joanne Beswick, 'Responsible Practice or Restricted Practice? An Empirical Study of the Use of Clinical Guidelines in Medical Negligence Litigation' (2021) 29(2) Medical Law Review 205.

[42] [1957] 2 All ER 118.

the other being that this only increased the risk. In this case, the judge ruled that a doctor would not be negligent if he acted 'in accordance with the practice accepted by a responsible body of medical men skilled in that particular art'. Negligence would not be inferred merely because there was a body of opinion which took a contrary view.[43]

Subsequent cases confirmed this approach. In *Maynard v West Midlands Regional Health Authority*, the trial judge had preferred an alternative medical approach to that which had been chosen by the defendant, notwithstanding the fact that this latter course found support in responsible medical opinion; both the Court of Appeal and the House of Lords confirmed that this was an unsatisfactory way of attributing negligence.[44] In *Muller v King's College Hospital NHS Foundation Trust*, the court held that while a court can prefer one expert's opinion over another when determining whether the conduct fell below the acceptable legal standard,[45] in diagnosis cases (i.e. whether the negligence lay in the failure to diagnose correct and/or on time), a court is not at liberty to reject a particular expert's view unless it is logically untenable or otherwise flawed in some way making it indefensible and impermissible.[46]

Bolam has been the object of sustained criticism from those who object to the implication that the medical profession itself can determine what is an acceptable level of care.[47] Critics have long argued that doctors themselves should not dictate whether conduct is negligent; this should be a matter for the courts.[48] This has been confirmed—albeit hesitantly—by the House of Lords' decision in *Bolitho v Hackney Health Authority*,[49] a case regarded by some commentators as representing a significant nail in *Bolam*'s coffin. *Bolitho* arose out of a failure on the part of a hospital doctor to examine and intubate a child experiencing respiratory distress. Negligence derived from a failure to attend the patient was not disputed; however, the problem of causation remained. Expert evidence was led by the claimant to the effect that a reasonably competent doctor would have intubated in such circumstances. The defendant, however, had her own expert witnesses prepared to say that non-intubation was a clinically justifiable response. The defendant argued that, had she attended the child, she would not have intubated her and her failure to attend would not, therefore, have made any difference to the outcome. The House of Lords accepted the truth of this evidence. The causation issue, here, is important from the jurisprudential aspect insofar as it was made clear that, while the *Bolam* test had no relevance as to the doctor's intention, it was central to the collateral question of whether the doctor would have been negligent in failing to take action. In other words, *Bolam* was applied to the question of causation when, in reality, the test is concerned only with standards of care. As a result, given that she had responsible support, the action failed on both counts.

However, the particular significance of *Bolitho* lies in the House of Lords' support for the Court of Appeal's departure from the certainties of *Bolam*. Rather than accepting

---

[43] There is potential conflict here with the existing authority. In *Hucks v Cole* (1968) [1993] 4 Med LR 393, it was held that an action that was clearly unreasonable could be negligent despite professional support.

[44] [1985] 1 All ER 635. *Maynard* was followed in *Hughes v Waltham Forest Health Authority* [1991] 2 Med LR 155, in which the court emphasised that the fact that a surgeon's decision was criticised by other surgeons did not amount in itself to an indication of negligence.

[45] *Penney v East Kent HA* [2000] Lloyd's Rep Med 41.   [46] [2017] EWHC 128 (QB).

[47] Particularly in the Commonwealth: *Reibl v Hughes* (1980) 114 DLR (3d) 1; *Rogers v Whittaker* (1992) 109 ALR 625. And see, in general, the discussion on information disclosure cases in Chapter 8.

[48] Sarah Devaney and Soren Holm, 'The Transmutation of Deference in Medicine: An Ethico-Legal Perspective' (2018) 26(2) Med L Rev 202.

[49] [1998] AC 232.

a 'body of opinion' simply because it was there, Lord Browne-Wilkinson held that the court must, in addition, be satisfied that the body of opinion in question rests on a logical basis. In particular, in cases involving, as they so often do, the weighing of risks against benefits, the judge, before accepting a body of opinion as being responsible, reasonable or respectable, will need to be satisfied that, in forming their views, the experts have directed their minds to the question of comparative risks and benefits and have reached a defensible conclusion on the matter.[50] This appears to be a clear rejection of the *Bolam* rule *simpliciter*,[51] but it must be read in the light of the strong caveat which Lord Browne-Wilkinson attached:

> In the vast majority of cases the fact that distinguished experts in the field are of a particular opinion will demonstrate the reasonableness of that opinion . . . But if, in a rare case, it can be demonstrated that the professional opinion is not capable of withstanding logical analysis, the judge is entitled to hold that the body of opinion is not reasonable or responsible . . . I emphasise that, in my view, it will very seldom be right for a judge to reach the conclusion that views genuinely held by a competent medical expert are unreasonable.[52]

Bolitho undoubtedly devalues the trump card which *Bolam* presented to the medical profession, but only in limited circumstances,[53] and, as to that, it is arguably undesirable to undermine the standard test beyond a certain point. *Bolam* provides some protection for the innovative or minority opinion or, indeed, the individual clinical judgement call.[54] If this protection is removed, then the opinion that the cautious medical practitioner will wish to follow will be that which involves least risk. This may have an inhibiting effect on medical progress: after all, many advances in medicine have been made by those who have pursued an unconventional line of therapy. Such doctors may quite easily be regarded as negligent by a judge given to favouring conventional medical opinion.

In this respect, we can look to the decision in *De Freitas* v *O'Brien*,[55] which, rather than bolstering a conservative approach in assessing the acceptability of a body of opinion, gives comfort to the so-called 'super-specialist' who may undertake procedures which others might regard as being inappropriate or even too risky. In this case, a spinal surgeon—said to be one of only 11 such specialists in the country—maintained that the surgery he performed was in line with what his fellow spinal surgeons would have considered clinically justified. In contrast, the claimants argued that run-of-the-mill orthopaedic surgeons would not have operated in the circumstances. The Court of Appeal confirmed that the *Bolam* test did not require that the responsible body of opinion be large, thus endorsing the acceptability of acting within limits defined by a sub-specialty. One criticism of the decision in *De Freitas* is that it licenses the taking of risks. Yet, the court clearly retains its ability to declare an opinion to be unreasonable, a power which is firmly endorsed by *Bolitho*.

---

[50] [1997] 4 All ER 771 [778].

[51] For an example of weighing the reasonableness and responsibleness of medical opinion post-*Bolitho*, see *M (a child)* v *Blackpool Victoria Hospital NHS Trust* [2003] EWHC 1744, in which an appeal on *Bolitho* terms was rejected. See also, *XYZ v Warrington and Halton NHS Foundation Trust* [2016] EWHC 331 (QB).

[52] [1997] 4 All ER 771 [779].

[53] For the correct approach for judges when dealing with expert evidence on accepted/acceptable practice, see *A v Burne* [2006] EWCA Civ 24.

[54] See e.g. *Zarb v Odetoyinbo* [2006] EWHC 2880 (QB).   [55] [1995] PIQR P281.

The Court of Appeal in *Bolitho* has been hailed as ushering in the 'new *Bolam*'[56] although there were many who viewed it with a modicum of distrust.[57] It is, therefore, interesting to consider its progress since its birth—and, certainly, the case has attracted its fair share of attention. A review of post-*Bolitho* clinical negligence cases involving a standard of care showed that, prior to November 2001, *Bolitho* was referred to in four cases in the Court of Appeal and in 25 cases at first instance.[58] There is no way in which all these cases, as well as those that since followed, could be aired in a book of this size and several of them were 'consent-based' and are considered under that heading.[59] Some do, however, merit mention—if only briefly.

Wisniewski v *Central Manchester Health Authority*[60] seems to us to be the most apposite case in that the 'logic' underlying the expert evidence was specifically considered. The case concerned a child who was born brain-damaged following 13 minutes' hypoxia during the birthing process; it was alleged that the midwife overestimated her ability and, as a result, the doctor failed to attend in appropriate time. As in *Bolitho*, negligence in relation to non-attendance was not in dispute; the problem, again, lay in causation—and in the two-stage definition of causation developed in *Bolitho* as to what would and should have happened in the absence of negligence. The establishment and the status of a 'responsible body of supporting opinion' were, therefore, of major importance and the conflict is illustrated in two quotations. Thomas J, at first instance, had this to say:

> where analysis of the expert evidence on the facts relating to a particular case shows that a decision made by a doctor and supported by experts cannot be justified as one that a responsible medical practitioner would have taken, then a judge should not preclude himself from reaching [a] conclusion simply because clinical judgment is involved.[61]

However, Brooke LJ said in the Court of Appeal:

> it is quite impossible for a court to hold that the views sincerely held by doctors of such eminence cannot logically be supported at all ... and the views of the defendants' witnesses were views which could be logically expressed and held by responsible doctors.[62]

The clear inference is that, had the doctor survived the first hurdle as to what he would have done had he attended, *Bolam* would have prevailed and the *Bolitho* exception would not have applied.[63] Logic is, however, a somewhat unusual criterion on which to assess what is, essentially, a matter of clinical judgement and it seems unlikely that the courts will be able to retain control over healthcare standards if they rely on 'logic' alone.[64]

---

[56] A phrase which we would attribute to Andrew Grubb, 'Commentary' (1998) 6 Medical Law Review 378.
[57] A most searching review is that of Margaret Brazier and Jose Miola, 'Bye-bye *Bolam*: A Medical Litigation Revolution?' (2000) 8(1) Medical Law Review 85; Harvey Teff, 'The Standard of Care in Clinical Negligence—Moving On From *Bolam*' (1998) 18(3) Oxford Journal of Legal Studies 473.
[58] Alasdair Maclean, 'Beyond *Bolam* and *Bolitho*' (2002) 5(3) Medical Law International 205. At the same time, there was judgment explicitly by way of the *Bolam* test in eight Court of Appeal and ten High Court cases; the author remarks that 'it would seem that *Bolam* is far from dead'.
[59] See also, Rachel Mulheron, 'Trumping *Bolam*: A Critical Legal Analysis of *Bolitho*'s "Gloss"' (2010) 69(3) Cambridge Law Journal 609.
[60] [1998] Lloyd's Rep Med 223, CA.   [61] Quoted [1998] Lloyd's Rep Med 223 [235].
[62] [1998] Lloyd's Rep Med 223 [237].
[63] For the appropriate application of the *Bolam* and *Bolitho* tests in determining what should or should not have been done, see *Gouldsmith* v *Mid-Staffordshire General Hospitals NHS Trust* [2007] EWCA Civ 397.
[64] For a discussion of the 'logical' approach, and the relatively innovative alternative of 'unreasonable risk', see: Rob Heywood, 'The Logic of *Bolitho*' (2006) 22(4) Journal of Professional Negligence 225.

It is, therefore, useful to turn to *Marriott*,[65] where a man sustained severe intra-cranial injury allegedly aggravated by his practitioner's failure to refer him back to hospital when his condition deteriorated. The health authority called expert evidence in support of the doctor, but the trial judge considered this not to be reasonably prudent and found for the claimant. The Court of Appeal dismissed the appeal on two main grounds. First, the Court questioned the acceptability of the evidence for both sides—'it is questionable whether either had given evidence from which it was reasonable to infer that their individual approaches were shared by a responsible body of others in their profession'[66]—a statement which seems to eliminate the single maverick from the *Bolam* equation. Even so, the judge was effectively dismissing the evidence of both sides—the Court's opinion suggests that the result might have been different had she chosen one expert's evidence in preference to the other, rather than substitute her own analysis. Second, however, the Court affirmed its entitlement to question whether an opinion was reasonably held given an analysis of the risks involved in following that opinion. On the face of things, then, *Marriott* moves the *Bolitho* test from one of logic to one of reasonableness, which is much more akin to the reasoning applied in other, non-medical standard of care decisions. Unfortunately, the situation is still not clear as, while the Court of Appeal supported the trial judge's approach, it still retained the language of 'logic'. *Marriott* does, however, open an alternative route to the 'new *Bolam*'. *Jones v Conwy and Denbighshire NHS Trust*[67] probably encapsulates the tenor of the emerging jurisprudence by collapsing the distinction between logicality and reasonableness in holding that in the absence of a clear bright-line rule about how to proceed in a given set of clinical circumstances—here the decision whether to order an immediate CT scan—it was neither illogical nor unreasonable to delay the procedure.

Penney v East Kent Health Authority[68] concerned three women who developed cancer of the cervix following a reported negative screening test. As with all screening tests, that for potential cervical cancer inherently involves both false positive and false negative tests, the latter being estimated as occurring in between 5% and 15% of cases examined. It was not, therefore, argued that a false negative report indicated negligence on the part of the screener per se; the issue was confined to what should have been done in 1993, given the agreed fact that there were abnormalities in the claimants' slides. The health authority maintained that the unusual abnormalities present were open to interpretation and disposal and that the outcome of the case should be decided on *Bolam* principles. The trial judge considered, and the Court of Appeal agreed, however, that the fact was that abnormal cells were present which no screener, acting with reasonable care, could have been certain were not pre-cancerous; the slides should, therefore, have been labelled at least as borderline—he found 'the *Bolam* principle ill-fitting to Mrs Penney's case'. It is not easy, however, to see why that should be so in respect of 'excusability'. Pepitt J was clearly conscious of this and further held that, if he was wrong, he would revert to *Bolitho* in that, given the facts, the contention of the health authority's experts that the slides could well have been reported as negative was inconsistent with the accepted principle of 'absolute confidence' and was, consequently, illogical—a conclusion with which it is difficult to disagree.

---

[65] *Marriott v West Midlands Regional Health Authority* [1999] Lloyd's Rep Med 23.
[66] At [27] (Beldam LJ).   [67] [2008] EWHC 3172 (QB).   [68] (2000) 55 BMLR 63.

Although subsequently revised on appeal,[69] in *Lillywhite* v *University College London Hospitals NHS Trust*,[70] a case involving radiological misdiagnosis, the main lesson of which seems to be that evidence adduced to refute an allegation of negligence must be that much more convincing when a specific diagnostic question has been posed. Penney was also considered and approved in *Manning* v *King's College Hospital NHS Trust*, the gist of which was that a case of doubtful malignancy should not be reported as negative.[71] Equally, a failure on the part of a judge to find illogicality (or indeed to have before them explicit findings of fact that would support such a conclusion) will mean that they are not in a position to reject expert medical opinion as unreasonable: see *Ministry of Justice* v *Carter*.[72] It has also been confirmed that a judge is not at liberty to choose between two responsible bodies of medical opinion unless on the basis that one is found to be illogical.[73]

We also have *Birch* v *University College London Hospital NHS Foundation Trust*.[74] This case is concerned largely with consent-based negligence and as such it is considered more fully in Chapter 8. Nevertheless, on the role of logic in negligence cases, the judge had this to say about *Bolitho*:

> Lord Browne-Wilkinson was indicating that such an opinion is not to be lightly set aside. The body of medical opinion must be incapable of withstanding logical analysis, in other words, cannot be logically supported at all. If there are different practices sanctioned by two bodies of medical opinion, both withstanding logical analysis, there is no basis for a finding of negligence against the doctor choosing one rather than the other. The matter may simply boil down to a different weighing of benefits and risks. If there is no failure to weigh the risks and benefits of each practice the *Bolitho* approach cannot be used to trump *Bolam*, even though the adherence to one body of medical opinion has led to the adverse outcome in the particular case . . . Not only am I bound by this view but I conceive it to be eminently sensible: it would be folly for a judge with no training in medicine to conclude that one body of medical opinion should be preferred over another, when both are professionally sanctioned and both withstand logical attack.[75]

An example of a successful outcome for a claimant based on the *Bolitho* authority is *Hearne* v *The Royal Marsden Hospital NHS Foundation Trust*.[76] Here, after extensive consideration of the competing medical evidence about whether and when a patient should have been started on heparin to avoid deep vein thrombosis following chemotherapy (the outcome that had eventuated and led to further physical injury), the court held the presence of clear NICE guidelines coupled with the relative ease with which a single contra-indication could have been ruled out, meant that there was 'no logic' in ruling out heparinisation for the patient in these circumstances. This case is also important for the emphasis placed on following the national guidelines, albeit recognised as non-mandatory. While it is unwise to generalise from a small number of selected cases, the impression gained thus

---

[69] [2006] Lloyd's Rep Med 268.   [70] [2004] EWHC 2452.

[71] [2008] EWHC 1838 (QB); affirmed in [2009] 110 BMLR 175.

[72] *Ministry of Justice* v *Carter* [2010] EWCA Civ 694, [22].

[73] *Hannigan* v *Lanarkshire Acute Hospital NHS Trust* [2012] CSOH 152, citing *Honisz* v *Lothian Health Board* (2008) SC 235. Note, although these are Scottish cases, it is well settled that the position on negligence is the same north and south of the border. For recent confirmation of the English position, see *Muller* v *King's College NHS Trust* [2017] EWHC 128 (QB) where the 'illogical' tenet is carried over to evidence about proper approaches to diagnosis.

[74] [2008] EWHC 2237 (QB).   [75] (2008) 104 BMLR 168 [55].   [76] [2016] EWHC 117 (QB).

far is that, while the courts are increasingly determined to see that the *Bolam* principle is not extended,[77] they still have an innate reluctance to abandon it in respect of medical opinion.[78] There is a sense that *Bolitho*, although welcome, is being used mainly in a 'back-up' position. What is certain is that *Bolam* can no longer be regarded as impregnable. Having said that, we await with interest the ruling of the Supreme Court in the case of *McCulloch & Ors v Forth Valley Health Board* which is pending at the time of writing.[79] In this case, the Scottish Inner House noted that in cases of disclosure to patients of reasonable alternative or variant treatments, it was the *Bolam* standard that was applicable in determining what was reasonable in the circumstances rather than what could be described as the more patient-centred approach in *Montgomery* (see Chapter 8).

12.3.3 CAUSATION

To be successful in a clinical negligence claim, it is also necessary that the claimant show that the defendant's wrongdoing was both the factual and legal cause of the alleged harm. This is often a particularly difficult aspect of the claim to establish for several reasons. For example, there may be several possible explanations available which explain the alleged harm include the defendant's actions and/or the claimant's pre-existing condition(s). In addition, there may be evidence available to the effect that it can be argued that the claimant's condition may have deteriorated in any case, regardless of any alleged negligence on the part of the defendant. In the circumstances, what has been lost is the chance of a being successfully treated (loss of a chance), and the threshold requirement of proof on the balance of probabilities must be satisfied in such cases.

Factual causation is concerned with establishing the physical connection between the defendant's conduct and the claimant's damage. In general terms, the burden of proof rests with the claimant to show that it is more likely than not that the wrongful conduct of the defendant in fact resulted in the damage of which they complain. This is known as the 'but for' test, which means that an act or omission is the cause in fact of harm suffered by the claimant when the injury would not have occurred *but for* the act. It is important that the claimant show that it is more than likely than not (balance of probabilities) that 'but for' the defendant's wrongdoing the damage would not have occurred. We can return to the *Barnett* case for authority on this point.[80] As noted, despite having proven the hospital owed her husband a duty of care and had breached that duty, Mr Barnett's widow was unable to recover damages for her husband's death from arsenic poisoning. Why? Because it is the nature of arsenic poisoning that even if Mr Barnett had been examined, he would have died anyway, there being no cure or treatment for the condition. In law, therefore, the doctor's negligence did not cause the death.

Under certain circumstances, however, the 'but for' test proves inadequate to determine factual causation, particularly where there may be a variety of possible independent explanations for the occurrence of a patient's medical condition. Thus, if a claimant brings an action for 'nervous shock', it may well be arguable that the symptoms complained of

---

[77] As, for example, into judging the patient's best interests: *Re S (adult patient: sterilisation)* [2001] Fam 15; [2000] 3 WLR 1288.

[78] See e.g. *Sutcliffe v BMI Healthcare Ltd* (2007) 98 BMLR 211, CA; *C v North Cumbria University Hospitals NHS Trust* [2014] EWHC 61 (QB). For critical commentary on post-*Bolitho* obstetric litigation, see Rob Heywood, 'Litigating Labour: Condoning Unreasonable Risk-taking in Childbirth?' (2015) 44(1) Common Law World Review 28.

[79] [2021] CSIH 21.   [80] [1969] 1 QB 428.

are those of a psychiatric state which existed before the claimed precipitating event.[81] Some assistance in this respect was provided to the claimant through the Scottish case of *McGhee* v *National Coal Board*,[82] in which it was held that liability will be imposed if it can be established that the negligence of the defender materially increased the risk of the pursuer being damaged in the way in question.[83] Another useful parameter is the 'but for' test: the harm would not have occurred but for the negligent conduct. The challenges are manifold.[84]

In *Ashcroft* v *Mersey Regional Health Authority*,[85] the claimant underwent a relatively straightforward and commonplace operation to remove granulation tissue—the result of chronic infection—from the ear; she sustained a severe paralysis of the facial nerve. Opinion was divided as to whether the surgeon had negligently pulled too hard on the nerve or whether the injury was an unfortunate accident. It was held by Kilner Brown J with obvious reluctance that on the balance of probabilities there was no negligence causing harm. The correctness of this view was later confirmed in *Wilsher*,[86] where the House of Lords went so far as to reverse the opinion of the Court of Appeal in the case and to order a retrial on the ground that the coincidence of a breach of duty and injury could not, of itself, give rise to a presumption that the injury was so caused: 'Whether we like it or not, the law . . . requires proof of fault causing damage as the basis of liability in tort.'[87]

The difficulty for the claimant in *Wilsher* lay in the fact that there were five possible causes for the condition with which he was afflicted. One of these was due to clinical negligence but it could not be established that this possible cause made a material contribution to the harm suffered.[88] It might have done so, but this fact still required to be proved by the claimant. A contrasting outcome was reached in *Bailey* v *Ministry of Defence*.[89] Again, the expert medical evidence available was unable to establish that 'but for' the negligent treatment the relevant harm would not have occurred, and the court was therefore entitled to apply a modified test for causation. It was deemed sufficient for the claimant to establish on a balance of probabilities that the defendants' lack of care had contributed to the injury in a way that was material or something more than negligible. Under this approach, the claimant was able to establish causation.

These issues are clearly matters of legal policy and justice. Causation is not a strict technical matter which can be 'solved' by the application of quasi-mathematical formulae.[90] Indeed, this is well reflected in two important House of Lords cases. In the non-clinical negligence case of *Fairchild* v *Glenhaven Funeral Services Ltd*,[91] the claimant had suffered multiple exposures to asbestos while working for various employers and could not, strictly, demonstrate who then had caused his disease. The court applied

---

[81] For other examples, see *Abada* v *Gray* (1997) 40 BMLR 116, CA (schizophrenia could not be precipitated by a road traffic injury); *Gates* v *McKenna* (1998) 46 BMLR 9 (it was improbable that taking part in a stage hypnosis programme could precipitate schizophrenia, and the possibility was unforeseeable).

[82] [1972] 3 All ER 1008.   [83] ibid. [1011] (Lord Reid).

[84] See *Bailey* v *Ministry of Defence* [2009] 1 WLR 1052. For commentary, see Stephen Bailey, 'Causation in Negligence: What is Material Contribution?' (2010) 30(2) Legal Studies 167. See also Per Laleng, '*Sienkiewicz v Greif (UK) Ltd and Wilmore v Knowsley Metropolitan Borough Council*: A Material Contribution to Uncertainty?' (2011) 74(5) Modern Law Review 777; Sandy Steel, *Proof of Causation in Tort Law* (CUP 2015).

[85] [1983] 2 All ER 245.

[86] *Wilsher* v *Essex Area Health Authority* [1988] AC 1074. See, too, a discussion of the scope and effect of the important decision in *Fairchild* v *Glenhaven Funeral Services Ltd and Others* [2002] 3 All ER 305 at 393–402.

[87] [1988] AC 1074 [1092] (Lord Bridge).

[88] For recent discussion on 'material contribution' in the Privy Council, see *Williams v Bermuda Hospitals Board* [2016] UKPC 4.

[89] [2008] EWCA Civ 883.

[90] For recognition of the policy considerations and the difficulty of shifting the onus of prof, see *McGlone* v *Greater Glasgow Health Board* (2011) CSOH 63.

[91] [2003] 1 AC 32.

Wilsher in holding that justice demanded a modified approach to the rules of causation; thus, so long as the claimant could show, on a balance of probabilities, that the wrong-doing of each employer had materially increased the risk to the employee that he might contract the disease, then this would be enough to establish that each employer had materially contributed to it, that is, each had caused his loss in legal terms.

Fairchild was then approved—and, perhaps, expanded—by the House in *Chester* v *Afshar*.[92] Again, as this case involved a dispute about information disclosure, it is discussed further in Chapter 8. It also demonstrates the House of Lords' willingness—albeit, in this case, by a majority only—to bend the rules of causation in the name of justice. Here a patient was not told of an inherent risk in a procedure to cure back pain. The risk materialised and the law of causation dictated that she had to prove that if she had known of the risk, she would never have had the operation. But the patient did not, and could not, prove that she would never have the operation; she only proved that she would not have had it on the day that she did.[93] All five of their Lordships agreed that she should therefore fail on a strict application of the law—but the majority could not accept this outcome and argued that the patient's right to self-determination demanded a remedy.

Following the ruling in *Fairchild*, the House of Lords considered another asbestos case: *Barker* v *Corus UK Ltd*[94] In this case, their Lordships held that employers who negligently exposed an employee to asbestos, thereby creating a material risk of mesothelioma, should be severally liable if that risk materialised, but only to the extent of the share of the risk created by their breach of duty. In other words, the attribution of liability would be apportioned according to the relative degree of contribution to the chance of the disease being contracted. The ruling prompted the inclusion of section 3 in the Compensation Act 2006, which enabled claimants who had contracted mesothelioma through asbestos exposure to receive full compensation from any 'responsible person'. Each responsible person who is successfully sued can then claim contributions from any other responsible person.[95] It is undoubtedly the case that these policy-driven decisions are a direct response to the considerable difficulties that claimants can face when attempting to clear the causation hurdle.

In *Schembri* v *Marshall*,[96] Mrs Marshall attended her GP complaining of chest pain and breathlessness. She had previously suffered a pulmonary embolism but had been successfully treated for that condition. The doctor examined her and stated the most probable cause of her symptoms was muscular strain affecting her hiatus hernia. She returned home and remained breathless overnight. The following morning, she suffered a cardiac arrest and died. It was agreed that there had been a breach of the duty of care by the GP, but what was in dispute was whether the breach had caused Mrs Marshall's death. There was debate among the experts who gave evidence as to what sort of treatment she would have received and whether it would have been timely in terms of preventing her death. The claimant could not prove on the balance of probabilities that Mrs Marshall would have been among the 64–75% who would have survived. Nevertheless, her chances would have been significantly

---

[92] [2005] 1 AC 134. We discuss the case in Ken Mason and Douglas Brodie, '*Bolam, Bolam*— Wherefore Art Thou, *Bolam*?' (2005) 9(2) Edinburgh Law Review 398. *Chester* was considered in two cases which address the question of a physician's duty to inform the patient of the risks and benefits of various alternative treatments: *Birch* v *University College London Hospital NHS Foundation Trust* [2008] EWHC 2237 (QB), and *Montgomery* v *Lanarkshire Health Board* [2015] UKSC 11.

[93] By contrast, establishing causation was more straightforward in *Montgomery* v *Lanarkshire Health Board* [2015] UKSC 11, as it was clear that the pursuer would have opted for an alternative procedure had she been informed properly of the comparative risks and benefits.

[94] [2006] UKHL 20.

[95] For an example of litigation under the Compensation Act 2006, see *Sienkiewicz* v *Greif (UK) Ltd* [2009] EWCA Civ 1159.

[96] [2020] EWCA Civ 358.

improved had she been in hospital overnight. At first instance, it was held by Mr Justice Stewart that it was a matter for the claimant to prove causation and that there was a need to show that Mrs Marshall would probably have survived had she been admitted to hospital in time. However, there was no need to prove the precise mechanism by which she would have survived if that had taken place. The first instance ruling was subsequently upheld on appeal. It was confirmed that Justice Stewart had been correct to first consider whether the claimant had established a specific train of events that would have avoided the death of Mrs Marshall. Having determined this to be in the negative, then it was legitimate to consider the statistical and other evidence and take a pragmatic and common-sense view of the evidence as a whole.

All of the judgments make for interesting reading as to how and how far abstract notions such as 'justice' and 'policy' can and should influence the direction of the law. *Chester* is one of the clearest examples we have of this to date, but it has been closely mirrored in *Rees v Darlington Memorial NHS Trust*.[97] As a result, causation rules were considered to be in a state of flux.[98] However, the Court of Appeal, for its part, has recently sought to limit too much drift away from the core principles upon which causation itself is built. In *Duce v Worcestershire Acute Hospitals NHS Trust*, following *Correia v University Hospital of North Staffordshire NHS Trust*,[99] the court agreed 'that if "the exceptional principle of causation" established by *Chester* was to be relied upon it was necessary to plead and prove that, if warned of the risk, the claimant would have deferred the operation'.[100] In *Duce*, the claimant had attempted to argue that *Chester* had made a special case of consent cases whereby the affront of suffering the harm at all, through inadequate information, was sufficient to ground a successful action.

An important variation on the causation theme was reintroduced in *Hotson*.[101] Here, the claimant was, admittedly, negligently treated following traumatic avulsion of the head of the femur and developed avascular necrosis. However, there was a 75% chance that this lesion would develop even in the event of correct diagnosis and treatment. The trial judge concluded that the matter was simply one of quantification of damages and the Court of Appeal upheld the view that the mistreatment had denied the claimant a 25% chance of a good recovery; damages were awarded and reduced accordingly. The House of Lords, however, declined to measure statistical chances and concluded that it was the original injury which caused the avascular necrosis, with Lord MacKay offering the following analysis:

> the probable effect of delay in treatment was determined by the state of facts existing when the plaintiff was first presented at the hospital . . . If insufficient blood vessels were left intact by the fall, he had no prospect of avoiding complete avascular necrosis whereas if sufficient blood vessels were left intact . . . he would not have suffered the avascular necrosis.[102]

---

[97] [2004] AC 309.

[98] For discussion, see Martin Hogg, 'Duties of Care, Causation and the Implications of *Chester v Afshar*' (2005) 9 Edinburgh Law Review 156; and Tamsyn Clark and Donal Nolan, 'A Critique of *Chester v Afshar*' (2014) 34 Oxford Journal of Legal Studies 659.

[99] [2017] EWCA Civ 356.   [100] [2018] EWCA Civ 1307 [70].

[101] *Hotson v East Berkshire Area Health Authority* [1987] AC 750. A similar claim was dismissed in the Scottish case of *Kenyon v Bell* 1953 SC 125.

[102] [1987] AC 750, [785].

On the balance of probabilities, the claimant fell into the larger group—there being no evidence that he was one of the fortunate 25% who could benefit from treatment—and, consequently, his injury could not be attributed to the negligence of the defendants. It would be different if 51% of people sustaining the type of injury which the claimant suffered could be treated with, say, a 20% chance of success. Then, on the balance of probabilities, the claimant would have fallen into that group of 51%, and, if a hospital negligently failed to offer him the treatment, he would have personally lost that 20% chance of a successful outcome. Whether that 20% loss is something which should attract compensation in the form of 20% damages was left open by the decision in *Hotson*.[103]

'Loss of a chance' was revisited by the House of Lords in *Gregg v Scott*,[104] where the whole percentage approach towards such cases was called into question. The facts related to what must be, sadly, a common occurrence. A patient presented to his doctor with an uncomfortable lump under his left arm. The doctor diagnosed this as benign and reassured the patient such that this was the patient's one and only visit to the GP. In truth, the lump was a malignant tumour for which aggressive treatment was required. This did not commence until some 14–15 months after the initial consultation, by which time the cancer had spread to the patient's chest. It was accepted that the cursory examination of the patient by his GP was negligent; the crux of the matter was whether this had caused a recognised legal harm. In the final analysis, the claimant argued that his 'harm' was the loss of the chance of survival for more than ten years,[105] or put slightly differently, the loss of the chance of a more favourable outcome to his prognosis.[106] Statistical evidence[107] indicated that while the claimant might have had a 42% chance of still being alive after ten years if there had been no negligence, this chance was reduced to 25% because of the negligence. There was, therefore, a significant drop in his statistical chances as a result of the misdiagnosis, but—crucially—at no point did he enjoy a more-than-50% chance of survival beyond ten years.[108] On a strict application of *Hotson* and the balance of probabilities test, the GP did not cause the alleged harm: it was not 'more probable than not' that but for the negligence the patient would be alive after ten years. Indeed, the trial judge found that he probably would not be. To put it another way, even without negligence, there would have been a 58% chance that the patient would not survive the decade.

This outcome was unacceptable to Lords Nicholls and Hope. Lord Nicholls, in particular, argued forcefully that the 'all-or-nothing' approach to what would have happened but for the negligence—that is, the application of the 49/51% rule from *Hotson*—was premised on a falsehood[109] and led to arbitrary and unjust outcomes: 'It means that a patient

---

[103] For a consideration of *Hotson* and *Bolitho* together, see *Bright v Barnsley District General Hospital NHS Trust* [2005] Lloyd's Rep Med 449.

[104] [2005] UKHL 2. For comment on the majority ruling and the apparent conflict of the decision with the previous authorities of *Hotson* and *Fairchild*, see Jane Stapleton, 'Loss of the Chance for Cure from Cancer' (2005) 68(6) Modern Law Review 996.

[105] [2005] UKHL 2, [87] (Lord Hoffman).

[106] ibid. [125] (Lord Phillips). Lady Hale seems to concur on this analysis, at [226]. *Cf.* Lord Hope who denied that this was a 'loss of a chance' case, at [117].

[107] Which was seriously questioned by Lord Phillips, ibid. [147].

[108] The significance of the criterion of 'survival at ten years' is that this is generally acknowledged in medical circles to amount to a 'cure'. The relevance of this to a legal concept of 'cure' was, however, rejected by Lady Hale, ibid. [197].

[109] Namely, that 'a patient's prospects of recovery are treated as non-existent whenever they exist but fall short of 50%', ibid. [43].

with a 60 per cent chance of recovery reduced to a 40 per cent prospect by medical negligence can obtain compensation. But he can obtain nothing if his prospects were reduced from 40 per cent to nil.'[110] Lord Hope found that the principle on which a patient's loss as a result of negligence is to be calculated—and, presumably, recompensed—is the same whether the prospects were better or worse than 50%.[111] The majority, however, rejected the appeal and did so largely to protect the integrity of legal principles. Lady Hale distinguished the House's rulings in *Fairchild* and *Chester* as cases 'dealing with particular problems which could be remedied without altering the principles applicable to the great majority of personal injury cases which give rise to no real injustice or practical problem.'[112]

She considered the instant case to be an invitation to introduce 'liability for the loss of a chance of a more favourable outcome' but refused to do so for the complexities involved and the consequences that this would have. Those consequences were largely summed up by Lords Phillips and Hoffmann in their view that a departure from *Hotson* would change the basis of causation from probability to possibility; that is, that some form of recovery would be due if it was shown that it was possible that negligence might affect a patient's case. Not only should this be a matter for Parliament, but as Lady Hale put it:

> it would in practice always be tempting to conclude that the doctor's negligence had affected ... [the claimant's] chances to some extent, the claimant would almost always get something. It would be a 'heads you lose everything, tails I win something' situation.

And, finally, we have Lord Phillips:

> it seems to me that there is a danger, if special tests of causation are developed piecemeal to deal with perceived injustices in particular factual situations, that the coherence of our common law will be destroyed.[113]

This rejection of the relevance of loss of a chance to claims for clinical negligence has been confirmed by the Court of Appeal in *Wright (a child)* v *Cambridge Medical Group*.[114] This is also an important case because it clarified the respective liabilities of GPs and those to whom patients are subsequently referred. In *Wright*, there were serial failures on the part of a GP and then a hospital to diagnose timeously an infant's bacterial superinfection. The GP's failure resulted in a two-day delay in referring the child to hospital, and the hospital's failure added three more days to the debacle, by which time the infection had reached the child's hip and resulted in permanent restricted movement. The overarching question was whether the GP's failure to refer was a causative factor, given the subsequent negligence of the hospital. In other words, even if the child had been referred on time, would it be the case that the harm would have resulted anyway, and so could the GP be said to have caused harm in their own right?

The Court of Appeal found that the trial judge had erred in both fact and law in rejecting the liability of the GP. The cumulative events were a 'synergistic reaction' that did not displace the existing legal principle that every tortfeasor should compensate the injured claimant in respect of that loss and damage for which he should justly be held responsible. The hospital's failures were not so egregious as to overwhelm the causative role of the GP's negligence. Moreover, the harms were separable as a matter of fact: the pain suffered in the two-day delay was different from any pain suffered after. Furthermore, and importantly, a GP cannot escape liability for a failure to refer even if there is subsequent

---

[110] ibid. [46].   [111] ibid. [121].   [112] ibid. [192].   [113] [2005] UKHL 2 [172].
[114] [2011] EWCA Civ 669.

negligence because such a failure will always deprive the patient of an opportunity to be treated properly. Finally, the Court revisited the loss of a chance arguments, albeit obiter, confirming their rejection by the House of Lords in *Gregg v Scott* and their failure to deliver a suitably responsive system of justice on the balance of probabilities.[115]

In addition to being a cause in fact, the defendant's actions must also be held to be a legal cause of the harm suffered by the claimant. Whereas factual causation is primarily concerned with how in fact the damage occurred, legal causation is concerned with whether it is fair and reasonable to hold the defendant liable for the harm which occurred. Legal causation can be characterised as about determining the scope of liability and is concerned with ensuring that liability is not imposed when dealing with what would be considered by the courts as remote or unusual consequences of actions. In direct consequences cases where there is an uninterrupted chain of events from the defendant's wrongful act to the harm suffered by the claimant, but unexpected or unusual damage occurs, then courts will rely upon the remoteness (or 'foreseeability of damage') test as was held in the famous *Wagon Mound* litigation.[116] Note that the remoteness test is concerned with the damage that occurred and it asks whether the defendant ought to have reasonably foreseen it. If physical injury of some kind is foreseeable then any physical injury will usually be regarded as sufficiently proximate, even if a particular type of injury was unexpected or unforeseeable. As long as it is the same type of harm, it will be deemed foreseeable.

As a default position, the defendant is usually held responsible for the sequence of events leading to the harm suffered by claimant, and an act of another person (without which the harm would not have occurred) intervenes between the defendant's wrongful act and the harm caused. Generally, the defendant will be liable for that harm unless the intervening act constitutes a *novus actus interveniens* (literally, a 'new act intervening'), i.e. whether it can be considered as breaking the chain of causation between the defendant's wrongful act and the damage. This usually takes one of three forms: (i) act of nature; (ii) intervening conduct of a third party; or (iii) the intervening conduct of the claimant. A recent case which addresses the question of legal causation and the scope of the defendant doctor's duty of care towards a patient claimant in a clinical negligence claim is *Khan v Meadows*.[117]

This was a wrongful birth claim that went on appeal to the Supreme Court and focused primarily on the issue of causation, which we deal with here. A more detailed analysis of the case as a wrongful birth claim is provided later in this chapter. While the negligence of the defendant towards the claimant was not an issue, the extent of recovery for harm caused was very much so. At first instance, damages had been awarded for the cost of raising the claimant's son who had been diagnosed with both haemophilia and autism. On appeal, the question was whether the defendant was liable for the costs of raising a child with haemophilia on its own, which was firmly within the scope of the negligent provision of information to the claimant by the defendant, or whether it extended to autism as well. This raised a scope of duty question on the part of the defendant doctor. In *South Australia Asset Management Corpn v York Montague Ltd*,[118] the House of

---

[115] 'Loss of a chance' arguments were similarly rejected by the High Court in *Oliver v Williams* [2013] EWHC 600 (QB) (delayed diagnosis of ovarian cancer). See further, Gordon Wishart and Andrew Axon, 'Proof of Causation: A New Approach in Cancer Cases' (2013) 19(6) Journal of Patient Safety and Risk Management 130.

[116] See *Wagon Mound (No.1) (Overseas Tankship v Morts Docks Engineering Co Ltd)* [1961] AC 388; *Wagon Mound (No. 2) (Overseas Tankship v The Miller Steamship Co Pty)* [1967] 1 AC 388.

[117] [2021] UKSC 21.   [118] [1997] AC 191.

Lords held that, 'a defendant is not liable in damages in respect of losses of a kind which fall outside the scope of his duty of care.' This has come to be known as 'the SAAMCO principle'. When *Khan* came before the Supreme Court, the matter under consideration was whether the SAAMCO principle applied to clinical negligence cases and, if so, how it should be applied. In their judgment, Lords Hodge and Sales (with whom Lords Reed and Kitchin, as well as Lady Black agreed) set out 'a helpful model for analysing the place of the scope of duty principle in the tort of negligence' which 'consists of asking six questions in sequence. It is not an exclusive or comprehensive analysis, but it may bring some clarity to the role of the scope of duty principle which SAAMCO highlighted'.[119] The questions are as follows:

1. Is the harm (loss, injury and damage) which is the subject matter of the claim actionable in negligence? (The actionability question.)

2. What are the risks of harm to the claimant against which the law imposes on the defendant a duty to take care? (The scope of duty question.)

3. Did the defendant breach his or her duty by his or her act or omission? (The breach question.)

4. Is the loss for which the claimant seeks damages the consequence of the defendant's act or omission? (The factual causation question.)

5. Is there a sufficient nexus between a particular element of the harm for which the claimant seeks damages and the subject matter of the defendant's duty of care as analysed at stage 2? (The duty nexus question.)

6. Is a particular element of the harm for which the claimant seeks damages irrecoverable because it is too remote, or because there is a different effective cause (including *novus actus interveniens*) in relation to it or because the claimant has mitigated his or her loss or has failed to avoid loss which he or she could reasonably have been expected to avoid? (The legal responsibility question.)[120]

In terms of application to the facts of the case in line with the approach set out previously, the court found that the costs of raising a child with a disability in a wrongful birth claim are clearly actionable. The provision of information by the defendant doctor to the claimant was concerned with a specific risk, that risk being that of having a child with haemophilia, and the defendant owed a duty of care to the claimant. The defendant was in breach of her duty to the claimant. Factual causation attributable to the defendant's negligence was established in relation to the birth of the claimant's son. The law did not impose any duty on the defendant in relation to unrelated risks such as autism which could be said to arise in any pregnancy. There was a lack of a sufficient nexus between the defendant's duty of care and the autism such that there was a lack of justification for imposing liability on the defendant for the condition. Finally, with there being no questions raised about remoteness, other effective cause or mitigation of loss, then the law only imposes liability on the defendant for the foreseeable consequences resulting from the (wrongful) birth of the claimant's son, that being haemophilia and the increased cost of raising a child with that condition.

Notwithstanding the joint judgment, there were clearly different points of view expressed by their Lordships Burrows and Leggatt on the value of the six-question approach, as set out. Commentary on the judgment has also questioned the likely reach of the approach with respect to defendants' scope of duty in clinical negligence claims,

---

[119] ibid [28].   [120] ibid.

querying whether it will be confined to information/advice claims or will have broader application.[121] Of particular interest (and indeed concern) is that the infringement of the claimant's autonomy and the invasion of her bodily integrity occasioned by what was a wrongful birth claim,[122] clearly did not merit sustained engagement by the Supreme Court, nor whether such issues might provide a justification for the modification of causation principles on broader policy grounds. We now turn in the next section of the chapter to consider different types of clinical negligence claims. They are offered by way of example to highlight some of the difficult and complex conundrums that are at stake in such claims.

12.4 TYPES OF NEGLIGENCE CLAIMS

12.4.1 DIAGNOSIS

Mistakes in diagnosing a condition can be considered an inevitable hazard of medical practice and will not usually be considered negligent as long as a doctor meets the usual standard of care.[123] Liability may, however, be imposed when a mistake in diagnosis is made because the doctor failed to take a proper medical history,[124] failed to conduct tests which a competent medical practitioner would have considered appropriate, or simply failed to diagnose a condition which would have been spotted by a competent practitioner.

Lower courts have suggested that *Bolam* and the subsequent authorities failed to distinguish between two different types of case, namely, (i) those where the patient's condition was known, and (ii) those where it was unknown, and a diagnosis was required. *Bolam* related to the former; the latter was not envisioned in that original decision, but it still remains subject to *Bolitho*, namely the conduct must have a logical basis.[125] As a minimum, the doctor must examine their patient and pay adequate attention to the patient's medical notes and to what the patient tries to tell them.[126] Telephone diagnosis or advice is hazardous, especially if the facts as related by the patient are such as to raise in the doctor's mind a suspicion that can only be allayed by proper clinical examination.[127]

---

[121] See e.g. Katie Gollop QC, '*Khan* v *Meadows* [2021] UKSC 21 And The New Approach To Negligence: Your Starter For 6' (UK Healthcare Law Blog, 21 June 2021) available at <https://www.ukhealthcarelawblog. co.uk/khan-v-meadows-2021-uksc-21-and-the-new-approach-to-negligence-your-starter-for-6/> accessed 07 December 2022.

[122] For commentary on this point, see Hale LJ in *Selby* v *Groom* [2002] PIQR P18, as discussed later in this chapter.

[123] For an example of a clinical negligence claim which failed because diagnosis and treatment were found to have been determined correctly, see *Meiklejohn* v *St George's Healthcare NHS Trust* [2014] EWCA Civ 1 20. For an example of a successful claim—based on negligent failure to diagnose meningitis—see *Coakley* v *Rosie* [2014] EWHC 1790 (QB).

[124] *Chin Keow* v *Government of Malaysia* [1967] 1 WLR 813 (failure to inquire as to the possibility of penicillin allergy); *Coles* v *Reading and District Hospital Management Committee* (1963) 107 Sol Jo 115 (failure to consider possibility of tetanus).

[125] See *Muller* (n 73).

[126] *Giurelli* v *Girgis* (1980) 24 SASR 264, discussed in Jones (n 2) 290.

[127] *Barnett* v *Chelsea and Kensington Hospital Management Committee* [1969] 1 QB 428; *Cavan* v *Wilcox* (1973) 44 DLR (3d) 42; *Burne* v *A* [2006] EWCA Civ 24 (failure to ask 'closed questions' in arriving at a diagnosis in relation to a child with a known medical condition and history). A number of 'failure to attend' cases have been discussed earlier. Although see the GP phone 'diagnosis' case of *Hewes* v *West Hertfordshire Hospitals NHS Trust* [2018] EWHC 1345 (QB) (no reasonable prospect of success in an action against a GP who advised a patient over the phone to go to A&E rather than to a specialist unit).

One of the problems in determining whether there has been a mistake in diagnosis turns on deciding what investigative techniques need to be used in a particular case. The answer to this is doubly difficult insofar as the decision is now dictated not entirely by medical intuition. Two factors bear heavily on accurate diagnosis. The fragmented nature of modern medicine means that many decisions about appropriate diagnosis and care depend as much on a timely referral than on the skills of an individual doctor.[128] In making their choice of diagnostic options, the doctor must be guided by the 'new *Bolam*'—that is, the test that the courts will read as incorporating an element of 'patient expectation' and also of what might count as a significant factor for the choice of the particular patient.[129] Ordinary laboratory tests must be used if symptoms suggest their use and, here, the situation is eased by the widespread introduction of automated 'battery' testing—the financial implications of doing several rather than a single biochemical analysis are now minimised.

The use of radiography provides a good example of the problem. Both professionals and the public are aware of the major contribution made by diagnostic radiography to the background radiation in developed countries and of the dangers to the individual of cumulative exposure. In *Lakey's* case,[130] the patient suffered a fall and it was agreed that she had sustained a pelvis fracture when she attended hospital. The casualty officer found no evidence of fracture and, since the patient had been exposed to X-irradiation on several previous occasions, he decided against X-ray examination before sending her home; the presence of fracture was, however, confirmed on readmission. The trial judge found that the original decision was taken after conscious deliberation and was not negligent, which was subsequently affirmed by the Court of Appeal. Equally, the Court of Appeal has confirmed the importance of first instance findings of fact that it will overrule only where they are plainly wrong. Disputes over diagnostic procedures can involve differing interpretations of events as between doctor and patient, and the judge is entitled to prefer one over another without an obligation to explain in detail his reasons for doing so,[131] but the rejection of expert opinion at this stage must be on the basis of it having 'no logic'.[132]

In cases where a doctor is doubtful about a diagnosis, good practice may require that the patient be referred to a specialist for further consideration. It may be difficult for a doctor to know when to seek specialist advice, a fact that was explicitly acknowledged in *Wilsher*. In case of doubt, it is certainly safer for a doctor to refer the patient.[133] In *Official Solicitor* v *Allinson*,[134] a GP was found liable in negligence when a patient died from breast cancer after he had examined her and reassured her there was nothing to worry about. His negligence was demonstrated by the failure at least to review his patient's condition within a short period of time given the asymmetry and localised abnormality of the lump in her breast and, on the probable findings at review, for failing to refer her to a specialist.[135]

---

[128] Note that a failure to refer (timeously) can be as much a breach of duty of care as an inappropriate diagnosis; see *Wright (a child)* v *Cambridge Medical Group* [2011] EWCA Civ 669.

[129] See *Birch* v *University College London Hospital NHS Foundation Trust* [2008] EWHC 2237 (QB); *Montgomery* v *Lanarkshire Health Board* [2015] UKSC 11.

[130] *Lakey* v *Merton, Sutton and Wandsworth Health Authority* (1999) 40 BMLR 18.

[131] *Burnett* v *Lynch* [2012] EWCA Civ 347.   [132] ibid.

[133] It is to be noted that access to a second opinion is now a matter of patient entitlement.

[134] [2004] EWHC 923 (QB).

[135] For the kinds of factors taken into account in assessing damages with delayed diagnosis, see *Woodward* v *Leeds Teaching Hospitals NHS Trust* [2012] EWHC 2167. For another 'failure to refer' case—this time in the context of allegation of sexual abuse—see *C* v *Cairns* [2003] Lloyd's Rep Med 90. Negligence was not found in the case.

In this context, it is also important to consider what have been described as 'pure diagnosis' claims. The cases of *Bolam* and *Bolitho* concerned the provision of medical treatment and whether the doctor had acted within a responsible range of medical opinion. In such circumstances, there is room for a genuine difference of opinion. There are, however, cases where a diagnosis is likely right or wrong, leaving little leeway for such a difference in opinion. A recent case of interest in this regard is that of *Brady v Southend University Hospital NHS Foundation Trust*.[136] The claimant had undergone a series of scans to determine the cause of pain in her abdomen, in which different diagnoses had been offered. Subsequently, she underwent a biopsy which confirm that she had an infection and abscess in her abdomen which required surgical drainage. The claimant alleged that had this specific diagnosis been made earlier then she would not have needed to undergo this surgical procedure. She argued that the radiologists who had performed the initial scans had breached their duty of care by failing to make the correct diagnosis. In the circumstances, where the central allegation of negligence focuses on diagnosis, it was further argued that questions of acceptable practice do not apply in line with the principles set out in *Bolam* and *Bolitho*. The High Court did not accept the claimant's arguments in this regard, finding that in fact such principles did apply and therefore that the defendant hospital was not negligent.[137] It has been suggested that the judgment should provide reassurance to clinicians that even if a diagnosis that they have made turns out to be wrong, they will not be found to be negligent if the court accepts that a responsible body of their peers would support the decision they made.[138]

12.4.2 TREATMENT

Where negligence is alleged to have taken place in treatment, the most important distinction to be made is between a medical mistake which the law regards as excusable[139] and a mistake which would amount to negligence.[140] In the former case, the court accepts that ordinary human fallibility precludes liability while, in the latter, the conduct of the defendant is considered to have strayed beyond the bounds of what is expected of the reasonably skilful or competent doctor. The issue came before the courts most classically in *Whitehouse v Jordan*, which still remains the authoritative example.[141] In this case, negligence was alleged on the part of an obstetrician who, it was claimed, had pulled too hard in a trial of forceps delivery and had thereby caused the claimant's head to become wedged, with consequent asphyxia and brain damage. The trial judge held that, although the decision to perform a trial of forceps was a reasonable one, the defendant had in fact pulled too hard and was therefore negligent. This initial finding of negligence was reversed in the Court of Appeal and, in a strongly worded judgment, Lord Denning emphasised that an error of judgement was not negligence.[142] When the matter came on

---

[136] [2020] EWHC 158.

[137] For an overview, see Samantha Schnabel, 'Brady v Southend University Hospital NHS Foundation Trust [2020] EWHC 158: "Pure Diagnosis" Claims and Setting the Professional Standard of Care' (2021) 29(2) Medical Law Review 373.

[138] DAC Beachcroft, 'Is It Always Negligent to Get it "Wrong"?' (20 February 2020) available at <https://www.dacbeachcroft.com/es/gb/articles/2020/february/is-it-always-negligent-to-get-it-wrong/> accessed 07 December 2022.

[139] See e.g. *E v Castro* (2003) 80 BMLR 14. For which, also see the rigid application of the *Bolam* test.

[140] For discussion, see Alan Merry and Warren Brookbanks, *Merry and McCall Smith's Errors, Medicine and the Law* (2nd edn, CUP 2017).

[141] [1981] 1 All ER 267.   [142] [1980] 1 All ER 650 CA [658].

appeal before the House of Lords, the views expressed by Lord Denning on the error of judgement question were rejected. An error of judgement could be negligence if it were an error which would not have been made by a reasonably competent professional man acting with ordinary care. As Lord Fraser pointed out:

> The true position is that an error of judgment may, or may not, be negligent; it depends on the nature of the error. If it is one that would not have been made by a reasonably competent professional man professing to have the standard and type of skill that the defendant holds himself out as having, and acting with ordinary care, then it is negligence. If, on the other hand, it is an error that such a man, acting with ordinary care, might have made, then it is not negligence.[143]

In the event, the House of Lords held that there had not, in any case, been sufficient evidence to justify the trial judge's finding of negligence.[144] Further examples of how circumstances can overwhelm a situation and tip the balance in favour of negligence include *Boustead v North West Strategic Health Authority*.[145] Here a child suffered brain damage due to hypoxia which was caused by a delay in deciding to opt for a Caesarean section. While much of the conduct of the HCPs in managing the childbirth was not judged to be negligent, eventually the failure to perform a caesarean section in light of the growing evidence of foetal distress amounted to a tragic and negligent error of judgement leading to compensation for the child. In *Mugweni v NHS London*,[146] brain damage was also in issue arising from a cardiac arrest suffered by a patient during open-heart surgery. The Court confirmed a breach of duty on the part of the anaesthetist for failing to notice early signs of distress, irrespective of the fact that the rest of the team was distracted preparing for the patient's removal. Indeed, particular vigilance was especially required during this time. The case however failed on causation.

Gross medical mistakes will almost always result in a finding of negligence. Operating mistakes such as the removal of the wrong limb or the performance of an operation on the wrong patient are usually treated as indefensible and settled out of court; hence the paucity of decisions on such points.[147] Use of the wrong drug or, often with more serious consequences, the wrong gas during the course of an anaesthetic will frequently lead to the imposition of liability, and in some of these situations the *res ipsa loquitur* principle (discussed going forward) may be applied.

Many historic cases deal with items of operating equipment being left inside patients after surgery. In these, generally known as the 'swab cases', the allocation of liability is made according to the principle laid down in the early decision in *Mahon v Osborne*.[148] In such cases, the courts have shown themselves unlikely to dictate the *exact* procedure that doctors should use to ensure that no foreign bodies are left in the patient. At the same time, however, the law requires that there should be some sort of set procedures adopted

---

[143] [1981] 1 All ER 267 [281]. See a very comparable case in which the obstetrician was found to have pulled on the forceps with a force beyond that which would have been used by a competent practitioner. The difficult issue of causation in cases of neonatal brain damage was also well aired: *Townsend v Worcester and District Health Authority* (1995) 23 BMLR 31.

[144] A misjudgement will also be negligent if it is in respect of something 'lying within the area where only a sound judgment measures up to the standard of reasonable competence expected': *Hendy v Milton Keynes Health Authority (No 2)* [1992] 3 Med LR 119 [127] (Jowitt J).

[145] [2008] EWHC 2375 (QB).   [146] [2012] EWCA Civ 20.

[147] An example is *Ibrahim (a minor) v Muhammad* (21 May 1984, unreported), QBD, in which a penis was partially amputated during circumcision; only the quantum of damages was in dispute.

[148] [1939] 2 KB 14.

in order to minimise the possibility of this occurring. Overall responsibility rests on the surgeon; he is not entitled to delegate the matter altogether to a nurse. This point was emphasised in *Mahon* by Lord Goddard, who said:

> As it is the task of the surgeon to put swabs in, so it is his task to take them out and if the evidence is that he has not used a reasonable standard of care he cannot absolve himself, if a mistake has been made, by saying, 'I relied on the nurse'.[149]

In *Urry* v *Bierer*,[150] the Court of Appeal confirmed that the patient was entitled to expect the surgeon to do all that was reasonably necessary to ensure that all packs were removed and that this duty required more than mere reliance on the nurse's count.

12.4.3 PROTECTING PATIENTS FROM THEMSELVES

In certain circumstances, it is part of the duty of care of doctors and nurses to predict that patients may damage themselves due to their medical condition.[151] The extent of the duty to safeguard against such damage is problematic, and the decisions have not all gone the same way. In *Selfe* v *Ilford and District Hospital Management Committee*,[152] the claimant had been admitted to hospital after a drug overdose. Although he had known suicidal tendencies, he was not kept under constant observation and climbed onto the hospital roof while the two nurses on duty were out of the ward; he fell and was injured. Damages of £19,000 were awarded against the hospital. In contrast, the claimant in *Thorne* v *Northern Group Hospital Management Committee*[153] failed to win an award of damages for the death of his wife who had left a hospital in suicidal mood. In this case, the patient had slipped out of the hospital when the nurses' backs were turned, returned home, and gassed herself. The court took the view that, although the degree of supervision which a hospital should exercise in relation to patients with known suicidal tendencies is higher than that to be exercised over other patients, they could not be kept under constant supervision by hospital staff.

A similar view was expressed by the Court of Appeal in *Dunn* v *South Tyneside Health Care NHS Trust*,[154] where a bipolar patient on one-hourly observations evaded detection and returned home to consume large quantities of anti-asthma tablets which resulted in severe brain damage. The subsequent negligence action claimed that an observation regime at 15-minute intervals was the appropriate standard of care; moreover, had this been implemented, the harm would not have resulted because the police would have been alerted sooner and would have found the patient. The action failed on both counts. The one-hour regime was a reasonable standard of care given the patient's history and mental state on detention and by reference to *Bolam* and *Bolitho*; furthermore, the Court found that it was not an established matter of 'fact' that the police would have intervened to prevent the harm even if they had been alerted earlier.

---

[149] [1939] 2 KB 14 [47]. Scott LJ qualified this by pointing out that it might be necessary to dispense with normal precautions in an emergency.

[150] (1955) *The Times*, 15 July, CA.

[151] For the nature and extent of the non-medical duty of care in such cases in respect of people in detention, see *Gary Smiley (through his litigation friend Raymond Smiley)* v *Home Office* [2004] EWHC 240, following *Reeves* v *The Commissioner of Police of the Metropolis* [2000] 1 AC 360.

[152] (1970) 114 Sol Jo 935.

[153] (1964) 108 Sol Jo 484. A similar decision was taken in the Scottish case *Rolland* v *Lothian Health Board* (1981, unreported), OH (Lord Ross).

[154] [2003] EWCA Civ 878. See also the approval of *Hunter* in *McHardy* v *Dundee Hospitals* 1960 SLT (notes) 19.

Whether suicide when under medical care is a human rights matter was discussed by the House of Lords in *Savage v South Essex Partnership NHS Trust*.[155] This case was brought as an alleged breach of Article 2 ECHR the right to life, by the daughter of a woman who escaped from a mental health unit and took her own life. Although the court questioned the *locus standi* of the daughter in such a case, they nonetheless let the case go to trial and, in doing so, clarified some of the parameters of the duty of care with respect to at-risk persons and the relationship with the ECHR. As pointed out by Lord Rodger, there is an overarching obligation to protect lives of patients in hospital, connected to which are ancillary obligations such as employing suitably trained staff and instituting safe working and security practices; failure to do so can lead to a finding of a violation of Article 2 ECHR. By the same token, if such systems are in place but, nevertheless, a patient kills themselves, then it is unlikely that Article 2 will be engaged although it is possible that an action might lie in professional negligence; for example, because an HCP failed to carry out surveillance properly.[156] While the obligations overlap, they are not entirely the same. More particularly, if staff know someone is a 'real and immediate' suicide risk, they must do all that is reasonable to prevent this, and failure to do so would result in the possibility of both the breach of duty of care and violation of human rights.

The Supreme Court has pronounced on the nature and scope of duties of care to voluntary mental health patients and their families in *Rabone and Another v Pennine Care NHS Foundation Trust*.[157] Here, the Trust had admitted a depressed patient on a voluntary basis; that is, not subject to mental health legislation, and assessed her as a high suicide risk. Subsequently, the patient was allowed to return home for two days whereupon she killed herself. The novel legal issues that arose were as follows: (1) whether a Trust owes a duty of care to protect an informal psychiatric patient in the same way as a sectioned patient in cases where there is a real and imminent risk of suicide, and (2) whether a duty was also owed to the parents of the patient who suffered non-patrimonial loss due to their daughter's death. The Supreme Court answered both questions in the affirmative. It is now clear that duties to voluntary and sectioned patients to be protected from themselves are substantially similar. In practice, it means that there should be an assessment of all such patients as to whether there is a real and immediate risk of suicide; if this is found to be the case then, for a voluntary patient, a Trust would be justified in moving to the Mental Health regime to detain the patient, even against their will. The duty to parents arose from Article 2 ECHR—and they counted as 'victims' under Article 34 of the Convention, as was well established by the European Court of Human Rights jurisprudence.[158]

In certain circumstances, a negligence claim against a healthcare provider can be defended partially on the grounds of contributory negligence. A court may reduce the amount of damages awarded if a patient's conduct is seen as irresponsible and contributing to the harm sustained. *Pidgeon v Doncaster HA* remains the classic application of the doctrine in the medical sphere.[159] In this case, the patient's cervical smear test had been diagnosed incorrectly as being negative. Nevertheless, the patient had refused to respond to numerous requests from her GP to submit to additional tests that would have

---

[155] [2009] 1 AC 681.
[156] See *Powell v United Kingdom* (admissibility) (Application 45305/99) [2000] Inquest LR 19 ECHR.
[157] [2012] UKSC 2.
[158] See, for example, *Yasa v Turkey* (1998) 28 EHRR 408. For commentary, see Mads Tønnesson Andenæs, 'Leading From the Front: Human Rights and Tort Law in *Rabone* and *Reynolds*' (2012) 128 LQR 323.
[159] [2002] Lloyd's Rep Med 130.

indicated pre-cancerous abnormalities. The patient's failure to present for further testing was viewed as blameworthy,[160] and she was held responsible for two-thirds of her injury. The doctrine of contributory negligence has also been invoked to reduce the award of damages in a case of suicide while under police custody.[161] It was held that the deceased had autonomous control over his own actions; responsibility for the suicide would therefore be shared equally between the deceased and the defendant.

12.5 WRONGFUL CONCEPTION, BIRTH, AND LIFE

Actions for wrongful conception, pregnancy, and wrongful birth are are particular types of clinical negligence claims. There may be circumstances where the birth of a child occurs that was unplanned and due to negligence on the part of an HCP, such as negligent provision of pre-conception advice or a failed sterilisation procedure. Such claims are often referred to as either wrongful conception or wrongful pregnancy claims (and we use the term wrongful conception). Wrongful birth claims usually arise where there has been a failure on the part of the HCP to inform of a genetic condition or disability where the mother would have terminated her pregnancy had she been informed. Subsequently, a child is born of that pregnancy with such a disability. Wrongful life claims are those brought on behalf of a child, where it is alleged that their birth arose due to the HCP's negligence. It goes without saying that the categories may overlap; a wrongful conception can also result in the wrongful birth of an unplanned child with a disability, for example.[162]

12.5.1 WRONGFUL CONCEPTION

Before discussing the nature of the duty of care in relation to a claim for wrongful conception, we must first consider to whom the duty is owed. Clearly, if a person seeks sterilisation independently of their partner, then the doctor's duty of care is limited to that person. By contrast, the doctor owes a duty to both partners if they both attend a medical consultation seeking a limitation on fertility that is of benefit to both. It follows from either premise that the doctor cannot be held liable to a potential present or future sexual partner of their patient of whom they have no knowledge.[163] Assuming, however, that a duty of care has been established, liability for a pregnancy resulting from an unsuccessful sterilisation will not be imposed unless it can be established that the doctor failed in their duty. Such failure can, in turn, be attributable either to incompetent clinical expertise or to an inadequate explanation of the inherent shortcomings of the procedure, in particular,

---

[160] For a contrasting outcome see *P* v *Sedar* [2011] EWHC 1266 (QB), where the patient's failure to present for further testing was not seen as blameworthy because letters had been sent to the wrong address.

[161] *Reeves* (n 151).

[162] We do recognise at times there is slippage between the use of the terms wrongful conception, wrongful pregnancy, and wrongful birth, as well as the principles underpinning such claims, in academic commentary and case law. We also note the observations by Yip J in *MNX* v *Meadows* [2017] EWHC 2990 (QB) at [10]–[11]: 'I cannot see that any sensible distinction can be drawn on the basis of whether it is the conception or the birth that is described as wrongful', who draws on earlier commentary made by Hale LJ in *Groom* v *Selby* [2002] PIQR P18, where she stated: 'The principles applicable in wrongful birth cases cannot sensibly be distinguished from the principles applicable in wrongful conception cases'. For further commentary on this point, see Graeme Laurie, Shaun Harmon, and Edward Dove, *Mason and McCall Smith's Law and Medical Ethics* (11th edn, OUP 2019) chapter 11.

[163] *Goodwill* v *British Pregnancy Advisory Service* [1996] 2 All ER 161.

the possibility that conception might still occur after the sterilisation procedure has been performed. As to what constitutes a breach of duty of care, this is still largely governed by the *Bolam/Bolitho* standard. The majority of actions based on the negligent performance of a sterilising operation will generally be of this relatively simple type and that liability may well be acknowledged prior to any court hearing. An exception would almost certainly lie when the patient has insisted on a modified operation in the anticipation of reversal at some time in the future,[164] but the situation would be far more doubtful where the individual doctor modified their surgical technique with this in mind.[165] A relatively specific aspect of negligent sterilisation in women is, however, to be found in a failure to diagnose pre-existing pregnancy at the time of the operation in question.

Common law actions in both negligence and contract have arisen based entirely on the grounds of inadequate provision of warning of the possibility of failure of a sterilisation operation. In such cases, the supposed deficit has proved to be no more than a matter of misunderstanding—in effect, providing good examples of the distinction to be made between consent that is based on information and that which is based on understanding of the information. In the case of *Thake* v *Maurice*,[166] the issue turned eventually on the definition of the word 'irreversible'—the defendant claiming that it implied no more than that the procedure could not be reversed by surgery, while the claimant contended that it represented a contract[167] to provide absolute sterility which was beyond recall by nature. After overturning the first instance decision that there was a breach of contract, it was held on appeal that the doctor had been negligent in his failure to warn of the possibility of natural reversal of vasectomy. A rather similar case turned on the interpretation of the words on the form signifying consent to the operation which stated, 'We understand that this means we can have no children' and which the claimants contended amounted to a representation that the operation was foolproof; the trial judge, however, held that the words merely acknowledged that the intended effect of the operation was that the couple should not have more children and found for the defendants.[168]

Damages following a wrongful pregnancy can be sought under two main heads. First, there are those that derive from the pregnancy itself, including damages for the pain and suffering of gestation and childbirth together with recompense for loss of earnings or additional expenses resulting from pregnancy and recovery—the bases of what can be loosely referred to as 'the mother's claim'. Second, and far more controversial, is the claim for the upkeep of the resulting child until, or even beyond, maturity. Put in simplest terms, the questions at issue have been whether damages for the upkeep of an unplanned child should ever be awarded and, if so, whether the health condition of the child or its mother should affect the quantum.

[164] As exemplified in the very early twin Canadian cases of *Doiron* v *Orr* (1978) 86 DLR (3d) 719 and *Cataford* v *Moreau* (1978) 114 DLR (3d) 585. Liability for a subsequent pregnancy was not imposed in the former in which the operation had been modified; the surgeon was found to have been negligent in the latter where there were no such extenuating conditions.

[165] In *Re M (a minor) (wardship: sterilisation)* [1988] 2 FLR 497, expert evidence preferred to look upon tubal ligation as being 'contraceptive in nature'. The sterilisation was, however, non-voluntary and the argument was based on different premises.

[166] [1986] QB 644. It was later said of the trial stage of this case: 'I, for my part, think that . . . the less we say about that decision, the better' (*Eyre* v *Measday* [1986] 1 All ER 488 [492] (Lord Slade)).

[167] Mr Thake was, in fact, a private patient.

[168] *Worster* v *City and Hackney Health Authority* (1987) *The Times*, 22 June. As a further hurdle, the claimants may have to convince the court that they would have continued contraceptive methods if they had been informed of a risk: *Newell* v *Goldenberg* [1995] 6 Med LR 371.

On the face of things, the issue is reasonably clear. A doctor owes a duty of care to a couple. They have failed in that duty and, as a result, the very circumstance their medical treatment was intended to avert has, in fact, occurred; therefore, the couple are entitled to recover damages as a result.[169] The fact that a child—and, particularly, a healthy child—is involved, however, introduces complications which are more of a moral than legal nature; in essence, objection to any award in such a context is based on the view that a child is a blessing and that the gift of a child should never be regarded as a matter for financial compensation. And we will see later how this view may have weathered over the years. In passing, though, we would highlight how strongly the 'child as a blessing' trope still holds sway over the courts. However, it should be kept in mind that there are four possibilities in the solution of actions for wrongful conception: damages should never be awarded; damages should always be awarded; the blessing of parenthood should be offset against the concurrent economic loss and the damages adjusted accordingly; and, finally, a distinction should be made between healthy children and those with a disability, and damages should be awarded only for the extra costs involved in the upkeep of the latter.

The validity of the wrongful conception action was upheld in *Udale* v *Bloomsbury Area Health Authority*,[170] in which damages were given for pain and suffering along with loss of earnings following a negligently performed operation; at the same time, an award in respect of the cost of bringing up the child was firmly rejected. In his judgment, Jupp J reiterated that the joy of having the child and the benefits it brought in terms of love should be set off against the inconvenience and financial disadvantages resulting from its birth: 'It is an assumption of our culture', he suggested, 'that the coming of a child into the world is an occasion for rejoicing'.[171]

The Court of Appeal opposed this view in the later case of *Emeh* v *Kensington and Chelsea and Westminster Area Health Authority*,[172] where, in addition, there was a strong rejection of the trial judge's view that the claimant's refusal of abortion was so unreasonable as to eclipse the defendant's wrongdoing.[173] Equally significantly, however, the Court of Appeal awarded damages for the cost of rearing the child and rejected the policy objections voiced in *Udale*. Despite the somewhat unsatisfactory nature of the case, *Emeh* became the leading authority in England and the practice of allowing damages for the costs of raising an unplanned healthy child was followed in a succession of cases. These included special damages for the costs associated with any disabilities and, even for the costs of private education when that seemed appropriate.[174] None of these costs were challenged on appeal. Indeed, the only remaining difficulty appeared to lie in the relationship between the two heads of damage—were they distinct or did one flow from the other?

---

[169] See, e.g. *Rees* v *Darlington Memorial Hospital NHS Trust* [2002] 2 All ER 177 [44] (Waller LJ) quoting previous concurrence.

[170] [1983] 2 All ER 522. Similar sentiments were expressed in an unreported negligence case, *Jones* v *Berkshire Area Health Authority*, first quoted in *Gold* v *Haringey Health Authority* [1986] 1 FLR 125; revsd [1988] QB 481.

[171] At All ER 531, WLR 1109.

[172] (1983) *The Times*, 3 January; revsd [1985] QB 1012.

[173] Also see *Crouchman* v *Burke* (1997) 40 BMLR 163, [176] (Langley J), where a woman who would have had an early termination refused one at 15 weeks 'for understandable reasons'. It is now doubtful if a different approach would be adopted in respect of an early abortion.

[174] *Benarr* v *Kettering Health Authority* [1988] 138 NLJ Rep 179; *Robinson* v *Salford Health Authority* (1992) 3 Med LR 270; *Allen* v *Bloomsbury Health Authority* [1993] 1 All ER 651; *Crouchman* (n 173).

The Court of Appeal later held that a wrongful conception is a personal injury which cannot be separated from its consequences.[175]

The Scottish case of *McFarlane* v *Tayside Health Board*[176] would prove to be seminal in the field. Mr and Mrs McFarlane already had four children when Mr McFarlane underwent a vasectomy. He was subsequently informed that he could safely resume sexual relations without undertaking contraceptive methods. When Mrs McFarlane became pregnant some two years later, she and her husband raised an action in negligence. In accordance with established practice, this was in two parts: the 'mother's claim' for pain and suffering during pregnancy and childbirth and the 'parents' claim' for the upkeep of the child until maturity.

At first instance, the Lord Ordinary in the Outer House of the Court of Session held that a pregnancy culminating in a healthy child could not be regarded as an injury and therefore could not provide the basis for an award of financial compensation. He also decided that the joys of the child's existence wholly compensated the financial cost of its upbringing. This decision was reversed in the Inner House, where the Lord Justice Clerk focused on the basic principles of Scots law.[177] An obligation to make reparation arises when there is concurrence of *injuria* (wrongdoing) and *damnum* (interference with the person's legal interests)—and these conditions were satisfied once the pregnancy was established.[178] The Inner House rejected the proposition that the blessing of a child was an overriding benefit, pointing out that the couple were relying on sterilisation to avoid the cost of raising another child. *Damnum* was therefore manifested in both the impact of pregnancy and childbirth on Mrs McFarlane's bodily integrity, and the pecuniary interests of both parents. The court went on to conclude that there was no overriding consideration of public policy which would be contravened by awarding damages.

Most commentators assumed that equilibrium between English and Scots law had been re-established, but *McFarlane* was appealed to the House of Lords.[179] The House decided by a 4:1 majority that the 'mother's claim' in respect of pain and suffering due to pregnancy and childbirth should stand, but the main appeal, related to the costs of bringing up an unplanned healthy child, was upheld unanimously. The reasoning behind this U-turn in the development of the jurisprudence has never been easy to unravel, given that the doctor's duty of care to the pursuers was admitted and acknowledged by way of the 'mother's claim'; each of the five Lords of Appeal gave different reasons for their decision.[180] Lord Slynn concluded that it would be neither just nor reasonable to impose liability on the doctor for the upkeep of a child until maturity and this is the theme which

---

[175] *Walkin* v *South Manchester Health Authority* [1995] 4 All ER 132; (1995) 25 BMLR 108. Which meant, in passing, that actions for wrongful pregnancy would be subject to the Limitation Act 1980, s 11—followed in *Godfrey* v *Gloucestershire Royal Infirmary NHS Trust* [2003] EWHC 549 (QB). But note the opposite view taken in the British Columbia Court of Appeal in the same year in a case of wrongful birth: *Arndt* v *Smith* [1996] 7 Med LR 108.

[176] 1997 SLT 211 (1996).

[177] *McFarlane and McFarlane* v *Tayside Health Board* 1998 SC 389 [393].

[178] Reiterated by Lord McCluskey 1998 SC 389 [398] who went so far as to hold that the right of a married couple to have sexual relations with each other without any likelihood that those relations will result in a pregnancy is a right that the law recognises. The House specifically held that the deliberate continuation of the pregnancy did not affect the chain of causation: *cf.* Slade LJ in *Emeh* v *Kensington and Chelsea and Westminster Health Authority*, n 172.

[179] *McFarlane* v *Tayside Health Board* [2000] 2 AC 59.

[180] See Victoria Chico, 'Saviour Siblings: Trauma and Tort Law' (2006) 14(2) Medical Law Review 180 and, covering much the same field from a different perspective, Nicolette Priaulx, *The Harm Paradox: Tort Law and the Unwanted Child in an Era of Choice* (Routledge 2007).

is adopted most often in the post-*McFarlane* case law.[181] Lord Steyn took refuge in some rather tenuous concepts of distributive justice. Lord Hope thought that, since the benefits associated with a healthy child were incalculable, it was illogical to attempt an assessment of the net economic loss sustained by the child's parents. Lord Clyde was struck by the disproportion between the damages available when based on the full costs of upbringing and the surgeon's degree of culpability. Finally, Lord Millett held that the law must accept the birth of a healthy baby as a blessing, not a detriment.

In essence, it could be argued that the problem does not lie in the value of a child but is simply that of whether two persons should be compensated if their financial resources are diverted due to the negligence of their treating doctor who had provided medical treatment to prevent that very outcome. Moreover, the House of Lords in *McFarlane* deliberately left open the possibility of recompense for the upkeep of an unplanned child with a disability. Since this was, apparently, still available by way of existing precedent, the resulting doubt had to be settled with some urgency. Efforts both to circumvent the decision and to clarify the situation were, therefore, to be expected. Attempts to undermine the 'healthy child = no maintenance' rule were disposed of summarily. In *Richardson v LRC Products Ltd*,[182] a burst condom case brought under section 3 of the Consumer Protection Act 1987, it was clearly held that the rule applied whether the claim was laid in negligence or in breach of a statutory duty. *Greenfield v Irwin (a firm)*[183] was a further case of missed pregnancy rather than failed sterilisation; otherwise, the conditions were very similar to those in *McFarlane*. The claimant sought to distinguish her case on the grounds that her loss was consequent on the physical injury of the pregnancy rather than on negligent advice and there was a difference between expenditure on a child and loss of earnings due to caring for that child. The Court of Appeal found both distinctions to be irrelevant; the suggestion that failure to provide financial support would contravene Article 8 ECHR—respect for family life—was also dismissed.

In contrast, attempts to entrench the possible exception for disabled children firmly within the law have, in general, been successful. In *Parkinson v St James and Seacroft University Hospital NHS Trust*,[184] a woman gave birth to a child with a disability following an admittedly negligent sterilisation operation. Brooke LJ pointed out that parents in a similar position had been able to recover damages for some 15 years following *Emeh* and that both the 'fair, just, and reasonable' test and the principles of distributive justice would be satisfied if the award was limited to the special costs associated with the disability. He was supported in a powerful speech by Hale LJ, who started from the premise that to cause a woman to become pregnant against her will was an invasion of her bodily integrity; she then listed the consequences of pregnancy which retained an invasive nature. She could find nothing unusual, or contrary to legal principle, in awarding damages in such a case on the ground that the caring role and therefore interference with the woman's personal autonomy persists throughout childhood. The admission of damages limited to the restitution of costs beyond those involved in bringing up a child without a disability gave no offence to those with disability and simply acknowledged the costs of raising a child with a disability.

---

[181] See *Caparo Industries plc v Dickman* [1990] 2 AC 605; *Robinson v Chief Constable of West Yorkshire* [2018] UKSC 4.

[182] [2000] PIQR P164.

[183] [2001] EWCA Civ 113, sub nom *Greenfield v Flather and Others* (2001) 59 BMLR 43.

[184] [2001] 3 WLR 376. It is to be noted that, even so, the child's disability in *Parkinson* (autism) only became apparent during infancy as opposed to at birth.

The importance of Lady Hale's opinion could be said to lie in her argument that the invasion of bodily integrity can be applied almost verbatim to the birth of an unplanned healthy child and, somewhat paradoxically, this leads one to question the logic of the *Parkinson* decision. It was, in fact, agreed that the child's disability was in no way attributable to a breach of duty on the defendant's part; that being the case, why is liability apportioned in *Parkinson* but not in *McFarlane*? The tenor of the *Parkinson* judgment leaves a strong impression of the court's dissatisfaction with the superior court's ruling in *McFarlane*[185] and the decision in the Court of Appeal in the former. It was not appealed to the House of Lords. In any case, the extent to which compensation for the unplanned birth of a child with a disability is available is not entirely settled which in the light of later litigation in the field, may have significant implications.

Hale LJ's innovative recognition of the invasive nature of the negligence involved in cases of unwanted pregnancy was further expressed in *Groom v Selby*,[186] which was tried at first instance before, and at appeal after, the Court of Appeal hearing in *Parkinson*. *Groom* arose from a sterilisation which was carried out in the presence of an unnoticed pregnancy. The claimant later consulted her GP who negligently failed to diagnose her pregnancy until her foetus was so far developed as to make a termination personally unacceptable. She subsequently gave birth to a healthy child, albeit born three weeks prematurely. Some three weeks after birth, the child developed meningitis due to infection by salmonella organisms derived from her mother's birth canal, leaving her with a degree of brain damage. Therefore, the facts of the case raise an interesting variation on wrongful conception cases: was the child born healthy and therefore subject to *McFarlane*, or was she born with a disability as a consequence of negligence during the birth process? At first instance, Clark J found the latter to be the case, and the Court of Appeal upheld the first instance judgment. Brooke LJ summarised the position:

> [The] birth of a premature child who suffered salmonella meningitis through exposure to a bacterium during the normal processes of birth was a foreseeable consequence of Dr Selby's failure to advise the claimant that, although she had been sterilised, she was in fact pregnant.[187]

At first glance, this seems harsh but acceptable in that a foetus is not 'born alive' until it is completely extruded from the mother; the infant's 'injury' here was clearly inflicted during the birth process. However, Brooke LJ went a stage further and considered that, although the child was apparently healthy at birth, 'it should not stand in the way of our doing justice, in a case like the present, in which a child's enduring handicaps, caused by the normal incidents of intra-uterine development and birth, were triggered within the first month of her life.' He went on to say that the longer the period before the disability becomes apparent, the more difficult it may be to establish a right to recover compensation. Whether it is right to undermine the *McFarlane* rule in such indefinite terms remains to be established.

In her judgment in *Groom*, Hale LJ repeated her view that the costs of bringing up a child who was born due to another's negligence are not 'pure' economic loss but, rather, economic loss consequent upon the invasion of a woman's bodily integrity. Her concept of unavoidable responsibility imposed by motherhood was, again, applied when she

---

[185] Described by Kirby J as a 'rebellion' in *Cattanach v Melchior* (2003) 215 CLR 1 [166]. See also *Rees v Darlington Memorial NHS Trust* [2003] 4 All ER 987 [143] (Lord Scott).
[186] (2002) 64 BMLR 47; [2002] Lloyd's Rep Med 1 [31], CA.   [187] ibid. [24].

extended the potential *McFarlane* exception from disability in the resultant child to disability in its mother. In *Rees v Darlington Memorial Hospital NHS Trust*,[188] a healthy child was born following a negligently performed sterilisation operation on a woman who was severely visually disabled. Hale LJ could see no essential difference between compensating for the extra costs of bringing up a child with a disability as opposed to one that did not have a disability (per *Parkinson*) and compensating a woman for the extra costs in supporting a healthy child that were dictated by her own disability. This continued and extended the concept of a persisting injury resulting from wrongful conception/pregnancy cases that she developed in *Parkinson*. Hale LJ thought that this did no more than put the mother in the same position as her 'able bodied fellows' who, by contrast, had no need for additional help in attending to a child's basic needs. Walker LJ, while rejecting the argument based on a 'deemed equilibrium' between the advantages and disadvantages of an unplanned healthy child, nevertheless agreed that the circumstances of the case were not covered by *McFarlane* and represented a legitimate extension of *Parkinson*. In a dissenting judgment, Waller LJ pointed to the unfairness of compensating a woman by virtue of her physical disability when other mothers in as great a need could not benefit. He also noted in McFarlane that a claim brought for damages for bringing up a healthy child born as a result of the negligence of a doctor would succeed under the established rules of tort law.[189] There is little doubt that a case that was decided to the contrary on what were, largely, moral principles, provides a less than satisfactory base from which to explore its various implications.

An influential Commonwealth case on point worth mentioning is *Cattanach v Melchior*,[190] which came before the High Court of Australia shortly after the House of Lords' judgment in *McFarlane*. The circumstances in *Cattanach* were comparable to *McFarlane*, save that it involved a negligent female sterilisation. The key issue at appeal was whether a court could award damages which would involve the doctor, whose negligence was responsible for the birth of a child, bearing the cost of raising and maintaining such child. The arguments in the judgment provide an interesting contrast to those deployed in *McFarlane*. In essence, they rested on whether the court should be governed by moral or legal principles: that is, is it wrong that the addition of a much loved, albeit unplanned, child to a family should be regarded as compensable damage, or should the legal principles of tort law be maintained in the face of such moral considerations? In the end, the High Court divided 4:3 in favour of legal principle and rejected the *McFarlane* ruling. As summarised by Heydon J:

> The various assumptions underlying the law relating to children and the duties on parents created by the law would be negated if parents could sue to recover the costs of rearing unplanned children. That possibility would tend to damage the natural love and mutual confidence which the law seeks to foster between parent and child ... It would permit conduct inconsistent with the duty to nurture children.[191]

The case for the majority was put most forcibly by Kirby J, who was highly critical of the *McFarlane* decision: 'Neither the invocation of Scripture nor the invention of a fictitious oracle on the Underground[192] ... authorises a court of law to depart from the ordinary principles governing the recovery of damages for the tort of negligence',[193] and 'the diverse

---

[188] [2002] EWCA Civ 88.   [189] ibid. [44].   [190] (2003) 215 CLR 1.   [191] ibid. [404].
[192] An allusion to Lord Steyn's commuter on the Underground as an assessor of distributive justice in *McFarlane*, AC 59 [62]; SLT 154 [165].
[193] ibid. [151].

opinions illustrate what can happen when judges embark upon the "quicksands" of public policy, at least when doing so leads them away from basic legal principle'.[194]

Noting this apparent collision course between two of the highest courts in the Commonwealth, many commentators would wonder if, given the opportunity, the House of Lords might reconsider its position. That opportunity arose when Ms Rees's case was appealed to them.[195] However, the *Cattanach* judgment was not considered in depth and *McFarlane* was confirmed unanimously, apparently on the grounds that it would be improper to reverse a decision within the short period of four years.[196] In the event, however, the House of Lords allowed the appeal in *Rees* by a majority of 4:3. It is unsurprising that their Lordships' reasons were, again, diverse.[197] The argument rested on whether, on the one hand, it was the exceptional costs dictated by disability in either the child or the parent which attracted recompense or whether the definitive factor was normality in the resultant child. In the event, the latter view held sway.

One interesting aspect of *Rees* lies in the fact that both the majority and minority accepted that *McFarlane* was an exception to the established rules in the tort of negligence, renewing concerns that justice was, at least, not being seen to be done. Lord Bingham's response, which was followed by the majority, was to make a conventional award of £15,000 to all victims of a negligent sterilisation in recognition of the affront to a woman's autonomy imposed by an unplanned pregnancy.[198] He was adamant that this was in no way compensatory but it is difficult to accept this at face value and, clearly, other members of the House were in some doubt, including those who supported the measure. Lord Steyn went so far as to question the power of the courts to make such an award. He maintained that to do so should instead be the prerogative of Parliament. It could be argued, however, that the 'conventional award' could be seen as recognition of a new head of damages: that is to say, a breach of autonomy or interference with the right to plan one's life as one wishes. Such an approach would then harmonise the apparent conflict between the Inner House of the Court of Session and the House of Lords in *McFarlane* and would be widely recognised as being a fair solution to an intense moral and legal dilemma. There has been some evidence that judicial policy is moving in such a direction,[199] although the Court of Appeal has refused more recently to accept the loss of personal autonomy as a free-standing head of loss.[200] The position therefore is that there should be no compensation for the costs of upkeep of a healthy, unplanned child and it is to be emphasised that it is the state of health of the child that determines the issue.[201]

12.5.2   WRONGFUL BIRTH

The parents of child with a disability may choose to raise an action in negligence against a doctor or antenatal counsellor who failed either to advise them of the risk of congenital illness in their children or to carry out, and interpret correctly, appropriate diagnostic procedures which would have disclosed abnormality in the foetus. The doctor or counsellor owes them a duty of care; the parents may contend that, as a result, they have been deprived of the opportunity to terminate the pregnancy and that they are now faced with

---

[194] ibid. [158].   [195] *Rees* v *Darlington Memorial Hospital NHS Trust* [2003] UKHL 52.
[196] ibid. [7] (Lord Bingham).
[197] See John K Mason, 'From Dundee to Darlington: An End to the *McFarlane* Line?' [2004] JR 365.
[198] *Rees* (n 195) [8].   [199] See, in particular, *Chester* v *Afshar* [2005] 1 AC 134 [24] (Lord Steyn).
[200] *Shaw* v *Kovac* [2017] EWCA Civ 1028.
[201] This was foreseen in *AD* v *East Kent Community NHS Trust* [2003] 3 All ER 1167.

the upkeep of a child with a disability. Such an action, brought by and on behalf of the parents, is generally known as one for 'wrongful birth'. Damages may be sought in respect of the distress caused to the parents, as well as for the extra costs which are entailed in bringing up a child with a disability.

The UK courts have allowed these types of legal action. Examples include the case of *Gregory v Pembrokeshire Health Authority*,[202] where the trial judge found that the doctor in question was in breach of their duty of care to their patient due to not informing her of the failure of an amniocentesis test. Nevertheless, the claim ultimately failed on the ground of causation with the claimant being unable to established that that she would have had a second investigation had she been offered one, nor that she would have then proceeded terminate the pregnancy. In the Scottish case of *Anderson v Forth Valley Health Board*,[203] a couple sought damages in respect of the alleged negligence on the part of the defendant health board which led to their two sons being born with muscular dystrophy. The pursuers averred that, had they been referred for genetic counselling and testing, the genetic disorder carried by the wife would have been discovered and the couple would have chosen to terminate both pregnancies. As it was, no tests were ever offered or carried out, despite the fact that the hospital had been informed of a history of X-linked Duchenne muscular dystrophy among the male members of the wife's family. The children's condition only came to light when one of the boys injured himself in a fall. After a very comprehensive review of the case law, Lord Nimmo Smith held that he could see 'no good reason' not to treat the pursuers as having suffered personal injuries 'in the conventional sense' and he accordingly awarded damages under the heads of both solatium (injury to feelings) and patrimonial loss.

Al Hamwi v Johnston[204] is a case which illustrates several of the problems associated with antenatal counselling and actions brought for wrongful birth. Mrs Al Hamwi already had one child and was aged 29 at the time she sought to have a second child. Four of her cousins, a niece, a nephew, and a half-sister all suffered from a rapidly fatal congenital condition which was considered to be Down's syndrome and she informed the hospital of this family background. At 11 weeks' gestation she was told by her GP that it was 'too late to have genetic tests' which was, in itself, a rather strange comment. It was not until she was 17 weeks' pregnant that she was referred for hospital antenatal care where preliminary maternal serum tests were carried out and the question of amniocentesis was raised. The evidence thereafter is less certain, but it is reasonably clear that, while she originally wanted to undergo what is an invasive investigatory procedure, she had changed her mind at the end of an hour-long consultation.

She had been informed that the risk of miscarriage following the procedure was 1:100; nonetheless, she believed adamantly that the risk was 75%. She was also told that her blood tests indicated the risk of her carrying a child with a disability was 1:8,396.[205] Mrs Al Hamwi eventually refused amniocentesis and, in due course, gave birth to a child suffering from the familial condition. She sued the GP on account of the delay involved in referring her for antenatal screening and the hospital for misinforming her of the hazards of amniocentesis. The combined effect of such alleged negligence was to deny her proper diagnostic facilities and therefore the opportunity to terminate her pregnancy, which she claimed she would have done given the right information at the right time. Simon J

[202] [1989] 1 Med LR 81.   [203] (1998) 44 BMLR 108.   [204] [2005] EWHC 206 (QB).
[205] The hospital was working on the assumption that the family history was one of Down's syndrome (trisomy-21); the fact that this was affected by a rare translocation type of chromosomal abnormality was discovered only in the postnatal follow-up.

dismissed the case against the GP on the factual evidence that the amniocentesis, or the alternative of chorionic villus sampling at another hospital, was not, in practice, delayed or voided by her admitted negligence. Accordingly, the breach of duty had not caused damage to the claimant. As to the hospital, he found that Mrs Al Hamwi had been given appropriate counselling by way of an information leaflet and interview with the obstetrician concerned.

He did, however, concede that she may have been confused about the information she received. In this respect, the judge made some interesting observations, taking the view that to hold that it is the clinician's duty to ensure that the information given to the patient is understood is 'to place too onerous an obligation on the clinician'. He continued:

> Clinicians should take reasonable and appropriate steps to satisfy themselves that the patient has understood the information which has been provided; but the obligation does not extend to ensuring that the patient has understood.[206]

It may be that to ensure success in achieving 'understanding consent' is an impossible goal in the circumstances. Given case law developments in relation to the disclosure of risk in healthcare settings (see Chapter 8), we may question whether Simon J's dictum is strictly in accord with professional guidelines and current medical practice in this regard. The latest in this line of authority is the *Khan v Meadows* litigation, mentioned previously.[207] Ms Meadows wanted to know whether she carried the haemophilia gene, a hereditary disease. Her GP arranged for a blood test which was designed to establish whether a person had haemophilia and not whether they carried the haemophilia gene. This required a referral to a haematologist for genetic testing. She had a consultation to discuss the blood test results with Dr Khan, another GP at the same practice, who informed her that the results were normal. As a result of the advice which she received in this and the earlier consultation, Ms Meadows was led to believe that any child she might have would not have haemophilia. She went on to give birth to her son Adejuwon, who was subsequently diagnosed with haemophilia and autism. It was following the birth that Ms Meadows underwent a genetic test, which showed that she was in in fact a carrier of the haemophilia gene. Had she been advised that she was a carrier of the haemophilia gene, Ms Meadows claimed that she would have terminated the pregnancy and her son would not have been born. She brought a claim for the costs of raising her child. In the statement of facts and issues, the parties agreed that it was 'reasonably foreseeable that as a consequence of [Dr Khan's] breach of duty, the appellant could give birth to a child that suffered from a condition such as autism, as well as haemophilia.'[208]

At first instance, Yip J found for the claimant and awarded £9 million plus interest in damages representing compensation for the costs of raising a child who had both haemophilia and autism.[209] In considering counsel for the defendant's submission that the additional losses associated with Adejuwon's autism fell outside the scope of the duty owed to the claimant, she 'did not accept that is so':

> The focus of the defendant's duty and the very purpose of the service the claimant sought was to provide her with the necessary information to allow her to terminate any pregnancy afflicted by haemophilia. The birth of [her son] resulted from a pregnancy which

---

[206] At [69]. Jose Miola, 'Autonomy Ruled OK?' (2006) 14(1) Medical Law Review 108 considered that, in giving preference to informing over understanding, Mrs Al Hamwi was denied an autonomous choice.
[207] *Khan v Meadows* [2021] UKSC 21.   [208] ibid. [12].
[209] *MNX v Khan* [2017] EWHC 2990 (QB).

was afflicted by haemophilia. His autism was bad luck, in the same way that the meningitis in Groom was bad luck. Equally, each condition was the natural consequence of a pregnancy that would not have continued if the doctor's duty had been performed correctly. The scope of the duty in this case extended to preventing the birth of [her son] and all the consequences that brought.[210]

On appeal by the defendant to the Court of Appeal, the scope of the defendant's duty of care was held to include haemophilia but not autism, with the facts of this case being distinguished from those in *Parkinson* and *Groom*. As a result, the award of damages was reduced to £1.4million.[211] On a further appeal by Ms Meadows, the Supreme Court confirmed the Court of Appeal ruling and dismissed her appeal. Several aspects of the court's judgment are worth noting. Regarding wrongful birth, counsel for Ms Meadows submitted that the court should prefer the ruling of Yip J, arguing that it was not appropriate to draw on case law which focused commercial transactions involving pure economic loss to limit the appellant's recovery of damages to haemophilia and not autism:

[Such an approach] was not suited to cases of clinical negligence in which there was an imbalance of knowledge and power between the clinician and the patient . . . Ms Meadows' claim should not be characterised as pure economic loss but as a mixed claim which combined her loss of autonomy through the continuation of the pregnancy and psychiatric damage incidental to her son's disability as well as her claim for the cost of caring for [her son]. It was also arbitrary and unfair to draw a distinction between a parent who did not want any pregnancy (as in *Parkinson* and *Groom*) and a parent who did not want a particular pregnancy . . . The court should bring cases of wrongful birth into line with cases in which clinical negligence causes direct physical injury . . . [They] did not give rise to the risk of indeterminate liability which can arise in commercial cases involving pure economic loss.[212]

The court agreed with counsel for the appellant that her son would not have been born but for the defendant's negligence in line with the facts established by Yip J. However, the Court also went to hold 'that conclusion as to factual causation does not provide any answer to the question as to the scope of the defendant's duty'.[213] The Court then stated:

Foreseeability of the possibility of a boy being born with both haemophilia and an unrelated disability, such as autism, which is a risk in any pregnancy, is a relevant consideration when addressing the scope of the duty of care undertaken by a defendant. That is because the absence of foreseeability would militate against there being a duty of care in relation to such a risk. But the foreseeability of such unrelated disability is in no sense determinative of the question of the scope of the duty of care. That is because the scope of duty question depends principally upon the nature of the service which the defendant has undertaken to provide to the claimant. One asks: 'what is the risk which the service which the defendant undertook was intended to address?' Where a medical practitioner has not undertaken responsibility for the progression of the pregnancy and has undertaken only to provide information or advice in relation to a particular risk in a pregnancy, the risk of a foreseeable unrelated disability, which could occur in any pregnancy, will not as a general rule be within the scope of the clinician's duty of care.[214]

---

[210] ibid. [60]–[61].   [211] [2019] EWCA Civ 152.   [212] ibid. [21].
[213] ibid. [64].   [214] ibid. [65].

The Court indicated that Yip J had been incorrect in directing herself to consider whether it was fair, just, and reasonable to impose liability in negligence for the totality of the son's disability. This was because the 'case did not concern a novel application of the law of negligence in which it was necessary for the court to address that question because established principles provide an answer'.[215] It concluded that the economic costs of caring for a child with a disability arising in a wrongful birth claim are clearly actionable. In the context of determining what range of costs are recoverable, the scope of duty question must be answered. This is addressed by considering the purpose for which Ms Meadows obtained the service of the GPs at their practice, where she had consulted them for a specific purpose of ascertaining if she was a carrier of the haemophilia gene. In the circumstances, 'Dr Khan owed her a duty to take reasonable care to give accurate information or advice when advising her whether or not she was a carrier of that gene.'[216] Although there was a causal link between Dr Khan's negligence and the birth of Ms Meadows' son, it was not relevant to the scope of Dr Khan's duty, which did not encompass unrelated risks which might arise in any pregnancy.

12.5.3　WRONGFUL LIFE

The basis of a parental claim for wrongful birth may be clear enough, but it could well be argued that it is misplaced. The parents of an unplanned child with a disability may be subject to both emotional and financial hardship, but it is the child who has the disability. Moreover, if the parents die before their own legal actions are fully settled, even in the presence of negligent action on behalf of their legal representatives, the child has no further recourse to recover costs in respect of their own upkeep as the duty of care is not owed to them.[217] This is commonly known as a legal action for wrongful life. This type of clinical negligence claim presents an interesting conundrum. The function of tort law is to restore the victim of negligence, so far as is possible, to the position they would have occupied absent that negligence. There can be no cause of action in this particular instance insofar as it is impossible to restore someone to the state of pre-existence. Moreover, when assessing the difference between an existence and non-existence, we have no known comparator. While there may be some sympathy with the logic of such a view, it could be argued that it represents an unduly formalistic way of disposing of what can be seen as a matter of justice.

In the case of *McKay* v *Essex Area Health Authority*,[218] the mother of a child with a disability contracted rubella while pregnant. A blood sample had been taken from her, but it was mislaid. After that, a second blood sample was taken and the mother was informed that neither she nor the foetus had been infected; however, the child was born with serious disabilities. The claimants, who included both the mother and the child, alleged negligence on the part of the defendants in that they either failed to carry out the necessary tests on the blood samples or failed to interpret them correctly. A number of claims were made as a result of this alleged negligence, including one by the child for damages for a life of distress and suffering. While recognising that there was no reason why a mother in such circumstances would not be able to claim in respect of

---

[215] ibid. [66]; see also *Robinson* (n 22) [27] (Lord Reed).　　　[216] ibid. [67].

[217] See *Whitehead* v *Searle* [2008] EWCA Civ 285; [2009] 1 WLR 549, where lawyers negligent in completing a wrongful birth case before the death of the mother were held to have no duty to the child who had been born as a result.

[218] [1982] QB 1166.

the negligent failure to advise her of her right to terminate her pregnancy grounded in a legal action for wrongful birth, the court was not prepared to recognise any legal action by the child for an award of damages for wrongful life. Having declined to find a duty basis to the claim, the court also struggled with the difficulties of assessing damages in such a case. Here, the impossibility-of-comparison argument was seen as a strong one: how could a court compare the value of a flawed life with non-existence or, indeed, with any 'after life' which an aborted child was experiencing? Even having accepted this conceptual difficulty, Stephenson LJ was of the opinion that it was better to be born with a disability than not to be born at all except, possibly, in the case of the most extreme cognitive and/or physical disability.

Mention must also be made of proposals for law reform that had been made in this area before this judgment, as well as the adoption of legislation that followed in support of such proposals. It should be noted that prior to *McKay*, the Law Commission had considered the merits of wrongful life actions and had come to the conclusion that it should not be allowed.[219] Subsequently, this led to the adoption of the Congenital Disabilities (Civil Liability) Act 1976, in which s 1(2)(b) of the Act excluded the right of a child to sue in such circumstances. The relevant provisions of the Act are set out in **Table 12.1**.

The scope of this Act was subject to legal challenge in the recent case of *Toombes v Mitchell*.[220] The claimant, Evie Toombes, was born in 2001 and was diagnosed with lipomyelomeningocele (LMM), a form of neural tube defect. She suffers from impaired mobility, double incontinence, and a gastrointestinal disorder. She alleged that the cause of her physical disability was her mother's failure to take folic acid before her conception, which it was alleged was due to the negligent advice provided by her GP prior to conception. Her mother had attended a consultation with her GP, Dr Mitchell, prior to Evie's conception. She had asked about the need for folic acid and claimed that her GP had reassured her that if she was eating a healthy diet, including cereals and bread (which she was), it was not necessary to take folic acid. The claim was brought through her mother and litigation friend where it was alleged that but for this negligence the mother would never have conceived and this led to the harm suffered by the claimant.

The proceedings came before the courts on two occasions. On the first occasion, it was heard by Lambert J in the High Court on a preliminary issue which focused on whether the

Table 12.1 Congenital Disabilities (Civil Liability) Act 1976, section 1

Civil liability to a child born disabled

(1) If a child is born disabled as the result of such an occurrence before its birth as is mentioned in subsection (2), and a person (other than the child's own mother) is under this section answerable to the child in respect of the occurrence, the child's disabilities are to be regarded as damage resulting from the wrongful act of that person and actionable accordingly at the suit of the child

(2) An occurrence to which this section applies is one which—

    (a) affected either parent of the child in his or her ability to have a normal, healthy child; or

    (b) affected the mother during her pregnancy, or affected her or the child in the course of its birth, so that the child is born with disabilities which would not otherwise have been present.

---

[219] Law Commission, *Report on Injuries to Unborn Children* (1974) Cmnd 5807.
[220] [2020] EWHC 3506 (QB).

claim disclosed a lawful cause of action on the basis of agreed facts between the parties.[221] The parties made the following separate submissions. The claimant submitted that her claim should be characterised as a claim for 'wrongful life'. While such legal actions in 'the strict sense of the term' were excluded under the Congenital Disabilities (Civil Liability) Act 1976, it was argued that this claim fell squarely within the scope of subsection 1(2)(a) of the Act which permitted recovery by children born disabled as a consequence of negligence affecting a parent in their ability to have a healthy child. As counsel for the claimant stated: 'A distinction needs to be made between "wrongful life" cases which are essentially "abortion cases" as distinct from cases in which it is alleged that, but for the negligence, the child would not have been conceived.'[222]

In contrast, it was the defendant's position that the mother had probably already been pregnant prior to the consultation and that the advice had not been negligent, being in line with the recommended guidance at the time. Although the defendant had no recollection of the consultation itself as it had taken place 20 years earlier, he had made a note in the mother's file to the effect: 'preconception counselling. adv. Folate if desired discussed'. He said that his usual advice at the time was to tell patients that guidance recommended daily folic acid supplementation for women preparing for pregnancy and during the first trimester. However, if the patient had very good folic acid intake from their normal diet, the benefit of taking additional supplementation would be less important. He therefore tended to leave the choice to the patient. On the preliminary issue, counsel for the defendant submitted that the claim was not brought on the basis of the claimant's disability but on the fact of her existence. It did not satisfy the requirements of 'occurrence' whether under section 1(2)(a) or (b) of the Act. In addition, there was no causal relationship between the harm suffered by the claimant and the alleged wrongful act because, but for that wrongful act, the claimant would never have been conceived. In the circumstances, this type of claim was expressly excluded under the provision of the Act. Relying on *McKay*, it was further submitted that the claim would not have been recognised at common law, even before the Act came into existence. As a consequence, whether under the Act or at common law, the agreed facts did not disclose a lawful cause of action.[223]

In delivering judgment, Lambert J noted in passing that it was common ground between the parties that, on the agreed facts, the claimant's mother would have had a 'valid' wrongful birth claim. Compensation payable in such a claim would have included the reasonable costs associated with the claimant's disability together with an award for pain and suffering arising from the pregnancy and childbirth. A key difference between the claims made by the mother's and the claimant, however, was that the mother's claim would have been limited to her life expectation, rather than the claimant's life expectation. No claim had been brought by the mother, however, as she had not wished to bring her own claim. The court then moved to consider the substantive legal issues at stake on the preliminary issue before the court, which she identified as a matter of 'proper interpretation' of the Act.

It was recognised that *McKay* was relevant for understanding the meaning of an action for wrongful life and to section 1(2)(b), where relevant. She agreed with the submission by the defendant's counsel that a cause of action under section 1 of the Act involved three components: a wrongful act, an occurrence (see section 1(2)(a) or (b)); and that a child is born disabled. In short, the occurrence must lead to a child born with disabilities.[224] The term 'occurrence' meant that something had happened, but the Act did not require a

---

[221] *Toombes* v *Mitchell* [2020] EWHC 3506 (QB).   [222] ibid. [4].   [223] ibid. [3].
[224] ibid. [41].

change or alteration in the mother's physiological state. The mother did not have to establish a legally recognised harm. Instead, it was sufficient that 'something may have altered her physical state but equally she may have been physically unaffected'.[225] In addition, where negligence actually causes the sexual intercourse which leads to the conception of a child with a disability, then this could be said to constitute an 'occurrence' for the purposes of the Act. In the circumstances, the court found that, on the agreed facts, the claimant mother had relied on the negligent advice given by the defendant GP which led her to having sexual intercourse without the benefit of folic acid and this was a 'relevant occurrence' under the terms of the Act.[226]

As to whether the claim should be viewed as a wrongful life claim in the 'strict sense', Lambert J stated that:

> On a plain reading of subsection 1(1) [of the Act] in conjunction with subsection 1(2)(a), all that a claimant must prove to come within the Act is a wrongful act or omission leading to an occurrence (as defined) which results in a child who is born with disabilities. Unlike in a post-conception case, there is no need for the claimant to prove that, but for the wrongful act, he or she would still have been born. It is sufficient that the claimant was, in fact, born with a disability resulting from the occurrence.[227]

On the question of causation, it was held that the causal link between the circumstances of the sexual intercourse and the disability must still be established in a pre-conception occurrence claim.[228] Lambert J went on to find in favour of the claimant, stating that she could bring a claim under the Act in respect of the pre-conception advice provided to her mother. The requisite elements under section 1(2) of the Act had been established on the basis of the agreed facts, with all three being present. This involved 'a wrongful act (negligent advice) leading to an occurrence (sexual intercourse in a folic acid deficient state) which resulted in a child born with disabilities due to that deficiency of folic acid'.[229]

The matter subsequently came before the court again for a trial hearing, in which a determination was made on key factual liability issues.[230] Drawing on the evidence presented, HHJ Coe QC found the defendant's note of the relevant consultation was 'completely inadequate'.[231] She further found that the GP's alleged usual practice of advising patients according to the relevant guidance was inconsistent with his evidence that he would not advise patients to delay attempting to conceive in order to take folic acid supplements, concluding that the mother 'was not advised appropriately by the defendant'.[232] Specific findings included the following: first, the defendant had failed to give the mother advice about folic acid in accordance with the relevant guidelines in which the advice was to take folic acid daily before conception; second, the mother was not pregnant at the time of the relevant consultation; third, had the mother received the correct advice she would have immediately begun to take folic acid at the recommended dose and waited about a month or so before trying to conceive; and finally, that taking all such matters into account, there would have been a later conception which would have resulted in a healthy child. She went on to find for the claimant on liability, with the quantum of damages to be assessed.

Although concerns have been expressed that this ruling would likely open the floodgates to similar claims against GPs, it has been suggested that such concerns are misplaced.[233]

---

[225] ibid. [45].   [226] ibid. [47]–[48].   [227] ibid. [53].   [228] ibid. [55].   [229] ibid. [56].
[230] *Toombes* v *Mitchell* [2021] EWHC 3234 (QB).   [231] ibid. [61].   [232] ibid. [66].
[233] Beth Walker, 'Commentary: A case of wrongful conception' (Medical Protection Society, 11 March 2022) available at <https://www.medicalprotection.org/uk/articles/commentary-a-case-of-wrongful-conception> accessed 07 December 2022.

Instead, it should be viewed as a 'salutary reminder' to HCPs of the importance of making clear and detailed notes in their patients' medical records with respect to consultations that take place.[234]

12.6 SPECIFIC CASES

12.6.1 THE PROBLEM OF THE NOVICE

The degree of expertise possessed by a medical practitioner obviously depends to a considerable extent on their experience, and the argument has been put forward that the standard of competence of a newly qualified doctor will be less than that expected of an experienced practitioner. Although this may be the day-to-day expectation, it is not that of the law. The strict application of the *Bolam* principle[235] would lead the courts to expect the doctor to show that degree of skill which would be shown by the reasonably competent professional. This is an objective standard and it is therefore irrelevant whether the doctor has qualified the day before or ten years before the alleged incident of negligence. In short, it should make no difference to the way in which their conduct is assessed.

The problem was considered in the *Wilsher* case.[236] The claimant had been born prematurely and had been admitted to a specialised neonatal intensive care unit. An error was made in the monitoring of arterial oxygen tension and, as a result, extra oxygen was administered by junior hospital doctors. It was claimed that this could have caused the virtually blinding condition of retrolental fibroplasia which occurred. It was argued by the defendants that the standard of care expected of the junior doctor was not the same as that of his experienced counterpart. Extensive use, it was said, had to be made of recently qualified medical and nursing staff and it was unavoidable that such staff should 'learn on the job'; it would be impossible for public medicine to operate properly without such arrangements and to do otherwise would, ultimately, not be in the best interests of patients. The judgments in the Court of Appeal are not free of ambiguity. The majority of the judges maintained that the public were entitled to expect a reasonable standard of competence in their medical attendants. The decision of Mustill LJ, however, makes it clear that he, at least, was prepared to define the standard of care according to the requirements of the post. An inexperienced doctor occupying a post in a unit which offered specialised services would, accordingly, need that degree of expertise expected of a reasonably competent person occupying that post; the defendant's actual hospital rank—house officer, registrar, etc.—would not be relevant in the determination.

Glidewell LJ also stressed the importance of applying an objective standard which would not take account of an individual doctor's inexperience. The apparent harshness of this conclusion was, nevertheless, mitigated by his suggestion that the standard of care is very likely to be met if the novice seeks advice from or consults with their more experienced colleagues when appropriate. Even so, this apparently simple solution does not answer the question which many juniors may ask, 'How am I to be so experienced as to know when I should be uncertain? And, if, I cannot tell this, am I to ask my seniors before I make any important decision?' These questions effectively force us back to accepting a standard of care test which is based on the doctor of similar experience irrespective of the

---

[234] NHS Resolution, 'Case of Note: *Evie Toombes v Dr. Mitchell* (High Court 21 December 2020 – Lambert J. and 1 December 2021 – Judge Coe QC)' (31 March 2022) available at <https://resolution.nhs.uk/2022/03/31/case-of-note-evie-toombes-v-dr-mitchell-high-court-21-december-2020-lambert-j-and-1-december-2021-judge-coe-qc/> accessed 07 December 2022.

[235] [1957] 2 All ER 118.   [236] [1987] QB 730.

post in which they operate. Conversely, an experienced doctor occupying a junior post would be judged according to their actual knowledge rather than by the lower standard of the reasonably competent occupant of that post—the rationale being that, by reason of their superior expertise, they would be more able to foresee the damage likely to arise from any negligent acts or omissions.[237] It is important to bear in mind that *Wilsher* was very much concerned with specialist units and there is no certainty that the judgments are applicable, say, to GPs insofar as delegation of responsibility, hierarchical organisation, and the like are particular features of hospital practice.

Hospital authorities cannot, of course, rely too much upon junior employees; the principles of vicarious liability will, by themselves, prevent this. As Lord Denning said in *Jones* v *Manchester Corporation*:

> It would be in the highest degree unjust that the hospital board, by getting inexperienced doctors to perform their duties for them, without adequate supervision, should be able to throw all the responsibility on to those doctors as if they were fully experienced practitioners.[238]

A junior to whom responsibility has been delegated must carry out their duties as instructed by their superior in order to avoid liability. If they choose to depart from specific instructions, they will be placing themselves in a risky position in the event of anything going wrong.[239] At the same time, there may be circumstances in which they are entitled to depart from instructions; obedience to manifestly wrong instructions might, itself, be construed as negligence in some cases.

12.6.2 INNOVATIVE TECHNIQUES

Resort to an innovative therapeutic technique may be appropriate in certain cases but should be approached with caution. Whether the use of such a technique could amount to negligence would depend on the extent to which its use was considered justified in the case in question. In assessing this, a court would consider evidence of previous trials of the treatment and would also, no doubt, take into consideration any dangers which it entailed. It is possible that a court would decline to endorse the use of an untried procedure if the patient was thereby exposed to considerable risk of damage.[240] Other factors might be the previous response of the patient to more conventional treatment, the seriousness of the patient's condition, and the attitude of the patient themselves towards the novelty and risk. In *Cooper* v *Royal United Hospital Bath NHS Trust*,[241] the Trust was held to have breached its duty of care to the claimant for abandoning a preferred course of medical care without adequately advising her as to the risks of implementing an alternative method. The standard of care to be applied in such circumstances would be that expected of a doctor who is reasonably competent in the provision of such treatment. A doctor should not, therefore, undertake procedures which are beyond their capacity.[242]

---

[237] See *Wimpey Construction UK Ltd* v *Poole* [1984] 2 Lloyd's Rep 499.

[238] [1952] 2 QB 852 at 871.   [239] *Junor* v *McNicol* (1959) *The Times*, 26 March, HL.

[240] Although, if the only alternative is serious harm or death, then the courts have endorsed the application of highly experimental techniques, see e.g. *Simms* v *Simms, A* v *A* [2002] EWHC 2734 (Fam); [2003] 1 All ER 669.

[241] [2005] EWHC 3381 (QB).

[242] In *Tomkins* v *Bexley Area Health Authority* [1993] 4 Med LR 235, the patient's lingual nerve was damaged in the course of an operation for the removal of wisdom teeth. Wilcox J observed: 'When fine movements and fine judgments are the order of the day, with surgery being conducted in the confined space of the mouth, a high degree of care is needed.'

A relevant Scottish case demonstrates the issues.[243] Here, the pursuer had suffered from abdominal pain for more than a year. In something of a last-ditch attempt, her doctor prescribed chloramphenicol as a result of which she developed aplastic anaemia from which she recovered only after receiving a bone marrow transplant. She sued her doctor in negligence on the grounds that he could have chosen another drug which was not known to carry the 1:8,000 to 1:30,000 risk of bone marrow dysplasia which was associated with chloramphenicol—it was claimed that the treatment given was, in effect, a 'shot in the dark'. In the event, Lord Johnston was not prepared to hold as negligent a decision which had been carefully arrived at, the doctor having weighed up all the possibilities.[244] Drawing from Lord Browne-Wilkinson in *Bolitho*, the Lord Ordinary held:

> Within the framework of a balanced judgment, I consider that the decision of Dr Todd can be rationally and responsibly supported . . . whatever may have been his alternatives. Furthermore, I consider that it should not be categorised even as an error of judgment . . . I am prepared to hold that, within the options reasonably available to him . . . it was a reasonable course to adopt.[245]

In *Walker-Smith* v *GMC*[246] the court recognised that the line between innovative treatment and experimental research is not a bright one and it confirmed, albeit obiter, that the matter falls to be determined by the intention of the HCP. This is important as a matter of which regulatory regime—care or research—governs an intervention.

In legislative terms, there has been an attempt to introduce a statutory framework for medical innovation through a Private Member's Bill presented to the UK Parliament House of Lords in 2014: the Medical Innovation Bill. However, it was blocked before it could reach debate in the House of Commons.[247] The Bill would have added a second system for determining the standard of care for using innovative treatments that would run parallel to the existing (*Bolitho*-modified) *Bolam* test. Under the proposed scheme, a doctor would not be negligent in departing from the existing range of accepted medical treatments for a condition if they obtained beforehand the views of one or more appropriately qualified doctors and took full account of the views obtained. Nevertheless, any objections from the consulted qualified doctor(s) could be overridden if the decision to do so was taken 'responsibly'. Many commentators took the view that the ambiguities within the proposed legislation would likely undermine—rather than promote—responsible medical innovation.[248] The Access to Medical Treatments (Innovation) Act 2016 provides a further development. In essence, this seeks to establish a database of innovative medical treatment, and to promote access thereto.[249] While such a model is to be welcomed, more questionable is

---

[243] *Duffy* v *Lanarkshire Health Board* 1998 SCLR 1142; 1999 SLT 906, OH.

[244] For related discussion of the possible negligence aspects of 'off-label prescription', see Rosie Harding and Elizabeth Peel, '"He was Like a Zombie": Off-Label Prescription of Antipsychotic Drugs in Dementia' (2013) 21(2) Medical Law Review 243.

[245] As a postscript, Ms Duffy's claim under the Administration of Justice Act 1982, s 8 for remuneration in respect of her sister's marrow donation was also rejected.

[246] [2012] EWHC 503.

[247] Medical Innovation Bill [HL] 2014–15.

[248] Nils Hoppe and José Miola, 'Innovation in Medicine through Degeneration in Law? A Critical Perspective on the Medical Innovation Bill' (2014) 14(4) Medical Law International 266; *cf.* Jo Samanta and Ash Samanta, 'Quackery or Quality: The Ethicolegal Basis for a Legislative Framework for Medical Innovation' (2015) 41(6) Journal of Medical Ethics 474.

[249] José Miola, 'Bye-Bye *Bolitho*: The Curious Case of the Medical Innovation Bill' (2015) 15 (2–3) Medical Law International 124.

the decision to put this on a statutory footing. For example, it is not clear upon whom the set-up and maintenance of the database falls, nor is participation in any way mandatory, nor whether there was sufficient public support for such legislative proposals.[250]

12.6.3 COMPLEMENTARY MEDICINE

By what standard should practitioners be judged in relation to the use of what may be termed 'alternative' or 'complementary' medicine? In *Shakoor v Situ*,[251] a patient died from an 'idiosyncratic' liver reaction after taking nine doses of a traditional Chinese remedy, prescribed by a herbal medicinalist. The skin condition from which the patient had been suffering could only be treated by surgery in orthodox medicine. His widow sued in negligence and the issue came down to the appropriate standard of care. The court held that an alternative medical practitioner could not be judged by the standard of orthodox medicine because they did not hold themselves out as professing that 'art'; rather, they would be judged by the prevailing standard in their own 'art' subject to the caveat that it would be negligence if it could be shown that that standard itself was regarded as deficient in the UK having regard to the inherent risks involved.

In the event, the negligence action failed because the court held that the practitioner had acted in accordance with the standard of care appropriate to traditional Chinese herbal medicine as properly practised in accordance with the standards required in the UK. It should be noted, however, that there is currently no statutory regulation of practitioners who offer herbal and traditional Chinese medicine in the UK. The Complementary and Natural Healthcare Council (CNHC) is a voluntary regulator of complementary HCPs, which has been established with UK government funding and support.[252] It has 'Accredited Register' status with the Professional Standards Authority (PSA), which oversees the regulation of a range of health and social care professional groups.[253] The Council undertakes a range of activities to facilitate standard setting in relation to the practitioner groups it covers, in addition to publishing a Code of Conduct, Ethics, and Performance.[254]

12.6.4 *RES IPSA LOQUITUR*

Because it may be difficult in many personal injury actions to establish negligence on the part of the defendant, claimants occasionally have recourse to the doctrine of *res ipsa loquitur*. This doctrine does not shift the onus of proof to the defendant, as is sometimes

---

[250] See José Miola, 'Postscript to the Medical Innovation Bill: Clearing Up Loose Ends' (2019) 11(1) Law Innovation and Technology 17. More generally, see Tsachi Keren-Paz, Tina Cockburn, and Alicia El Haj, 'Special Issue: Regulating Innovation Treatments, Information, Risk, Allocation and Redress' (2019) 11(1) Law Innovation and Technology 1.

[251] [2001] 1 WLR 410.

[252] The CNHC covers the following complementary therapies: Alexander technique teaching, aromatherapy, Bowen therapy, colon hydrotherapy, craniosacral therapy, healing, hypnotherapy, kinesiology, massage therapy, microsystems acupuncture, naturopathy, nutritional therapy, reflexology, reiki, shiatsu, sports massage and therapy, and yoga therapy. See CNHC, 'About Us' (2022) available at <https://www.cnhc.org.uk> accessed 07 December 2022.

[253] Professional Standards Authority, 'About Accredited Registers' (2022) available at <https://www.professionalstandards.org.uk/what-we-do/accredited-registers/about-accredited-registers> accessed 07 December 2022. For further details on the work of the PSA, see Chapter 4.

[254] Complementary and Natural Healthcare Council, 'The CNHC Code of Conduct – Ethics and Performance' (2022) available at <https://www.cnhc.org.uk/code-conduct-registrants> accessed 07 December 2022.

suggested; it gives rise to an inference of negligence on the defendant's part.[255] If the defendant cannot then rebut this inference of negligence, the claimant will have established his case. As such, it is considerably easier for the claimant to succeed in his claim when *res ipsa loquitur* applies. The classic case is that of *Cassidy v Ministry of Health*,[256] in which the claimant went into hospital for an operation to remedy Dupuytren's contracture of two fingers and came out with four stiff fingers. Denning LJ (as he then was) expressed the view that the claimant was quite entitled to say:

> I went into hospital to be cured of two stiff fingers. I have come out with four stiff fingers and my hand is useless. That should not have happened if due care had been used. Explain it if you can.[257]

The doctrine has been found most useful in cases where damage has occurred in an incident involving machinery or in the context of damage suffered while the claimant was involved in some sort of complex process. It can apply only where the claimant is unable to identify the precise nature of the negligence which caused his injury and where no explanation of the way in which the injury came to be inflicted has been offered by the defendant. The injury itself must be of such a kind as 'does not normally happen' in the circumstances unless there is negligence, and cannot simply be an inherent risk of the procedure.[258]

The doctrine's application in medical cases may be useful to claimants because of the difficulty that they may experience in unravelling the cause of an injury sustained during technical procedures of which they may have little understanding; indeed, they may well have been unconscious at the relevant time. However, courts are generally reluctant to apply *res ipsa loquitur* and that this is certainly evident in clinical negligence cases. As Megaw LJ said:

> [if] one were to accept the view that negligence was inevitably proved if something went wrong and it was unexplained], few dentists, doctors and surgeons, however competent, conscientious and careful they might be, would avoid the totally unjustified and unfair stigma of professional negligence probably several times in the course of their careers.[259]

In order to rely on the doctrine, claimants must establish facts which, if unexplained, would give rise to an inference of negligence,[260] or if no explanation for the events which transpired is available.[261] For example, in *Glass v Cambridge Health Authority*,[262] the patient suffered brain damage as a result of suffering a heart attack under a general anaesthetic. The court held that this was not an event which normally would be expected to happen in the circumstances and that the onus therefore transferred to the defendant to provide an explanation of the event which was consistent with the absence of negligence.

[255] There has been some debate as to the precise effect of *res ipsa loquitur*, but the weight of opinion favours the view outlined here: see *Ng Chun Pui v Lee Chuen Tat* [1988] RTR 298, PC.
[256] [1951] 2 KB 343.
[257] ibid. [365]. Other medical cases in which *res ipsa loquitur* has applied include: *Saunders v Leeds Western Health Authority* (1984) 129 Sol Jo 225; *Cavan v Wilcox* (1973) 44 DLR (3d) 42; and *Holmes v Board of Hospital Trustees of the City of London* (1977) 81 DLR (3d) 67.
[258] See e.g. *O'Malley-Williams v Board of Governors of the National Hospital for Nervous Diseases* (1975, unreported), cited in [1975] 1 BMJ 635.
[259] *Fletcher v Bench* (1973, unreported), CA cited in [1973] 4 BMJ 117.
[260] See e.g. *Ludlow v Swindon Health Authority* [1989] 1 Med LR 104, an unsuccessful attempt to raise the doctrine.
[261] *Hay (Gill's curator bonis) v Grampian Health Board* 1995 SLT 652 (OH).   [262] [1995] 6 Med LR 91.

At times however, the courts have upheld claims on the basis of lack of explanation but without direct recourse to the *res ipsa loquitur doctrine*. For example, in *Thomas* v *Curley*,[263] the court found for the claimant on the basis that, on the balance of probabilities, the defendant had failed to explain how '[the] injury could have been occasioned in an uncomplicated procedure conducted some distance from the site of the common bile duct injury other than a want of care'. This position and the finding for the claimant were upheld by the Court of Appeal.[264]

The courts' general antipathy to *res ipsa loquitur* was however re-emphasised in *Ratcliffe* v *Plymouth and Torbay Health Authority*,[265] which involved paraesthesia following a spinal anaesthetic. The Court of Appeal affirmed that it could not be inferred that the untoward symptoms could not have occurred in the absence of negligence.[266] The courts, it was said, would do medicine a considerable disservice if, because a patient suffered a grievous and unexpected outcome, a careful doctor was ordered to pay compensation as if the doctor had been negligent:

> If the untoward outcome was extremely rare, or was impossible to explain in the light of the current state of medical knowledge, the judge will be bound to exercise great care in evaluating the evidence before making such a finding, but if he does so, the prima facie inference of negligence is rebutted and the claim will fail.[267]

These cases suggest, and as expressed by Hobhouse LJ, that *res ipsa loquitur* is no more than a convenient phrase to describe the proof of facts which are sufficient to support an inference—based on ordinary human experience with no need for expert evidence—that a defendant was negligent and, therefore, to establish a prima facie case against them.[268]

Indeed, subsequent to *Ratcliffe*, questions of explanation and evidence continue to arise, notably in obstetric cases. *Smith* v *Sheridan*,[269] concerned a who child suffered serious brain damage as a result of a doctor's negligent 'hard pull' during forceps delivery. The court rejected the case as an example of *res ipsa loquitur* on a confusing basis: 'it is clear that the defendant must have used excessive force in delivering Jake and was thus negligent in the absence of any other explanation'. It would seem that the basis of this is that, having excluded all other causes on the basis of expert argument, it was probable—perhaps a near certainty—that, despite his protestations, the obstetrician was at fault. Similarly, in *Richards* v *Swansea NHS Trust*,[270] the court held that the considerable delay in performing a Caesarean section placed an onus on the Trust to adduce evidence to explain why it took 55 minutes to deliver the child. Its failure to do so led to an inference that there were no such constraints on the management of the case and it followed that the claimant had proven, on the balance of probabilities, a breach of the duty of care owed to him.

The application of the doctrine to medico-legal cases was revisited by the Court of Appeal in *O'Connor* v *The Pennine Acute Hospitals NHS Trust*,[271] which concerned a patient injured while under anaesthetic. A core question was whether *res ipsa loquitur* was being invoked, and whether the trial judge had erred in any of the inferences drawn (because the claimant's evidence was, naturally, indirect). The Court of Appeal took the

---

[263] [2011] EWHC 2103.   [264] [2013] EWCA Civ 117.   [265] (1998) 42 BMLR 64.

[266] For a similar Scottish ruling, see *T* v *Lothian NHS Board* [2009] CSOH 132.

[267] BMLR 80, (Brooke LJ).

[268] *Ratcliffe* was followed in *Gray* v *Southampton and South West Hampshire Health Authority* (2000) 57 BMLR 148; affirmed [2001] EWCA Civ 855.

[269] [2005] EWHC 614.   [270] [2007] EWHC 487 (QB).   [271] [2015] EWCA Civ 1244.

opportunity to revisit the principles of the doctrine, and it held both that it had not been invoked and that the trial judge had not acted incorrectly. In reiterating the legal position, the Court said the following:

> More recent authority has tended to the view that res ipsa loquitur is not a principle of law at all. There is no reversal of the burden of proof. The so-called res ipsa loquitur cases are merely cases in which, on the totality of the evidence, the court was able to make a finding of negligence. It has always been the position that courts can make findings of fact by means of inference when there is no direct evidence of the events in issue.[272]

We note the apparent paradox that the doctrine will be rejected yet negligence accepted, simply because there is unassailable evidence of it. It would appear, based on this authority, that the preferable approach today would be for a court make a finding of negligence based on the 'totality' of evidence, rather than recourse to the doctrine alone.[273]

12.7 CRIMINAL NEGLIGENCE

Clinical negligence is predominantly a civil matter, but an increase in prosecutions in the 1990s in England and Wales served to remind doctors and other HCPs that the death of a patient may sometimes lead to criminal prosecution.[274] Such prosecutions used to be rare; however, their increase points to heightened interest in the external regulation of medicine and to a diminution in the professional immunity which it may have previously enjoyed. The principle that doctors, and indeed all HCPs, should be accountable for their failures is entirely acceptable; what is more dubious is that the criminal law, and particularly prosecutions for gross negligence manslaughter (GNM) should be the instrument chosen to perform that task.

In England and Wales, questions of criminal liability for HCPs are essentially limited to GNM prosecutions. Empirical research has shown that between 1970 and 1999, there were 17 such prosecutions, of which 13 arose in the 1990s; seven cases resulted in conviction, excluding those where an appeal was successful.[275] More recent research published in 2019 revealed that over the previous 25-year period, the deaths of 38 patients had led to GNM prosecutions of 47 HCPs (37 doctors, 9 nurses and 1 optometrist). This resulted in 23 convictions, with 4 subsequently being overturned on appeal. In recent years though, there has been a marked decline in obtaining successful convictions. Since 2013, GNM prosecutions brought against 15 HCPs resulted in only 6 convictions, of which 2 were subsequently overturned on appeal.[276] A review of a sample of Crown Prosecution Service

---

[272] ibid. [60] (Jackson LJ). The Court also reiterated and reaffirmed the seven principles laid down in *Ratcliffe* v *Plymouth & Torbay Health Authority* [1998] PIQR 170, 184.

[273] See also, *Hussain* v *King Edward VII Hospital* [2012] EWHC 3441 (QB).

[274] Note that this has not been in the case in Scotland, which has an offence of culpable homicide rather than a GNM offence which operates in England, Wales, and Northern Ireland. See GMC, 'Independent Review of Gross Negligence Manslaughter and Culpable Homicide (Hamilton Review)' (June 2019) available at <https://www.gmc-uk.org/-/media/documents/independent-review-of-gross-negligence-manslaughter-and-culpable-homicide---final-report_pd-78716610.pdf> accessed 07 December 2022, para 39.

[275] Robin Ferner, 'Medication Errors That Have Led to Manslaughter Charges' (2000) 321 BMJ 1212, See also Oliver Quick, 'Prosecuting "Gross" Clinical Negligence: Manslaughter, Discretion and the Crown Prosecution Service' (2006) 33(3) Journal of Law and Society 421.

[276] Department of Health, 'Williams Review into Gross Negligence Manslaughter in Healthcare' (2018) available at <https://www.gov.uk/government/publications/williams-review-into-gross-negligence-manslaughter-in-healthcare> accessed 07 December 2022, paras 4.5–4.6.

(CPS) files showed that there were 192 GNM investigations referred to the CPS between 2007 and 2018. There was a noticeable increase in the years 2011–17, which they attributed to greater awareness on the part of the police regarding the need to refer such cases to the CPS, alongside better recordkeeping in such cases on the part of both the police and the CPS. Despite such increase, however, it had only resulted in 12 prosecutions, representing 6% of the total number of referrals. Apart from a spike observed in 2014, they noted that the rate of GNM prosecutions against HCPs in the sample reviewed remained relatively stable at one per year during this period.[277]

The requisite elements of the GNM offence are similar to those in the civil law: namely, that there is a duty of care; there is a breach of that duty of care; and the breach amounts to gross negligence. The need for resultant harm is, of course, a given and here it is the death of the patient. The level of negligence which the accused must have manifested is considerably above that at which civil liability may be incurred. Traditionally, such negligence has been defined as 'gross' and, sometimes, somewhat tautologically, as 'criminal negligence'. In essence, the central concern is that it surpasses the civil test, as was stressed in *R v Bateman*:

> In order to establish criminal liability, the facts must be such that . . . the negligence of the accused went beyond a mere matter of compensation between subjects and showed such disregard for the life and safety of others as to amount to a crime against the State and conduct deserving punishment.[278]

Of course, this does not answer the question of when conduct goes beyond the level of financial compensation, but it is probably impossible to be much more specific. What is required is conduct which gives rise to a sense of outrage, or to the conclusion that the accused deserves punishment for what they did. Such a conclusion, though, is likely to be articulated in terms of a lack of regard for the patient's welfare or safety and therein lies the problem. If criminal negligence is defined in terms of a deliberate exposure of the patient to some form of risk, then we are in the realms of recklessness rather than negligence.[279] It is one thing to punish a person for subjective recklessness; it is quite another to punish for objective negligence. In the former case the accused has effectively said, 'I knew of the risk of harm but did not care'; in the latter, they may have been quite unaware of any risk at all. The damage caused may have been the result of incompetence or ignorance, neither of which qualities necessarily deserve criminal punishment.

The leading authority on GNM remains *R v Adomako*,[280] in which an anaesthetist failed to notice the fact that his patient was in distress when this would have been glaringly obvious to any competent medical practitioner. There was conflicting evidence on the question of whether the accused was out of the operating theatre at the time; if he had been, and if there had been a failure on his part to make adequate arrangements for the monitoring of the patient, then that would surely have amounted to a degree of recklessness which was strongly deserving of punishment. If, however, he was merely incompetent, it

---

[277] Danielle Griffiths and Oliver Quick, 'Managing Medical Manslaughter Cases: Improving Efficiency and Transparency?' (University of Bristol Law Research Paper Series 2019) available at <https://research-information.bris.ac.uk/en/publications/managing-medical-manslaughter-cases-improving-efficiency-and-tran> accessed 07 December 2022.

[278] [1925] All ER Rep 45 [48] (Lord Hewart LCJ).

[279] A difficulty which the courts have acknowledged in those decisions where GNM appears to have been replaced by reckless manslaughter: *R v Seymour* [1983] 2 AC 493; *Kong Cheuk Kwan v R* (1986) 82 Cr App R 18.

[280] *R v Prentice, R v Adomako* [1993] 4 All ER 935, sub nom *R v Holloway, R v Adomako, R v Prentice and Sulman* [1993] 4 Med LR 304. See C Dyer, 'Manslaughter Verdict Quashed on Junior Doctors' (1993) 306 BMJ 1432.

might be more difficult to argue for his conviction of manslaughter, although, undoubtedly, professional sanctions would still be needed. The case eventually went on appeal to the House of Lords. The House considered that gross negligence requires 'an egregious failure' to exhibit a minimum standard of competence (judged objectively) or a gross dereliction of care: 'Conduct so bad in all circumstances as to amount to a criminal act or omission.'[281] Lord Mackay explained that the test for gross negligence depends 'on the seriousness of the breach of duty committed by the defendant in all the circumstances in which the defendant was placed ... [and] the extent to which the defendant's conduct departed from the proper standard of care incumbent upon him ... was such that it should be judged criminal.'[282]

As the criminal law now stands, a grossly incompetent doctor is liable to conviction despite the fact that there is no element of subjective wrongdoing on his part. This might well be considered inappropriate.[283] The alternative view is that the law should protect the public and that prosecution represents one way of controlling those who cannot meet minimal professional standards. Surely, however, the law should, at the same time, recognise the difference between the reckless and the inadequate practitioner. The ruling in *Adomako* has remained controversial since it was delivered and there have been various attempts to have the House of Lords revisit their decision. The application for appeal was rejected in *R v Mark*, for example, because it was said that the law is perfectly clear and no decision since *Adomako* has questioned its validity.[284] It was, indeed, applied to uphold the convictions of two doctors in *R v Misra* and *R v Srivastava*,[285] in which a patient died after developing a staphylococcal infection following routine surgery. The prosecution arose not because the doctors had failed to diagnose the particular infection, but because they failed to notice that their patient was ill at all, despite his high fever, high pulse rate, and low blood pressure. They did nothing to diagnose his condition until it was too late and the patient succumbed to toxic shock syndrome. The importance of the appeal lay in the questions it raised as to the compatibility of GNM with the Human Rights Act 1998.

Two essential arguments were made: (i) that there was no 'fair trial' (Article 6 ECHR) in such cases because they involve juries that are not required to articulate the reasoning behind their verdict, and (ii) there was a breach of Article 7 ECHR which requires a clear pre-existing criminal offence in law. The argument here was that the English law lacked clarity because of its circularity: the jury should convict if they consider the defendant's behaviour to be 'criminal'; so what is 'criminal' is what the jury considers to be such. Dismissing the appeals, however, the Court of Appeal held that the elements of the offence are very clearly defined in *Adomako* and involve no uncertainty. A doctor can easily be apprised of his obligation to his patients within the limits of the criminal law. Nor is there any valid human rights argument that can call into question the operation of the present jury system: it has, indeed, been accepted as valid by the ECtHR itself. The Court, once again, refused a request for leave to appeal to the House of Lords. As an addendum to the *Misra* case, the NHS Trust was subsequently prosecuted under section 3 of the Health and Safety at Work etc. Act 1974 on an indictment of five charges. In January 2006, the Trust pleaded guilty to an amended charge of failing to adequately manage and

---

[281] [1995] 1 AC 171 [187] (Lord Mackay).   [282] ibid.

[283] For expansion of this argument, see Alexander McCall Smith, 'Criminal Negligence and the Incompetent Doctor' (1993) 1(3) Medical Law Review 336.

[284] *R v Mark (Alan James)* [2004] EWCA Crim 2490.

[285] [2004] EWCA Crim 2375; (2004) *The Times*, 13 October.

supervise the doctors. The Trust was initially fined £100,000, but this was reduced on appeal to £40,000.[286]

More recent case law has raised a range of troubling concerns about the use of the GNM offence to prosecute doctors arising out of the death of their patients. In *Rudling* v *R*,[287] the Court of Appeal confirmed no case to answer in a prosecution of a GP after the death of a 12-year-old boy from a rare condition who had had intermittent symptoms over a series of months. Symptoms had been recounted over the telephone to the GP on the eve of the child's death, albeit the specific details were disputed on both sides. Determining factors were that the expert witness at no point had stated that there was a serious risk of death, and moreover his interpretation of the medical facts did not support such a conclusion.

In *Rose* v *R*,[288] Ms Rose, a registered optometrist, carried out a sight test on a young child. Retinal images had been taken prior to the testing taking place. Following the consultation, Ms Rose recorded no issues of concern and advised that the child did not need glasses. In the clinical notes, she recorded: 'Reasons for visit: routine check / had few H/ ache over Xmas 2011, but now all gone'. Five months later, the young child became ill and subsequent died. Following a post-mortem investigation, it was revealed that the main cause of death was acute hydrocephalus (i.e. acute build-up of cerebrospinal fluid within the normal ventricles of the brain because its normal outlet had been blocked). Following further investigations, Ms Rose was subsequently charged with GNM. The prosecution argued that GNM was established because Ms Rose had failed, without good reason, to properly to examine the back of the child's eyes during his sight test, as she was required to do by reason of her statutory duty of care. Therefore, she had failed to refer the child for urgent medical treatment as a result of the significant findings shown on the retinal images which she should have viewed. Had she not breached her statutory duty of care to examine his eyes properly and had she referred him, the young child in question could have been successfully treated in hospital and would not have died. In July 2016, Ms Rose was convicted of GNM and was sentenced to two years' imprisonment, suspended for two years. She then appealed to the Court of Appeal, which subsequently quashed her conviction. In the course of its judgment, the Court highlighted the following 'relevant principles' which should be taken into account in GNM prosecutions:

(1) The offence of GNM requires breach of an existing duty of care which it is reasonably foreseeable gives rise to a serious and obvious risk of death and does, in fact, cause death in circumstances where, having regard to the risk of death, the conduct of the defendant was so bad in all the circumstances as to go beyond the requirement of compensation but to amount to a criminal act or omission.

(2) There are, therefore, five elements which the prosecution must prove in order for a person to be guilty of an offence of manslaughter by gross negligence:

(a) the defendant owed an existing duty of care to the victim;

(b) the defendant negligently breached that duty of care;

(c) it was reasonably foreseeable that the breach of that duty gave rise to a serious and obvious risk of death;

---

[286] *R v Southampton University Hospital NHS Trust* [2006] EWCA Crim 2971. For a discussion, see Jo Samanta, 'Charges of Corporate Manslaughter in the NHS' (2006) 332 BMJ 1404.
[287] [2016] EWCA Crim 741.　　[288] [2017] EWCA [2017] EWCA Crim 1168.

(d) the breach of that duty caused the death of the victim;

(e) the circumstances of the breach were truly exceptionally bad and so repre-
     hensible as to justify the conclusion that it amounted to gross negligence and
     required criminal sanction.

(3) The question of whether there is a serious and obvious risk of death must exist at,
     and is to be assessed with respect to, knowledge at the time of the breach of duty.

(4) A recognisable risk of something serious is not the same as a recognisable risk of
     death.

(5) A mere possibility that an assessment might reveal something life-threatening is
     not the same as an obvious risk of death: an obvious risk is a present risk which
     is clear and unambiguous, not one which might become apparent on further
     investigation.[289]

Fundamentally, at the time of the breach of the duty of care, there must be an objectively
foreseeable risk of death and this could not be established on the facts of this case. On this
basis, the accused optometrist was not guilty of the GNM of a boy when she had breached
her duty of care to examine the internal structure of his eyes as part of a routine eye examination, albeit that this then involved a failure to identify an abnormality on the optic
nerve and ultimately led to his death.[290] The judgment has been criticised on the grounds
that it has served to undermine the 'objective nature of the test set out in *Adomako*',[291]
in addition to concerns being expressed that in effect unless 'wilful blindness' is shown,
'even the most truly, exceptionally bad negligence resulting in ignorance will excuse one
suspected of GNM'.[292]

In the wake of the increase in GNM prosecutions involving HCPs in England and
Wales, as well as continuing concerns over the lack of clarity as to when such prosecutions
would be pursued, the Crown Prosecution Service (CPS) published legal guidance setting
out its approach to GNM in 2019. The guidance identified conduct that would meet the
'evidential test for grossness', drawing on relevant case law to date. Examples included
where there was evidence of a course of conduct by an individual and a series of serious
breaches; deliberately overriding or ignoring of systems which were designed to be safe
and had proved to be safe; and ignoring warnings from other members of staff; or acting against the advice of other members of the team alerting them to serious dangers or
risk. It was also emphasised that 'all relevant circumstances in which that individual was
working' would be taken into account by prosecutors in assessing whether the conduct in
question satisfied the test.[293]

In addition to persisting uncertainty as to type and range of negligent conduct that
would satisfy the evidential test for grossness, sentences for HCPs convicted of GNM
have also increased in severity in recent decades. In the case of *Adomako*, the doctor in

---

[289] ibid. [77].   [290] ibid. [94].

[291] Karl Laird, 'Case Comment – Manslaughter: *R v Rose* (Honey Maria) Court of Appeal (Criminal
Division): Sir Brian Leveson P, Haddon-Cave J and Judge Inman QC: 31 July 2017; [2017] EWCA Crim 1168'
(2018) 1 Criminal Law Review 76 [81].

[292] Alexandra Mullock, 'Gross Negligence (Medical) Manslaughter and the Puzzling Implications of
Negligent Ignorance' (2018) 26(2) Medical Law Review 346, 354.

[293] Crown Prosecution Service, 'Gross Negligence Manslaughter' (CPS, 14 March 2019) available at
<https://www.cps.gov.uk/legal-guidance/gross-negligence-manslaughter#:~:text=The%20offence%20
of%20gross%20negligence%20manslaughter%20requires%20breach%20of%20an,so%20bad%20in%20
all%20the> accessed 07 December 2022.

question received a six month suspended sentence despite his conduct being described as 'abysmal' and a 'gross dereliction of care',[294] whereas those convicted in recent years have received custodial sentences spanning a number of years.[295] With updated sentencing guidelines for the GNM offence published for England and Wales in 2018, convicted HCPs are now likely to face a custodial sentence in the range 1–18 years, with provision for sentencing in the upper year range in cases identified as involving a (very) high level of culpability.[296]

Professional regulators have also exhibited a more interventionist approach to dealing with HCPs in the wake of such convictions. This was highlighted by the approach taken by the General Medical Council (GMC) in the *Bawa-Garba* litigation. The regulatory proceedings brought against Dr Hadiza Bawa-Garba are dealt with in detail in Chapter 4. Here we focus primarily on the GNM prosecution and the consequences that followed from the doctor's conviction. To recall, Dr Bawa-Garba had been convicted of GNM, following the death of a six-year-old child, Jake Adcock, who was under her care as a junior paediatrics doctor. Following her GNM conviction, the Medical Practitioners Tribunal Service (MPTS), initially imposed a 12-month suspension from medical practice. Its reasoning for this approach was based on what the Tribunal described as the need to balance 'mitigating and aggravating factors' in her case, which meant that 'erasure would be disproportionate'.[297] Nevertheless, the GMC decided to appeal the MPTS decision to the High Court, arguing that it had been 'wrong' to allow Dr Bawa-Garba to continue to practise, as a GNM conviction was evidence of the fact that her professional failings, which had resulted in the death of her patient, 'were truly exceptionally bad'.[298]

At first instance, Ouseley J agreed with the GMC, holding that the MPTS had failed to give the 'required' weight to the jury's verdict 'when considering the need to maintain public confidence in the profession and proper standards'. In the circumstances, what followed from this was erasure from the medical register.[299] Following a successful appeal by Dr Bawa-Garba, the Court of Appeal ruled that the first instance ruling should be set aside with the Tribunal's decision reinstated. In doing so, the Court recognised that the Tribunal was an expert body which had been satisfied on the evidence that the risk of future harm to patients under Dr Bawa-Garba's care was low, and on a par with other doctors of similar standing and experience.[300] Following this judgment, Dr Bawa-Garba's case again came before the MPTS in April 2019. Having reviewed all the evidence, the Tribunal determined that a cumulative 18-month suspension from medical practice had served the public interest in the circumstances.[301] From July 2021, Dr Bawa-Garba was permitted to return to unrestricted medical practice.[302]

---

[294] *R v Adomako* (n 280).

[295] See e.g., *Garg v R* [2012] EWCA 2520; *Sellu v R* [2016] EWCA Crim 1716.

[296] The Sentencing Council for England and Wales, 'Manslaughter: Definitive Guideline (Crown Court), effective 1 November 2018' (2018) available at <https://www.sentencingcouncil.org.uk/offences/crown-court/item/gross-negligence-manslaughter/> accessed 07 December 2022.

[297] Referred to in *General Medical Council v Bawa-Garba* [2018] EWHC 76 (Admin) [19]–[24] (Ouseley J).

[298] ibid. [38] (Ouseley J); [55] (Gross LJ).

[299] ibid. [53]–[54].

[300] *Bawa-Garba v General Medical Council & Ors* [2018] EWCA Civ 1879 [93].

[301] Medical Practitioners Tribunal Service (MPTS), Record of Determination: Dr Hadiza Bawa-Garba, GMC Ref No 6080659, 9/4/2019, paras 23, 27.

[302] Kim Pilling, 'Dr Hadiza Bawa-Garba Can Return to Unrestricted Practice' (Medscape UK, 2 July 2021) available at <https://www.medscape.co.uk/viewarticle/dr-hadiza-bawa-garba-can-return-unrestricted-practice-2021a1001wcg> accessed 07 December 2022.

There was significant concern expressed by doctors and other HCPs in the wake of the *Bawa-Garba* litigation. In response to such concerns, reviews were commissioned by the GMC (Hamilton Review)[303] and the UK Department of Health (Williams Review).[304] Both called for the embedding of a more just culture in response to the criminalisation of cases of substandard care by HCPs. This would involve the development of 'systems, procedures and processes surrounding the criminal law and medical regulation being applied', in circumstances where HCPs would be able to learn 'without fear of retribution'.[305] At the same time, they should be encouraged to admit to medical errors, against a background where they, and all parties involved, were dealt with in a 'fair and compassionate manner'.[306] Recommendations made included taking steps to minimise professional perceptions of arbitrariness and inconsistency in the conduct of police and prosecutorial investigations into alleged cases of GNM; promoting greater trust between doctors and the GMC through removing its right to appeal fitness to practice decisions; providing greater support to bereaved families through increased transparency of investigative processes; and engaging in professional and systems learning to prevent a reoccurrence of the events that led to the death of patients.[307]

The *Bawa-Garba* litigation served to re-ignite longstanding concerns about the pursuit of GNM prosecutions against individual HCPs. This is particularly so where a range of existing legal options are rarely used—and with little success where they are so used—to prosecute NHS bodies for facilitating unsafe workplace environments where episodes of (grossly) substandard care occur leading to the death of patients.[308] For example, the Corporate Manslaughter and Homicide Act 2007 created the offence of corporate manslaughter which applies to any organisation that owes a duty of care and explicitly covers NHS bodies providing medical treatment. Penalties under the Act include unlimited fines, remedial orders, and publicity orders. Notwithstanding the existence of this legislation, there has only been one successful corporate manslaughter prosecution to date.[309] The lack of successful prosecutions under the Act against NHS bodies has been attributed to difficulties in establishing 'a direct causal link between high level policy decisions and the death of an individual patient'.[310]

Increasingly, England and Wales now present as an outlier in terms of the rate of GNM prosecutions when compared to other Commonwealth jurisdictions.[311] The approach to prosecutions and sentencing are also seen as more punitive than rehabilitative in approach, which arguably is mirrored in the approach taken by professional regulators,

---

[303] Hamilton Review (n 274).

[304] Williams Review (n 276).

[305] ibid. para 3.4.

[306] ibid. para 2.1.

[307] ibid. 5–6.

[308] For a successful prosecution of another NHS Hospital Trust under health and safety legislation, see the case of Swindon Advertiser, 'Court Date Set for Epidural Death Case' (28 December 2009) available at <https://www.swindonadvertiser.co.uk/news/4822073.court-date-set-for-epidural-death-case/> accessed 07 December 2022.

[309] *R v Cornish and another* [2016] EWHC 779 (QB).

[310] Hamilton Review (n 274) para 76. For a successful prosecution of another NHS Hospital Trust under health and safety legislation, see Swindon Advertiser (n 308).

[311] For an overview of the approach taken in other Commonwealth jurisdictions towards the criminalisation of healthcare malpractice, see Anne-Maree Farrell, Amel Alghrani, and Melinee Kazarian, 'Gross Negligence Manslaughter in Healthcare: Time for a Restorative Justice Approach?' (2020) 28(3) Medical Law Review 526, 534–537.

such as the GMC, which was criticised for its pursuit of Dr Bawa-Garba's erasure from the medical register (as we discuss further in Chapter 4).[312] It also leads us to consider whether it might be appropriate for HCPs to receive some form of special immunity from such prosecutions, or indeed whether the criminal law should be invoked at all in cases of medical error.[313] If it is to be invoked, then it could be argued that specific criminal offences should be created which recognise the socially vital work that HCPs undertake which often involve quick, high-pressure decision-making in complex institutional environments. However, it could be counterargued that this set of workplace circumstances also apply to other professional occupations, so it is not clear why HCPs should be singled out for special treatment in this way.

12.8 ALTERNATIVES TO CLINICAL NEGLIGENCE LITIGATION

Clinical negligence is more than a matter between two parties. It is also a serious political and economic issue. For injured patients or families where their loved one has died as a result of alleged negligence by HCPs, what published empirical research tells us about their experiences is that the decision to pursue a clinical negligence claim is not taken lightly.[314] It usually comes at the end of a process where (in)formal complaints have been made,[315] there has been poor or unsatisfactory communication and a lack of follow up on the part of treating HCPs and institutions over concerns expressed by injured patients and/or families.[316] When things go wrong in the provision of health care and harm is caused, what patients have indicated they want is an explanation as to what went wrong; an apology; financial compensation where appropriate; and that lessons are learned and

---

[312] ibid. 543–544.

[313] Margaret Brazier and Amel Alghrani, 'Fatal Medical Malpractice and Criminal Liability' (2009) 25(2) Professional Negligence 5; Oliver Quick, 'Expert Evidence and Medical Manslaughter: Vagueness in Action' (2011) 38(4) Journal of Law and Society 469.

[314] Alexy Buck, Pascoe Pleasance, and Nigel Balmer, 'Do Citizens Know How to Deal with Legal Issues? Some Empirical Insights' (2008) 37(4) Journal of Social Politics 661.

[315] Each of the UK's four health systems have different approaches to managing patient complaints: NHS England, 'Complaint Policy' (16 November 2021) available at <https://www.england.nhs.uk/publication/nhs-england-complaints-policy/> accessed 07 December 2022; NHS Wales, 'Complaints and Concerns: Putting Things Right' (14 September 2020) available at <https://gov.wales/nhs-wales-complaints-and-concerns-putting-things-right> accessed 07 December 2022; Scotland, NHS Inform, 'Making A Complaint About Your NHS Care Or Treatment' (2022) available at <https://www.nhsinform.scot/care-support-and-rights/health-rights/feedback-and-complaints/making-a-complaint-about-your-nhs-care-or-treatment/> accessed 07 December 2022; Northern Ireland, 'HSC Complaints – Standards and Guidelines' (1 April 2022) available at <https://www.health-ni.gov.uk/publications/hsc-complaints-standards-and-guidelines> accessed 07 December 2022. See also Chapter 4 for details of how patients can also make complaints to professional regulators (e.g. General Medical Council).

[316] Frank Stephen, Angelia Melville, and Tammy Krause, 'A Study of Medical Negligence in Scotland' (Scottish Government Social Research, 2012) available at <https://www.escholar.manchester.ac.uk/api/datastream?publicationPid=uk-ac-man-scw:162603&datastreamId=FULL-TEXT.PDF> accessed 07 December 2022; NHS Resolution, 'Behavioural Insights Team and NHS Resolution, Behavioural Insights Into Patient Motivation To Make A Clinical Negligence Claim' (August 2018) available at <https://resolution.nhs.uk/resources/behavioural-insights-into-patient-motivation-to-make-a-claim-for-clinical-negligence/> accessed 07 December 2022.

those responsible are held to account for the harm caused so that it does not happen again.[317] From the point of view of those in medical and governmental circles, there are longstanding concerns about the increased rate of clinical negligence claims, as well as the accompanying costs to the NHS as a result. This is quite apart from the time and resources that HCPs must devote to defending such claims, in addition to reputational concerns and the general stress of being involved in such litigation. It is argued that monies spent on clinical negligence litigation could be better spent on the provision of vital healthcare resources, as well as on treating patients. In addition, it is argued that the adversarial nature of the litigation process is harmful to all involved parties as its focuses on blame, rather than promoting a culture of learning from clinical error.[318]

The costs of clinical negligence litigation have increased at a steady rate in recent decades in the UK, but a range of strategies have been employed to manage the process. This is exemplified in the approach taken by NHS Resolution which runs a number of schemes as part of managing the defence of clinical negligence claims in England.[319] This includes the Clinical Negligence Scheme for Trusts (CNST), which is by far the largest scheme.[320] The high-value claims within this scheme are obstetric claims (otherwise known as maternity claims), which account for '62% of the total estimated value of new claims', despite being only 12% of all such claims. In order to reduce the rate of such claims, NHS Resolution operates an Early Notification Scheme which it states has provided for ongoing feedback on safety improvements, as well as early admissions of liability and interim payments, where appropriate.[321] Another key scheme managed by NHS Resolution is the Clinical Negligence Scheme for General Practice, covering clinical negligence liabilities arising in general practice in relation to incidents that occurred on or after 1 April 2019. Claims prior to this date are managed as part of the Existing Liabilities Scheme for General Practice (ELSGP), many of which were previously managed by a range of Medical Defence Organisations (MDOs).[322]

---

[317] For a seminal paper on the topic, see Charles Vincent, Magi Young, and A Phillips, 'Why Do People Sue Their Doctors? A Study of Patients and Relatives Taking Legal Action' (1994) 343(8913) BMJ 1612.

[318] For a recent overview of such arguments, see UK Parliament Health and Social Care Committee, 'NHS Litigation Reform, Thirteenth Report of Session 2021-22' HC740 (28 April 2022).

[319] While we draw on the defence of clinical negligence claims in England by NHS Resolution by way of example, it is important to recognise that different bodies and protocols exist for managing the defence of these claims in other UK jurisdictions. In the case of Scotland: NHS National Services Scotland, Central Legal Office, Clinical Negligence and Other Risks Scheme (CNORIS), see Central Legal Office, 'CNORIS' (2022) available at <https://clo.scot.nhs.uk/our-services/cnoris.aspx> 07 December 2022. In Wales: NHS Wales, Shared Services Partnership, Legal & Risk Services, Clinical Negligence, see NWSSP, 'Clinical Negligence' (2022) available at <https://nwssp.nhs.wales/ourservices/legal-risk-services/areas-of-practice/clinical-negligence/> accessed 07 December 2022. In Northern Ireland: Health and Social Care, Directorate of Legal Services, Clinical Negligence, see HSC Business Services Organisation, 'Clinical Negligence and Inquests Team' (2022) available at <https://hscbusiness.hscni.net/services/1950.htm> accessed 07 December 2022.

[320] NHS Resolution, 'Clinical Negligence Scheme for Trusts (CNST)' (2022) available at <https://resolution.nhs.uk/services/claims-management/clinical-schemes/clinical-negligence-scheme-for-trusts/> accessed 07 December 2022. Note: From 1 April 2013, independent sector providers of NHS care have been able to join CNST and cover under CNST was extended to include the cost of representation at inquests.

[321] NHS Resolution, 'Early Notification Scheme' (2022) available at <https://resolution.nhs.uk/services/claims-management/clinical-schemes/clinical-negligence-scheme-for-trusts/early-notification-scheme/> accessed 07 December 2022.

[322] For further details on this scheme, see NHS Resolution, 'General Practice Indemnity' (2022) available at <https://resolution.nhs.uk/services/claims-management/clinical-schemes/general-practice-indemnity/> accessed 07 December 2022.

The management of such schemes forms part of NHS Resolution's overarching pro-active approach to the resolution of clinical negligence claims, which it has argued has been successful in both preventing claims, and contributing to their early resolution without the need for court proceedings:

> A record 77% of claims were resolved in 2021/22 without court proceedings, continu-ing the year-on-year reduction for the last five years, and in line with NHS Resolution's strategy to keep patients and healthcare staff out of court. This was achieved by the delivery of a range of dispute resolution approaches described in the report and contin-ued cooperation across the legal market, which continued to gain momentum during the pandemic. The reduction in litigation has not, however, been at the expense of a less rigorous approach to investigation. NHS Resolution's flagship Early Notification Scheme for maternity incidents is reported in detail as it entered its fifth year of accel-erating the investigation of brain injury sustained at birth, supported by a new patient advisory group.[323]

NHS Resolution's latest Annual Report revealed that payments against all its clinical schemes for 2021/22 were £2,402.8 million in total (up from £2,209.3 million in 2020/21). This comprised damages paid to claimants of £1,775.3 million (up by 10.3% from 2020–21), with claimant legal costs at £470.9 million (up 5.1% from 2020–21); and defendant legal costs at £156.6 million (up from 3.4% in 2020–21). NHS Resolution has acknowl-edged that a contributing factor to the increase in defence legal costs was in 'in part attrib-uted to increased spending on the general practice indemnity schemes, mainly the Existing Liabilities Scheme for General Practice (ELSGP).'[324] NHS Resolution also noted that the provision (not compensation payouts) for claims arising in relation to incidents in 2021/22 under the CNST scheme stood at £13.3 billion, which it referred to as the 'annual cost of harm'. Although recognising that this was 'a very significant sum', it acknowledged that the more accurate provision was in fact £8.7 billion (once account was taken of the UK Government's Treasury discount rate change during 2021–22).[325]

It has long been acknowledged that clinical negligence litigation is one of the most dif-ficult and complex areas of personal injury law, particularly with regard to establishing liability (see earlier in this chapter).[326] The litigation system has been criticised on the basis of excessive costs, lack of accessibility, and a failure to improve patient safety at a systemic level. This has been combined with concerns about the adverse psycho-social impact on both injured patients and HCPs resulting from the litigation process.[327] As a result, this has led to successive proposals for reform in the area, many of which have

---

[323] NHS Resolution, 'Annual Report and Accounts 2021/22' (2022) available at <https://resolution.nhs.uk/corporate-reports/> accessed 07 December 2022.

[324] ibid.   [325] ibid 9.

[326] Note that clinical negligence often warrants separate consideration in any proposals for law reform in personal injury litigation, see e.g. 'Royal Commission on Compensation for Personal Injury' (Pearson Report) Cmnd 7054–1, 1978; 'Access to Justice: Final Report to the Lord Chancellor on the Civil Justice System in England and Wales' (1996) (Woolf Report); 'Review of Civil Litigation Costs: Final Report' (TSO 2009) (Jackson Report), Part 4, 23.

[327] In relation to clinical negligence claiming, see e.g. Kelly Dickson et al., 'No-Fault Compensation Schemes: A Rapid Realist Review', (EPPI-Centre, 2016) available at <https://eppi.ioe.ac.uk/cms/Publications/Systematicreviews/No-faultcompensationschemesArapidrealistreview/tabid/3687/Default.aspx> accessed 07 December 2022; Arpan Mehta, Tamás Szakmany, and Annie Sorbie, 'The Medicolegal Landscape Through the Lens of COVID-19: Time for Reform' (2021) 114(2) Journal of the Royal Society of Medicine 55–59.

recommended either partial or wholesale replacement of clinical negligence claiming with a no-fault scheme arising from harm caused in healthcare settings.[328] In the alternative, calls have also been made for the granting of specific immunity for HCPs in relation to clinical litigation processes, most recently arising from the demands created by working during a public health emergency, such as the Covid-19 pandemic.[329]

Notwithstanding recommendations for reform in this regard, there has been little success in implementing a UK-wide scheme in this regard (with a notable exception in Wales, see below). In the past two decades, the publication of National Audit Office (NAO) reports on the increasing costs of clinical negligence litigation has provided the political catalyst for proposals for reform. Following the publication of an NAO Report in 2001,[330] the then Chief Medical Officer for England proposed that an NHS redress scheme be established.[331] This subsequently led to the adoption of legislation in 2006 to establish NHS redress schemes in England and Wales for small value claims up to £25,000, where redress would involve the provision of explanations, apologies and lesson-learning.[332] In the end, it was never implemented in England; however, it was subsequently adopted in Wales. The Welsh NHS redress scheme covers small value claims up to a maximum of £25,000, where a 'qualifying liability' is established. This eligibility criterion essentially mirrors tort-based liability and requires that where a patient has suffered harm as a result of a breach of a duty of care from an organisation or healthcare professional, then they must inform the complainant, provide copies of the records and any expert evidence and offer access to free legal advice.[333] Notwithstanding the implementation of the redress scheme in Wales, concerns have been expressed that it has operated to increase, rather than decrease, the cost of claiming in practice.[334]

In 2011, the No-Fault Compensation Review Group published its findings, recommending the adoption of a no-fault scheme in Scotland.[335] The Group laid out what it considered to be essential features of such a scheme, focusing on the cause of harm from medical (in)action rather than proof of fault, and including a need to have an efficient, equitable and affordable scheme. The proposal involved ten recommendations and would

---

[328] For a recent reform proposal regarding a partial no-fault scheme focused on obstetric claims in England, see UK Department of Health, 'Rapid Resolution and Redress Scheme for Severe Birth Injury' (1 December 2017) available at <https://www.gov.uk/government/consultations/rapid-resolution-and-redress-scheme-for-severe-birth-injury> accessed 07 December 2022.

[329] For commentary on the advantages of granting immunity to HCPs from clinical negligence claims, see (Christine Tonkins—Yes) and disadvantages (Jose Miola et al.—No), see Christine Tomkins et al., 'Should Doctors Tackling Covid-19 Be Immune from Negligence Liability Claims?' (2020) 370 BMJ m2487.

[330] National Audit Office, 'Handling Clinical Negligence Claims in England, Report by the Comptroller and Auditor-General' (03 May 2001) HC 403, Session 2000–2001.

[331] Department of Health, 'Making Amends: A Consultation Paper Setting Out Proposals for Reforming the Approach to Clinical Negligence in the NHS: A Report' (2003).

[332] NHS Redress Act 2006, c. 44; Anne-Maree Farrell and Sarah Devaney, 'Making Amends or Making Things Worse? Clinical Negligence Reform and Patient Redress in England' (2007) 27(4) Legal Studies 630. Note also the Compensation Act 2006, c.29, s 2 which states: 'an apology, an offer of treatment or other redress, shall not of itself amount to an admission of negligence or breach of statutory duty'.

[333] National Health Service (Concerns, Complaints and Redress Arrangements) (Wales) Regulations 2011 (SI 2011/704).

[334] See Vivienne Harpwood, 'Clinical Negligence and Poor Quality Care: Is Wales Putting Things Right?' in Pamela Ferguson and Graeme Laurie (eds.), *Inspiring a Medico-legal Revolution: Essays in Honour of Sheila McLean* (Ashgate 2015). In relation to current concerns about the increasing cost of clinical negligence claims in Wales, see Mark Smith, 'The Astronomical Sums the Welsh NHS Has Paid Out in Compensation Claims' (Cymru Online, 28 September 2022) available at <https://www.walesonline.co.uk/news/health/astronomical-sums-welsh-nhs-paid-25124997> accessed 07 December 2022.

[335] No-Fault Compensation Review Group, Report and Recommendations: Volumes I-III (February 2011) (McLean Report).

cover all medical treatment injuries in Scotland and awards would be based on need (not tariffs). The Report also explored the relationship between the scheme and the right to litigation and would involve an independent appeal process. The Scottish Government conducted a consultation on the proposal, and subsequently published its own preferred approach in 2016.[336] To date, however, no further steps have been taken to implement its preferred no fault scheme.[337]

In 2017, the NAO again published a report outlining concerns about the costs of clinical negligence claims, which it noted were rising at a faster rate than NHS funding on a year-on-year basis. The report concluded that the UK Government lacked 'a coherent cross-government strategy, underpinned by policy, to support measures to tackle the rising cost of clinical negligence'.[338] This led to a further round of parliamentary reports,[339] as well as government consultations and proposals for reform designed to bring down the costs of clinical negligence litigation.[340] More recently, the Cumberlege Review, which investigated a range of concerns arising out of the administration of various medicines and medical devices that subsequently harmed patients, recommended an independent redress agency be established that would focus on 'a no-blame, systems-based approach to delivering redress as a substitute for litigation'.[341] The advantages of the proposed redress agency were identified as offering easier access and 'one fixed point of contact; it would be flexible to adapt and respond to situations as they arise.' The Cumberlege Review also suggested that the redress agency would 'operate in line with the ombudsman model. It will listen to both sides, investigate impartially and reach a decision.'[342]

In 2021, the UK Parliament's House of Commons Health and Social Care Committee published the findings from its inquiry into the safety of maternity services in England. The report emphasised the need for clinical negligence reform, which it stated would involve a shift away from 'adversarial court-based dispute resolution to administrative compensation schemes', resulting in lower costs. As part of such reform, it was recommended that a no-fault compensation scheme be established in relation to avoidable harm arising in maternity cases.[343] In 2022, the Committee published a further report

---

[336] Scottish Government, 'Consultation Report—Consultation on Recommendations for No-fault Compensation in Scotland for Injuries Resulting from Clinical Treatment' (4 April 2014) available at <https://www.gov.scot/publications/consultation-report-consultation-recommendations-fault-compensation-scotland-injuries-resulting-clinical-treatment/> accessed 07 December 2022.

[337] Carolyn Jackson and Laura Dodson, 'No-Fault Compensation for Medical Negligence? Watch This Space' *The Scotsman* (26 September 2022) available at <https://www.scotsman.com/news/opinion/columnists/no-fault-compensation-for-medical-negligence-watch-this-space-carolyn-jackson-laura-dodson-3852591> accessed 07 December 2022.

[338] National Audit Office, 'Managing the Costs of Clinical Negligence in Trusts (2017–19)' HC 305, 7 September 2017.

[339] See e.g. UK Parliament, House of Commons, Committee on Public Accounts, 'Managing the Costs of Clinical Negligence in Hospital Trusts' (2017–19) HC 397 (01 December 2017).

[340] For an overview of government initiatives in relation to clinical negligence reform in the period 2017–2021, see Charley Coleman, 'Negligence in the NHS, Liability Costs' (House of Lords Library, 29 November 2021) available at <https://lordslibrary.parliament.uk/negligence-in-the-nhs-liability-costs/> accessed 07 December 2022.

[341] 'First Do No Harm: The Report of the Independent Medicines and Medical Devices Safety Review', 8 July 2020 (Cumberlege Review) para. 2.51.

[342] ibid. Appendix 3, para 16.

[343] UK Parliament, House of Commons, Health and Social Care Committee, 'The Safety of Maternity Services in England, Fourth Report of Session 2021-22' HC 19 (6 July 2021) paras 91–92.

examining in detail the need for reform of clinical negligence litigation in England, with a view to addressing rising costs, learning from error, and improving patient safety. The Committee's 'central recommendation' was as follows:

> the NHS adopt a radically different system for compensating injured patients which moves away from a system based on apportioning blame and prioritises learning from mistakes. An independent administrative body should be made responsible for investigating cases and determining eligibility for compensation in the most serious cases. Reconstituting the new Special Health Authority, which will take over maternity investigations from HSSIB, would be an efficient way for the Government to implement our recommendation. This would be the most effective long-term way to reduce both the number of tragedies and the cost to the NHS. Changing from a blame culture to a learning culture is not easy but can be accelerated by some simple but important changes to current NHS processes which we encourage the Government to adopt.[344]

There has been stakeholder criticism of the Report, which has ranged from its findings being 'ill-informed', to concerns that any attempt to abolish a fault-based approach will be unworkable in practice, and that patient-claimants will not receive appropriate remedial or 'top-up' care for injuries suffered through avoidable treatment incidents.[345] More broadly, patient advocacy groups remain concerned that the reform proposals may in fact reduce 'access to justice for the very people that the NHS has harmed and is incompatible with a "just culture and a false economy".'[346] The current UK Government has indicated that it is committed to a programme of reform in relation to clinical negligence litigation (England only), which includes proposals for implementing fixed recoverable medico-legal fees in lower-value claims, as well as supporting initiatives to facilitate the quicker resolution of claims.[347] At the time of writing, it remains to be seen whether it is committed to pursuing the recommendation from the Health and Social Care Committee with regard to establishing a no-fault (or administrative) scheme as an alternative to the current clinical negligence litigation system.

With no-fault schemes often expressed in policy, academic, and practitioner literatures as a preferred option for clinical negligence reform, what has been identified as the key features of such schemes, as well as their advantages and disadvantages? By way of example, a report commissioned by the No-Fault Compensation Review Group in Scotland provided a cross-jurisdictional review of such schemes in New Zealand, Sweden, Denmark,

[344] UK Parliament, House of Commons, Health and Social Care Committee, 'NHS Litigation Reform, Thirteenth Report of Session 2021-22' HC740 (28 April 2022) para 8.

[345] See e.g. Exchange Chambers, 'Barristers from Exchange Chambers Criticise Proposed Reforms to Clinical Negligence Litigation' (6 May 2022) available at <https://www.exchangechambers.co.uk/barristers-criticise-proposed-reforms-clinical-negligence-litigation/> accessed 07 December 2022.

[346] AvMA, 'Health and Social Care Committee Inquiry: NHS Litigation Reform' (18 November 2021) available at <https://www.avma.org.uk/news/health-and-social-care-committee-inquiry-nhs-litigation-reform/> accessed 07 December 2022.

[347] See e.g. UK Department of Health and Social Care, 'Fixed Recoverable Costs in Lower Value Clinical Negligence Claims' (31 January 2022) available at <https://www.gov.uk/government/consultations/fixed-recoverable-costs-in-lower-value-clinical-negligence-claims> accessed 07 December 2022; Zoë Grunëwald, 'Government Publishes Proposals for NHS Litigation Reform' New Statesman (2 February 2022) available at <https://www.newstatesman.com/spotlight/healthcare/2022/02/government-publishes-proposals-for-nhs-litigation-reform> accessed 07 December 2022.

Norway, and Finland, and Virginia and Florida in the United States.[348]Although the basis for such schemes varies, they often include the following common features:

- All have eligibility and threshold disability criteria which need to be satisfied before cover is accepted.
- There may be caps on certain categories of compensation and compensation for non-pecuniary losses, such as pain and suffering, may not be available.
- Levels of financial compensation/entitlements tend to be lower for comparative injuries in clinical negligence claims brought under tort-based systems.
- There is simpler and broader 'access to justice' in no-fault schemes, particularly in relation to the cost of initiating or submitting claims, as well as time to resolution.
- Access to the courts may be restricted.
- Clinical staff remain accountable for their actions through other regulatory systems.

The Review also identified the following advantages of no-fault compensation schemes, with particular reference to the schemes operating in New Zealand and Sweden:

- A principled social/community response to personal injury which includes a recognition of community responsibility; comprehensive entitlement; full rehabilitation; fair and adequate compensation; and administrative efficiency.
- More patients are eligible for compensation than under tort-based schemes.
- A clear and faster road map towards obtaining redress for patients who have suffered medical injury, than that available from litigation.
- Promotion of better, as well as less defensive, relationships between patients and health practitioners when medical injury has occurred.
- Greater efficiency in terms of both time and costs than would be the case in relation to the management of clinical negligence claims brought under tort-based systems.
- Much-reduced threat of litigation for clinicians and reduced insurance premiums.

The positive features of no-fault compensation are considerable and such schemes are well established in a number of countries. However, it is important to recognise that they are not a panacea and cannot meet all the needs of injured patients and their families. No-fault schemes still require that causation be established which, as we have seen earlier in this chapter, is one of the most difficult aspects of bringing a successful clinical negligence claim. Eligibility thresholds may also vary across no-fault schemes and they may change over time depending on scheme preferences and the ongoing financial viability of the scheme. The effect of widening access to justice which is seen as a clear advantage of such schemes may also impact downstream in terms of lower value awards of compensation being made, than would otherwise have been the case in the courts.

In order to ensure quality of justice for injured patients who seek to access such schemes, it is also vital that appropriate medico-legal expert advice is available to them to assess eligibility and causation issues. In the circumstances, medico-legal experts need to be remunerated appropriately for advice in relation to what can often be complex issues

---

[348] Anne-Maree Farrell, Sarah Devaney, and Amber Dar, 'No-Fault Compensation Schemes for Medical Injury: A Review' (2013) available at <https://papers.ssrn.com/sol3/papers.cfm?abstract_id=2221836> accessed 07 December 2022; Michael Bichard et al., 'Expert Report to the Infected Blood Inquiry on Public Health and Administration' (Infected Blood Inquiry, 4 August 2022) 63–64.

arising from substandard care and causation of harm in healthcare settings. Low fixed recoverable medico-legal fees will necessarily impact on the preparedness of such experts to provide such advice. We also cannot assume that the establishment of no-fault schemes will necessarily enhance safety learning or have a major impact on the blame culture, and this will require significant investment in terms of institutional, professional, and financial support for this to be effective.

Drawing on the example provided by Nordic no-fault schemes, it is also important to keep in mind that no fault schemes are likely to work best in conjunction with well-established and well-funded national social security systems. With relatively low levels of social security provision in the UK, higher levels of compensation would be required to adequately support injured patients in any no-fault scheme.[349] There is no doubt that no-fault schemes have some significant advantages over clinical negligence claiming, as outlined. No-fault schemes have the potential to compensate more injured patients, provide compensation more quickly, with less stress to all concerned. They may also be particularly suited to dealing with the impact of new technologies, such as artificial intelligence (AI) systems, on the delivery of health care.[350] However, in designing, implementing, and funding such a scheme, it must always be kept in mind that account must be taken not only of access but also of the quality of justice provided, to injured patients and their families.

12.9 CONCLUSION

In this chapter, we examined key elements involved in bringing a claim in clinical negligence with a focus on England and Wales, where a patient alleges that they have suffered harm in a healthcare setting, including duty of care, breach of the duty of care, and factual and legal causation. We also highlighted the contested issues and policy conundrums that have arisen in different types of clinical negligence claims, such as where innovative techniques and complementary medicine are used and there is misdiagnosis and negligence in treatment. This is in addition to considering how best to address the problem of the novice HCP, where responsibility should lie for protecting patients from themselves, and the thorny ethical and legal issues raised by wrongful conception, birth, and life claims. The doctrine of *res ipsa loquitur* was also briefly considered, as well as the issues faced by HCPs where the death of a patient may lead to engagement with the criminal law. Alternatives to the current clinical negligence litigation system were also considered, including recent government and parliamentary proposals for reform in the area. It was recognised that this is a difficult and complex area of personal injury litigation, but also one which is highly politically sensitive given that it takes place in the context of a publicly funded health system. While reform based on a

---

[349] For a detailed overview of the principles that should be taken into consideration in designing no-fault schemes for medical injury, see McLean Report (n 335); Anne-Maree Farrell, 'No Fault Compensation for Medical Injury: Principles, Practice and Prospects for Reform' in Pamela Ferguson and Graeme Laurie (eds), *Inspiring a Medico-Legal Revolution: Essays in Honour of Sheila McLean* (Ashgate 2015) 155–170. See more generally, Sonia McLeod and Christopher Hodges, *Redress Schemes for Personal Injuries* (Hart 2017).

[350] It has also been argued that such schemes may also be more appropriate for dealing with difficulties in establishing liability created by the use of AI systems in healthcare, see Søren Holm, Catherine Stanton, and Benjamin Bartlett, 'A New Argument for No-Fault Compensation in Health Care: The Introduction of Artificial Intelligence Systems' (2021) 29(3) Health Care Analysis 171–188.

no-fault (or other administrative) scheme appears to be the preferred option, important justice-based issues are at stake for injured patients and their families. Such issues must necessarily be taken into account in the event that reform proposals are taken forward towards implementation in the future.

FURTHER READING

1. Tom Douglas, 'Medical Injury Compensation; Beyond "No-Fault"' (2009) 17(1) Medical Law Review 30–51.

2. Danielle Griffiths and Andrew Sanders (eds), *Medicine Crime and Society, Bioethics, Medicine and the Criminal Law, Volume 2* (CUP 2013).

3. Rob Heywood, '"If the Problem Persists, Come Back To See Me . . . ." An Empirical Study of Clinical Negligence Cases Against General Practitioners' (2019) 27(3) Medical Law Review 406.

4. Alan Merry and Warren Brookbanks, *Errors, Medicine and the Law* (2nd edn, CUP 2017).

5. Ash Samanta, Jo Samanta, and Joanne Beswick, 'Responsible Practice or Restricted Practice? An Empirical Study of the Use of Clinical Guidelines in Medical Negligence Litigation' (2021) 29(2) Medical Law Review 205.

6. Gemma Turton, 'The Scope of a Doctor's Duty of Care to their Patient' (2022) Medical Law Review available at <https://academic.oup.com/medlaw/advance-article-abstract/doi/10.1093/medlaw/fwac031/6671816?redirectedFrom=fulltext> accessed 08 December 2022.

13

ORGAN DONATION FOR TRANSPLANTATION

13.1 INTRODUCTION

In the twenty-first century, advances in scientific research, biotechnology, and clinical care have greatly expanded the potential for organ and tissue donation and transplantation. There have been recent successes with uterine and reconstructive transplants,[1] and research continues into xenotransplantation, although safety and regulatory challenges remain.[2] Work also continues into potential clinical applications arising from organoids research, as well as 3D bioprinting or bio-inks of organs.[3] Notwithstanding such developments, deceased human donors remain the main source of organ donation, although rates of living organ donation continue to rise, particularly involving kidneys. In addition, organ donors with a disclosed history of increased risk behaviour (IRB) are now considered as part of the range of deceased donors whose organs are made available for transplantation purposes.[4] As things stand, there remains a significant gap between demand and supply of solid human organs for transplantation purposes, including hearts, lungs, kidneys, livers, intestines, and pancreases. There are over 6,800 people on transplant waiting lists in the UK at the time of writing, and over 420 people died while on the waiting list in the 2021–22 financial year.[5] The situation is worse for people from Black and Asian backgrounds, who are more likely to suffer from an illness that may lead to them needing a transplant.[6]

---

[1] See Ben Peyton-Jones et al., 'Uterine Transplantation: Scientific Impact Paper No. 65' (Royal College of Obstetricians and Gynaecologists, April 2021) 128(1) BJOG: An International Journal of Obstetrics & Gynaecology e51.

[2] See Koko Kwisda, Tobias Kantz, and Nils Hoppe, 'Regulatory and Intellectual Property Conundrums Surrounding Xenotransplantation' (2021) 39 Nature Biotechnology 796.

[3] Madhuri Dey and Ibrahim Ozbolat, '3D B of Cells, Tissues and Organs' (2020) 10(1) Science Reports 14023; Jihoon Kim, Bon-Young Koo, and Jurgen Knoblic, 'Human Organoids: Model Systems for Human Biology and Medicine' (2020) 21(10) Nature Reviews Molecular Cell Biology 571.

[4] Patrick Trotter et al., 'Deceased Organ Donors with a History of Increased Risk Behavior for the Transmission of Blood-Borne Viral Infection: The UK Experience' (2017) 101(7) Transplantation 1679.

[5] NHSBT, 'Statistics about Organ Donation' (2022) available at <https://www.organdonation.nhs.uk/helping-you-to-decide/about-organ-donation/statistics-about-organ-donation/> accessed 29 December 2022.

[6] Note that 'Black patients wait almost a year longer for a kidney transplant when compared to White patients. One year after being listed for a kidney transplant, 35% of White patients had received their transplant whereas only 19% of Black, Asian, Mixed Race or minority ethnic patients had received a transplant ... This shows the continued imbalance between the need for transplants in our Black and Asian communities and the availability of suitable organs'. See NHSBT, 'Organ Donation and Transplantation data for Black, Asian, Mixed Race and Minority Ethnic (BAME) Communities Report for 2020/2021' (23 May 2022) available at <https://www.organdonation.nhs.uk/helping-you-to-decide/about-organ-donation/statistics-about-organ-donation/transplant-activity-report/#bame> accessed 29 December 2022.

In order to address this persisting problem of organ shortage, national legislative reform has also recently taken place, involving a shift towards opt-out organ donation regimes which is designed to encourage higher rates of deceased organ donation.[7] We provide an overview of such reform in this chapter, as part of an examination of key legal and ethical issues arising in relation to both deceased and living organ donation for transplantation. In the final section of the chapter, we also briefly consider scientific, legal, and ethical issues arising in xenotransplantation. By way of introduction, we now turn to provide a brief overview of key organisations, as well as key legal frameworks that inform the approach taken to organ donation for transplantation in the UK.

13.2 KEY LEGISLATION AND ORGANISATIONS

There are two main legislative instruments in the UK which provide the legal framework for organ donation. The Human Tissue Act 2004 (HTA 2004) covers England, Wales, and Northern Ireland (NI), and the Human Tissue (Scotland) Act 2006 (HTA 2006) covers Scotland only. Both Acts have been subject to amendment since they were passed, with a range of statutory instruments being adopted to support them. Prior to Brexit, organ donation for transplantation in the UK was also subject to EU laws. Specifically, this included the EU Organs Directive, which was transposed into UK law in 2012.[8] The Directive provided for the setting of quality and safety standards involving human organ donation for transplantation for transposition into the laws of EU Member States. Legislation was subsequently passed to ensure that these standards remained in place in the UK post-Brexit from 1 January 2021 onwards.[9]

In general terms, the Acts set out the arrangements for donor consent or authorisation, with both being fundamental principles underpinning the lawful removal, storage, and use of body parts, organs, and tissue. In addition, they set out how organs and tissues may be acceptably used, as well as the data that must be recorded to ensure compliance. Different consent requirements apply when dealing with 'tissue' from the deceased and the living, including organs intended for transplantation. Both pieces of legislation provide for certain organisations to regulate activities concerning the removal, storage, use and disposal of human tissue. In the case of the HTA 2004, the Human Tissue Authority was established as the nominated regulator for England, Wales, and NI, and is a non-departmental public body (otherwise known as an 'arms-length body') of the UK Department of Health and Social Care.[10]

---

[7] For a short summary of the changes brought about this legislative reform in the UK, see NHSBT, 'Organ Donation Laws' (2022) available at <https://www.organdonation.nhs.uk/helping-you-to-decide/organ-donation-laws/> accessed 29 December 2022.

[8] Directive 2010/53/EU of the European Parliament and of the Council of 7 July 2010 on standards of quality and safety of human organs intended for transplantation [2010] OJ L 207/14–29. The EU Directive was transposed into UK law via the Quality and Safety of Organs Intended for Transplantation Regulations 2012.

[9] See the Quality and Safety of Organs Intended for Transplantation (Amendment) (EU Exit) Regulations 2019, which apply on a UK-wide basis. From 1 January 2021, it has also been necessary to treat suppliers outside the UK as third country suppliers in relation to the import or export of organs, tissues and cells, necessitating the obtaining of a relevant import/export licence and where it involves an import, then an import agreement with the third country supplier. See UK Government, 'Quality and Safety of Human Organs, Cells and Tissue' (28 September 2021) available at <https://www.gov.uk/guidance/quality-and-safety-of-human-organs-tissues-and-cells> accessed 29 December 2022.

[10] Human Tissue Authority, 'Who Are the HTA?' (2022) available at <https://www.hta.gov.uk/about-hta/who-are-hta> accessed 29 December 2022.

The Human Tissue Authority regulates organisations that remove, store, and use human tissue for research, medical treatment, post-mortem examination, education and training, and display in public. It is charged with licensing the quality and safety of organs intended for transplantation, which was originally part of the UK's obligations under EU laws, and these powers have continued in the post-Brexit period (see previously). The Authority also gives approval for organ and bone marrow donations from living organ donors and ensures that consent processes in relation to this form of donation are complied with. In relation to deceased organ donation, it ensures compliance with legal consent requirements under the HTA, providing advice and guidance to professionals. In this regard, the Authority issues a range of regularly updated Codes of Practice to expand upon the way in which the HTA 2004 should be interpreted and applied in practice,[11] some of which will be examined later in this chapter. As noted by the Authority, the Codes have the following standing:

> Code A: Guiding principles and the fundamental principle of consent, is the overarching Code and contains information that is applicable to all establishments and professionals operating under our governing legislation. In combination, this Code and the sector-specific Codes aim to provide anyone undertaking activities relevant to each sector with a reference source which gives practical advice on the minimum steps necessary to comply with the relevant legislation and HTA policy.[12]

NHS Blood and Transplant (NHSBT) is a Special Health Authority within the NHS. It is not a regulator and is subject to oversight by the Human Tissue Authority.[13] In general terms, NHSBT provides a blood and transplantation service to the NHS, looking after blood donation services in England and transplant services across the UK. In relation to organs, this includes managing the donation, storage, and transplantation of organs and undertaking research into new treatments and processes in the area.[14] UK-wide responsibilities include managing the NHS Organ Donor Register and National Transplant Register, ensuring the fair and equitable allocation of organs, managing the National Organ Retrieval Service (NORS)[15] which provides a national 24 hour service for retrieving organs from deceased donors, promoting community awareness to encourage organ donation, and the managing, collection, and publication of data on organ donation and transplantation outcomes.[16] In June 2021, NHSBT published a new ten-year strategy for organ donation and transplantation in the UK, offering a joined up approach for the first time to both deceased and living donation and transplantation and focusing on areas for research and innovation.[17] The Strategy notes that while there have been significant increases in the rates of both deceased and living organ donation in recent years, this

---

[11] For an overview, see Human Tissue Authority, 'Codes of Practice' (2022) available at <https://www.hta.gov.uk/guidance-professionals/codes-practice-standards-and-legislation/codes-practice> accessed 29 December 2022.

[12] ibid.

[13] NHSBT, 'Who We Are' (2022) available at <https://www.nhsbt.nhs.uk/> accessed 29 December 2022.

[14] NHSBT, 'Transplantation Services' (2022) available at <https://www.nhsbt.nhs.uk/what-we-do/transplantation-services/> accessed 29 December 2022.

[15] NHSBT, 'National Organ Retrieval Services' (2022) available at <https://www.odt.nhs.uk/retrieval/> accessed 29 December 2022.

[16] NHSBT, 'Statistics and Reports' (2022) available at <https://www.odt.nhs.uk/statistics-and-reports/> accessed 29 December 2022.

[17] NHSBT, 'Organ Donation and Transplantation 2030: Meeting the Need' (1 June 2021) available at <https://www.odt.nhs.uk/odt-structures-and-standards/key-strategies/> accessed 29 December 2022.

has not corresponded to a similar increase in organs transplanted, primarily because the organs available are not of suitable quality. Factors attributed to this situation include an expansion of eligible donors, including older donors, as well as the adverse impact of donor lifestyle factors. Therefore, there will now be a particular focus on better organ utilisation driven by research and technological advances, designed to boost and maintain organ quality during the retrieval process. The six identified areas for action are set out below.[18]

NHSBT—key areas for action

1. For living and deceased donation to become an expected part of care, where clinically appropriate, for all in society.

2. For optimal organ utilisation in every organ group, benefitting from new technologies and techniques.

3. To make the most effective use of a precious donor organ, ensuring that recipient outcomes are amongst the best in the world.

4. To enable people of all backgrounds and circumstances to have timely access to the organ they need.

5. To secure a sustainable service across the UK, making the most of every opportunity for a donation and a transplant, as donation numbers increase due to the new legislation.

6. To build a pioneering culture of research and innovation in donation and transplantation in the UK.

The UK's devolved administrations also have their own organ donation and transplantation plans, which complement the NHSBT strategy identified previously. The Scottish Government's current plan runs from 2021 to 2026 and identifies seven priorities.[19] The plan was developed with strategic input from the Scottish Donation and Transplant Group (SDTG) (formerly the Scottish Transplant Group), which was established over 20 years ago to provide a forum for the discussion of policy in the area and is comprised of representatives from the donation and transplant communities in Scotland. The SDTG provides expert advice to the Scottish Government within its remit and oversees the implementation of the plan (noted previously). Its work is seen as complementary to that undertaken by the HTA.[20] Organ Donation Scotland is charged with implementing the

[18] ibid. For a summary overview of the Strategy, see NHSBT, 'New UK Strategy Sets Out Ambition To Be World Leaders in Organ Donation and Transplantation' (1 June 2021) available at <https://www.nhsbt.nhs.uk/news/new-uk-strategy-sets-out-ambition-to-be-world-leaders-in-organ-donation-and-transplantation/#:~:text=This%20new%20strategy%20sets%20the,donation%20and%20increase%20organ%20transplantation> accessed 29 December 2022.

[19] The Scottish plan involves seven identified priorities: (1) implementation of the Human Tissue (Authorisation) (Scotland) Act 2019; (2) increasing organ transplantation; (3) removing missed opportunities for deceased donation; (4) increasing living donation and the wait for a kidney transplant; (5) transplant recipient support and aftercare; (6) research and innovation; and (7) public health improvement. See Scottish Government, 'Donation and Transplantation: Plan 2021-2026' (24 March 2021) available at <https://www.gov.scot/publications/donation-transplantation-plan-scotland-2021-2026/pages/10/> accessed 29 December 2022.

[20] Scottish Government, 'Scottish Donation and Transplant Group' (2022) available at <https://www.gov.scot/groups/scottish-donation-and-transplant-group/> accessed 29 December 2022.

plan and working towards encouraging higher rates of organ donation, as well as education activities designed to increase awareness of the potential for organ donation.[21]

In Wales, a new plan was published in 2022 and runs through to 2026, which is seen
as complementary to and supportive of the UK plan.[22] Recognising the impact of the
Covid-19 pandemic in terms of contributing to a decrease in donors and an increase in
organ waiting lists, the plan focuses on actions that are likely to increase organ and tissue
transplantation; reduce inequalities and improve access to transplantation for patients;
and improve outcomes from transplantation. Similarly to the Scottish plan, it sets out
specific actions to be taken forward in line with six identified priorities.[23]

In NI, consultations on the future of organ donation policy and transplantation took
place between 2017 and 2018, but the collapse of power sharing institutions in NI during
this period no doubt made it difficult to progress strategic policy in the area. A further
consultation in 2021 explored whether there was support for a shift to an opt-out system
for organ donation to bring NI in line with the rest of the UK.[24] This subsequently led
to the adoption of new legislation to facilitate this shift, which will come into force in
2023 and will be discussed later in this chapter. Ahead of its implementation, the Organ
Donation Service, which is run under the auspices of the NI Public Health Agency, is
running a community awareness campaign about the change.[25] As things stand, NI will
likely act in support of the UK-wide strategy published by NHSBT in 2021.

13.3 DIAGNOSIS OF DEATH AND ORGAN DONATION

It is important to have a diagnosis of death which is recognised for legal purposes, such
as the transfer of property or the granting of probate, for example. In the case of deceased
organ donation for transplantation, it is imperative that such a diagnosis has been established in accordance with legally acceptable criteria before any organs can be removed.
This is known as the 'dead donor rule'.[26] In the past, it used to be the case that where a
person's heart had stopped, they ceased to breathe, and a diagnosis of death could then be
made. Advances in medicine and technology have now made the situation more complex.
For example, if a person's heart stops, they may be able to be resuscitated and/or placed
on mechanical ventilation to assist with breathing. In the context of organ donation, such
advances have necessitated a 'rethink' about how death is diagnosed, particularly as time
may be of the essence where organs need to be preserved for transplantation purposes.[27]

---

[21] See Organ Donation Scotland, 'Organ & Tissue Donation' (2022) available at <https://www.orgando-
nation.scot/> accessed 29 December 2022.
[22] Welsh Government, 'Donation and Transplantation Plan 2022 to 2026 (WHC/2022/12)' (16 June
2022) available at <https://gov.wales/donation-and-transplantation-plan-2022-2026-whc202212> accessed
29 December 2022.
[23] ibid., p. 2. These priorities are as follows: (1) increasing deceased organ donation; (2) increasing tissue
and eye donation; (3) increasing living donation and transplantation; (4) increasing access to transplantation; (5) improving transplant outcomes; and (6) ensuring a sustainable, supported, and diverse workforce.
[24] Department of Health NI, 'Public Consultation Document on the Introduction of a Statutory Opt-Out
System for Organ Donation for Northern Ireland' (19 February 2021) available at <https://www.health-ni.
gov.uk/consultations/organ-donation> accessed 29 December 2022.
[25] Organ Donation Northern Ireland, 'You Could Be a Lifesaver – Organ Donation Law is Changing
in Spring 2023' (2022) available at <https://www.organdonationni.info/changes-to-the-law> accessed
29 December 2022.
[26] Robert Truog and Franklin Miller, 'The Dead Donor Rule and Organ Transplantation' (2008) 369 (14)
New England Journal of Medicine 1287.
[27] See Anne-Maree Farrell et al., *Health Law: Frameworks and Context* (CUP 2017) 228.

13.3.1 DONATION AFTER BRAIN STEM DEATH

In the UK, the diagnosis of death for the purposes of deceased organ donation for transplantation is based on brain stem death. It is important to keep in mind that brain stem death does not inevitably involve death of the whole body where ventilation is in place. In such circumstances, it offers a prognosis, but actual death is dependent upon the withdrawal of treatment. At common law, there has long been judicial support for a definition of death being brain stem death. For example, in *R v Malcherek; R v Steel*,[28] the Court of Appeal dealt with two joined cases in order to consider the issue. In the first case, the defendant had stabbed his wife. She was taken to hospital and put on a life support machine. She was found to have irreversible brain damage and so the machine was disconnected and shortly thereafter her bodily functions ceased. In the second case, the defendant had assaulted a girl, causing multiple skull fractures and severe brain damage. The girl was taken to hospital and also put on a life support machine. The machine was disconnected when doctors concluded that her brain had stopped functioning. The defendants argued that they were not guilty of murder as they had not killed the victims in question and that instead it was the hospital team which had disconnected the life support machines from them. Although not directly engaging with the issue of defining death, the Court held that it was the original criminal acts by the defendants that were the continuing, operating, and substantial causes of the death of the victims. Where treatment was given in a bona fide manner by healthcare professionals (HCPs) but failed to result in the survival of the victims in question, then they could not be said to have caused their death.

In the later case of *Re A*,[29] a two-year-old boy was placed on artificial ventilation following severe head injuries. His condition deteriorated and he was determined to have suffered brain stem death. His parents objected to the removal of their son's ventilator. The hospital sought a declaration from the court that the doctors would not act unlawfully if they switched off the ventilator. The judge in the case found that the boy was for all purposes legally dead, relying on the definition of death now set out in the then UK Code of Practice for diagnosing death. In *Airedale NHS Trust v Bland*, Lord Browne-Wilkinson in the House of Lords acknowledged that medical professionals now defined death 'in terms of brain stem death, i.e., the death of that part of the brain without which the body cannot function at all without assistance.'[30]

In legislative terms, a number of other jurisdictions provide for a statutory definition of death, such as various states in the United States and in Australia.[31] More recently, there have also been attempts by the World Health Organization (WHO) to develop an international consensus with regards to harmonised standards for determining brain death; however, this has proved difficult to achieve to date.[32] In the UK, definition of death is contained in guidance, 'A Code of Practice for the Diagnosis and Confirmation of Death

---

[28] [1981] 2 All ER 422.   [29] [1992] 3 Med LR 303.   [30] [1993] 1 All ER 821 [878].

[31] In the United States, many states have adopted the Uniform Determination of Death Act which sets out a statutory definition of death as involving whole brain death (e.g. the irreversible cessation of the functioning of the entire brain, including the brain stem). For an overview, see Nikolas Nikas, Dorinda Bordlee, and Madeline Moreira, 'Determination of Death and the Dead Donor Rule: A Survey of the Current Law on Brain Death' (2016) 41(3) Journal of Medical Philosophy 237. For an overview of a similar approach in Australia, see Farrell et al., (n 27) 228–230.

[32] James Bernat, 'Is International Consensus on Brain Death Achievable?' (2015) 84(18) Neurology 1878.

(Code of Practice)', the last edition of which was published in 2008.[33] The Code of Practice, which defines death as brain stem death, states:[34]

> The irreversible cessation of brain-stem function whether induced by intra-cranial events or the result of extra-cranial phenomena, such as hypoxia, will produce this clinical state and therefore irreversible cessation of the integrative function of the brainstem equates with the death of the individual and allows the medical practitioner to diagnose death.

In these circumstances, a person is considered dead whether or not the function of some organs (such as a heartbeat) is still maintained by artificial ventilation, for example.

In terms of diagnosing death, this must be undertaken by way of brain-stem testing by at least two medical practitioners who have been registered for more than five years and are competent in the conduct and interpretation of brain-stem testing. At least one of the doctors must be a consultant. Those carrying out the tests must not have, or be perceived to have, any clinical conflict of interest and neither doctor should be a member of the transplant team. Testing should be undertaken by the nominated doctors acting together and must always be performed on two occasions.[35] A complete set of tests should be performed on each occasion, i.e. a total of two sets of tests will be performed. Doctor A may perform the tests while Doctor B observes; this would constitute the first set. Roles may be reversed for the second set. If the first set of tests shows no evidence of brain-stem function, there need not be a lengthy delay prior to performing the second set.[36] A short period of time will be necessary after reconnection to the ventilator to allow return of the patient's arterial blood gases and baseline parameters to the pre-test state, rechecking of the blood sugar concentration and for the reassurance of all those directly concerned. Although death is not confirmed until the second test has been completed, the legal time of death is when the first test indicates death due to the absence of brain-stem reflexes.[37] The Code of Practice emphasises that there is a need for declaration of brain stem death to occur before any discussion takes place with regard to organ donation.[38]

Since 2015, there has been an upsurge in legal challenges that have come before the UK courts concerning diagnosis of brain stem death. While the courts have affirmed that the diagnosis of brain stem death in accordance with the Code of Practice constitutes legal death, some commentators have suggested that a distinct jurisprudence may be emerging in the area in light of such challenges.[39] The UK courts' position on the matter was recently affirmed in the Court of Appeal judgment in *Re M (Declaration of Death of Child)*.[40] The facts of the case involved a baby, M, who was deprived of oxygen for a significant period of time during the birth process and had no detectable heartbeat at birth. He was resuscitated and then ventilated in the neonatal intensive care unit. Two weeks following his birth, M was diagnosed as being brain stem dead according to the Code of Practice. His parents did not accept the diagnosis and the treating hospital subsequently sought a declaration from the court that it was lawful to withdraw mechanical

---

[33] Academy of Medical Royal Colleges, 'A Code of Practice for the Diagnosis and Confirmation of Death' (10 August 2008) available at <https://www.aomrc.org.uk/reports-guidance/ukdec-reports-and-guidance/code-practice-diagnosis-confirmation-death/> accessed 29 December 2022.

[34] ibid., para 2.1.   [35] ibid., para 6.3.   [36] ibid., Appendix 2.

[37] ibid., para 6.2.   [38] ibid., Appendix 2.

[39] For an overview of UK and international jurisprudence concerning the diagnosis of death by neurological criteria, see Mary Donnelly and Barry Lyons, 'Disputing Death: Brain Death in the Courts' (2023) Legal Studies (doi:10.1017/lst.2022.45).

[40] [2020] EWCA Civ 164.

ventilation. The declaration sought by the treating hospital was granted at first instance, as well as on appeal. In giving judgment in the Court of Appeal, McFarlane P noted 'as a matter of law, it is the case that brain stem death is established as the legal criteria in the UK by the House of Lords' decision in *Bland*. It is therefore not open to this court to contemplate a different test.'[41] He also confirmed that 'once death had been established, then the concept of "best interests" no longer has any legal relevance.'[42] In making a declaration of legal death in this case, he also noted with approval the words used by Justice Hayden in *Re A* that the purpose in doing so is to allow the individual who has died 'dignity in death'.[43]

The *Battersbee* litigation has also highlighted difficulties that may arise with diagnosing brain stem death according to the current Code of Practice. This litigation focused on a range of issues, including best interests at the end of a child's life, which we examine in more detail in Chapter 9. For present purposes, we refer only to those rulings which touch on the issue of diagnosing death in the case of Archie Battersbee. He was 12 years of age when he suffered traumatic brain injuries in April 2022 and fell into a coma. A dispute arose between his parents and treating doctors over whether life support treatment should be continued in his case. His treating doctors viewed Archie's brain damage as so extensive that they considered him to be brain stem dead. In light of this, they asked his parents whether brain stem death testing could be conducted in accordance with the Code of Practice in order to confirm their views; however, the parents refused to provide consent. In May 2022, this led the NHS Hospital Trust where Archie was being treated to seek a declaration from the High Court for permission to carry out such testing, which was subsequently granted. When the doctors attempted to administer brain stem function testing in accordance with the Code of Practice, they were unable to complete such testing because Archie did not respond to a peripheral nerve stimulation test (a precursor to the brain stem test), meaning that there would be a danger of a false negative. Following results from further MRI scans, treating and second opinion doctors considered it was likely that Archie was already brain dead. However, no doctor was suggesting that a declaration of death should be made without testing being done in accordance with the Code of Practice.

The matter returned to court for further consideration. In a ruling in the High Court by Mrs Justice Arbuthnot on 13 June 2022, she found that Archie was 'probably' dead and had died on the day of his MRI scan on 31 May 2022 and his life support treatment could now cease. The ruling on the declaration of death was decided that it was more likely than not that Archie had died (i.e. balance of probabilities). It was further stated that even if no declaration of death had been made, then it would have been in Archie's best interests for ventilation to be withdrawn.[44] The parents appealed the ruling to the Court of Appeal. On 6 July 2022, the Court of Appeal handed down judgment, criticising the reasoning in the first instance judgment and remitted the case to Mr Justice Hayden for a more detailed best interests assessment as to whether medical treatment should be withdrawn in Archie's case.

In giving judgment, the Court confirmed that the Code of Practice governs the practice for the diagnosis and confirmation of death in the UK. This said, they also noted a submission by counsel that there is a caveat in the Code which in effect contemplates

---

[41] ibid. [91].   [42] ibid. [49].
[43] ibid. [60], drawing on *Re A (A Child)* [2015] EWHC 443 (Fam).
[44] *Barts Health NHS Trust* v *Dance & Battersbee* [2022] EWHC 1435 (Fam).

'diagnosing death in the context of irreversible cessation of brain stem function in circumstances where the six-stage test cannot be undertaken'. Although not tested at hearing, the Court observed that 'it is a submission which must, at least, be open to question'.
Yet, it recognised that there was no 'alternative basis for diagnosing death on the basis
of cessation of brain stem function other than by conducting the test'.[45] In the circumstances, there had been no diagnosis of death made in Archie's case in line with the Code
of Practice. The Court went on to state:

> No authority has been produced in which previous judges have declared that death has
> occurred in an individual whose bodily functioning is being mechanically maintained
> by a ventilator and where death is said to be established on evidence other than testing
> undertaken in accordance with the Code, or where the judge does not have any medical
> witness who has diagnosed death. The course that the judge was invited to follow in the
> present case was, it seems, unprecedented . . . It would have been better for the judge to
> have proceeded to consider best interests once it was clear that a brain stem test could not
> be undertaken, it is not necessary for this court to go further and hold that the parents'
> fourth ground is established and that it was wrong for the judge to diagnose death on a
> basis which is not compliant with the Code. We do, however, strongly caution judges in
> future cases of this kind from being drawn into attempting to declare death on a basis
> outside the Code where none of the medical witnesses has themselves made a diagnosis
> of death.[46]

The rise of a diagnosis of death being based on brain stem death needs to be seen alongside
developments in intensive care and in addition, organ transplantation. If a diagnosis of
death is based on brain stem death, then it was argued that this provided a sounder, more
appropriate basis on which a decision could be made about organ donation. Of course,
this has not stopped ethical and legal debate on the issue, with differing arguments being
put forward about the competing interests between demand for organs and the need for
a scientifically and legally recognised definition of death.[47] One of the contentious issues
is the fact that brain stem death does not inevitably involve the death of the whole body,
even where ventilation was in place. For example, there are cases of brain-dead pregnant
women being kept alive via ventilation for months and thereafter giving birth to healthy
children. There are also published reports of brain-dead children being kept alive for up
to 14 years with ventilator and nutritional support.[48] What is clear though is that brain-
dead patients will not recover. Therefore, brain stem death provides the prognosis, but
actual death is dependent upon the withdrawal of treatment.

Accepting this type of prognosis may be difficult for families, particularly if their
family member is still breathing. After all, they are pink and warm; their hearts continue to beat and they continue to breathe with ventilator support. Although they will
not recover, there are cases of brain-dead persons being kept alive via ventilation and
nutritional support, often for extended periods. This liminal state appears to blur the
distinction between what it means to be alive and what we might commonly understand

---

[45] ibid. [33].

[46] ibid., [35] and [37].

[47] See e.g. Robert Truog and Walter Robinson, 'Role of Brain Death and the Dead-Donor Rule in the Ethics
of Organ Transplantation' (2003) 31(9) Critical Care Medicine 2391; Michael Nair-Collins and Franklin
Miller, 'Do the "Brain Dead" Merely Appear to Be Alive? (2017) 43(11) Journal of Medical Ethics 747.

[48] See e.g. David J Powner and Ira M Bernstein, 'Extended Somatic Support for Pregnant Women After
Brain Death' (2003) 31(4) Critical Care Medicine 1241.

from a layperson's point of view to be death. And again, although brain-dead patients will not recover, withdrawal of treatment may nevertheless be required to bring about the cessation of heartbeat.[49] In the circumstances, it has been suggested that death should be defined by reference to cardiorespiratory criteria, as this would be well understood by the public. Patients who are assessed as being brain dead could then be accepted as dying, rather than dead. Withdrawal of treatment would be initiated on the basis that they have no hope for recovery on the grounds of brain stem death and thereafter they could be considered as potential organ and tissue donors. Given such concerns, it has been argued this offers a principled way forward that would be publicly acceptable and would also allow deceased organ donation to proceed.[50]

Yet other concerns have been raised about the appropriate ethical framework that should operate when managing perceived or real conflicts of interest for those HCPs involved in end-of-life care, and those involved in organ donation for transplantation. In order to clarify this matter, professional guidance requires HCPs with clinical responsibility for patients who are potential donors to exercise a duty to consider organ donation as part of end-of-life care.[51] While it is outside the scope of this chapter to consider this issue in more detail,[52] highlighting these select concerns serves as a reminder of the importance of recognising that death is a medical, legal, and cultural issue: getting the diagnosis of death right is vital to maintaining public trust and confidence in national organ donation for transplantation programmes.

13.3.2 DONATION AFTER CIRCULATORY DEATH

As the need for organ transplantation has increased in recent decades, there has been an expansion of the categories in which there will be a diagnosis of death, as a prerequisite for organ donation. This has led to the development of organ procurement based on what is known as donation after circulatory death (DCD).[53] For example, in the financial year to 31 March 2022, deceased organ donation in the UK via the DCD route involved 612 donors, and this represented an increase of 48% (after usual criteria for DCD donation were reinstated following the first wave of the Covid-19 pandemic).[54] All in all, 44% of all deceased organ donation in 2021–22 was via the DCD route.[55] What this means is that it essentially allows the declaration of death for the purposes of organ donation after a specified period of period of absent heart activity. Where death is diagnosed by traditional cardio-respiratory criteria, there is usually a need to move quickly to remove organs for the purposes of transplantation as otherwise they would rapidly decay and not be usable

---

[49] Truog and Miller (n 26).

[50] Ian Kerridge et al., *Ethics and Law for the Health Professions* (4th edn, Federation Press 2013), 760–761.

[51] General Medical Council, 'Treatment and Care Towards the End of Life: Good Practice in Decision-Making' (15 March 2022) available at <https://www.gmc-uk.org/ethical-guidance/ethical-guidance-for-doctors/treatment-and-care-towards-the-end-of-life> accessed 29 December 2022; see also Intensive Care Society, et al., 'Donation Actions Framework: A Professional, Ethical and Legal Framework for Deceased Organ Donation Actions (for use in England, Wales and Northern Ireland)' (June 2022) available at <https://ics.ac.uk/resource/donation-actions-framework.html> accessed 29 December 2022.

[52] For a detailed consideration of the medico-legal and ethical issues at stake, see Graeme Laurie, Shaun Harmon, and Edward Dove, *Mason and McCall Smith's Law and Medical Ethics* (11th edn, OUP 2019) ch 17.

[53] Note that previous terms used included donation after cardiac death and non-heart beating donation.

[54] NHSBT, 'Organ and Tissue Donation and Transplantation, Activity Report, 2021–22' (2022) 2, available at <https://www.organdonation.nhs.uk/helping-you-to-decide/about-organ-donation/statistics-about-organ-donation/transplant-activity-report/> accessed 29 December 2022.

[55] NHSBT, 'Donation after Circulatory Death' (2022) available at <https://www.odt.nhs.uk/deceased-donation/best-practice-guidance/donation-after-circulatory-death/> accessed 29 December 2022.

for these purposes.[56] The Maastricht Classification has become the accepted approach to determining the clinical circumstances in which DCD can take place.[57] Within this classification scheme, DCD is recognised as taking place in either controlled or uncontrolled environments. In the UK, controlled DCD takes place and is understood as arising in the following circumstances:

> [There is] a mechanically ventilated patient with overwhelming single organ failure, usually the brain, [and] a decision is made to withdraw life-sustaining treatment. Once consent for organ donation is confirmed following discussion with the patient's family by a Specialist Nurse for Organ Donation (SNOD), a surgical retrieval team is mobilised. Withdrawal of life sustaining treatment only commences once the surgical team is prepared in theatre and recipients for the organs have been identified. This type of DCD is called 'controlled' DCD because the death is expected, and the surgical team are already prepared.[58]

In contrast, it is considered uncontrolled where cardiac arrest was unexpected and treating doctors consider that the patient cannot or should not be resuscitated in the circumstances. This form of DCD has been carried out in a range of other countries,[59] but currently does not take place in the UK. At the time of writing, a framework for uncontrolled DCD is in the process of being developed.[60] Although we discuss the new opt-out systems for deceased organ donation in the UK later in this chapter, we would note for present purposes that consent to DCD can be deemed under the Human Tissue Acts in the UK.[61]

Despite the increasing growth in this source of organ donors, there is a range of ethical issues to be considered in the context of DCD. First and foremost, the dead donor rule must be respected: that is to say, the individual must be diagnosed as dead and confirmed using cardio-respiratory criteria before any donation can take place. Given that controlled DCD is the preferred option in the UK, this usually takes place after the planned withdrawal of life-sustaining medical treatment which is considered to be of no overall benefit to the patient in question. In doing so, this requires that due respect be shown for the patient's autonomy and dignity and that DCD must be grounded in best interests considerations.[62] In terms of any medical interventions that may be contemplated in this context, the principle of non-maleficence must be adhered to, as well as beneficence, which requires that account be taken of the need to maximise the benefits and minimising the risks of any medical interventions that are contemplated with respect to preserving organs through the DCD route for the purposes of transplantation.[63]

---

[56] There are several options for preserving organs in such circumstances, with significant positive developments taking place with machine perfusion technologies. See Annemarie Wiessenbacher et al., 'The Future of Organ Perfusion and Reconditioning' (2019) 32(6) Transplant International 586.

[57] See Gerrit Koostra, John Daemen, and APA Oomen, 'Categories of Non-Heart-Beating Donors' (1995) 27(5) Transplant Proceedings 2893. For an overview of developments in relation to DCD, see Robert Langer, 'Donation After Cardiac Death - From Then to Now' (2023) 8(1) Transplantation Reports 100119.

[58] Intensive Care Society et al. (n 51) 7.

[59] Uncontrolled DCD currently takes place in France, Spain, and the Netherlands, for example; see NHSBT, 'Donation after Circulatory Death' (2022) available at <https://www.odt.nhs.uk/deceased-donation/best-practice-guidance/donation-after-circulatory-death/> accessed 29 December 2022.

[60] Intensive Care Society et al. (n 51) 8.

[61] See Human Tissue Authority, 'Codes of Practice' (n 11).

[62] See British Transplantation Society and Intensive Care Society, 'Consensus Statement on Donation After Circulatory Death' (June 2010) available at <https://nhsbtdbe.blob.core.windows.net/umbraco-assets-corp/1360/donation-after-circulatory-death-dcd_consensus_2010.pdf> accessed 29 December 2022; Alex Manara, Paul Murphy, and Gerry O'Callaghan, 'Donation After Circulatory Death' (2012) 108 (suppl 1) British Journal of Anaesthesia i108; Intensive care Society et al (n 51).

[63] Anji Wall et al., 'Applying the Ethical Framework for Donation after Circulatory Death to Thoracic Normothermic Regional Perfusion Procedures' (2022) 22(5) American Journal of Transplantation 1311.

13.4 DECEASED ORGAN DONATION

A person has very limited rights as to the future disposal of their dead body in common law,[64] and the wishes of the executors would normally be supported, rather than those of the deceased, in the event of conflict. Statute law has, however, largely replaced common law, and the collection and use of organs from deceased donors has been regulated in the UK since 1961. Initially, human tissue legislation was fairly sparse and reflected the fact that organ donation for transplantation, as well as human tissue donation and related technologies, were in their infancy. Over subsequent decades, there were substantial advances in the field which combined with some egregious examples of breaches of the law and poor medical practice. This led to comprehensive legal reform in the area, resulting in the adoption of the HTA 2004 and the HTA 2006. While these Acts share many common features, the most important conceptual difference is that when adopted, the HTA 2004 was dominated by the concept of 'appropriate consent', while the HTA 2006 used the term 'authorisation' for removal and use of tissues from the deceased person.[65] In contrast to the HTA 2004, the HTA 2006 also refers to transplantation in detail.[66] In the final analysis, however, the provisions of both Acts are similar in many respects and the Scottish Ministers may call upon other UK bodies, including the Human Tissue Authority and NHSBT (see earlier), for assistance in many functions relating to organ donation for transplantation, which is important for the coordination of transplant services across the UK.[67]

There are several aspects of the Human Tissue Acts that are worth highlighting before we go on to examine recent legislative reforms. Under the HTA 2004, little detail is provided about the legal framework underpinning the therapeutic use of organs from deceased donors, with transplantation being no more than one of 12 'scheduled purposes' for the use of human tissues with which the act is concerned.[68] The Act regulates 'relevant material' which is defined as 'material, other than gametes, which consists of or includes human cells', but this does not include 'embryos outside the human body, or hair and nail from the body of a living person.'[69] In addition, 'material' that is not regarded as being from a human body where 'it is created outside the human body'.[70] When initially adopted, consent was at the centre at the HTA 2004, with transplantation only being lawful if it was done with 'appropriate consent',[71] which, in the case of an adult, meant their consent.[72] In the absence of an advance directive, consent could be given or withheld by a person or persons nominated by a living adult to act in their interests after death.[73] If neither of these options was available, authority was vested in a person who stood in a qualifying relationship to the deceased.[74]

---

[64] On this point, see Chapter 14.

[65] See Sheila McLean (Chair), 'Independent Review Group on Retention of Organs at Post-Mortem, Final Report' (2001) s 1, para 17. For comment see Margaret Brazier, 'Retained Organs, Ethics and Humanity' (2002) 22(4) Legal Studies 551; Shawn Harmon and Aisling McMahon, 'Banking (on) the Brain: From Consent to Authorisation and the Transformative Potential of Solidarity' (2014) 22(4) Medical Law Review 572.

[66] See generally HTA 2006, Part 1.

[67] HTA 2006, Part 6, s 54. NHSBT, 'Organ Donation and Transplantation 2030' (n 17); note that the Human Tissue Authority is, in fact, responsible for assessing and approving all organ transplants from living donors in Scotland (see later in this chapter).

[68] HTA 2004, Sch 1, Pts 1 and 2.   [69] HTA 2004, Part 3, s 53.   [70] HTA 2004, Part 3, s 54(7).
[71] HTA 2004, Part 1, s 1(1)(b)(c).   [72] HTA 2004, Part 1, s 3.

[73] An appointment, if made orally, is valid only if it is made before two witnesses together, see HTA 2004, Part 1, s 4(4). A written appointment must be attested by at least one witness or may be part of a will, see HTA 2004, Part 1, s 4(5).

[74] HTA 2004, Part 2, s 27(4) and (5). The definition and scope of what constitutes a 'qualifying relationship' in relation to the deceased adult, for example, is set out in ranking order as follows: (a) spouse, civil partner, or partner; (b) parent or child; (c) brother or sister; (d) grandparent or grandchild; (e) child of a person falling within paragraph (c); (f) stepfather or stepmother; (g) half-brother or half-sister; and (h) friend of long standing. Note that relationships in the same paragraph (a)–(h) are accorded equal ranking (see HTA 2004, Part 1, s 2).

Under the HTA 2006, the preferred terminology was grounded in the notion of 'express authorisation' for organ donation, rather than consent (albeit with similar effect).[75] Instead of using the term 'qualifying relationship', the HTA 2006 uses the term 'nearest relative' to refer to a person who is eligible in specified circumstances to make a decision to authorise the donation of organs by a deceased adult.[76] In relation to a child, defined as a person under the age of 18,[77] it would ordinarily be the person with parental responsibility for the child who would have authority to consent to organ donation after the child's death;[78] failing that, the consent of a person who stood in a qualifying relationship to the child at that time would be considered sufficient.[79] In contrast to the HTA 2004, a child aged 12 years and over could authorise the remove and use of a part of their body after their death for the purposes of transplantation.[80] Both the Human Tissue Acts provide for steps to be taken to preserve a body lying in a hospital or similar institution, which may be suitable for organ donation, those steps being minimally invasive to preserve the parts and to retain the body for the purposes of transplantation until it is established that consent or authorisation has not been, and will not be, given.[81]

13.4.1 DEEMED CONSENT/AUTHORISATION

In recent years, consideration has been given to whether reform was needed to the Human Tissue Acts in the UK in order to promote greater rates of organ donation, while at the same time ensuring that potential donors' autonomy, grounded in the notion of consent, was preserved. Initial attempts to introduce an opt-out system for deceased organ donation were met with resistance on the part of UK policymakers, with concerns about the lack of sufficient evidence that such a reform on its own would increase rates of deceased organ donation. Instead, the firm policy preference in the early 2000s was to focus on reforming institutional arrangements within the NHS to increase such rates.[82] A focus on institutional reform yielded a good deal of initial success, with the number of organ donors increasing by 75%, in addition to transplants from deceased organ donation increasing by 56%. Nevertheless, a persistent gap remained with respect to supply and demand for donors,[83] and the issue of family veto remained stubbornly high in the UK.[84] The reasons for family veto in relation to deceased organ donation were attributable to a number of factors. One such factor included uncertainty on the part of families as to whether their family member would have wanted to donate their organs after death.[85]

---

[75] See e.g. HTA 2006, Part 1, s 6 in relation to express authorisation by an adult.

[76] HTA 2006, Part 4, s 50. The nearest relatives is set out as follows: (a) the adult's spouse or civil partner; (b) living as husband or wife or in a relationship which had the characteristics of the relationship between civil partners and had been so living for a period of not less than six months; (c) the adult's child; (d) the adult's parent; (e) the adult's brother or sister; (f) the adult's grandparent; (g) the adult's grandchild; (h) the adult's uncle or aunt; (i) the adult's cousin; (j) the adult's niece or nephew; and (k) a friend of long standing of the adult.

[77] HTA 2004, Part 3, s 54(1).   [78] HTA 2004, Part 1, s 2(2).   [79] HTA 2004, Part 1, s 2(7).

[80] HTA 2006, Part 1, s 8(1). Note subsequent legislative amendments via the Human Tissue (Authorisation) (Scotland) Act 2019 regarding authorisation which can be provided by those with parental rights and parental responsibilities. See HTA 2006, Part 1, s 8D.

[81] See HTA 2004, Part 3, s 43; HTA 2006, Part 1, s 13.

[82] See Organ Donation Taskforce, 'Independent Report: The Potential Impact of an Opt-out System for Organ Donation in the UK' (Department of Health 2008).

[83] See NHSBT, Statistics About Organ Donation (n 5).

[84] See e.g. David Shaw and Bernice Elgar, 'Persuading Bereaved Families to Permit Organ Donation' (2014) 40(1) Intensive Care Medicine 96.

[85] Other factors that have been identified for family refusal to deceased organ donation including not wanting their family member to be subject to any more invasive procedures, false beliefs and cognitive biases. See Magi Sque, Sheila Payne, and Jill Macleod Clark, 'Gift of Life or Sacrifice? Key Discourses to Understanding Organ Donor Families' Decision-Making' (2006) 11(2) Mortality 117; David Shaw et al., 'ELPAT Working Group on Deceased Donation, Family Over Rules? An Ethical Analysis of Allowing Families to Overrule Donation Intentions' (2017) 101(3) Transplantation 482.

Against this background, there was a gradual sea-change in policy terms, with growing support for a shift towards establishing an opt-out system for deceased organ donation. Under such a system, persons are presumed (or deemed) to have consented to or authorised the removal of their organs in the event of death unless they have registered an objection to this taking place. Such objection is usually formally registered by way of a national organ donor database or perhaps at a local town hall, for example. What evidence was available from a range of jurisdictions as to the success or otherwise of such schemes, was mixed. This was particularly so in the absence of institutional reforms to facilitate higher rates of organ procurement. In any case, many such jurisdictions operated a soft opt-out system, where families were ordinarily consulted before deceased organ donation took place in any case.[86]

In contemplating reform involving a shift to an opt-out system, UK policymakers recognised that there had long been widespread public support for organ donation with around 80% of people in England saying that they supported organ donation in principle, though only 38% had actually recorded their decision to donate. When asked, the majority said, 'they just hadn't got around to it'.[87] Therefore, legislative reform was designed not only to increase rates of deceased organ donation but also to emphasise the importance of letting family members know of their individual preference or wishes for such donation to take place in the event of their death. Legislation to establish opt-out systems for deceased organ donation has now been passed in all four UK jurisdictions. The term that is used is 'deemed consent' in England, Wales, and NI, and 'deemed authorisation' in Scotland. More broadly, this has resulted in changes to the Human Tissue Acts, which we now turn to consider in more detail.

Wales was the first jurisdiction in the UK to shift from an opt-in to an opt-out system for organ donation, having initially passed legislation to this effect in 2013 (HWTA 2013).[88] It subsequently came into force on 1 December 2015, amending a number of sections of the HTA 2004 to establish a deemed consent system for Wales.[89] The gap between the passage of the legislation and the majority of its provisions coming into force was primarily to allow time for local awareness-raising activities to take place about the change. This was underpinned by a legislative duty imposed on the Welsh Ministers to 'promote transplantation as a means of improving the health of the people of Wales; to provide information and increase awareness about transplantation; and to inform the public of the circumstances in which consent to transplantation activities is deemed to be given in the absence of express consent'.[90] At least once every 12 months, Welsh Ministers are required to 'promote a campaign for the purpose of informing the public throughout Wales about the circumstances in which consent to transplantation activities is deemed to be given in the absence of express consent'.[91] As required under the HWTA 2013,[92] the HTA also issued

[86] See e.g. Alberto Abadie and Sebastien Gay, 'The Impact of Presumed Consent Legislation on Cadaveric Organ Donation: A Cross-Country Study' (2006) 25(4) J Health Econ 599; Amber Rithalia et al., 'Impact of Presumed Consent For Organ Donation on Donation Rates: A Systematic Review' (2009) 338 BMJ a3162; John Fabre, Paul Murphy, and Rafael Matesanz, 'Presumed Consent: A Distraction in the Quest for Increasing Rates of Organ Donation' (2010) 341 BMJ c4973; Melissa Palmer, 'Opt-Out Systems of Organ Donation: International Evidence Review' (Welsh Government Social Research 2012).

[87] NHSBT, 'Family and Public Support Helping Save Lives One Year on From the Introduction of Max and Keira's Law' (20 May 2021) available at <https://www.organdonation.nhs.uk/get-involved/news/family-and-public-support-helping-save-lives-one-year-on-from-the-introduction-of-max-and-keira-s-law/> accessed 29 December 2022.

[88] Human Transplantation (Wales) Act 2013 (HTWA 2013).

[89] ibid., s 16.   [90] ibid., s 2(1).   [91] ibid., s 2(2).   [92] ibid., s 15.

a Code of Practice to support this legislative reform and assist with its interpretation.[93] **Table 13.1** highlights the deemed consent provisions of the Act in relation to adults.

In summary, the HWTA 2013 allows for consent to deceased organ donation to be deemed in circumstances where 'there is no record of a person's decision on organ dona-tion . . . unless a person with a close relationship provides evidence that the person did not want to be an organ donor.'[94] The new system applies where a person both lived and died in Wales, unless the person is one of the following: a person under the age of 18 (a child);[95]

Table 13.1 HWTA 2013 section 4 Consent: Adults

(1) This section makes provision about consent for the purposes of section 3 in relation to a transplantation activity involving the body, or relevant material from the body, of a person who is not—

    (a) an excepted adult (see section 5), or

    (b) a child (see section 6).

(2) Consent is deemed to be given to the activity unless—

    (a) the case is one mentioned in the first column of Table 13.1a in subsection (3); in which case express consent is required, or

    (b) the case is not one mentioned in the first column of Table 13.1a in subsection (3) and subsection (4) applies.

(3) For each case mentioned in the first column of Table 13.1a the meaning of express consent in relation to an activity is as provided in the second column of the table—

(4) This subsection applies if—

    (a) a relative or friend of long standing of the deceased objects on the basis of views held by the deceased, and

    (b) a reasonable person would conclude that the relative or friend knows that the most recent view of the deceased before death on consent for transplantation activities was that the deceased was opposed to consent being given.

Table 13.1a

Case	*Meaning of express consent*
1. The person is alive.	The person's consent.
2. The person has died and a decision of the person to consent, or not to consent, to the activity was in force immediately before his or her death.	The person's consent.
3. The person has died, case 2 does not apply, the person had appointed a person or persons to deal with the issue of consent in relation to the activity and someone is able to give consent under the appointment.	Consent given by the person or persons appointed.
4. The person has died, case 2 does not apply and the person had appointed a person or persons to deal with the issue of consent in relation to the activity, but no one is able to give consent under the appointment.	Consent of a person who stood in a qualifying relationship to the person immediately before death.

[93] Human Tissue Authority, 'Code of Practice on the Human Transplantation (Wales) Act 2013' (May 2020) available at <https://www.hta.gov.uk/guidance-professionals/codes-practice-standards-and-legisla-tion/codes-practice> accessed 29 December 2022.

[94] Human Tissue Authority, 'Code of Practice on HTWA 2013' (n 93) para 11.

[95] In relation to specific provisions in relation to children, see HTWA 2013, s 6; HTA, 'Code of Practice on HTWA 2013' (n 93) paras 30–43.

an adult who has lived in Wales for less than 12 months; an adult who has lived in Wales for more than 12 months but is not ordinarily resident there; and an adult who lacked the capacity to understand the notion of deemed consent for a significant period before their death.[96] Where a person falls into one of these categories, then a person's consent cannot be deemed, and express consent should be established or sought.[97] 'Excluded relevant material' for the purposes of deemed consent for transplantation are specified in regulations,[98] but examples specified in the legislation include 'composite tissues and other types of material the removal and use of which is considered to be novel'. In such circumstances, express consent is required.[99] The Wales deemed consent system has been in place longer than the other jurisdictions in the UK and differing views have been expressed as to the success or otherwise of the scheme. Public policymakers have claimed the reform as successful, stating that rates of consent to deceased organ donation rose from 58% to 72% between 2015 and 2017.[100] Other commentators have pointed to a lack of published empirical research within a similar time period showing it has made a (significant) difference with regards to increasing such rates.[101] What is clear is that further longitudinal studies area required over the medium to longer term to properly assess the success or otherwise of the scheme.[102]

In England, a public campaign was led by families of children who had been involved in donating and receiving organs for transplant. Colloquially known as 'Max and Keira's Law', the Organ Donation (Deemed Consent) Act 2019 (ODDCA 2019) was passed in 2019 and came into force in 2020. The amended section 3 of the HTA 2004 may be summarised as follows.

Section 3 HTA 2004 Appropriate consent: adults

(6A) This subsection applies to the following activities done in England unless the body is the body of an excepted adult—

   (a) the storage of the body of a deceased person for use for the purpose of transplantation;

---

[96] HTWA 2013, s 5(3). In terms of what constitutes a 'significant period', it means a sufficiently long period as to lead a reasonable person to conclude that it would be inappropriate for consent to be deemed to be given.

[97] For an overview, see HTA, 'Code of Practice on HTWA 2013' (n 88) para 9. With regards to how to interpret the legislative provisions with regards to persons assessed as lacking capacity, see paras 62–74 of the Code.

[98] See The Human Transplantation (Excluded Relevant Material) (Wales) Regulations 2015 (WSI 2015/1775) (W.247). These Regulations may be updated from time to time, and further information can be obtained from the HTA website.

[99] HTWA 2013, ss 7(2) and (3).

[100] See Organ Donation (Deemed Consent) Act 2019, Explanatory Notes, Policy Background, para 7; Welsh Government, 'Evaluation of the Human Transplantation (Wales) Act: Impact Evaluation' (30 November 2017) available at <https://gov.wales/evaluation-human-transplantation-wales-act-impact-evaluation> accessed 29 December 2022.

[101] See Jane Noyes et al., 'Short-Term Impact of Introducing a Soft Opt-Out Organ Donation System in Wales: Before and After Study' (BMJ Open, 2019) available at <http://dx.doi.org/10.1136/bmjopen-2018-025159> accessed 29 December 2022.

[102] For an overview of the success or otherwise of the deemed consent regime in Wales, see Jordan Parsons, 'Ensuring Appropriate Assessment of Deemed Consent in Wales' (2019) 45(3) Journal of Medical Ethics 210.

(b) the removal from the body of a deceased person, for use for the purpose of transplantation, of any permitted material of which the body consists or which it contains;

(c) the storage for use for the purpose of transplantation of any permitted material which has come from a human body;

(d) the use for the purpose of transplantation of any permitted material which has come from a human body.

(6B) The person concerned is to be deemed, for the purposes of subsection (6)(ba), to have consented to the activity unless a person who stood in a qualifying relationship to the person concerned immediately before death provides information that would lead a reasonable person to conclude that the person concerned would not have consented.

In summary, the purpose of the ODCCA 2019 was to change the way in which consent is to be given for organ and tissue donation in England, for the purposes of transplantation. It provides that, in the absence of a deceased adult having made express provision in relation to consent before their death or having appointed someone to make a decision on consent for them, the default position in most cases will be that consent will be deemed to have been given. This means that, after death, a person will be considered to have consented to organ donation in their lifetime unless: they made specific provision to the contrary in their lifetime; they appointed someone to make the decision on their behalf; there is evidence that would lead a reasonable person to conclude that they would not have consented; or an exception applies. Such exceptions include where a person is younger than 18 years of age, then their parents will still be asked to consent on their child's behalf before organ donation will proceed;[103] individuals who lack mental capacity to understand the new arrangements and take the necessary action; and people who have lived in England for less than 12 months or who are not living here voluntarily.[104] It is also important to note that the ODCCA 2019 was intended to apply to the donation of organs for routine transplant purposes (e.g. heart, lung, kidney, liver).[105] It does not apply to organ donation for what is considered rare or novel transplantation purposes, such as those involving a limb, face, or uterus, for example. In such circumstances, an individual's family would be required to give their explicit consent to such donation before it could take place.[106]

In NI, legislative reform involving a shift towards deemed consent was adopted in 2022 via the Organ and Tissue Donation (Deemed Consent) Act (Northern Ireland) 2022 (OTDDCA 2022), and came into force in 2023. This followed a lengthy period of political and public debate on the issue. The eventual political catalyst for legislative reform in the area was largely driven by a public campaign conducted by the family of a young

---

[103] Having said that, any person can sign up the NHS Organ Donor Register, so if a young person had so registered then this information would be shared with the family to assist them in their decision-making with regards to organ donation. See NHSBT, 'Organ Donation, Own Your Decision' (2022) available at <https://www.organdonation.nhs.uk/uk-laws/organ-donation-law-in-england/under-18/#:~:text=If%20you%20are%20under%2018%20you%20can%20still%20decide%20whether,your%20decision%20at%20any%20time> accessed 29 December 2022.

[104] see HTA 2004, Part 1, s 3(9).

[105] On this point, see UK Department of Health and Social Care, 'Organs and Tissue to be Excluded from the Opt-Out Organ Donation System: Government Response' (2022) available at <https://www.gov.uk/government/consultations/opt-out-organ-donation-organs-and-tissues-excluded-from-the-new-system/outcome/quick-read-organs-and-tissues-to-be-excluded-from-the-opt-out-organ-donation-system-government-response> accessed 29 December 2022.

[106] ibid.

organ recipient and in his honour, the legislative reform is known colloquially as 'Dáithí's law'.[107] In many ways, the OTDDCA 2022 mirrors English legislative reform on deemed consent, except the imposition of a statutory duty on NI Ministers to promote deceased organ donation, which mirrors the Scottish and Welsh approaches.[108] The OTDDCA 2022 also drew on the definition of 'excepted persons' from the Welsh legislation. Such persons include an adult who has died and who was not resident in NI for a period of at least 12 months before death; and an adult who has died and who for a significant period before dying lacked capacity to understand the effect of the new law on deemed consent for organ donation.[109] With the adoption of the Act, the Human Tissue Authority published a revised draft version in September 2022 of Code of Practice F, Part Two: Deceased Organ and Tissue Donation. The revised Code incorporates and interprets legislative provisions establishing deemed consent for deceased organ donation for the purpose of transplantation in England, Wales and NI. This followed on from a public consultation that took place regarding the proposed changes to the earlier Code, and which was taken on board in revising the guidance.[110] The revised Code has now been published in its final form, with the NI legislation coming into force in 2023.[111]

As we have already highlighted, the legal position in Scotland under the HTA 2006 differs from the other UK jurisdictions. Legislative reform was adopted via the Human Tissue (Authorisation) (Scotland) Act 2019 (HTASA 2019) to amend the HTA 2006 and establish a system for deemed authorisation for deceased organ donation. The Act was only brought into force in 2021; implementation was delayed due to the Covid-19 pandemic in order to allow time for local education awareness activities to take place to facilitate the shift to the opt-out system.[112] The key legislative provisions for deemed authorisation under the new Scottish system are provided below.

Deemed authorisation for transplantation: adult

Section 6D HTA 2006

(1) An adult is deemed to have authorised the removal and use of a part of the adult's body after the adult's death for transplantation where there is in force at the relevant time—

   (a) no express authorisation by the adult of removal and use of any part of the adult's body for transplantation, and

   (b) no opt-out declaration by the adult as respects removal and use of the part of the adult's body for transplantation

---

[107] For an overview of the campaign for 'Dáithí's law', as well as NI political and public debates over the legislative reform, see Ruby Reed-Berendt et al., 'The Regulatory Shift to Opt-Out Organ Donation Across the UK' (forthcoming, 2023).

[108] Organ and Tissue Donation (Deemed Consent) Act (Northern Ireland) 2022, s 1(7) (OTDDCA 2022). This statutory obligation on the part of NI Ministers to promote local awareness of organ donation was originally introduced via the Health (Miscellaneous Provisions) Act (Northern Ireland) 2016, Part 4, s 15.

[109] OTDDCA 2022, s 1(4), which amends HTA 2004, Part 1, s 3(9), inserting a new s 3(9A).

[110] Human Tissue Authority, 'Review of Code of Practice F: Part Two for Deemed Consent' (2 September 2022) available at <https://www.hta.gov.uk/news/review-code-practice-f-part-two> accessed 29 December 2022.

[111] Human Tissue Authority, 'Code of Practice F: Donation of Solid Organs and Tissue for Transplantation; Part Two: Deceased Organ and Tissue Donation' (2022) available at <https://www.hta.gov.uk/guidance-professionals/codes-practice-standards-and-legislation/codes-practice> accessed 29 December 2022.

[112] HTA 2006, Part 2, s 2. This was similar to the approach taken under the HTWTA 2013 (see earlier in this chapter).

(2) Subsection (1) does not apply in relation to—

    (a) a person who was not ordinarily resident in Scotland for a period of at least 12 months ending immediately before the relevant time (a 'non-resident adult'),

    (b) an adult who is incapable of understanding the nature and consequences of deemed authorisation,

    (c) an excepted body part,

    (d) a part of the adult's body (that is not an excepted body part), if a person provides evidence to a health worker that would lead a reasonable person to conclude that—

        (i) the adult's most recent view was that the adult was unwilling for the part to be used for transplantation, or

        (ii) if the adult were capable of making a decision about removal and use of the part, the adult would be unwilling in the circumstances for the part to be used for transplantation.

(3) In this Part, an adult is incapable of understanding the nature and consequences of deemed authorisation if, over a significant period ending immediately before the relevant time, the person was incapable of understanding—

    (a) that an adult may be deemed to have authorised removal and use of a part of the adult's body after the adult's death for transplantation, and

    (b) that if authorisation is so deemed, after the adult's death part of the adult's body may be removed from the body and used for transplantation.

Scotland's new deemed authorisation system is primarily focused on adults aged 16 years and over.[113] Where they have not confirmed whether they want to be a donor, then they are considered to be willing to donate their organs and tissue when they die. This will apply unless they choose to opt out. A specific duty is imposed on healthcare professionals to inquire when organ donation is being considered as to whether an authorisation or opt-out exists, and, in consultation with the family, what the adult's most recent views would be in relation to organ donation.[114] Excluded groups from the new scheme in Scotland include children under the age of 16 years, unless specific steps are taken to register their decision to donate or this decision is taken in specified circumstances by those with parental rights and responsibilities;[115] adults who are assessed as lacking the capacity to understand the new laws and to take the necessary actions;[116] and adults who have lived in Scotland for less than 12 months before their death (non-resident adult).[117] Where a non-resident adult dies in circumstances in which it may be possible to donate their organs, but they have not recorded their views on such a donation, then their 'nearest relative' will be asked whether they wish to authorise organ donation in the circumstances.[118] As in other UK jurisdictions, there are a number of organs which are excluded from the deemed authorisation system in Scotland.[119]

---

[113] As noted previously, the HTA also makes clear that any child or young person aged 12 years or older may also register an authorisation for organ donation following their death, see HTA 2006, Part 1, s 8.

[114] HTA 2006, Part 1, s 16H (in relation to adults); s 16I (in relation to children).

[115] HTA 2006, Part 1, ss 8 and 8D; not also the position under s 10 in relation to persons with parental rights and responsibilities for children under the age of 12 years.

[116] HTA 2006, Part 1, s 6D(2)(b), (3)–(4).   [117] HTA 2006, Part 1, s 6D(2)(a).

[118] HTA 2006, Part 1, s 6E.

[119] HTA 2006, Part 1, ss 6D and 6G(1). These excepted body parts are specified in The Human Tissue (Excepted Body Parts) Scotland Regulations 2020 (SSI 2020/388), reg 2.

Of particular concern in the Scottish context was the need to make clear what pre-death procedures were legally permitted in the circumstances. The 2019 Act provided a new statutory framework for such procedures, which are defined as a medical procedure which is carried out on a person for the purpose of increasing the likelihood of successful transplantation of a part of their body after their death and which is not for the primary purpose of safeguarding or promoting the physical or mental health of the person. These procedures must be followed up until the point at which the individual has been confirmed to have died so do not need to be taken into account where individuals have been declared dead according to brain stem death testing.[120]

There are two different types of pre-death procedures: Type A and Type B procedures: Type A procedures are those which are generally considered routine procedures which would be needed to enable deceased donation to progress, whereas Type B procedures are less routine and are generally more invasive. In relation to the former, the donor will be considered to have authorised Type A procedures when they have either expressly authorised deceased organ donation for transplantation (such as where they had opted in on the Organ Donor Register); where their authorisation for donation is deemed under the new scheme; or where they have expressly authorised pre-death procedures under the new statutory framework.[121] Type B procedures are not usually routine in the context of organ transplantation and are generally of a more invasive nature. As a result, additional authorisation and further criteria need to be met before they can be performed.[122]

Finally, it is important to note that an eligible individual can register to be an organ donor via the NHS Organ Donor Register, which is operated on a UK-wide basis.[123] If an individual does not want to be an organ donor under new opt-out schemes, then they will need to register the decision to opt out via the Register.[124] There are also other choices available in the registration process. These include making clear that only some organs should be donated. An individual can also record their decision to withdraw their name from the register although it is made clear that this is not the same as recording a decision not to donate. A withdrawal only applies if an individual has previously recorded their decision regarding deceased organ donation.[125]

As has been highlighted in this section of the chapter, the approach taken to establishing opt-out systems for deceased organ donation in the UK's four jurisdictions have been broadly similar in terms of legislative approach, with an attempt to find 'something of a middle ground' between a 'hard' and a 'soft' opt-out system.[126] There are some interesting differences, however, including variation in what organs are 'excluded' from the opt-out

---

[120] For an overview, see Scottish Government, 'Organ and Tissue Donation - Authorisation Requirements: Guidance' (11 March 2021) available at <https://www.gov.scot/publications/guidance-deceased-organ-tissue-donation-scotland-authorisation-requirements-donation-pre-death-procedures-1st-edition-published-march-2021-1st-ed/> accessed 29 December 2022.

[121] Human Tissue (Authorisation) (Specified Type A Procedures) (Scotland) Regulations 2020 (SSI 2020/80).

[122] Human Tissue (Authorisation) (Specified Type B Procedures) (Scotland) Regulations 2021 (SSI 2021/110).

[123] NHSBT, 'NHS Organ Donor Register, Register a Decision to Donate' (2022) available at <https://www.organdonation.nhs.uk/register-your-decision/donate/> accessed 29 December 2022.

[124] NHSBT, 'NHS Organ Donor Register, Register a Decision Not to Donate' (2022) available at <https://www.organdonation.nhs.uk/register-your-decision/do-not-donate/> accessed 29 December 2022.

[125] NHSBT, 'Register Your Decision: About Your Choices on the NHS Organ Donor Register' (2022) available at <https://www.organdonation.nhs.uk/helping-you-to-decide/about-your-choices/> accessed 29 December 2022.

[126] On this point, see Jordan Parsons, 'Deemed Consent for Organ Donation: A Comparison of the English and Scottish Approaches' (2021) 8(1) Journal of Law and the Biosciences lsab003.

system.[127] It remains to be seen whether this shift towards an opt-out system will have the desired outcomes of promoting greater awareness of the importance of making one's views known about organ donation in the event of death and increasing the rates of organ donation from deceased donors. Any conclusions in this regard must necessarily await detailed evaluation in the medium to longer term.

13.4.2 DIRECTED DECEASED ORGAN DONATION

While it is hoped that the shift towards establishing opt-out systems for deceased organ dona-tion in the UK will have a positive effect on reducing rates of family veto over time, it has also been suggested that the anonymity of deceased organ donation may exert a negative influence and contribute to family veto. It could be argued that more organs might be donated if families were allowed more control with regards to their intended future use. Therefore, the possibility exists that a form of directed deceased organ donation might be a matter to take into consider-ation. Various terminology has been used over time in order to describe this form of donation, with the term 'conditional donation' being used to refer to a situation where an organ is either offered or withheld from a specific class of recipient. Instead, directed donation is a term that is most often used to refer to an organ that is directed to a specific person, where a particular individual is given priority to receive that organ for transplant.[128]

This policy option has been raised on several occasions in the UK, usually following high-profile instances where a request for a directed deceased organ donation was made by individuals and/or families.[129] This led to the UK Government convening two expert groups to consider the issue. In the year 2000, the first group's conclusion was to reject decision making on this basis by reference to individual cases, and to condemn all condi-tional organ donation as being contrary to the principles of altruism.[130] This was recon-sidered some ten years later in 2010. The group stated it was important to recognise that the fundamental principle of all deceased organ donation, was that it must be uncondi-tional. Having first established that the consent or authorisation to such donation was unconditional, it recommended that 'a request for the allocation of a donor organ can be considered in exceptional cases,' and only where the seven principles apply, as set out below.[131]

Principles Guiding Consideration of Directed Donation in the UK

- There is appropriate consent, or authorisation in Scotland, to organ donation.

- The consent or authorisation for organ donation is not conditional on the request for the allocation of a donor organ to the specified relative or friend of long standing going ahead.

- There are no others in desperately urgent clinical need of the organ who may be harmed by a request for the organ to be allocated to a named individual going ahead.

---

[127] Nicola Williams, Laura O'Donovan, and Stephen Wilkinson, 'Presumed Dissent? Opt-out Organ Donation and the Exclusion of Organs and Tissues' (2022) 30(2) Medical Law Review 268.

[128] See Michael Volk and Peter Ubel, 'A Gift of Life: Ethical and Practical Problems with Conditional and Directed Donation' (2008) 85(11) Transplantation 1542.

[129] See e.g., BBC News, 'Racist Organ Donation Condemned' (24 February 2000) available at <http://news.bbc.co.uk/1/hi/health/652132.stm> accessed 29 December 2022; Aidan Jones, 'Mother Denied Dead Daughter's Organ Transplant' The Guardian (12 April 2008) available at <https://www.theguardian.com/society/2008/apr/12/health.nhs> accessed 29 December 2022.

[130] Department of Health, 'An Investigation into Conditional Organ Donation' (2000).

[131] Department of Health, 'Requested Allocation of a Deceased Donor Organ' (March 2010) paras 3–4.

- In life the deceased had indicated a wish to donate to a specific named relative or friend of long standing in need of an organ; or, in the absence of that indication, the deceased's family expresses such a wish.

- The specific named relative or friend of long standing is on the transplant waiting list or could be considered to be placed on the waiting list in line with 2005 Directions to NHS Blood and Transplant as amended or subsequent directions.

- The need for a transplant is clinically indicated for the intended recipient.

- Priority must be given to a patient in desperately urgent clinical need over any requested allocation of deceased donor organ.

This is a highly restrictive protocol for allowing conditional donation to proceed and it is not clear that it does much to resolve the issue, although it remains established policy for organ transplantation programmes in the UK.[132] Academic commentators have critiqued this approach from various angles. Some have argued that under the HTA 2004, this form of deceased organ donation is not unlawful, but instead it is a policy matter that has achieved legal status through usage.[133] Others have suggested that just as there are many faces of discrimination, so are there also many ways in which we can measure altruism. Directed deceased organ donation may have its difficulties and contradictions, but a blanket rejection of any motive to donate an organ, other than indifference as to the outcome, might well be considered a perverse position to take.[134] Yet others have argued that the policy on rejecting this form of deceased organ donation sits uneasily with the existing directed donation policy involving living organ donors.[135] We now turn in the next section of the chapter to examine the legal position in relation to living organ donation for transplantation in the UK.

13.5 LIVING ORGAN DONATION

Up until the late 1980s, organ transplantation from living donors was limited to kidneys, but this situation has changed rapidly in recent decades. The first living related segmental liver transplant was performed in Brazil in 1988. Over the next ten years, more than 700 such transplants were performed around the world.[136] Since the 1990s, partial lung transplants, known as lobar lung transplantation, have also been undertaken successfully in relation to recipients suffering from diseases, such as cystic fibrosis.[137] The donation of

---

[132] In Scotland, see HTA 2006, Part 3, s 49.

[133] Antonia Cronin and James Douglas, 'Directed and Conditional Deceased Donor Organ Donations: Laws and Misconceptions' (2010) 18(3) Medical Law Review 275.

[134] Tom Martin Wilkinson, 'What's Not Wrong with Conditional Organ Donation?' (2003) 29(3) Journal of Medical Ethics 163.

[135] See Human Tissue Authority, 'Types of Living Organ Donation' (2022) available at <https://www.hta.gov.uk/guidance-public/body-organ-and-tissue-donation/living-organ-donation/types-living-organ-donation> accessed 29 December 2022.

[136] Amadeo Marcos et al., 'Right Lobe Living Donor Liver Transplantation' (1999) 68(6) Transplantation 798.

[137] Margaret Hodson, 'Transplantation Using Lung Lobes from Living Donors' (2000) 26(6) Journal of Medical Ethics 419. For an overview of current approaches in the UK, see NHSBT, 'Organ Transplantation – Lung' (2022) available at <https://www.nhsbt.nhs.uk/organ-transplantation/lung/> accessed 29 December 2022.

uteruses by living donors is also now possible, although it currently remains an experimental programme in the UK.[138]

As a result of medical and scientific advances, transplantation from organs from living donors has become the preferred clinical option, resulting in longer life expectancy and lower mortality rates in the recipient. Tissue compatibility is ordinarily much closer, the damage done to the functioning organ is minimised, there is a reduced need for immunosuppression, and the organs of living donors are generally in a much better shape than organs from a deceased organ donor.[139]

Living donor kidney transplantation 'accounts for 97% of living donation activity in the UK and for 28% of kidney transplants across both adult and paediatric recipients'.[140] It has also been reported that in the first decade of the 2000s, such activity 'trebled in the UK',[141] with encouragement and greater support provided for this form of living organ donation.[142] In general terms, the risks to the living organ donor from the surgical removal of the kidney in a procedure known as a nephrectomy, for example, have been shown to be minimal, with end-stage renal disease being remote. Nevertheless, published data does point to evidence of both minor and major complications from the surgical procedure for living donors. While there are also many benefits for the recipient from receiving a donated kidney, transplant surgery is not risk-free and there are also recognised complications that do arise from such surgery.[143]

When it comes to the legality of living organ donation (for non-regenerative tissue), the starting point under the common law is the principle that a person cannot consent to being killed or seriously injured; therefore, living transplantation of a heart is necessarily prohibited in legal terms.[144] Apart from this extreme case, legality depends upon the presumed risk-benefit ratio. This assessment is difficult because technological advances in transplantation medicine are always expanding and there is variation in medical expertise in the area. Given that the relative risks and benefits of a given procedure are both assessable and acceptable, both the ethical and common law position of living organ donation has long been settled: consent to a surgical procedure which is, in itself, non-therapeutic will be valid so long as the consequent infliction of harm can be shown not to be against the public interest.[145] The risk-benefit assessment is not uncomplicated, however, as the ratio may change over time, particularly where individual circumstances of the donor and/or the recipient mean a likely increase in the risk of complications and

---

[138] For an overview of this research programme, see Womb Transplant UK, 'Home' (2022) available at <https://wombtransplantuk.org/> accessed 29 December 2022.

[139] Eghlim Nemati et al., 'Does Kidney Transplantation with Deceased or Living Donors Affect Graft Survival?' (2014) 6(4) Nephro-Urology Monthly e12182; Mary Amanda Dew et al., 'Long-Term Medical and Psychosocial Outcomes in Living Liver Donors' (2017) 17(4) American Journal of Transplantation 880.

[140] NHSBT, 'Living Donor Kidney Transplantation' (2022) available at <https://www.odt.nhs.uk/living-donation/living-donor-kidney-transplantation/> accessed 29 December 2022.

[141] ibid.

[142] In order to encourage further advances in the area, NHSBT has launched a new policy strategy, 'Living Donor Kidney Transplantation 2020: A UK Strategy' (2020) available at <https://www.odt.nhs.uk/odt-structures-and-standards/key-strategies/archived-strategies/living-donor-transplantation-strategy-2020/> accessed 29 December 2022.

[143] For an overview, see NHSBT, 'Risks of Kidney Transplant' (2022) available at <https://www.nhsbt.nhs.uk/organ-transplantation/kidney/benefits-and-risks-of-a-kidney-transplant/risks-of-a-kidney-transplant/> accessed 29 December 2022. Note that the UK has established a vigilance framework to facilitate donor safety and welfare and to monitor outcomes in relation to living donor transplantation, see NHSBT, 'Living Donor Kidney Transplantation 2020' (n 142) 6.

[144] R v Coney (1882) 8 QBD 534.   [145] A-G's Reference (No 6 of 1980) [1981] QB 715.

disease post-surgery.[146] Where consent is possible, it is subject to the same principles as any other medical procedure under the common law and mental capacity legislation (see further in the next section, and more generally Chapter 8).

Both the HTA 2004 and the HTA 2006 also deal with this form of transplantation in broad terms,[147] supplemented through guidance, statutory regulations,[148] and Codes of Practice, which are regularly updated by the Human Tissue Authority.[149] Both Human Tissue Acts criminalise living organ donation for transplantation if performed other than in accordance with the legislation.[150] The Human Tissue Authority assesses and approves applications for living organ donation, with a specific remit for Scotland.[151] For the Authority to grant approval, it is necessary to show that no reward has been given or is to be given; and when organs are removed, consent for its removal for the purpose of transplantation has been given, or its removal for that purpose is otherwise lawful.[152]

13.5.1 LIVING ORGAN DONORS WHO LACK CAPACITY

The common law position is that there is no automatic legal prohibition on a donor who lacks capacity being a living organ donor. Indeed, it has been highlighted that consent to a surgical procedure on a child below the age of 16 years should normally be obtained from the parents, subject only to the possible *Gillick*-rights of the child.[153] Valid parental consent, however, refers to treatment for the advantage of the child whereas more

---

[146] On this, see Walter Glannon, 'Underestimating the Risk in Living Kidney Donation' (2008) 34(3) Journal of Medical Ethics 127. In relation to support for the risk/benefit consensus in relation to living organ donation for transplantation in the UK, see Antonia Cronin, 'Allowing Autonomous Agents Freedom' (2008) 34(3) Journal of Medical Ethics 129.

[147] HTA 2004, Part 2, ss 33–34; HTA 2006, Part 1, ss 17–18.

[148] See e.g. Human Tissue Act 2004 (Persons Who Lack Capacity to Consent and Transplants) Regulations 2006 (SI 2006/1659) (HTA 2004 Regulations 2006); Human Organ and Tissue Live Transplants (Scotland) Regulations 2006 (SSI 2006/390) (HTA 2006 Regulations 2006).

[149] See e.g., Human Tissue Authority, 'Codes of Practice' (n 11).

[150] HTA 2004, Part 2, ss 32(1), 32A and 33; HTA 2006, Part 1, ss 17, 20(1), s 20A. Note recent amendments inserted via the Health and Care 2022, Part 6, s 170, which address the commission of extra-territorial offences by a person from the UK in relation to living organ donation outside the UK. These new offences were created because there were 'concerns' that the existing Human Tissue Acts 'did not cover all scenarios in which a person from the UK might engage in the purchase and sale of organs.' This has now been addressed via the insertion of a new s 32A in the HTA 2004 and a new s 20A in the HTA 2006. These new sections 'make it an offence to pay for the supply of an organ, pay for an offer to supply an organ, or seek somebody willing to supply an organ for payment anywhere in the world. It would also make it an offence to supply, or offer to supply, an organ for payment anywhere in the world. This includes initiating or negotiating any arrangement involving the giving of a reward for the supply of, or for an offer to supply, an organ, and taking part in the management of a body that does so', see Health and Care Act 2022, Explanatory Notes, paras 232, 1199–1200.

[151] The Human Tissue Authority's remit in Scotland is set out in a letter entitled 'Human Tissue (Scotland) Act 2006: A guide to its implications for NHS Scotland', which the Scottish Health Department issued on 20 July 2006 (updated March 2017). The Authority assesses applications for living organ donation and donation of bone marrow and peripheral blood stem cells (PBSCs) on behalf of the Scottish Ministers who delegated this responsibility to the Authority. See also Human Tissue Authority, 'Code of Practice F: Donation of Solid Organ and Tissue for Transplantation, Part One: Living Organ Donation' (20 May 2020) paras 10–11.

[152] Human Tissue Authority, 'Code of Practice F, Part One' (n 151) para 35.

[153] It is reasonable to argue that s 8 of the Family Law Reform Act 1969 has no application to non-therapeutic procedures. The statutory position in Scotland under s 2(4) of the Age of Legal Capacity (Scotland) Act 1991 is unclear but organ donation is not positively excluded as being within the 'understanding' of the child's remit.

troublesome questions arise in relation to medical procedures which are not calculated
to be to the child's benefit. In this regard, it is useful to note the case of *Re W (A Minor)
(Medical Treatment: Court's Jurisdiction)*,[154] where the Court of Appeal made clear that
the 'medical age of majority' of 16 years of age as stated under the Family Law Reform
Act 1969 did not mean that young people can consent to or authorise organ donation.
In his judgment, Lord Donaldson doubted that the courts would find a young person
sufficiently *Gillick*-competent to give an independent assessment to any non-therapeutic
procedure, such as organ donation. In the circumstances, consent from the parent/guard-
ian and the young person must be advisable.

It is arguable that the principle that a person who lacks capacity cannot legally be subjected to any medical procedure which is not medically to their advantage is not an absolute one. It is therefore possible that a court might consider the donation of an organ by
such a donor to be not only in the public interest but also in the interests of the person in
question, who will almost certainly be a member of the donor's immediate family (e.g.
sibling, parent). In such circumstances, it might be supposed that it is in the interests of
the potential donor that a member of their family should be saved rather than die. This
line of argument was successfully pursued in the early US case of *Strunk v Strunk*.[155] In
this case, the donor who was an adult, but who had been assessed as having a mental age
of six years, was eligible to donate a kidney to his critically ill brother. The court held
that it would be in the donor's best interests for his brother's life to be saved, given the
evidence of the close relationship which they shared. Consequently, the operation was
allowed although the donor was not in a position to give consent.

In practice, while the donation of regenerative tissue is permissible under stringent
conditions, most jurisdictions are reluctant to allow the taking of non-regenerative tissues from those who lack capacity.[156] For example, the WHO advocates for a prohibition
on living organ donation involving minors for the purpose of transplantation, other than
narrow exceptions allowed under national law.[157] In addition, the Additional Protocol
to the Council of Europe's Convention on Human Rights and Biomedicine envisages
the donation of 'regenerative tissue' involving a living donor who lacks capacity as being
exceptional and subject to 'protective conditions prescribed by law', provided the following conditions are met: there is no compatible donor available who has the capacity to
consent; the recipient is a brother or sister of the donor; the donation has the potential
to be life-saving for the recipient; approval in writing has been given by the appropriate
oversight body; and the donor does not object.[158]

Certainly, there are significant reasons why limits should be placed on the use of persons who lack capacity as organ donors, with extreme caution being exercised in cases
where there is unlikely to be any significant understanding of what the donation entails
both at the time and, most significantly, in the future. Under both the common law and

[154] [1992] 4 All ER 627.
[155] 445 SW 2d 145 (Ky, 1969). Note that *Strunk* received a mixed reaction in the US courts and is unlikely
to represent the current preferred approach.
[156] See Kristof Thys et al., 'Could Minors Be Living Kidney Donors? A Systematic Review of Guidelines,
Position Papers and Reports' (2013) 26(10) Transplant International 949; Jenny Prüfe, 'Decision Making in
the Context of Paediatric Solid Organ Transplantation Medicine' (2022) Transplant International available
at <https://doi.org/10.3389/ti.2022.10625> accessed 29 December 2022.
[157] WHO, 'Guiding Principles on Human Cell, Tissue and Organ Transplantation' (2010) Guiding
Principle 4, available at <https://apps.who.int/iris/handle/10665/341814> accessed 29 December 2022.
[158] Council of Europe, Additional Protocol to the Convention on Human Rights and Biomedicine on
Transplantation of Human Organs and Tissues of Human Origin (2002), Strasbourg, 24.I.2002, Art 14(2).
Neither the Convention nor this Additional Protocol has been signed or ratified by the UK to date.

legislation in the UK, however, there is no blanket prohibition on organ donation by those who lack capacity, and decisions are made on a case-by-case basis. In relation to the common law position, this was highlighted in the case of *Re Y*,[159] an English case involving a bone marrow transplantation between two sisters. The older sister, aged 36 years, was dying of leukaemia and her younger sister (Y), aged 25 years, who had an intellectual disability, was the only match for a bone marrow transplant for her older sister. The sisters were not particularly close, although the mother was close to both daughters. The older sister sought a declaration that a bone marrow donation from Y would be lawful. It was held by Justice Cornell that if the older daughter had died, her death would have an adverse impact on the mother. She would be less able to visit Y and she would be much occupied in caring for her older daughter's child, if she died. If the transplant went ahead, then the positive relationship between Y and her mother would be enhanced, as would the relationship between the sisters. The risk and discomfort to Y would be minimal, so it was in Y's best interests to allow the bone narrow transplant to go ahead. The judge made it clear that in deciding the case the aim was not to set a precedent for kidney donation by a person who had an intellectual disability.

The position in *Re Y* was recently confirmed in *A NHS Foundation Trust v MC*,[160] which involved a young woman who lacked capacity and was aged 18 years of age. An order was sought in the Court of Protection to permit the donation of her stem cells to her mother who had leukaemia. In giving judgment, Justice Cohen confirmed that in line with *Re Y*, it can be in the best interests of a person to donate stem cells, applying the test set down in section 4 of the Mental Capacity Act 2005. It was noted that this was the first time that this type of application by someone lacking capacity had come before the Court of Protection and the first time the Human Tissue Authority had been involved in such a case.[161]

Under the HTA 2004, it is only in extremely rare circumstances that a child (under 18 years of age) will be able to be a living organ donor.[162] Court approval should be obtained before the removal of a solid organ or part organ from a living child for the purposes of donation for transplantation. It is only when court approval is obtained, that any such application could be referred to the Human Tissue Authority for consideration. Any approval would be given by a panel consisting of at least three members of the Authority.[163] The HTA 2004 does not elaborate upon the criteria to be applied in considering whether an adult who lacks capacity should be able to act as a living organ donor. While separate provisions are made in Wales and NI in this regard, we highlight the English position, by way of example. Although the HTA 2004 does not specify what constitutes appropriate consent for the removal of an organ from a living adult who lacks capacity to consent for themselves,[164] the Human Tissue Authority recognises in its relevant Code of Practice that there are four accepted routes by which such an adult could consent to being a living

---

[159] *Re Y (Mental Patient: bone marrow donation)* [1997] Fam 110.   [160] [2020] EWCOP 33.

[161] See Alex Ruck Keene, 'Stem Cell Donation, Altruism and the Court of Protection' (Mental Capacity Law and Policy Blog, 30 June 2020) available at <https://www.mentalcapacitylawandpolicy.org.uk/stem-cell-donation-altruism-and-the-court-of-protection/> accessed 29 December 2022; Bonnie Venter, '*A NHS Foundation Trust v MC* [2020] EWCOP 33: Revisiting Best interests and "Altruistic" Incapacitous Stem Cell Donation' (2021) 29(2) Medical Law Review 337.

[162] See HTA 2004 Regulations 2006 (n 148) reg 12.

[163] ibid., reg 12(1); Human Tissue Authority, 'Code of Practice F: Part One' (n 151) paras 44–46; 102–103; see also Human Tissue Authority, 'Code of Practice G: Donation of Allogeneic Bone Marrow and Peripheral Blood Stem Cells for Transplantation' (3 April 2017).

[164] However, note the HTA 2004 Regulations 2006 (n 148), reg 12.

organ donor.[165] Reference will be made to the Mental Capacity Act 2005 (MCA 2005), as well as general common law principles governing capacity to consent to medical procedures. Further, the MCA 2005 Code of Practice states that where an adult lacks the capacity to consent to the removal of an organ for transplantation, the case must be referred to the Court of Protection for a declaration that the removal would be lawful. Donation may then only proceed if court approval has been obtained and, following court approval, the case is referred to a three-person Authority panel for consideration and approval, where appropriate.[166]

On behalf of the Scottish Ministers, the Authority also assesses applications for living organ donation in relation to children (under 16 years of age) and adults lacking capacity who are based in Scotland. For both groups, there are only two forms of living organ donation which can be considered under the HTA 2006. First, the donation of regenerative tissue, which in terms of how this is defined in the Act means that only bone marrow, peripheral blood stem cells, and skin.[167] Second, the donation of an organ or part of an organ as part of a domino organ procedure.[168] Further details regarding the approach to be taken to living organ donation by children and adults who lack capacity are set out in the Human Organ and Tissue Live Transplants (Scotland) Regulations 2006.[169] By virtue of these Regulations, the Authority must be satisfied that the donor is an adult with incapacity or a child, the organ is being removed as part of a domino transplant operation or the tissue being removed is regenerative tissue, there is no unwillingness on the part of the donor, information has been given to the donor and there is no evidence of reward. The donor will be interviewed in all cases where approval is sought from the Authority for this type of donation. Where it is possible to do so, the adult's proxy or a parent/guardian of the child will also be interviewed to obtain their views as to the adult or child's past wishes and feelings on the issue of organ donation.[170] In sum, the circumstances in which the Authority will approve living organ donation for those who lack capacity is clearly subject to strict regulation, where it is permitted at all.

13.5.2 TYPES OF LIVING ORGAN DONATION

The Human Tissue Acts also distinguish several different concepts in living organ donation, including directed donation; directed altruistic donation; non-directed altruistic donation; paired and pooled donation; non-directed altruistic donor chains, and domino donation, with a summary of these differing types of donations provided in **Table 13.2**.[171]

---

[165] Human Tissue Authority, 'Code of Practice F: Part One' (n 151) paras 54–55.

[166] ibid., para 56.

[167] See HTA 2006, Part 1, s 17(10) where 'regenerative tissue' is defined as 'tissue which is able to be replaced in the body of a living person by natural processes if the tissue is injured or removed'. For a definition of what constitutes 'tissue', see HTA 2006, Part 7, s 60(1).

[168] See HTA 2006, Part 1, s 17(10) where a 'domino organ transplant operation' means a transplant operation performed on a living person by a registered medical practitioner (a) which is designed to safeguard or promote the physical health of the person by transplanting organs or parts of organs into the person; and (b) by so doing, necessitates the removal of an organ or part of an organ from the person which in turn is intended to be used for transplantation in respect of another living person.

[169] See HTA 2006 Regulations 2006 (n 148) Parts 3 and 4.

[170] See Scottish Executive, Health Department, 'Human Tissue (Scotland) Act 2006: A Guide to its Implications for NHS Scotland' NHS HDL (2006) 46, paras 27–29.

[171] Human Tissue Authority, 'Code of Practice F: Part One' (n 151), Glossary; see also British Transplantation Society, 'Guidelines for Living Donor Kidney Transplantation' (4th edn, 2018).

Table 13.2 Types of Living Organ Donation

Type	Description
Directed donation	Where a person donates an organ to a specific, identified recipient with whom they have a genetic or pre-existing emotional relationship (e.g. parent to child, brother to sister or friend to friend).
Directed altruistic donation	Where a person donates an organ to a specific individual and there is no evidence of a qualifying genetic or pre-existing emotional relationship between the donor and recipient. These cases tend to be characterised by a third party—either a person or other mechanism such a social networking website—bringing the donor and recipient together for the purpose of transplantation.
Non-directed altruistic donation	Where a person donates an organ to an unknown recipient. This may involve a non-directed altruistic donor donating into a paired/pooled arrangement to a 'chain' of organ transplants.
Altruistic donor	Where a person donates an organ on an altruistic basis to an unknown recipient. This type of donor will be assessed in the first instance by the local transplant unit, which includes medical tests and a mental health assessment. If a person is assessed as clinically suitable as a donor, they will be referred to an HTA Independent Assessor (IA). The IA will interview the potential altruistic donor to ensure the requirements of the HTA 2004 have been met and will submit a report of their interview to the HTA. A decision on the case is then made by a panel of the HTA board members. Following HTA approval, the donor's name will be put forward to a national allocation scheme and matched to a suitable recipient.
Paired/pooled donations	A person wishes to donate an organ but is unable to (or chooses not to) donate because they are either incompatible with their recipient or prefer a better match. They can be matched with another donor and recipient in the same situation under the UK Living Kidney Sharing Scheme. The donor organs are then swapped between recipients. When two donor-recipient pairs are involved, this is known as a paired donation. Where more than two donors and two recipients are involved in the swap, then this is known as a pooled donation. This type of arrangement is currently only available for kidney transplants in the UK.
Domino donation	A person donates an organ that has been removed for the primary purpose of the person's medical treatment. The organ removed may prove suitable for transplant into another person. The Human Tissue Authority does not regulate domino donations.

To some, the (increased) availability of living organ donation may represent a significant means of improving the supply of available organs for transplant; for others, it may be a Pandora's box full of moral pitfalls, largely related to the potential for the emergence of markets and trade in organs by living donors. To address such concerns, it is required that all non-directed altruistic donations, as well as paired and pooled donations, be approved by a suitably constituted Human Tissue Authority panel.[172] This is in addition to strict rules regarding living donor consent, counselling of both donors and recipients, as well as a prohibition on commercial transactions involved in living organ donation for transplantation.[173]

The clinician responsible for the donor must refer the matter to the Human Tissue Authority, which, before making a decision, must consider reports from independent qualified persons (known as Independent Assessors) who have interviewed both the donor and the recipient,[174] with specific points required to be covered. The donation by the living donor must be approved by a panel of at least three members of the Human Tissue Authority, if the donor is an adult who lacks capacity or a child, or when the donation is paired, pooled, or non-directed and altruistic (as noted previously).[175] These requirements, other than those associated with non-payment, are waived in the event that the donation is part of the treatment of the donor.[176] This may arise in the context of what is known as the 'domino donation' (see **Table 13.2**). An example of this type of situation is where a person who has cystic fibrosis receives a heart-lung transplant from a deceased donor, rather than just receiving a lung transplant on its own. This will mean that the heart of the person with cystic fibrosis would be available for donation following the heart-lung transplant, which will most likely be offered to a non-related recipient.[177]

13.5.3 TRADE AND COMMERCE

The commercialisation of transplant surgery remains one of the most divisive issues in the context of living organ donation. Its acceptability involves a complex amalgam of public policy and the validation of individual consent in exceptional circumstances. On the latter score alone, it is to be distinguished from payment for organs from deceased donors, a matter which is better considered as an aspect of the availability of organs rather than of ethical principle. Clearly, the legislative intention is to distinguish altruism from commercialism and to approve the former while condemning the latter.[178] In general terms, the Human Tissue Acts prohibit commercial dealings, other than the provision of legitimate expenses, in the supply of human material for the purpose of transplantation both by the living and the dead.[179]

Under the sub-heading 'trafficking', section 32 of the HTA 2004 states that the giving or receiving of reward for the supply of, or offer to supply, any 'controlled material',[180] or advertising to that effect, are criminal offences. Specifically, a person commits an offence if they give, offer, or receive any reward (financial or other material advantage) for the supply or offer of supply of any organ or part organ; look for a person willing to supply any

---

[172] Human Tissue Authority, 'Code of Practice F: Part One' (n 151) paras 103–104.
[173] ibid., para 35.   [174] HTA 2004 Regulations 2006 (n 148), reg 11.
[175] ibid., reg 12.   [176] ibid., reg 10(2).
[177] See Human Tissue Authority, 'Code of Practice F: Part One' (n 151) para 34.
[178] see Greg Moorlock, Jonathan Ives, and Heather Draper, 'Altruism in Organ Donation: An Unnecessary Requirement?' (2014) 40(2) Journal of Medical Ethics 134; Leonard Fleck and Arthur Ward, 'Altruistic Organ Donation: On Giving A Kidney To A Stranger' (2022) 31(3) Cambridge Quarterly of Healthcare Ethics 395.
[179] HTA 2004, Part 2, s 32; HTA 2006, Part 1, s 17(3).
[180] Pursuant to HTA 2004, Part 2, s 32(8), 'controlled material' is defined as 'any material which consists of or includes human cells; is or is intended to be removed, from a human body; and is intended to be used for the purpose of transplantation'. Under s 32(9), it does not include gametes, embryos and material which is the subject of property because of an application of human skill. Cell lines do not come within the remit of the HTA 2004, see Part 3, s 54(7). For a detailed examination of what is meant of the exception based on the application of human skill, see Chapter 14.

organ or part organ for reward; offer to supply any organ or part organ for reward; initiate or negotiate any arrangement involving the giving of a reward for the supply of, or for an offer to supply, any organ or part organ; take part in the management or control of any type of group whose activities consist of or includes the initiation or negotiation of such arrangements; cause to be published or distributed, or knowingly publish or distribute, an advertisement inviting people to supply, or offering to supply, any organ or part organ for reward, or indicating that the advertiser is willing to initiate or negotiate any such arrangements. This covers all and any types of advertising, including via social media.[181]

It should be noted that it is not illegal under the HTA 2004 to use advertising or social media per se to seek a living donor provided there is no offer of reward/payment or material advantage to a potential living organ donor who is found by such means. It is, however, an offence to offer a reward as part of any such advertisement.[182] The Human Tissue Authority has issued guidance to assist individuals who wish to use social media to seek a matching living organ donor, or conversely for those individuals who may have been approached by such a potential donor via social media. In the first instance, those seeking to find a living organ donor in this way should liaise with their transplant centre. Transplant units are not obliged to consider any potential donors who may be referred in this way which may in any case raise logistical difficulties. For example, a transplant unit may not have the capacity or resources to test all of those who may come forward as potential donors as a result.[183]

The use of 'transplantable material' from living donors is controlled by section 33 of the HTA 2004, which makes it an offence either to remove and/or to implant any such material from a living person, unless regulations provide otherwise.[184] Each case of living organ donation will be decided by the Human Tissue Authority which must, in turn, be assured that consent has been given and that no reward is involved in the procedure (see later in this chapter).[185]

In Scotland, section 20 of the HTA 2006 prohibits commercial dealings in relation to living organ donation for transplantation. It is a criminal offence to engage in such dealings, unless certain conditions are met, including that the living donor has given consent, and there must have been no coercion or reward in relation to the removal of organs.[186] Restrictions on the circumstances in which living organ donation for transplantation can take place are set out in section 17 of the HTA 2006, including what constitutes 'reward' for the purposes of section 20 of the Act.[187] Pursuant to an agreement reached between

---

[181] This summary draws on the Human Tissue Authority, 'Code of Practice F: Part One' (n 151) para 42.

[182] For clarification on this point, see Human Tissue Authority, 'Code of Practice F: Part One' (n 151) paras 33, 40–43.

[183] Human Tissue Authority, 'Living Organ Donation Matching Websites and Social Media' (2022) available at <https://www.hta.gov.uk/guidance-public/living-organ-donation/living-organ-donation-matching-websites-and-social-media> accessed 29 December 2022.

[184] In the HTA 2004 Regulations 2006 (n 148), reg 9, 'transplantable material' is defined as (a) the whole or part of any of the following organs if it is to be used for the same purpose as the entire organ in the human body: (i) kidney, (ii) heart, (iii) lung or a lung lobe, (iv) pancreas, (v) liver, (vi) bowel, (vii) larynx; (b) face, or (c) limb. Note that a more restricted definition of the term is provided where it involves a child or an adult lacking capacity (see reg 10). For further details, see under the section on living organ donors who lack capacity in this chapter.

[185] ibid., reg 11(3). See also Human Tissue Authority, 'Code of Practice F: Part One' (n 151) paras 35–39.

[186] See HTA 2006, Part 1, s 20.

[187] These restrictions may be waived in certain circumstances involving adults who have capacity, the details of which are set out in the HTA 2006 Regulations 2006 (n 143) Part 2. Note that this is also the case in relation to potential donors who are children and adults lacking capacity (Parts 3 and 4). For further details in relation to such donors, see under the sub-heading 13.5.1 Living Organ Donors who Lack Capacity in this chapter.

the Scottish Ministers and the Human Tissue Authority, potential living donors are assessed by the Human Tissue Authority to ensure that there is no evidence of coercion or financial reward.[188]

The term 'reward' is defined similarly under the Human Tissue Acts as involving 'financial or other material advantage'.[189] It is also made clear in both Acts that what does not come within the definition of reward are costs associated with transporting, removing, preparing, preserving, or storing the body of a deceased person, or organs or tissue in relation to such body, as well as any liability incurred in respect of expenses (or loss of earnings) incurred by a third party in relation to such costs.[190] In practice, the term 'reward' means any money, gift, or other benefit with a financial value which influences the decision to donate an organ. However, reimbursement of legitimate expenses to a living donor, including loss of earnings that are directly attributable to the organ donation, does not contravene the Human Tissue Acts and is supported by all of the UK's health services (see Chapter 3). The overarching aim in developing this type of policy is to remove potential financial disincentives which may arise as a result of being a living organ donor and therefore to reimburse the donor for a range of expenses incurred as a result.[191] For present purposes, we focus on the policies for reimbursement of expenses by living organ donors in England and Scotland by way of example.[192]

NHS England now operates a single pathway for its reimbursement policy, rather than having a separate approach based on the type of organ involved (e.g. kidney and livers).[193] The policy confirms that reimbursement of expenses will be in line with eight principles as set out in **Table 13.3**, and covers loss of earnings, travel and accommodation, retention of tax working and child tax credits, as well as miscellaneous expenses on a case-by-case basis. A time frame of 6–12 weeks is allowed for such expenses to be incurred, with some flexibility for an extension depending on individual circumstances. Provided that the transplant which is derived from the living organ donation is approved in line with the HTA 2006, the Scottish policy on reimbursement of expenses confirms that it does not prohibit the reimbursement of reasonable expenses to a living donor if they are directly attributable to their organ donation.[194] This includes loss of earnings (within a specified time frame), travel, accommodation and miscellaneous expenses, in line with a number of key principles which are similar but not identical to the approach taken in England (see **Table 13.3**).[195]

---

[188]   See Human Tissue Authority, 'Code of Practice F: Part One' (n 151) para 35.

[189]   HTA 2004, Part 2, s 32(11); HTA 2006, Part 1, s 17(10).

[190]   HTA 2004, Part 2, s 32(7). In the Explanatory Notes to the HTA Act 2004, it also notes that s 32(6) provides for the 'possibility of commercial tissue banks by allowing licence-holders to receive more than just expenses in relation to these activities.'

[191]   See NHS England, 'Commissioning Policy on Reimbursement of Expenses for Living Donors, Ref: NHS England A06/P/a' (revised August 2018) paras 3, 4a. For commentary on the importance of removing financial disincentives to facilitating living organ donation for transplantation, see e.g. Daniel Salomon et al., 'AST/ASTS Workshop on Increasing Organ Donation in the United States: Creating an "Arc of Change" From Removing Disincentives to Testing Incentives' (2015) 15(5) American Journal of Transplantation 1173; Frank McCormick et al., 'Removing Disincentives to Kidney Donation: A Quantitative Analysis' (2019) 30(8) Journal of the American Society of Nephrology 1349.

[192]   See also Welsh Health Specialised Services Committee, 'Specialised Services Policy: CP30 Live Donor Expenses' (Version 2.0, February 2021).

[193]   NHS England (n 191) paras 8–11.

[194]   Scottish Government, 'Health Directorate, Policy on Reimbursement of Living Solid Organ Donor Expenses by NHS Boards in Scotland, DL' (2016) para 1.2.

[195]   NHS National Services Scotland, National Services Division, NHS Scotland Financial Operating Procedure for Reimbursement of Living Solid Organ Donor Expenses, NSD607003 V4, para 2.

Table 13.3 Key Principles for Reimbursement of Expenses for Living Organ Donors in England and Scotland

England	Scotland
a) The principle of reimbursement is founded on the premise that there should be no financial incentive or disincentive in becoming a living donor.	a) The principle of reimbursement is founded on the premise that there is no financial incentive or disincentive in becoming a living donor.
b) A robust, stratified claims assessment process based upon the level of risk and proportionality is required i.e. in line with the donor's earnings, in order to assess claims accurately across the spectrum of costs.	b) All individual claims must be submitted and settled in a timely manner to prevent unnecessary hardship to the donor as a consequence of the donation.
c) The financial reimbursement will reflect the loss of earnings and other relevant expenses, except where exceptions apply.	c) The financial reimbursement will reflect the loss of earnings and other relevant expenses.
d) The calculation of reimbursement will be agreed in a transparent and consistent manner before donation so that donors receive reimbursement with the minimum of delay post donation.	d) The principles of reimbursement will be communicated clearly to the donor in a transparent and consistent manner before donation, as set out in the NHS Scotland Financial Operating Procedure for Reimbursement of Living Donor Expenses.
e) Special arrangements for retrospective consideration of claims may apply where there is insufficient time prior to donation for prospective agreement, e.g., donors who are non-resident in the UK, urgent lobe of liver donation, non-directed altruistic donors and where a subsequent claim is made for previously unforeseen expenses.	e) Special arrangements (e.g., retrospective consideration of claims) may need to be considered where donors who are non-resident in the UK are involved or those that relate to the National Living Kidney Sharing Schemes, if the timeframe prior to donation precludes prospective agreement.
f) Reimbursement is funded by NHS England. Mechanisms must be in place to process payments to avoid delay.	f) NHS Boards will reimburse donors directly and will make every effort to avoid delayed payment.
g) Potential donors who are unsuitable to proceed to donation are eligible to claim for reimbursement of travel expenses, including parking costs.	g) Potential donors who are deemed unsuitable to proceed to donation may be eligible to claim for reimbursement of certain expenses such as travel expenses, including parking costs.
h) Under exceptional circumstances, additional reimbursement costs may be considered on a case-by-case basis at the discretion of NHS England.	h) NHS Boards may consider additional reimbursement costs on a case-by-case basis.

We now turn in the next section of the chapter to consider in more detail a range of ethical issues which may arise in the context of considering options for trade and commerce, as well as payments for living organ donors for transplantation purposes.

13.5.4 ETHICAL ISSUES

Notwithstanding the legislative prohibition on trade and commerce in organ donation for transplantation in the Human Tissue Acts, there has been ongoing policy and academic debates about whether trade, incentives, and markets to manage supply and demand for organs can be ethically justified and should be legally permitted in certain circumstances.[196] There have been a wide range of proposals in this regard, including forms of insurance policies, taxes, and priority organ allocation.[197] In the case of deceased organ donation in particular, this has included proposals for payment of a specified amount for funeral expenses to families who consented to donate organs after the death of a family member.[198] In addition, proposals for broader structural reform have included establishing a single (state-sponsored) provider to manage supply and demand for organs in what has been described as a 'monopsonistic market';[199] facilitating a partnership between the state and not-for-profit organisations to manage the process;[200] and promoting a futures market in organs.[201]

For those who object to markets for organs, the use of direct financial payments is ethically problematic on a number of grounds, including their likely adverse impact upon the altruistic motivation to donate: this is a particularly influential argument given the long-standing commitment to the gift relationship in organ (and tissue) donation in the UK.[202] This also needs to be set in the context of the prohibition against the commodification of the body in human rights instruments, which is accompanied by longstanding concerns about the potential for donor exploitation.[203] It has also been suggested that financial incentives will likely entrench power, wealth, and race disparities, with donors suffering from socio-economic disadvantage servicing a more wealthy recipient population.[204]

Living organ donation raises particular ethical concerns and has been the subject of detailed examination in the relevant literature. These concerns may differ depending on whether the donation is directed to a relative or friend (most common) or non-directed donation with the donor unknown to the recipient. Clearly, there is a need to consider the respective interests of the donor and recipient. Within the principlist ethical framework, for example, this could involve respecting the autonomy of the individual donor

---

[196] This section draws in part on Anne-Maree Farrell et al. (n 27) ch 18.

[197] See e.g. Shawn Harmon, Chunshui Wang, and Jing Bai, 'Organ Transplantation in China and Beyond: Addressing the "Access Gap"' (2010) 11(1) Medical Law International 191; Thomas Petersen and Kasper Lippert-Rasmussen, 'Ethics, Organ Donation and Tax: A Proposal' (2012) 38(8) Journal of Medical Ethics 451; Nuffield Council on Bioethics, 'Human Bodies: Donation for Medicine and Research' (2011) paras 3.68–3.74.

[198] David Rodriguez-Arias et al., 'Success Factors and Ethical Challenges of the Spanish Model of Organ Donation' (2010) 376(9746) The Lancet 1109.

[199] Charles Erin and John Harris, 'An Ethical Market in Human Organs' (2003) 29(3) Journal of Medical Ethics 137.

[200] Ahad Ghods and Shekoufeh Savaj, 'The Iran Model of Paid and Regulated Living-Unrelated Kidney Donation' (2006) 1(6) Clinical Journal of the American Society of Nephrology 1136.

[201] Lloyd Cohen, 'Increasing the Supply of Transplant Organs: The Virtues of a Futures Market' (1989) 58(1) George Washington Law Review 1.

[202] See Richard Titmuss, *The Gift Relationship: From Human Blood to Social Policy* (George Allen & Unwin 1970). For an analysis of the importance of the gift relationship in human tissue donation in the UK, see Anne-Maree Farrell, 'Altruism, Markets and the Importance of the Social Contract in Healthcare: Richard Titmuss's The Gift Relationship' in Sara Fovargue and Craig Purshouse (eds.) *Leading Works in Health Law and Ethics* (Routledge 2023).

[203] Nuffield Council on Bioethics (n 197) para 22.

[204] Francis Delmonico et al., 'Ethical Incentives – Not Payment – For Organ Donation' (2002) 346(25) New England Journal of Medicine 2002.

to consent to such procedure on the one hand, but could also be said to infringe upon the 'do no harm' principle on the other hand, given it could be argued that there is no therapeutic benefit to them. A consequentialist perspective would instead support living organ donation. In the case of kidney donation, for example, it could be argued from this perspective that there would no need for ongoing dialysis in the event of a successful transplant outcome. This would outweigh the risks faced by living donors due to having to undergo the medical procedure to remove the kidney, as well as living with one kidney in the longer term. In contrast, those arguing from a deontological perspective would express concern about a living organ donor being used as a means to an end.[205] Added to this perspective would be broader concerns about fairness and justice, particularly in circumstances where there were concerns about donor exploitation or trafficking.

Those in favour of financial payments in living organ donation have focused on individual donor autonomy and the right to decide to donate in circumstances where no harm is caused to another, provided that obtaining informed consent is possible. It has been argued that many individuals are happy to become organ donors and it should therefore be a matter for them if they want to use the monies received from the donation to alleviate their difficult financial situation or to help their family, for example. In such circumstances, it is not clear that financial payments for organs are against the interests of donors.[206] Objections to payment for organs from living donors could also be said to be Western-centric and may not be objectionable in other cultures. At a broader level, it has been argued that there are significant benefits to using financial payments to encourage higher rates of living organ donation and transplantation, as it will result in significant cost savings for national health services in the long term.[207]

The main arguments put forward against the use of financial payments or incentives in organ donation identify key issues as being the need to avoid commodification of the body, and the problem of donor exploitation. Such exploitation is said to be exacerbated by the lack of any medical follow-up post-transplant and monitoring of donors' long-term health. The lack of donor protection has been raised as a matter of particular concern in the case of Iran, which is one of the few countries in the world which operates a compensated and regulated living unrelated donor renal transplant program.[208] In addition, it has been argued that providing direct financial payments to living organ donors would mean that governments would be less likely to provide proper funding and support to encourage deceased organ donation.[209] A summary overview of key arguments put forward in support of, as well as against, living organ donation for transplantation are set out in **Table 13.4**.

---

[205] See Chapters 1 and 2 for a more detailed overview of these ethical perspectives.

[206] See Julian Savulescu, 'Is the Sale of Body Parts Wrong?' (2003) 29(3) Journal of Medical Ethics 138.

[207] For an overview of the arguments highlighted in this paragraph see Janet Radcliffe Richards et al., 'The Case for Allowing Kidney Sales' (1998) 351(9120) The Lancet 1950; Erin and Harris (n 199); James Taylor, 'Autonomy and Organ Sales, Revisited' (2009) 34(6) Journal of Medicine and Philosophy 632.

[208] Ghods and Savaj (n 195) 1137; Dianne Tober, 'Kidneys and Controversies in the Islamic Republic of Iran: The Case of Organ Sale' (2007) 13(3) Body & Society 151, 165–166.

[209] See Samuel Kerstein, 'Kantian Condemnation of Commerce in Organs' (2009) 19(2) Kennedy Institute of Ethics Journal 147; Kate Greasley, 'A Legal Market in Organs: The Problem of Exploitation' (2014) 40(1) Journal of Medical Ethics 51; Julian Koplin, 'Assessing the Likely Harms to Kidney Vendors in Regulated Organ Markets' (2014) 14(10) American Journal of Bioethics 7.

Table 13.4 Arguments Surrounding the Role of Trade and Commerce in Living Organ Donation

Arguments in favour	Arguments against
• Question of the vendor's individual rights where no harm caused to another. • Living organ donation is more expensive and intensive in the short term but a cheaper, more effective option in the long term. • The continuing gap between supply and demand for organs causes ongoing pain and death to those awaiting transplant. • Many vendors wish to sell as options restricted due to poverty: if vendor wants to use money to alleviate poverty, help family, etc., why should such a worthy cause not be permitted? • Informed consent of vendor is possible. • To prohibit commercialism, there is a need to show that payment for organs is always against the interests of vendors. • Objections to payment for organs is a Western concept. • There is growing public support for payment for human organs.	• Human organs should not be treated as a commodity to be bought and sold in marketplace. • There is potential for vendor exploitation, particularly of those in poverty. • Vendors from resource-poor settings receive little, if any, health checks/follow-up in the medium to long term. • Consent of vendors is not genuine because of the financial incentive. • Exploitation by rich against poor is not just or fair. • It must be an altruistic donation to be acceptable on socio-cultural level. • If payment is allowed, there will be a consequent reduction in altruism. • Allowing payment will lead to a 'slippery slope' and a rise in deceptive, fraudulent, criminal practices. • Establishing a market in organs would reduce incentives for governments to provide proper funding and resources for deceased organ donation or to provide for dialysis for (end-stage) renal patients.

13.6 XENOTRANSPLANTATION

Xenotransplantation refers to 'any procedure that involves the transplantation, implantation, or infusion into a human recipient of either live tissues or organs retrieved from animals, or human body fluids, cells, tissues, or organs that have undergone ex vivo contact with live non-human animal cells, tissues, or organisms.'[210] Although offering much promise, it is not yet a practical solution to the shortage of organs available for transplantation. Nevertheless, scientific research continues to increase the viability of xenotransplantation with better immunosuppression options, in addition to the use of the CRISPR-Cas9 gene editing technique to remove viruses from DNA, thus lessening the risk of transmission of disease between the animal organ and the human recipient.[211] In 2015, for example, a pig's kidney that had been edited to get rid of the antigen that would cause a human to reject a pig's heart, was transplanted into a baboon, which lived for 136 days.[212]

---

[210] UK Department of Health, 'Xenotransplantation Guidance' (12 December 2006) para 1.
[211] See David KC Cooper, et al., 'Xenotransplantation—The Current Status and Prospects' (2018) 25(1) British Medical Bulletin 5; Richard Pierson et al., 'Progress Toward Cardiac Xenotransplantation' (2020) 142 Circulation 1389.
[212] Kelly Servick, 'Xenotransplant Advances May Prompt Clinical Trials' (2017) 357(6358) Science 1338.

In 2021, a genetically modified pig's kidney was successfully transplanted into a recipient who was brain-dead. Permission had been granted by the patient's family for the experimental procedure to go ahead and it had been sanctioned by the US regulator, the Food and Drug Administration (FDA). The procedure was designed to ascertain whether the organ would be accepted or rejected in a human being as part of ongoing research in the area.[213] In January 2022, the first animal-to-human heart transplant took place in the US, with the heart coming from a pig which had been genetically engineered to reduce the risk of passing on infectious disease to the recipient.[214] The patient had given their consent to the experimental procedure as they had been refused a human organ transplant and there were few, if any, other treatment options available.

By way of background, xenotransplantation research initially came to prominence in the 1990s in the UK, which prompted government authorities to establish the Xenotransplantation Interim Regulatory Authority (UKXIRA). The Authority was charged with overseeing the development of xenotransplantation and its coordination, pending the introduction of legislation. One of the first actions of the UKXIRA was to declare a moratorium on human clinical trials of xenografting until further research was conducted. By the mid-2000s, such research had tapered off and UKXIRA was subsequently disbanded in 2006. The decision to do so was criticised at the time on the grounds that a centralised agency such as the Authority would have been best placed to deal with the ongoing contested scientific, ethical, and regulatory issues at stake in xenotransplantation research.[215] Oversight of such research was thereafter diverted to NHS research ethics committees, with the conduct of any clinical trials to be overseen by the Medicines and Healthcare Products Regulatory Agency (MHRA).[216]

In terms of considering the advantages and disadvantages of xenotransplantation involving animal-to-human organ transplants, there are several ethical issues to consider.[217] It has long been recognised that a number of scientific obstacles need to be overcome in terms of managing risk to the human recipient arising from xenotransplantation: first, there is a need to minimise the risk of transmission of disease from the donor animal to humans; second, there is a need to prevent rejection of the animal organ in humans; and third, being able to demonstrate evidence that the animal organ functions effectively in humans is vital. The availability of gene editing has clearly shifted the risk calculus in more recent times, with more of a focus on the animal donor, with the technique being employed to remove genes in animal donor to minimise the risk of infection in the human recipient.[218]

---

[213] Michelle Roberts, 'US Surgeons Test Pig Kidney Transplant in a Human' (BBC News, 21 October 2021) available at <https://www.bbc.com/news/health-58993696> accessed 29 December 2022.

[214] BBC News, 'Man Gets Genetically-Modified Pig Heart in World-First Transplant' (11 January 2022) available at <https://www.bbc.co.uk/news/world-us-canada-59944889> accessed 29 December 2022. Note that the patient subsequently passed away in March 2022. See BBC News, 'Man Given Genetically Modified Pig Heart Dies' (9 March 2022) available at <https://www.bbc.com/news/health-60681493> accessed 29 December 2022.

[215] See Lorna Williamson, Marie Fox, and Sheila McLean, 'The Regulation of Xenotransplantation after UKXIRA: Legal and Ethical Issues' (2007) 34(4) Journal of Learning Sciences 441.

[216] See UK Department of Health, 'Xenotransplantation Guidance' (12 December 2006) para 3.

[217] See e.g. John Loike and Alan Kadish, 'Ethical Rejections of Xenotransplantation? The Potential and Challenges of Using Human-Pig Chimeras to Create Organs for Transplantation' (2018) 19(8) EMBO Reports e46337.

[218] Emma Nance, 'Could Genetically Modified Animal Organs Solve the Human Transplant Crisis?' (24 May 2022) available at <https://eusci.org.uk/2022/05/24/could-genetically-modified-animal-organs-solve-the-human-transplant-crisis/> accessed 29 December 2022.

In addition, understanding the risk posed to the human recipient from xenotrans-plantation requires that we reflect upon whether they can consent to what is a highly experimental procedure involving much uncertainty with regards to outcome.[219] Given its experimental nature, it could be argued that the recipient is consenting to not just the xenotransplant procedure itself, but also to continuing surveillance post-transplant surgery. In the circumstances, it would be better to characterise what is being asked of the recipient as involving 'contracts to undergo treatment', rather than simply a one-off consent to do so.[220] While not applicable to all individual recipients, a further concern may arise about using pigs for the purposes of xenotransplantation, due to existing religious beliefs. This may be a problematic issue for those of the Jewish and Muslim faiths, given how the animal is viewed within these religions. This may be so, notwithstanding the fact that the use of such animal material may be considered permissible on religious grounds, especially where it involves a life-saving medical procedure.[221]

Taking account of the risks posed by xenotransplantation also means taking account of the potential for the transmission of animal micro-organisms, including viruses, to humans and the fact that such organisms could adapt and contribute to human-to-human spread. This risk remains very real and constitutes the main reason why xenotransplan-tation continues to be viewed with a good deal of concern.[222] This is not least because of recent experience involving the Covid-19 pandemic, which was caused by SARS-CoV-2, a zoonotic virus which spreads between animals and humans.[223] Given the potential broader risk to public health, the question needs to asked as to whether the public is entitled to dissent from a programme of xenotransplantation research (including clinical trials) which is likely to pose a potential threat to collective well-being, and which is likely to have impact at both national and global levels.[224]

In considering the ethics of xenotransplantation, we also need to consider the impor-tant issue of animal welfare. In conducting such research, we should reflect on whether animals should be bred for this purpose;[225] whether they are likely to suffer more than minimal harm; and how we should balance human advantage over animal disadvantage

[219] Sara Fovargue, '"Oh Pick Me, Pick Me"—Selecting Participants for Xenotransplant Clinical Trials' (2007) 15(2) Medical Law Review 176.
[220] Tim Caulfield and Graeme Robertson, 'Xenotransplantation: Consent, Public Health and Charter Issues' (2001) 5(2) Medical Law International 81; Sara Fovargue, 'Consenting to Bio-risk: Xenotransplantation and the Law' (2005) 25(3) Legal Studies 404; Jonathan Hughes, 'Justice and Third-Party Risks: The Ethics of Xenotransplantation' (2007) 24(2) Journal of Applied Philosophy 151.
[221] Jack Hunter, 'Three Ethical Issues Around Pig Heart Transplants' (BBC News, 11 January 2022) avail-able at <https://www.bbc.co.uk/news/world-59951264> accessed 29 December 2022.
[222] See Nuffield Council on Bioethics, 'Animal-to-Human Transplants: The Ethics of Xenotransplantation' (Nuffield Council on Bioethics, 1996), ch 6; Fritz Bach, Adrian Ivinson, and Christopher Weeramantry, 'Ethical and Legal Issues in Technology: Xenotransplantation' (2001) 27(2–3) American Journal of Law & Medicine 283; Sara Fovargue and Suzanne Ost, 'When Should Precaution Prevail? Interests in (Public) Health, the Risk of Harm and Xenotransplantation' (2010) 18(3) Medical Law Review 302.
[223] Edward Holmes, 'Covid-19 – Lessons for Zoonotic Disease' (2022) 375(6585) Science 1114.
[224] For differing positions on this debate, see Margaret Clark, 'This Little Piggy Went to Market: The Xenotransplantation and Xenozoonose Debate' (1999) 27(2) Journal of Law and Medical Ethics 137 and Harold Vanderpool, 'Commentary: A Critique of Clark's Frightening Xenotransplantation Scenario' (1999) 27(2) Journal of Law & Medical Ethics 153. On broader ethical questions involving the risk/benefit calculus arising from xenotransplantation in terms of the divide between the poor and the rich, see Robert Sparrow, 'Xenotransplantation, Consent and International Justice' (2009) 9(3) Developing World Bioethics 119.
[225] See Marie Fox and Jean McHale, 'Xenotransplantation: The Ethical and Legal Ramifications' (1998) 6(1) Medical Law Review 42.

in such circumstances.[226] For animal rights advocates, the risk of harm and suffering to animals, particularly in light of the use of gene editing techniques, makes xenotransplantation ethically unacceptable, in addition to being a poor use of resources.[227] Even if we agree that it is acceptable to use animals in this way, one must ask, 'What sort of animals?' Tissue rejection would be minimised if non-human primates were used, but it is widely accepted that primates have special characteristics which exclude them as organ donors.[228] Typically, baboons are used for solid organ xenotransplantation research, as their larger size makes it easier to transplant pig organs. However, xenotransplantation research tends to make use of pigs as organ donors, due to the ease with which they are bred and can be subject to gene editing in which graft rejection has been minimised. Although there has been little progress in xenotransplantation research for over 15 years,[229] the recent pig-to-human heart transplant in the US has led to renewed calls to re-start such research and clinical trials in the UK.[230] What this means is that genetically modified pig organs are likely to be used in the conduct of clinical trials that may take place in the future.[231]

13.7 CONCLUSION

This chapter examined key legal and ethical issues arising in deceased and living organ donation for transplantation. An initial overview was provided of key legislation and organisations with respect to organ donation for transplantation in the UK. Having provided this background, we identified what constitutes a diagnosis of death, including what criteria must be fulfilled before consideration can be given to the question of organ donation. We then examined key aspects of law and regulation in relation to deceased organ donation, with analysis provided of recent law reform to establish deemed consent/authorisation systems in the UK's four jurisdictions. An overview of key aspects of living organ donation for transplantation was also provided, which included an examination of the similarities and differences on this issue as between the two Human Tissue Acts in

---

[226] That such a balance exists was accepted by UK Department of Health, 'Animal Tissue into Humans: A Report by the Advisory Group on the Ethics of Xenotransplantation' (The Stationery Office, 1996) and the Nuffield Council on Bioethics (n 222).

[227] Following the first animal to human heart transplant in January 2022 (see Roberts (n 208)), a range of ethical concerns have been highlighted by animal rights advocates. See People for the Ethical Treatment of Animals (PETA), 'First Heart Transplant from Genetically Altered Pig: PETA Statement' (10 January 2022) available at <https://www.peta.org/media/news-releases/first-heart-transplant-from-genetically-altered-pig-peta-statement/> accessed 29 December 2022; FRAME, 'Xenotransplantation: Why Animals Do Not Provide the Best Ethical or Scientific Solution to Organ Donation' (1 April 2022) available at <https://frame.org.uk/latest/history-ethics-xenotransplants/> accessed 29 December 2022.

[228] Note that the UK Department of Health Advisory Group (n 226) did state that primates could, in strictly circumscribed conditions, be used for research into xenotransplantation. They would, of course, be protected by the Animals (Scientific Procedures) Act 1986. For a current overview, see UK Research and Innovation, 'Regulation and Policy, UK Legislation, The Animals (Scientific Procedures) Act 1986' (2022) available at <https://www.ukri.org/about-us/mrc/our-policies-and-standards/research/research-involving-animals/regulation-and-policy/> accessed 29 December 2022.

[229] See UK Department of Health, 'Xenotransplantation Guidance' (n 216).

[230] Joe Pinkstone, 'Doctors Urge NHS to Restart Animal Organ Transplants on Humans' (The Telegraph, 22 January 2022) available at <https://www.telegraph.co.uk/news/2022/01/22/doctors-urge-nhs-restart-animal-organ-transplants-humans/> accessed 29 December 2022.

[231] Douglas Anderson and Allan Kirk, 'Primate Models in Organ Transplantation' (2013) 3(9) Cold Spring Harbour Perspectives in Medicine a015503.

the UK. We then turned to explore the legal and ethical parameters of the prohibition on trade and commerce in organ donation, before concluding with a brief examination of the scientific, legal, and ethical issues arising in xenotransplantation. In recent decades, scientific and technological advances in the field have not only expanded access but also the range of treatment options, to those in need of an organ transplant. In light of such advances, this chapter highlights the importance of offering a principled way forward in managing contested legal and ethical issues in the field, particularly in the context of persisting organ shortage.

FURTHER READING

1. Jessie Cooper, 'Organs and Organisations: Situating Ethics in Organ Donation After Circulatory Death in the UK' (2018) 209 Social Science & Medicine 104.

2. Anne-Maree Farrell, David Price, and Muireann Quigley (eds.) *Organ Shortage: Ethics Law and Pragmatism* (CUP 2011).

3. Mélanie Levy, 'State Incentives to Promote Organ Donation: Honoring the Principles of Reciprocity and Solidarity Inherent in the Gift Relationship' (2018) 5(20) Journal of Law and the Biosciences 398.

4. Amy Lewis, et al., 'Organ Donation in the US and Europe: The Supply vs Demand Imbalance (2021) 35(2) Transplantation Reviews 100585.

5. Stephen Wilkinson, 'The Sale of Human Organs' in Edward Zalta (ed.), *The Stanford Encyclopedia of Philosophy* (Winter 2016 Edition) available at <https://plato.stanford.edu/archives/win2016/entries/organs-sale/> accessed 29 December 2022.

14

THE BODY AS PROPERTY

14.1 INTRODUCTION

As a result of advances in scientific research and biotechnology, there is increasing demand for human material for research, therapeutic, and commercial purposes. The changing dynamics of supply and demand have contributed to ongoing academic and policy debates about broader issues around value, (self-)ownership, and control over our bodies, and bodily material that has been separated from the body. The centrality in health and medical law of the principle of autonomy offers the individual patient the ultimate right to control their body and what is done with (or to) it. That control is most often exercised through the concept of consent or refusal of consent to treatment. As we have seen in Chapter 12, failure to respect a refusal of surgery can result in actions in negligence or assault; equally in Chapter 16, we see that the use and storage of gametes is strictly controlled according to the written consent of the donor. Having said that, we do not have an absolute right, either ethically or legally, to do whatever we want with our bodies. For example, under the Human Tissue Act 2004 (HTA 2004), 'trafficking' in human material is prohibited,[1] and UK appellate courts have been categorical in stating that ritual physical abuse of the body for sexual pleasure remains criminal, even when undertaken with the full and informed consent of the parties.[2] The question, therefore, arises as to what limits are set on the right to control our bodies and what we are able to do with our separated material. In recent years, this debate has centred on the status of the body as property, key aspects of which are examined in this chapter.

The chapter proceeds with first identifying key terms relevant to understanding the parameters of the debate, before moving on to examine key concepts such as ownership, control, and commodification; various property models in human tissue; and a comparative overview of jurisprudence involving trade and property in human tissue. Thereafter, an examination is provided of key UK case law which engages with the property approach in human tissue, covering reproductive material, the embryo, and the dead body, by way of example. The final section briefly examines intellectual property in human tissue.

14.2 KEY TERMS

In examining this topic, we first note that UK property law can be a difficult and complex area of study, with jurisdictional differences as between the UK nations. For present purposes, we therefore have adopted a narrow focus on identifying key aspects that are relevant to understanding how the common law and legislation addresses the

---

[1] Human Tissue Act 2004, s 32. The Human Tissue (Scotland) Act 2006, s 20 prohibits commercial dealing in 'any part of the human body. . .'.

[2] R v Brown [1994] 1 AC 212.

ownership and control of human material. Before we examine the topic in more detail, it is worth noting some key terms that are relevant to examining the property approach to the human body and its parts/tissue.[3] The focus in this chapter is predominantly on English case law and legislation. With this in mind, **Table 14.1** outlines the terms as they are understood in property law in England and Wales. We note the jurisdictional differences with Scots property law, and reference is made to select Scottish case law, by way of example.

Table 14.1 Key Property Law Terms Surrounding Ownership/Control of Human Material

Personal property	Items which are subject to the control of a person (in contrast, real property covers land and anything attached to the land under common law annexation rules). Intellectual property deals with the right to reproduce an idea, invention or process that comes from the mind or intellect of the person who produced it.
Possession	An intent to control an item, plus physical control,[4] whereas ownership should be viewed as a bundle of rights, rather than just a single right.[5]
Bailment	Recognises that an owner can divest themselves of possession of goods, but still retain ownership of them. Where this occurs, the owner is the bailor and the person who currently possesses the goods is the bailee.
Alienability	Property rights can be alienable in the sense that they can be transferred to others. For example, if a hospital had property rights in human tissue samples, it could transfer them to a pharmaceutical company for a fee. That company would then have the right to use the samples to manufacture a product and would be entitled to any income that was generated by such activity.[6]
Abandonment	Under the common law, a person who owns personal property can relinquish all rights to its control and a person who finds abandoned property may claim it. Where the principle applies, it extinguishes any property interest that would otherwise operate. Examples of human tissue that could be said to have been abandoned include cut hair, amputated limbs and tissue excised during surgery. Where scientific researchers use such tissue to later develop a new diagnostic test or cell line, for example, they could argue that they now have a proprietary interest in such tissue, given it has been abandoned by the source.[7]

[3] The section on key terms is taken from Anne-Maree Farrell, 'Property and Human Tissue' in Anne-Maree Farrell et al., *Health Law: Frameworks and Context* (CUP 2017) 246–247.

[4] See generally *Powell* v *McFarlane* (1979) 38 P & CR 452.

[5] See Anthony Honoré, 'Ownership' in *Making Law Bind: Essays Legal and Philosophical* (Clarendon Press 1987), originally published in Anthony Guest (ed.), *Oxford Essays in Jurisprudence* (OUP 1961).

[6] ibid.

[7] For a critique on the notion of abandonment in relation to excised human material, see Imogen Goold, 'Abandonment and Human Tissue' in Imogen Goold et al., (eds.), *Persons Parts and Property: How Should We Regulate Tissue in the 21st Century* (Hart 2014) 125–155.

Causes of action	Where property rights have been infringed, three causes of action may arise under the law of torts: trespass, conversion and detinue. Trespass to goods protects against any unauthorised interference with the possession of goods, provided that the person had actual possession at the time of the interference.[8] Conversion involves a serious interference with a person's goods or assuming the rights of an owner of goods, provided there is a right to immediate possession on the part of the person alleging such interference.[9] A person may sue in detinue where there has been wrongful detention of goods.[10]

14.3 KEY CONCEPTS

Intuitively, a person might naturally speak of 'my body', and consider that because it is 'their' body, they can determine what is done to it or its parts. For most individuals, this is bound up with the proprietary notion that, because their body is their own, they 'own' their body. Historically, it was considered that there could be no property interest in the human body, whether living or dead.[11] There were a number of historical factors that led to the development of this principle. Christian religious traditions involving the human body were important, and common law courts considered that jurisdiction over a dead body was a matter for the religious courts.[12] In addition, the activities of 'body snatchers' who secretly removed corpses from burial sites to supply the burgeoning demand for bodies for anatomical examination also played an influential role.[13] In relation to the living body, no person can own another person and there can be no buying or selling of another, as otherwise that would constitute slavery, which is illegal.[14] Over time, this legal prohibition has also been extended to cover separated human body parts and tissue, although the justification for this extension has been the subject of debate.[15] Nevertheless, the position in common law jurisdictions is that there is no property in a whole human body, nor in separated parts or tissue, in favour of an individual who is the source.[16]

In ethical terms, no single principle or imperative exists on which one can ground a property right in oneself,[17] and, it would therefore be wrong to conclude that because

[8] See *Bailiffs of Dunwich v Sterry* (1831) 1 B and ad 831; *Tharpe v Stallwood* (1843) 5 Man and G 760; *Barker v Furlong* (1891) 2 Ch 172.
[9] See *Penfolds Wines v Elliott* (1946) 74 CLR 204; *Healing Sales Pty Ltd v Inglis Electrix* (1968) 121 CLR 584.
[10] See *Lloyd v Osborne* (1899) 20 LR (NSW) 190.
[11] Shawn Harmon and Graeme Laurie, '*Yearworth v North Bristol NHS Trust*: Property, Principles, Precedents and Paradigms' (2010) 69(3) Cambridge Law Journal 476, 480.
[12] *Hayne's case* (1614) 12 Co Rep 113; *Exelby v Handyside* (1749) 2 East PC 652.
[13] Harmon and Laurie (n 11) 480–481.
[14] See for example Art 4, ECHR, which prohibits slavery, servitude and forced labour. This Article has been incorporated into UK domestic law via the Human Rights Act 1998, Sch 1. For an overview of more recent anti-slavery legislation, see UK Government, Modern Slavery Act 2015 available at <https://www.gov.uk/government/collections/modern-slavery-bill> accessed 13 January 2023.
[15] See Chapter 13 for a detailed examination of this legislative prohibition. For an overview of academic debates on the issue, see Muireann Quigley, 'Property in Human Biomaterials – Separating Persons and Things?' (2012) 32(4) Oxford Journal of Legal Studies 659.
[16] See generally Farrell (n 3) 246–247.
[17] However, for argument to this effect, see Derek Beyleveld and Roger Brownsword, *Human Dignity in Bioethics and Biolaw* (OUP 2001) ch 8; Rohan Hardcastle, *Law and the Human Body: Property Rights, Ownership and Control* (Hart 2007).

no one can own my body, I necessarily own it myself.[18] This is in part because the very idea of property is a legal one; a construct which allows us to order our society according to a worldview which facilitates the achievement of certain social goals, such as the encouragement of commerce and the sanctioning of commodification.[19] The role of ethics lies not in grounding a property right, but in determining whether it is appropriate to commodify the human body, which has a particular moral status deserving of respect. For many, a commodity approach would lead to buying and selling body parts, and this is viewed as repugnant in that it shows a fundamental disrespect for the status of the human body.[20]

Trade in human bodies, material, and related products gives rise to the spectre of donor exploitation, which it has been argued is ethically questionable because it has the potential to harm. On this basis, the Medical Research Council (MRC) has stated that:

> The human body and its parts shall not, as such, give rise to direct financial gain. Researchers may not sell for profit samples of human biological material they have collected as part of MRC funded research, and research participants should never be offered any financial inducement to donate samples. Payment of reasonable expenses or costs is, however, acceptable.[21]

It is widely assumed that the interposition of commercial interests between the source of valuable material and its user is unacceptable because it leads necessarily to exploitation.[22] Therefore, our main concern about allowing both property and greater freedom in trade in human material might be that it could lead to (greater) exploitation of (weaker) individuals. This is undoubtedly true, but the same might be said of those who donate materials for research or transplantation—emotional coercion can be as great or greater than economic coercion; exploitation and commerce do not necessarily go hand-in-hand. Undue coercion should always be guarded against irrespective of the context or motivation. Similarly, as we discuss in the context of surrogacy (Chapter 16), it is not necessarily exploitative to offer financial incentives or rewards to individuals to use their bodies in certain ways. Indeed, it has been argued that it may be more devaluing to persons *not* to recognise their worth (in monetary terms) for the contributions they can make to society from the use of their bodies, than it is to protect them from potential predators. This is provided that the value that they represent is not entirely reducible to those terms.[23] In short, because something is potentially exploitative does not mean that it must always be so.

---

[18] James Harris, 'Who Owns My Body?' (1996) 16 Oxford Journal of Legal Studies 5, 71.

[19] For a classic account, see Honoré (n 5). For a more recent examination of such issues, see Muireann Quigley, 'Property and the Body: Applying Honoré' (2007) 33(11) Journal of Medical Ethics 631; Jesse Wall, 'The Legal Status of Body Parts: A Framework' (2011) 31(4) Oxford Journal of Legal Studies 783.

[20] See Loane Skene, 'Arguments Against People Legally "Owning" Their Own Bodies, Body Parts and Tissue' (2002) 2 MacQuarie Law Journal 165; Stephen Munzer, 'An Uneasy Case Against Property Rights in Body Parts' (1994) 11(2) Social Philosophy and Policy 259. A good account of the relevant arguments is provided by the Nuffield Council on Bioethics, *Human Bodies: Donation for Medicine and Research* (Nuffield Council on Bioethics 2011), which also includes examples of current commercialisation practices with respect to human material.

[21] UK Research and Innovation, 'Human Tissue and Biological Samples for Use in Research: Operational and Ethical Guidelines' (2019) 6; see also Art 21, Council of Europe, Convention for the Protection of Human Rights and Dignity of the Human Being with regard to the Application of Biology and Medicine: Convention on Human Rights and Biomedicine, Oviedo, 4.IV.1997 (Convention on Human Rights and Biomedicine).

[22] For discussion see Peter Halewood, 'On Commodification and Self-Ownership' (2008) 20(13) Yale Journal of Law and Humanities 131.

[23] Lori Andrews, 'Beyond Doctrinal Boundaries: A Legal Framework for Surrogate Motherhood' (1995) 81(8) Virginia Law Review 2343.

The counterargument that can be made regarding concerns about exploitation is that while no one would sanction forced participation in the trade of human material, it is unduly paternalistic to disregard the consent of individuals who would willingly sell their bodily tissues.[24] In the HTA 2004, for example, it is concerned not just with 'organs', but with 'controlled material', which is defined as 'any material which (a), consists of or includes human cells, (b) is, or is intended to be removed, from the human body, excepting (a) gametes, (b) embryos, or (c) material which is the subject of a property right because of the application of human skill'.[25] This definition is considerably wider—and extends the application of the no-trade rule—although, ironically, it simultaneously recognises not only that property rights *can* accrue in human material but also that these can endure. The HTA 2004 was the first piece of legislation to expressly recognise the potential existence of property rights in human material, although it does so merely by repeating the pre-existing common law position.[26] The HFEA 1990, as amended, relies on the expressed written wishes of donors in controlling the use and storage of gametes, which falls short of acknowledging a property right.[27] In short, the distinction between persons and things remain strong.[28]

The issue at the heart of this debate, of course, is that of control. Property, through the bundle of rights that it confers, is a powerful control device which also carries a particular message offering the potential for commerce and trade. To recognise a 'quasi-property' claim is to support a normatively strong connection to that item and, accordingly, to establish a strong, justiciable legal interest. 'Full' property rights will only be recognised where there is little or no prospect of exploitation or other harm, which can include the 'harm' of disrespect for the dignity of the human organism. In sum, there is a widespread ambivalence about property in the body and its parts and products.[29]

In fact, many legal instruments draw a distinction between property in the body and its parts *as such* and 'inventions' using human material, which may be subject to intellectual property rights.[30] Similarly, although the HTA 2004 imposes a prohibition on commercial dealings in human material for transplantation,[31] it recognises property in materials in some circumstances. Accordingly, the Act excepts from this prohibition 'material which is the subject of property because of an application of human skill'.[32] Indeed, the Act gives enables the Human Tissue Authority (HTA) to authorise financial returns beyond mere expenses for the handling of, or trade in, human tissue.

[24] Julian Savulescu, 'Is the Sale of Body Parts Wrong?' (2003) 29(3) Journal of Medical Ethics 138; Shawn Harmon, 'A Penny For Your Thoughts, A Pound For Your Flesh: Implications of Recognizing Property in Human Body Parts' (2006) 7 Medical Law International 329. For an argument that failure to recognise property can lead to exploitation, see Radhika Rao, 'Genes and Spleens: Property, Contract or Privacy Rights in the Human Body?' (2007) 35(3) Journal of Law, Medicine and Ethics 371.

[25] Human Tissue Act 2004, s 32(8) and (9). The Human Organ Transplants Act 1989, s 7(2) defined 'organ' as 'any part of the human body consisting of a structured arrangement of tissues which, if wholly removed, cannot be replicated by the body'.

[26] Human Tissue Act 2004, s 32(9).

[27] Jessica Berg, 'Owning Persons: The Application of Property Theory to Embryos and Fetuses' (2005) 40 Wake Forest Law Review 159.

[28] For a philosophical challenge to this position, see Muireann Quigley, *Self-Ownership, Property Rights and the Human Body: A Legal and Philosophical Analysis* (CUP 2018).

[29] For a more detailed examination of current debates, see e.g. Remigius Nwabueze, *Biotechnology and the Challenge of Property: Property Rights in Dead Bodies, Body Parts, and Genetic Information* (Routledge 2016) and Donna Dickenson, *Property in the Body: A Feminist Analysis* (CUP 2017).

[30] See Christian Lenk et al. (eds.), *Human Tissue Research: A European Perspective on the Ethical and Legal Challenges* (OUP 2011).

[31] Human Tissue Act 2004, s 32.   [32] Human Tissue Act 2004, s 32(9)(c).

For example, s 32(6) of the Act allows licence terms for the transporting, removing, preparing, preserving, and storing of controlled material to include payments on a commercial basis. The reality is that the trading of bodily materials, products, or by-products inside and outside the National Health Service (NHS) is an essential part of the Service.[33] Mixed messages abound, however, about the role of property and commercialisation in relation to these endeavours.

There is also the all-important principle of respect for autonomy and freedom of choice. Undue regulatory interference cannot be justified. In the case of commercial cord blood banks for autologous use, for example, it has been argued that while the therapeutic options for the use of such human material remains limited, a strict ban on such banks would represent an undue restriction on the freedom of enterprise and the freedom of choice of individuals or couples who wish to make use of their services.[34] As to the entitlement of donors of cord blood to make any claims with regards to the patenting of such material, it was suggested that apart from justified compensation, they should not receive any type of reward that would contravene the prohibition on commodification of the human body.[35]

What is important to remember as this debate rumbles on is that there is arguably nothing inherently valuable in an appeal to property itself, save when such an appeal can furnish rights or solutions to disputes which escape other legal concepts. Other devices, such as consent or contract, can be used instead of property to establish rights and resolve conflicts. Indeed, Sperling has concluded that:

> Whatever the case may be, proprietary interest does not provide any necessary procedural advantage to claimants in the post-mortem context, and cases that deal with interference with dead bodies can be perfectly well decided and remedied without the fictional and unnecessary appeal to the right to property in the body of the deceased.[36]

Whether this is also true of property claims from living individuals remains to be seen.[37] It is with this in mind that we now turn to critically examine the range of legal solutions that are, and have been, employed in the medico-legal sphere.

14.4 MODELS OF PROPERTY IN HUMAN TISSUE

It is important to note that some jurisdictions do grant direct recognition of property rights in human material.[38] For example, the German *Bundesgerichtshof* has ruled that excised body parts that are not intended for another (such as transplant organs), and are not for return to the individual (such as stored sperm), are subject to the normal rules of personal

---

[33] See Nuffield Council on Bioethics (n 20).

[34] European Group on Ethics in Science and New Technologies (EGE), Opinion No 19: Opinion on the Ethical Aspects of Umbilical Cord Blood Banking (2004), available at <https://ec.europa.eu/archives/bepa/european-group-ethics/publications/opinions/index_en.htm> accessed 13 January 2023, paras 2.01–2.02.

[35] ibid. 5.

[36] Daniel Sperling, *Posthumous Interests: Legal and Ethical Perspectives* (CUP 2008) 142; see also Harmon and Laurie (n 11).

[37] For an argument that appeals to dignity can do the necessary work (and far better) see Charles Foster, 'Dignity and the Use of Body Parts' (2014) 40 Journal of Medical Ethics 44–47. For further contributions to the debate, see Niels Hoppe, *Bioequity: Property and the Human Body* (Routledge 2016); Roger Brownsword, 'Biobank Governance: Property, Privacy and Consent' in Christian Lenke and Nils Hoppe (eds.), *Ethics and Law of Intellectual Property* (Routledge 2016).

[38] For a comparative and philosophical account see Sperling, (n 36).

property.[39] Often, however, the courts appeal to property rights as a means to other legal ends. For example, in the Australian case of *Roche* v *Douglas*,[40] it was held that human tissue taken from a deceased person was 'property' for the purposes of the court rules; this allowed the court to claim dominion over the sample and authorise testing to settle a paternity dispute. Similarly, in *Bazley* v *Wesley Monash IVF Pty Ltd*,[41] and *Re Edwards*,[42] the Australian courts held that the women applicants were entitled to a right to possession of the sperm of their deceased husbands by virtue of the 'work done' on extracting and storing the semen and turning it into property, thereby differentiating it from the dead body per se.[43]

In the United States, older case law set the precedent for these kind of succession cases. For example, in *Hecht* v *Superior Court (Kane)*,[44] the Court of Appeal of California's Second District held that a deceased man who had previously deposited sperm for the use of his partner had an interest 'in the nature of ownership' of the samples such as to render them 'property' within the meaning of the Probate Code, and, accordingly, disposable property on his death.[45] In *Davis* v *Davis*,[46] the Tennessee Supreme Court held that the embryo occupied an 'interim category' as neither 'person' nor 'property', yet which entitled it to a special respect. Although the parties were denied 'a true property interest', they retained an interest—'in the nature of ownership'—in relation to the use and disposal of their pre-embryos.[47]

In Canada, this position was echoed and extended by the Supreme Court of British Columbia in the case of *JCM* v *ANA*.[48] The facts of this case involved a dispute over the disposal of sperm 'straws' obtained from a sperm bank in the United States. On dissolution of the litigants' marriage, the question arose as to what should happen to the sperm, with one party wishing to obtain and use it, the other seeking that it be destroyed. Drawing heavily from English precedent, the Court held that the law must keep pace with medical science and that, as a matter of fact and practice, the sperm had long since been treated as an artefact of property. As such, it belonged to both parties equally with the pragmatic solution being that each should receive half to dispose of as they saw fit, or a 7/6 split of the straws in favour of the woman if there were practical difficulties. It is worth noting that the use of the sperm did not create a genetic relationship of paternity since these were anonymised donor samples. Note that this ruling stood despite a prohibition in the Canadian Assisted Human Reproduction Act, which reads: 'No person shall purchase, offer to purchase or advertise for the purchase of sperm or ova from a donor or a person acting on behalf of a donor.'[49]

---

[39] Bundesgerichtshof, 9 November 1993, BGHZ, 124, 52. See also Christian Lenk and Katharina Beier, 'Is the Commercialisation of Human Tissue and Body Material Forbidden in the Countries of the European Union?' (2012) 38(6) Journal of Medical Ethics 342.

[40] [2000] WAR 331 (SC).   [41] [2010] QSC 118.   [42] [2011] NSWSC 478.

[43] Loane Skene, 'Proprietary Interests in Human Bodily Material: *Yearworth*, Recent Australian Cases on Stored Semen and Their Implications' (2012) 20(2) Medical Law Review 227.

[44] 16 Cal App 4th 836 (1993).

[45] On the issues from an ethical perspective, see Leslie Cannold, 'Who Owns a Dead Man's Sperm?' (2004) 30(4) Journal of Medical Ethics 386.

[46] 842 SW 2d 588 (1992).

[47] See also *In the Matter of X* [2002] JRC 202, where the Jersey Royal Court relied on the 'interest in the nature of ownership' on the part of a minor in respect of her aborted foetus as the reason to respect her refusal to release fetal tissue to the police which was sought in the pursuit of a prosecution for under-age intercourse against the minor's sexual partner. In the final analysis the Jersey Court of Appeal overrode the refusal in the interests of justice: [2003] JCA 050.

[48] [2012] BCSC 584.

[49] Section 7(1). The court's reasoning on this point is thin and seems to amount to no more than a reiteration of the point that the sperm had de facto been serially treated as property on the facts of the case: *JCM*, ibid., para 70.

Statutory attempts or proposals to embody property rights in human material have been equally equivocal. In the state of Oregon in the United States, a property right in genetic samples was granted to citizens in 1995. However, after several years of intensive lobbying by the pharmaceutical industry and research institutes, this right was removed by legislation and replaced with more stringent privacy protection.[50] Although the claim was made that Oregon would now have the most far-reaching privacy legislation of its kind in the United States, it is doubtful if the Oregon experiment was given sufficient time for the promise and the pitfalls of a property paradigm to be addressed and explored. Similar antipathy to property rights in human material was also to be found in Australia. In the late 1990s, a legislative bill addressing matters of genetic privacy came before the Commonwealth (federal) Parliament which proposed that authorisation should be obtained from individuals either to waive or to receive economic benefits deriving from their human tissue samples.[51] Although the bill was subsequently defeated, it led to a consultation by the Australian Law Reform Commission (ALRC) regarding the use of human genetic material. Part of the consultation considered whether individuals should have a form of property right in their own genetic material. As the ALRC noted with concern in its consultation documentation:

> The recognition or creation of donor property rights might allow donors to negotiate with researchers for the use of their genetic samples and contract to share in any resulting commercial benefits.[52]

Of course, the UK has also grappled with the matter of property rights in human material. In 1995, the Nuffield Council on Bioethics (NCB) produced a report exploring the issue.[53] While the report's findings have been superseded by subsequent legal developments in many respects, it remains valuable for its treatment of the cultural and philosophical considerations. Indeed, many of the NCB's conclusions remain as valid today as they were when the report was first published, including, for example, that the medical/institutional expectation is that any material given or taken from individuals is received free of all claims.

Empirical research on the topic presents a mixed picture. There is also some sociological evidence supporting a similar belief on the part of some sectors of the public;[54] conversely, there is also evidence that the prospect of profit from research involving donated human material is not favoured and research participants expect there to be some 'profit pay-off', even if this does not involve any personal return.[55]

In short, attitudes and expectations are diverse and changing, and the existence of diversity raises the spectre of conflict. The NCB recommended that any disputed claim over material should be determined with regard to the nature of the consent given to

[50] See Oregon Health Authority, 'Genetics and Privacy', available at <https://www.oregon.gov/oha/ph/diseasesconditions/geneticconditions/pages/research.aspx> accessed 13 January 2023.
[51] See Parliament of Australia, Senate Legal and Constitutional Legislation Committee, *Provisions of the Genetic Privacy and Nondiscrimination Bill 1998* (Commonwealth of Australia 1999).
[52] Australian Law Reform Commission, *Protection of Human Genetic Information*, Issues Paper 26 (ALRC 2001), available at <https://www.alrc.gov.au/publication/protection-of-human-genetic-information-ip-26/> accessed 13 January 2023, para 7.47.
[53] Nuffield Council on Bioethics, *Human Tissue: Ethical and Legal Issues* (Nuffield Council on Bioethics 1995).
[54] Mary Dixon-Woods et al., 'Tissue Samples as "Gifts" for Research: A Qualitative Study of Families and Professionals' (2008) 9(2) Medical Law International 131.
[55] Gill Haddow et al., 'Tackling Community Concerns about Commercialisation and Genetic Research: A Modest Interdisciplinary Proposal' (2007) 64(2) Social Sciences and Medicine 272.

the initial procedure for removal. It was the NCB's view that it should be implied in any consent to medical treatment which involves the removal of human tissue that the tissue has been abandoned by the person from whom it was removed.[56] A similar perspective informed the NCB's later report, *Human Bodies*, where the property paradigm was not entirely eschewed but a distinction was drawn between property rights as a vehicle to recognise more deep-rooted interests in recognition and control, and property claims that are motivated by income rights. The latter was rejected for their overall potential to lead to exploitation.[57]

14.5 TRADE AND PROPERTY IN HUMAN TISSUE

Ultimately, trade in material exists and property rights *are* generated; but in many cases property rights flow to parties other than the persons from whom the material has been taken. Why should this be so? The NCB's 1995 report was based, in the main, on the premise that people see no value in their excised body parts. This premise has long dominated, yet it has always been questionable, and now perhaps more than ever.[58] 'Value' exists in a variety of forms. The advent of the biotechnological age has meant that there can be considerable economic value which accrues to products produced using human material. To suggest that patients should be deemed to have abandoned their tissues is to ignore the potential values which they may well and rightly hold in retaining control over such material. A system of consents does not permit that control to be exercised as fully as might be desirable. This is not to ignore, however, the consequentialist concerns which could flow from granting individualistic rights of property in human material when the public benefit of that material is derived from its collective and aggregate value. However, it is important to note that there have been a number of high-profile cases across various jurisdictions which have suggested that the denial of property claims can leave claimants without adequate recourse, and that law and policymakers should think again about the *no property* rule.

The case which most clearly reveals the skewed attitude of the judiciary towards these matters is *Moore v Regents of the University of California*.[59] Although now dated, this judgment remains one of the most clearly illustrative of the contested issues that can arise in this area. The facts of the case involved Mr Moore, who suffered from hairy cell leukaemia. His spleen was removed at the UCLA Medical School. His treating doctor, Dr Golde, discovered that cells from the spleen had unusual and potentially beneficial properties and developed an immortal cell-line from them without Mr Moore's knowledge or consent. Moreover, Dr Golde sought and obtained a patent over the cell-line, which he subsequently sold to a drug company for $15m and it has been reported that the drugs and therapies which were developed from the patented product are now worth in excess of $3bn.[60] Moore brought legal proceedings against the researchers, the University, and the drug company when he discovered the truth of what had happened following the removal of his spleen. He filed 13 causes of action in total, but those concerning property and consent are of most direct interest. He alleged *conversion*: that is to say, as the 'owner'

---

[56] Nuffield Council on Bioethics (n 53) ch 9, in particular para 9.14.

[57] Nuffield Council on Bioethics (n 20) chs 5 and 7 and esp para 7.20.

[58] For the National Council on Bioethics' 'evolution' in thinking, see Muireann Quigley, 'From Human Tissue to Human Bodies: Donation, Interventions and Justified Distinctions?' (2012) 7(2) Clinical Ethics 73.

[59] 793 P 2d 479 (Cal 1990). See also *Brotherton v Cleveland* 923 F 2d 661 (6th Cir 1991).

[60] B Merz, 'Biotechnology: Spleen-Rights' *The Economist* (11 August 1990) 30.

of the cells, his property right had been compromised by the work carried out on the cells by the defendants. He also alleged breach of fiduciary duty and lack of informed consent, arguing he had never been told of the potential use of his cells and, correspondingly, he had never given his full and informed agreement to the initial operation which had involved the removal of his spleen from which the cells were taken.

The Californian Supreme Court upheld these two last claims by Mr Moore but rejected the argument in conversion. By a majority, the court held that it was inappropriate to recognise property in the body for a number of reasons. First, no precedent could be found on which to ground such a claim; and second, the recognition of individual property rights in body parts would hinder medical research 'by restricting access to the necessary raw materials'. Indeed, the Court appeared to be particularly concerned that a contrary decision would '[threaten] to destroy the economic incentive to conduct important medical research' because, 'If the use of cells in research is a conversion, then with every cell sample a researcher purchases a ticket in a litigation lottery'. The irony of this decision is pointed out in the dissent of Broussard J:

> the majority's analysis cannot rest on the broad proposition that a removed part is not property, but . . . on the proposition that a patient retains no ownership interest in a body part once the body part has been removed.

Put another way, while persons are denied recognition of a property interest in excised parts of their bodies, third parties may not only gain such an interest but can go on to protect it using forms of property law such as the law of patents.[61]

This example demonstrates precisely the type of value which individuals could retain in their excised parts. Without the cells from Mr Moore's spleen, there would have been no patentable immortal cell-line to be created by Dr Golde. While no one would deny that much time and money would need to be expended in turning the raw human material into a patentable product, is the view of the Supreme Court in *Moore* not something of an over-reaction to the *possible* consequences of applying property law to the human body? It is entirely reasonable to hold that some financial reward should be given to the source of the valuable sample while, at the same time, accepting that the majority of the spoils should return to those who have done the work in creating a patentable invention. It is *not* reasonable to exclude completely from the equation the one person who can make everything possible.

Policy is not always on the side of the researchers, as another US dispute demonstrated. In *Greenberg et al. v Miami Children's Hospital Research Institute Inc*,[62] an action was brought by parents of children affected by a rare, fatal, and incurable genetic disorder called Canavan disease. The defendant researchers had worked closely with afflicted families, receiving samples and gaining access to registers containing details of other affected groups around the world. However, when the Canavan gene was eventually identified, the researchers sought a patent over the gene and the related test, and proceeded to restrict access to the latter save through tightly controlled exclusive licences. The plaintiffs objected and, in much the same way as happened in *Moore*, mounted an action on a number of grounds, including lack of informed consent, unjust enrichment, breach of

---

[61] For comment, see Erik Seeney, '*Moore* 10 years later—Still Trying to Fill the Gap: Creating a Personal Property Right in Genetic Material' (1998) 32(4) New England Law Review 1131; Bernard Dickens, 'Living Tissue and Organ Donors and Property Law: More on Moore' in David Price (ed.), *Organ and Tissue Transplantation* (Routledge 2006).

[62] *Greenberg v Miami Children's Hospital Research Institute* 264 F Supp 2d 1064 (SD Fla 2003), settled action.

fiduciary duty, and conversion. In this last respect, the plaintiffs claimed a property interest in their samples, the genetic information therein, and information contained in the Canavan register.

Paradoxically, here policy favoured the plaintiffs, in that the families wanted information about the disease and the test to be freely available, while it was the patent holders who wished to restrict access and so potentially hinder research. The case was eventually abandoned after a preliminary hearing in which the judge rejected the property claim, but suggested that the argument made on the grounds of unjust enrichment might succeed. While the precise basis for this is unclear, the outcome revealed the continuing antipathy to property approaches to individual rights in human material.

This approach was confirmed at the federal level in *Washington University* v *Catalona et al.*[63] In this case, the US District Court was asked to declare on the ownership of samples provided by research participants enrolled in cancer research, which was conducted by Dr Catalona during his employment with Washington University, Missouri.[64] Dr Catalona had written to all of his participants informing them of his move to Northwestern University, Illinois, his intention to continue his valuable cancer research, and asking that they sign an authorisation for release with respect to their samples held by the university for delivery to him. Around 6,000 participants did so but the University refused to release the samples and sought declaratory relief. As the Court put it: 'the sole issue determinative of this permanent injunction; in fact in this lawsuit; is the issue of ownership'.[65] In finding for the University, the Court held that exclusive possession and control had come to the University after the provision of samples; that all legal, regulatory, and compliance risks fell on the University; that the University had continually exerted its ownership claims to materials in its repository, notably through the informed consent materials, and in its intellectual property policy; that the participants had freely given consent to donate samples for research at the University; and that Dr Catalona had willingly signed up to the ownership policy of his employers.

Dr Catalona and the research participants argued, inter alia, that there had been no intent to donate the samples to the University but rather to Dr Catalona; that the participants had retained control through the 'right to discontinue participation' (which is standard in research protocols); and alternatively, that participants made a bailment of property and not a gift at all. Each claim was found to be meritless. The Court held that on the evidence the intent was to donate to the University and this was made sufficiently clear in the consent forms, especially the repeated use of the University logo to indicate the body under whose auspices the work would be carried out. Second, the right to discontinue participation did not imply a right to continued control; rather, the Court suggested that a right to withdraw is nothing more than a right not to provide any more samples. Expert testimony went as far as to suggest that researchers would be operating within the law either if they were to destroy samples after withdrawal, store them indefinitely with no further use, or anonymise samples and continue in their use.[66] The bailment claim failed because it required a continuing expectation of return of property at some time, and the Court found no evidence that participants had informed the university of such an expectation, nor was such an expectation reasonable in the circumstances. Furthermore, it was relevant that the medical community had never considered

[63]   437 F Supp 2d 985 (US Dist 2006).

[64]   For comment, see Lori Andrews, 'Rights of Donors: Who Owns Your Body? A Patient's Perspective on *Washington University* v *Catalona*' (2006) 34(2) Journal of Law, Medicine and Ethics 398.

[65]   *Catalona* v *Washington University* 128 S Ct 1122, 169 L Ed 2d 949 (2008).

[66]   ibid. 999.

the relationship between research institution and research participant to be one of bail-ment. The Court of Appeals for the Eighth Circuit affirmed the District Court's judgment in all respects,[67] stating: 'If left unregulated and to the whims of research participants, these highly-prized biological materials would become nothing more than chattel going to the highest bidder.'[68]

Despite initial impressions, *Catalona* might be viewed as moving the debate forward in some respects. For one thing, it proceeds on the premise of property in the samples them-selves and finds evidence of a transfer of ownership, albeit not where the initial 'own-ers' might have wanted. Washington University won because it could show prima facie evidence of absolute possession and control of the samples, and because the participants could *not* show that they had any expectations other than outright gift. As a postscript, we should not be distracted from the property debate by the illusion that consent is the sole, or optimal, ethico-legal solution to the dilemmas thrown up by modern medicine, as many official bodies would have us believe.[69] A consent model disempowers individu-als to the extent that the single 'right' that it gives is a right to refuse. How does this help the person who is willing to participate in research but has qualms about the subsequent use of their samples towards undesirable ends? It does not, for their only option is to not participate. A property right would offer an opportunity for an element of continuing control over samples after surrender and would allow for a legally recognised voice in how they are used.[70] The same is not true once an initial consent has been obtained, for so long as the requisite information is disclosed at the time the sample is provided, the sample source's 'rights' have been exhausted.[71]

14.6 PROPERTY IN HUMAN MATERIAL: UK CASE LAW

14.6.1 REPRODUCTIVE MATERIAL

Let us begin with the beginning of life and its elemental constituents: the gametes. Whereas once the position was that the common law in the UK was unclear and static, case law developments in recent decades suggest the opposite. We consider the statutory provisions which apply to the obtaining, storage, and use of gametes in the UK in Chapter 16, but the question to be considered in light of such developments is whether common law property claims trump these regulatory provisions, or instead do such claims now provide rights not recognised in the legislation. We now turn to consider relevant case law in this regard.

---

[67] *Catalona* (n 65).

[68] ibid. 1002. In contrast to this position, we would point once again to the irony borne out by the motives in *Greenberg*, and to the mounting social science evidence that research participants do not necessarily see property as a device for selfish gain but rather as a means to engage more fully in the research enterprise, and/or to curb some of its worst commercial excesses.

[69] Nuffield Council on Bioethics (n 53).

[70] Imogen Goold, 'Why Does It Matter How We Regulate the Use of Human Body Parts?' (2014) 40(1) Journal of Medical Ethics 3; Remigius Nwabueze, 'Body Parts in Property Theory: An Integrated Framework' (2014) 40(1) Journal of Medical Ethics 33.

[71] For further comments on the limits of consent in the commercialisation context, see Graeme Laurie, 'Patents, Patients and Consent: Exploring the Interface between Regulation and Innovation Regimes' in Hans Somsen (ed.), *The Regulatory Challenge of Biotechnology Human Genetics, Food and Patents* (Edward Elgar 2007) 214–237.

In *L v The Human Fertilisation and Embryology Authority, Secretary of State for Health*,[72] the claimant sought a lawful basis to preserve, store, and use her deceased husband's sperm in circumstances where his prior written consent had not been obtained and for use of the sperm abroad if fertility services were not available in the UK. As noted in Chapter 16, the lawfulness of this is in serious doubt under the Human Fertilisation and Embryology Act 1990, as amended (HFE Act 1990); the distinguishing feature of *L*, however, was a submission that the common law, which recognises that in certain circumstances property rights can accrue in human materials, could be a lawful basis for the claimant's proposed course of action. Although this was rejected by the court—which distinguished the existing legal authorities from the case as dealing with the position *after* authorised or unauthorised removal—the point was made nonetheless that the common law 'does not stand still'.

No better illustration of this can be found than the decision in *Yearworth v North Bristol NHS Trust*.[73] Here, the Court of Appeal acknowledged the challenge for the common law as represented by the expanding frontiers of medical science. In this case, six men were due to receive aggressive cancer treatment which, they were advised, might damage their fertility. Accordingly, before treatment each man provided sperm samples to the hospital's fertility clinic for possible future use. Unfortunately, the storage facility suffered a technical malfunction and the sperm perished. A range of actions was brought, including negligent loss of a chance of becoming a father, psychiatric injury, and, in one case, mental distress. Of interest here is that while the judge at first instance dismissed a claim that there had been damage to the men's 'property', this was accepted by the Court of Appeal.[74] The relevance of the property claim was twofold: first, if it can be shown that there was damage to or loss of property through breach of a duty of care, an action would lie in negligence; and second, wrongful interference with property per se is actionable in its own right through bailment.

The Court of Appeal fully acknowledged that the law has remained 'noticeably silent' about property in parts or products of the living human body, postulating that, until recently, medical science did not endow them with any value or significance. This has changed. Although the Court was invited to leave the matter to Parliament and to avoid piecemeal development, it declined to do so. Rather, it began its analysis by rejecting the argument that the HFEA 1990 eliminates common law rights of ownership. The Court's view was that the Act must be confined to its original purposes (see Chapter 16), which are to regulate the storage and use of reproductive material outside the human body and in the hands of third parties who are subject to rigorous licensing requirements. No such licences apply to individuals with respect to their own gametes or embryos produced without artificial assistance. Furthermore, the legislation requires 'informed consent' from persons with respect to their reproductive materials, and a large part of this is about respecting the individual's wishes about disposition.[75] The pivotal paragraph in the ruling merits repetition in full:

> In this jurisdiction developments in medical science now require a re-analysis of the common law's treatment of an approach to the issue of ownership of parts or products of a living human body, whether for present purposes (viz. an action in negligence) or otherwise.[76]

---

[72] [2008] EWHC 2149 (Fam).   [73] [2009] 3 WLR 118.

[74] The claim that damage to the sperm itself once excised from the body could nonetheless still constitute a personal injury was rejected by the Court of Appeal at paras 19–24: 'To do otherwise would generate paradoxes, and yield ramifications, productive of substantial uncertainty, expensive debate and nice distinctions in an area of law which should be simple, and the principles clear.'

[75] This is not to imply that those wishes have paramountcy in all cases: compare, for example, requests *not* to use gametes with requests to make *specific* uses of gametes, but this is to say little because few rights are absolute.

[76] *Yearworth* (n 73) [45].

The basis of confirming ownership in the sperm for the purposes of their claims in negligence was as follows:

   (i)   provenance: they alone generated the sperm from their own bodies;

  (ii)   purpose: the object of ejaculation was for storage with a view to future use;

 (iii)   control: the 1990 Act confirms a negative right to require destruction of gametes (albeit not a correlative positive right of absolute control);

 (iv)   exclusivity: no other person, human or corporate, has any rights over gametes held under the Act;

  (v)   correlation: there was a direct link between the claims of the men to control use of their sperm and the preclusion of that use by the Trust's breach of duty.

This is a difficult ruling to untangle.[77] There is a complex mix of references to common law and statutory provision, and the Court of Appeal was emphatic in pointing out that its decision as to property claims must be seen as context-specific: that is to say, referrable to the circumstances of a negligence action relating to materials produced and designated for future use. As such, it might be claimed that any precedent should be confined to the facts of this case, but this sits uneasily with the pivotal paragraph quoted previously. It ignores the further cause of action considered by the Court, namely, bailment. The Court in *Yearworth* distinguished *Catalona* as a case where the tissue was clearly donated free of all claims, whereas here there was an equally clear expectation of (and obligation to) return of the sperm.[78] Bailment can be gratuitous, as in the present case, and carries with it a duty to take reasonable care of the goods.[79] Moreover, the Court found the measure of damages to be more akin to breach of contract than in tort, and to include reasonably foreseeable injuries such as psychiatric injury and mental distress.

For all of its qualifications and uncertainty, this decision is an important turning point in case law examining a property approach in human tissue. While it lacks any consideration of the (counter) policy considerations that we have seen in US case law previously referred to,[80] it signals a sea change in judicial attitude in UK courts towards patients' rights. It suggests, for example, that property claims might bring a range of remedies not available through other legal routes, and it offers a degree of empowerment for patients over material taken from their bodies should they choose to exercise it.[81]

Warren v Care Fertility (Northampton) Ltd[82] is further evidence of this willingness to support gamete-originators' wishes. Here, W sought a declaration that it was lawful for the sperm of her late husband, H, which had been taken prior to his failed cancer

---

[77] For deeper analysis see Harmon and Laurie (n 11); Shawn Harmon, 'Yearworth v North Bristol NHS Trust: A Property Case of Uncertain Significance?' (2010) 13(4) Medicine, Heath Care and Philosophy 343; Luke David Rostill, 'The Ownership That Wasn't Meant To Be: Yearworth and Property Rights in Human Tissue' (2014) 40(1) Journal of Medical Ethics 14.

[78] The Court of Appeal did not consider it necessary to address the legal basis for a property claim in bailment because it was of the view that this flowed naturally and a fortiori from the finding with respect to their claims in tort, see *Yearworth* (n 73) para 47.

[79] *Port Swettenham Authority* v *T W Wu and Co* (M) Sdn Bhd [1979] AC 580.

[80] It is easy to confirm that property rights are not absolute; what remains to be seen is how and how far limits can or will be placed on them in the name of other claims, most notably claims by scientists.

[81] And it has been applied in many jurisdictions, including Australia (*Bazley* v *Wesley Monash IVF Pty Ltd* [2010] QSC 118, and *Jocelyn Edwards; Re the Estate of the Late Mark Edwards* [2011] NSWSC 478) and Canada (*JCM* v *ANA* [2012] BCSC 584), the latter of which extended it to both parties in the IVF enterprise. For a Scots law perspective, see *Holdich* v *Lothian Health Board* [2013] CSOH 197.

[82] [2014] EWHC 602.

treatment, to be stored beyond the statutory period, and for her use. In granting the declaration, the court noted that certain information had not been furnished to H as stipulated under the law, and that given that there was no conflict of rights as between W and H, it should take a purposive approach to statutory interpretation. The UK Parliament intended to enable a deceased man's sperm to be used by a named person, provided that it was the deceased's wish. While not all of the statutory conditions were met, the husband's intentions were known, so W's rights under Article 8 of the ECHR should be vindicated.

When we consider the union of gametes to produce a human embryo, matters become still more complicated. As discussed in Chapter 16, the moral significance of embryos is sufficiently disputed even before property claims are added to the mix. But embryos are used and discarded in healthcare settings, and the law must deal with this in an appropriate fashion. The Human Fertilisation and Embryology Authority (HFEA) faces the dilemma of the disposal of embryos which are created for assisted reproduction, but which are not used.

As previously noted, the HFE Act 1990 avoids any recognition of property rights, and control over the use and disposal of frozen embryos falls to be determined by the will of the parties contributing to their formation. However, unlike gametes, two parties provide the genetic material contained in embryos, which themselves are indivisible entities. Who, then, has the power to dispose of them? Schedule 3 to the HFE Act 1990 provides that effective written consent must be given by each person whose gametes have contributed to the embryo.[83] In practice, this gives either contributor a veto over use of the embryo but it provides neither with positive rights of disposition—the embryos must be allowed to perish if the gamete providers cannot agree and the storage time for the embryo has exceeded the statutory limit.[84]

As discussed in Chapter 16, this system involving agreement between parties who may be in conflict is almost designed for stalemate.[85] The English courts in the case of *Evans* v *Amicus Healthcare Ltd and Others* stuck rigidly to the letter of the law, holding that the refusal to cooperate by the estranged partners of two women who sought possession of their frozen embryos meant that there was no other legal option but to deny access to the embryos, effectively condemning the organisms to destruction.[86] The Grand Chamber of the European Court of Human Rights (ECtHR) rejected Ms Evans's appeal and confirmed that the UK's approach to regulation in this area, based as it is on written informed consent(s), was justifiable and not a breach of human rights.[87]

The outcome of the *Evans* litigation highlights that, in the absence of any property right in embryos, the aim for which they have been created can be thwarted by the absence or withholding of consent by a potentially disinterested, bitter, or uncontactable contributor. The Canadian case of *SH* v *DH* dealt with such a situation,[88] wherein DH sought an order naming her the owner of an embryo created from gametes purchased by her and her estranged husband during their marriage so that she could have it implanted. The purchase of the embryo from the US was handled via contract and the court approached the matter as a matter of marital property to be divided under the Family Law Act. Given

---

[83] Sch 3, para 6(3), HFE Act 1990, as amended.

[84] For a detailed examination of this point, see Chapter 16.

[85] For a challenge to the consent model, see Malcolm Parker, 'Response to Orr and Seigler—Collective Intentionality and Procreative Desires: The Permissible View on Consent to Posthumous Conception' (2004) 30(4) Journal of Medical Ethics 389.

[86] [2004] 3 WLR 681.

[87] *Evans* v *United Kingdom* [2007] 1 FLR 1990. For a detailed overview of this case, see Chapter 16.

[88] In this regard, note the Canadian case of *S.H.* v *D.H.* (2018) ONSC 4506.

the clause in one of the relevant contracts that 'the agent shall respect the patient's [in this case, woman's] wishes,' and in contrast to *Evans*, the embryo was released to DH.

While it is not suggested that that a property system would be problem-free, the failure to recognise such a property right, which vests, in the first instance, in the person who is to receive treatment as part of assisted conception, would go a long way to resolving the current controversies surrounding these issues.[89] The ruling in *Yearworth* might provide a basis for such an argument. Indeed, conflicts of claims, as between the partners involved in such treatment, are neither unique nor insurmountable.[90]

14.6.2 THE DEAD BODY

For a long time the 'no property in a dead body' rule was thought to exclude all possibility of property in a dead body or its parts, at least in England and Wales.[91] In *Yearworth*,[92] the Court of Appeal speculated that the general basis for the rule might be: (i) a matter of logic;[93] (ii) a matter of religious conviction; and (iii) a matter of public health. The case of *R v Kelly*,[94] however, established that there are serious limitations to any such rule which have important consequences for the users of human tissue removed from deceased persons. In *Kelly*, the question was whether it was theft for a junior technician of the Royal College of Surgeons (RCS) to remove body parts for use, and ultimate disposal, by an artist who was interested in employing them as moulds for his sculptures. The defendants relied on the 'no property' rule as their defence. The Court held that the rule refers only to a dead body or its parts which remain in their natural state, but that:

> parts of a corpse are capable of being property . . . if they have acquired different attributes by virtue of the application of skill, such as dissection or preservation techniques, for exhibition or teaching purposes.[95]

Here, work had indeed been done on the body parts in question such that they became specimens owned by the RCS. To remove them without authority was, therefore, theft. The Court went on to hold that the 'no property' rule is so deeply entrenched in English jurisprudence that legislative action would be required for it to be changed *in se*. That having been said, the Court speculated that the common law might recognise property in body parts from a deceased person even when those parts had not acquired different attributes, but if they had attracted a 'use or significance beyond their mere existence'.[96]

What we are not told is who would be the holder of any such right. An answer is found, however, in the earlier case of *Dobson v North Tyneside Health Authority*,[97] which was

[89] Acknowledging the preeminent position of the woman here is important for a variety of reasons: Donna Dickenson, 'Disappearing Women, Vanishing Ladies and Property in Embryos' (2017) 4(1) Journal of Law and Biosciences 175.
[90] Mary Ford, '*Evans v United Kingdom*: What Implications for the Jurisprudence of Pregnancy?' (2008) 8(1) Human Rights Law Review 171; Mary Ford, 'A Property Model of Pregnancy' (2005) 1(3) International Journal of Law in Context 261.
[91] Nuffield Council on Bioethics (n 53) para 10.02. There is some authority in Scotland that property can exist in a dead body, at least until it is buried or otherwise disposed of: *Dewar v HM Advocate* 1945 JC 5, at 14.
[92] *Yearworth* (n 73) para 31.
[93] If ownership did not vest in the living person, why should it do so in the dead? On connectedness between our obligations to the living and to the dead, see Sheelagh McGuiness and Margaret Brazier, 'Respecting the Living Means Respecting the Dead Too' (2008) 28(2) Oxford Journal of Legal Studies 297.
[94] [1998] 3 All ER 741 (CA).   [95] ibid. 749–750.   [96] ibid. 750.   [97] [1996] 4 All ER 474 (CA).

noted with approval in the case of *Kelly*. In *Dobson*, the relatives of a woman who had died from brain tumours brought an action in negligence against the health authority for failure to diagnose the nature of the condition properly and in time. In order to succeed, however, it was important to establish whether the tumours were malignant or benign, and this could only be done by examining samples from the deceased's brain, which had been removed by the hospital at an autopsy directed by the coroner and subsequently disposed of.[98] The relatives therefore brought a further action against the hospital, alleging that it had converted 'property' to which the relatives were entitled, and that it acted as a bailee having no right of unauthorised disposal. In rejecting these claims, the Court of Appeal held that no right of possession or ownership of the brain, or indeed of the dead body, vested in the relatives. At best, a limited possessory right to the dead body is enjoyed by the executor or administrator of a deceased person, but this right is only to possess the body with a view to its burial or disposal.[99]

It also held that property rights could arise in respect of body parts from the deceased person where some work or skill differentiates the body or its parts from a corpse in its natural state. It quoted, with halting approval, the following passage from the Australian decision *Doodeward* v *Spence*,[100] which involved a dispute over the 'ownership' of a two-headed foetus:

> when a person has by lawful exercise of work or skill so dealt with a human body or part of a human body in his lawful possession that it has acquired some attributes differentiating it from a mere corpse awaiting burial, he acquires a right to retain possession of it, at least as against any person not entitled to have it delivered to him for the purposes of burial.

Two elements from this passage are worth noting. First, any property right which accrues does so to the person who does the work. Second, the property right which springs into existence is subject to the right of those with the right to possession for burial.[101] We have already seen that no possessory right for burial existed in *Dobson*. But had the brain become property? Gibson LJ did not seem to think so; the brain had not been preserved for the purposes of teaching or exhibition, nor was the case analogous to a stuffing or embalming, which displays an intention to retain the part as a specimen. The brain had been removed and preserved only under the obligation to remove material bearing on the cause of death imposed by the Coroners Rules 1984.[102] The hospital intended to abide by these rules and was at liberty to destroy the brain once the material was no longer required by the coroner.

Dobson is as interesting for the questions that it does not answer as it is for those that it does. For example, as to the possessory right of executors, must the dead body and *all* of its parts be returned? Similarly, what is the role of intention in creating property rights? Reading *Dobson* and *Kelly* in conjunction, it seems that property rights can arise if work is done on a tissue *with the intention* of retaining the sample as a specimen or for some other purpose. But just how much, or little, work needs to be done? In *Kelly*, the Court indicates that dissection or preservation techniques are enough to make a sample 'property'.[103] If so, then merely to carry out an autopsy or to place a sample in formaldehyde is enough

---

[98] The case reports that it had been preserved in paraffin, though normal procedure would be to preserve the brain in formaldehyde and remove pieces which would be processed into small 'paraffin blocks' for examination.

[99] No executor or administrator had been appointed in the present case until after the body had been disposed of.

[100] (1908) 6 CLR 406 (Griffith CJ) [414].

[101] Confirmation of this right and of the *Kelly* rule can be found in *Re St Andrew's Churchyard, Alwalton* [2012] PTSR 479 [52].

[102] Coroners Rules 1984 (SI 1984/552), r 9.   [103] ibid. [749]–[750].

to create 'property'.[104] As we have seen from *Dobson*, that property belongs to those who would 'use' the goods and certainly not to the source or their significant others.

If the Court of Appeal in *Kelly* is correct and the common law does one day move to the position that property rights may arise because of the 'inherent' valuable attributes in human tissue samples, it is undoubtedly the case that such rights will vest in the 'discoverer' of those properties. As has been previously mentioned, the HTA 2004, for example, leaves open the position on accrual of property rights, but also leaves the common law's 'no property' rule untouched. This includes the attribution of property because of 'an application of human skill'. At the same time, the Act extends the consent model by allowing third parties, such as next of kin, to authorise, or veto, dealings with the remains of a loved one.[105] Consent and property are not mutually exclusive concepts; indeed, to the extent that they are both a means of furnishing respect, they should perhaps be made to work together towards a common end.[106]

Litigation brought by aggrieved parents in respect of post-mortem examinations performed on their dead children has shed more light on the legal position. In *AB v Leeds Teaching Hospital NHS Trust*,[107] claims were made, inter alia, in negligence for psychiatric injury and for wrongful interference with the body, which was a tort not previously recognised under English law.[108] It was argued that inadequate care and attention was exercised when obtaining parental consent to the post-mortems and that body parts of the children should not have been retained without express authority. Gage J confirmed the 'no property in a corpse' rule, but followed *Kelly* in holding that parts of a body may acquire the character of property provided sufficient work and skill has been expended. In the particular case of the work undertaken by the pathologist, it was stated: 'to dissect and fix an organ from a child's body requires work and a great deal of skill . . . The subsequent production of blocks and slides is also a skilful operation requiring work and expertise of trained scientists'.[109]

Moreover, the Court held that the post-mortem examinations were lawfully executed and therefore capable of giving rise to possessory rights on the part of the pathologists; any possessory rights of the parents for the purposes of burial could not, from a pragmatic stance, be a right to return of every part of the body after post-mortem.[110] But what if parents make it an express stipulation of their consent to post-mortem that all body samples be returned? Here, Gage J refused to create a new common law tort where none had existed—namely, a tort of wrongful interference with the body or of conversion in the body. Rather, he held that such matters fall to be considered as a matter of negligence: the doctor who receives such instructions from parents has a duty of care to pass these on to

---

[104] There is a world of difference between placing a brain in preservative and preparing blocks for microscopic examination; the precise conditions obtaining in *Dobson* are, therefore, of some significance.

[105] Human Tissue Act 2004, ss 27(4) and 54(9). For a case law example on point, see *CM v EJ's Executor* [2013] EWHC 1680.

[106] See John Kenyon Mason and Graeme Laurie, 'Consent or Property? Dealing with the Body and Its Parts in the Shadow of Bristol and Alder Hey' (2001) 64(5) Modern Law Review 710.

[107] [2004] 2 FLR 365. The circumstances of this case arose from the concerns generated by the practices at Alder Hey and Bristol which became the subject of two public inquiries. This also saw the establishment of the Retained Organs Commission which issued Recommendations on the Legal Status of Tissue Blocks and Slides (ROC 17/6, 2003), which supported the suggestion that 'straightforward legal ownership was not a preferred option . . . tissue blocks and slides should be subject to some form of custody or stewardship'.

[108] But probably recognised in Scotland: *Pollok v Workman* [1900] 2 F 354, and *Hughes v Robertson* [1930] SC 394, discussed in Niall Whitty, 'Rights of Personality, Property Rights and the Human Body in Scots Law' (2005) 9(2) Edinburgh Law Review 194.

[109] *AB v Leeds Teaching Hospital* (n 108) [148].   [110] ibid. [158] and [160].

the pathologist; in turn they are obliged to heed such a condition lest they be found to be in breach of their duty of care.[111]

An alternative route is available in Scotland. *Stevens v Yorkhill NHS Trust and another*[112] emerged out of similar post-mortem circumstances. In this case, the pursuer (claimant) argued that, despite authorising a post-mortem on her daughter, it was never explained to her that this would involve removal and retention of organs, particularly the brain, and, as a result, this led to severe depression and loss of employment. The legal proceedings were based on two grounds: (1) that a duty of care in negligence was owed to her such that she should have been informed and provided with the opportunity to give appropriate consent to the procedure, and, separately, to the removal and storage of tissue; (2) that under Scots common law wrongful interference with a dead body was actionable in its own right as an affront to human dignity. While legal authority was sparse, there was support in the ancient *actio injuriarum* (reflecting Scots law's roots in Roman law) which allowed recovery in the terms averred and in particular for recovery for *solatium* (hurt to feelings, as opposed to psychiatric injury). This had never been superseded by statute nor was the English ruling in *Leeds Teaching Hospital* binding on a Scottish court. That case was followed, however, with respect to the negligence claim in that it was accepted that a duty of care could be owed to the pursuer and its scope could include information about organ removal and retention when seeking consent to post-mortem examination. These conclusions were reached without the need to rely on a property paradigm.

Once again, we see that a range of legal devices is employed to protect the interests at stake. It is helpful, however, to consider the differences here. While recognition of a property-type claim would entitle the right-holder to control (and return) of the thing itself,[113] which is what parents have often sought in cases such as these, a negligence action is for financial compensation and requires proof of causation of a recognised form of harm, which can be difficult to establish in legal terms. Remedies in negligence, privacy, autonomy, or *actio injuriarum* undoubtedly serve their purpose, but a property model reveals different aspects to the rights currently enjoyed by individuals and their families, which cannot wholly be subsumed within other concepts or under these other rights of legal action.

14.7 INTELLECTUAL PROPERTY IN HUMAN TISSUE

In this section, we offer a brief consideration of the role of intellectual property (IP) in the products that are generated with the application of knowledge and skill from human tissue from both living and deceased persons. In doing so, we recognise that IP law is a complex and specialised area of law to which we could not do justice here. However, it is important to recognise its importance in offering legal protection to companies and researchers who apply knowledge and skill to make such products. IP law has had to adapt rapidly in the last few decades to meet the demands of the biotechnology industry.

---

[111] ibid. [161]. The court also recognised the relevance of human rights arguments to the circumstances where body parts are retained for research purposes, namely unauthorised retention with a view to research ends is capable of engaging the right to respect for private and family life under Art 8(1) ECHR, and that the circumstances in which this could be justified by the public authority under Art 8(2) 'will probably be rare', see paras 287–300.

[112] 2007 SCLR 606.

[113] Absent its destruction or the operation of other supervening property rights such as commixtion, confusion, or specification (to use the Scottish terminology).

Astronomical sums are invested in research and development, and the pharmaceutical industry, for example, has fought hard to ensure that its products receive patent protection with a view to facilitating legal certainty and ensuring an adequate degree of return on the investment.

Crucial to continued success and growth, it is still felt, is a healthy IP system, and the search for patents is central to this (which is not the same as saying that more patents means a healthier system). A patent offers a monopoly for up to 20 years over an invention, to the extent that all others can be excluded from competing in the marketplace with the same, or a substantially similar, product.[114] Strict criteria must be met to obtain protection, but once secured, a patent can protect a commercial enterprise against all-comers. Patenting is not, however, a morally neutral exercise and the biotechnology industry has faced problems in obtaining protection.[115] In Europe, for example, there have been issues with regards to recognising patents where it involves the manipulation of living organisms. The policy concern about such recognition lies in the attempt to patent a biotechnological invention in such circumstances, which may be viewed as being akin to patenting 'life' itself.[116]

Standard criteria for patentability are accepted in most countries of the world.[117] While terminology varies slightly, to be patentable, an invention must:

(1) be new or novel;

(2) involve an 'inventive step'—in the sense that the development should not be obvious to a person skilled in the particular field; and

(3) have utility or be made or used in some kind of industry.

In general terms, a broad and permissive approach to these criteria is adopted. However, when it comes to living organisms, there have been noticeable differences in approach between the US and Europe. In the case of *Diamond v Chakrabarty*,[118] the US Supreme Court held that 'anything under the sun that is made by man' could be patented. This permissive approach was highlighted in the case of OncoMouse, where Harvard University sought a patent for a mouse that had been genetically engineered with a human cancer gene in such a way that it developed cancer as a matter of course. The position of the US Patent and Trademark Office was to grant the patent without question. In contrast, the approach taken in Europe was quite different. Although an application for a patent over OncoMouse was filed in 1985, it was not granted until 1991,[119] and even then, its validity was in constant doubt, with further restrictions on its scope being imposed in 2001[120] and 2004.[121] While the monopoly was originally granted to cover 'transgenic mammals',

---

[114] See Graeme Laurie, 'Patenting and the Human Body' in Jean McHale et al. (eds.), *Principles of Medical Law* (3rd edn, OUP 2010).

[115] For useful historical accounts, see Nuffield Council on Bioethics, *The Ethics of Patenting DNA* (Nuffield Council on Bioethics 2002) Appendix 2; Aurora Plomer and Paul Torremans (eds.), *Embryonic Stem Cell Patents: European Patent Law and Ethics* (OUP 2010).

[116] Justine Pila, 'Adapting the *Ordre Public* and Morality Exclusion of European Patent Law to Accommodate Emerging Technologies' (2020) 38 Nature Biotechnology 555–557.

[117] See World Trade Organization, TRIPS Agreement—Trade Related Aspects of Intellectual Property Rights (2022) available at <https://www.wto.org/english/tratop_e/trips_e/trips_e.htm> accessed 13 January 2023. In the UK, see Patents Act 1977, s 1(1).

[118] 447 US 303, 66 L Ed 2d 144 (1980).   [119] [1991] EPOR 525.

[120] Alison Abbott, 'Harvard Squeaks Through Oncomouse Patent Appeal' (2001) 414 Nature 241.

[121] T0315/03 *Transgenic Animals/HARVARD*, 6.7.2004, ECLI:EP:BA:2004:T031503.20040706, European Patent Office (2004), available at <https://www.epo.org/law-practice/case-law-appeals/recent/t030315ex1.html> accessed 13 January 2023.

it was ultimately restricted to 'transgenic mice'. The problem of patent protection faced by the industry in Europe stems from the 'morality provisions' of the European Patent Convention.[122]

Ethical and legal concerns over the patenting of human material have been highlighted in particular by the increased use of human embryonic stem cells (hESCs) in research and product development. While it has been possible to derive stem cells from adults for more than 60 years, and from animals, including animal embryos, for over 40 years, hESCs were first isolated only 25 years ago.[123] As noted (and discussed in Chapter 16 in more detail), the contested moral status of the human embryo makes research on it problematic. The concern surrounding hESC technologies is that, at present, we must both use and destroy a human embryo to produce valuable embryonic stem cell cultures. This has meant that hESC technologies are unpatentable in the EU due to the operation of Article 6 of the EC Directive on the legal protection of biotechnological inventions, which prohibits the patenting of 'uses of human embryos for industrial or commercial purposes' for reasons of *order public* or morality.[124] Alternatives to hESC are now in use, including 'induced pluripotent stem cells' (iPSCs), which are produced from reprogrammed adult somatic cells,[125] and are therefore said to avoid the ethical dilemmas of hESCs.[126] Although much progress has been made in iPSC research with a view to developing viable therapies, the use of hESCs remains the 'gold standard'.[127]

If one is concerned by the acts of creation/destruction of hESCs, then arguably attention should be turned not to the point at which patent protection is offered, but the point at which the creation takes place.[128] This cannot be done through the law of patents, but rather through other mechanisms such as regulatory schemes or authorities which monitor the industry. Making morality part of patent law does nothing to regulate the biotechnology industry, except perhaps in a very indirect way of removing an incentive; allowing patent law to drive the regulatory and innovation systems is a dangerous formula. Some insight into the problems of failing to maintain some sort of boundary between patent law and regulatory regimes can be gained by considering the possible effect of the current stem cell patent rulings on countries where hESC research is both legal and encouraged. The UK is one such country that has invested heavily in the science and constructed a robust regulatory framework for embryo research administered by the HFEA.

---

[122] See Art 53, European Patent Convention, 17th edn (2020), available at <https://www.epo.org/law-practice/legal-texts/epc.html> accessed 13 January 2023.

[123] For an overview, see David Cyranoski, 'How Human Embryonic Cells Sparked A Revolution' (2018) 555(7697) Nature 428.

[124] Directive of the European Parliament and of the Council on the Legal Protection of Biotechnological Inventions, No 98/44/EC of 6 July 1998; C–34/10 *Brüstle v Greenpeace eV* [2011] ECR I-09821 (Grand Chamber, 18 October 2011). For academic commentary on point, see Myrthe Nielen, Sybe de Vries, and Niels Geijsen, 'European Stem Cell Research in Legal Shackles' (2013) 32(24) *The EMBO Journal* 3107.

[125] See Sharif Moradi et al., 'Research and Therapy with Induced Pluripotent Stem Cells (iPSCs): Social, Legal, and Ethical Considerations' (2019) 10 Stem Cell Research & Therapy 341.

[126] Tetsuuya Ishii, Renee Reijo Pera, and Henry Greely, 'Ethical and Legal Issues Arising in Research on Inducing Human Germ Cells from Pluripotent Stem Cells' (2013) 13(2) Cell Stem Cell 145.

[127] For an overview of the issues at stake, see Dusko Ilic and Caroline Oglivie, 'Concise Review: Human Embryonic Stem Cells—What Have We Done? What Are We Doing? Where Are We Going?' (2017) 35(1) Stem Cells 17. For a more recent reference supporting the 'gold standard' point, see Paul De Sousa, 'Human Embryonic Stem Cell Banking for Clinical Applications: 20 Years From Their Isolation' in George Galea, Marc Turner, and Sharon Zahra (eds.), *Essentials of Tissue and Cells Banking* (Springer 2021).

[128] This is argued more fully in Graeme Laurie, 'Biotechnology: Facing the Problems of Patent Law' in Hector MacQueen (ed.), *Innovation, Incentive and Reward: Intellectual Property Law and Policy* (Edinburgh University Press 1997) 46; see Graeme Laurie, 'Patenting Stem Cells of Human Origin' (2004) 26(2) European Intellectual Property Review 59.

As discussed in Chapter 16, the HFEA operates a licensing system whereby research is only authorised provided certain conditions are met and approved by the Authority. To date, it has granted licences in respect of numerous hESC research projects.[129] Any ambitions to commercialise the results of such projects could run into challenges due to the difficulty in obtaining patent protection in the EU.

Indeed, commercial interests arguably suffered another blow in this regard in the US case *Association for Molecular Pathology* v *Myriad Genetics, USPTO et al.*,[130] wherein a group of claimants alleged that Myriad's patents on two human genes associated with early onset of breast and ovarian cancer—the BRCA1 and BRCA2 genes—hampered scientific research, limited accessibility to health care, were invalid on patent law criteria, and were unconstitutional. The patents, which cover the genes themselves (composition patents) and the processes making use of them (process patents), gave Myriad a lucrative monopoly to conduct or license medical tests relating to the genes, and Myriad had become notorious for its aggressive business model and enforcement practices, particularly within the US. The case eventually made its way to the US Supreme Court, which held that genes and the information that they encode are not patent-eligible simply because they have been isolated from the surrounding genetic material. Overturning decades of lower court precedent, it invalidated Myriad's patents on isolated genomic human DNA on the basis that a naturally occurring DNA segment is a 'product of nature', but it upheld some of Myriad's claims directed towards complementary DNA molecules, determining that synthesising these molecules creates something new.[131] Although it has been cited and extended in two California district court cases,[132] and other litigation is proceeding apace,[133] the extent of the fallout from Myriad IV has yet to be determined, especially outside the US.

In light of this brief discussion, there are numerous responses that we might have to the challenges raised by by IP involving the use of human tissue, including hESCs. For example, one could:

- *Deny patent protection*: but this is a generally unrealistic prospect and may be counter-productive if venture capitalists are to be believed—they would simply cease funding the research necessary to produce the products in the first place.

- *Improve the patent system*: standards of drafting patent applications could be strengthened to ensure that (1) inventions are properly described, and (2) unsustainable claims to protection are not made. This, in turn, would facilitate a more rigorous examination process that should ensure that protection is granted only to innovations that are truly inventive and which have never been made available to the public.

- *Move to open science*: advocates of this approach wish to free-up the sharing of scientific and medical knowledge through various mechanisms such as the use of IP rights to require sharing rather than to police exclusivity.[134]

---

[129] HFEA, 'Applying for a Research Licence', available at <https://www.hfea.gov.uk/about-us/applying-for-a-research-licence/> accessed 13 January 2023.

[130] 133 S Ct 2107 (2013).

[131] *Myriad IV*, at 2111 and 2119–2120.

[132] *Ariosa Diagnostics Inc* v *Sequenom Inc*, No C 11–06391 SI, 2013 WL 5863022; *Genetic Technologies Ltd* v *Agilent Technologies Inc*, No CV 12–01616 RS, 2014 WL 941354.

[133] Tup Ingram, '*Association for Molecular Pathology v. Myriad Genetics, Inc.*: The Product of Nature Doctrine Revisited' (2014) 29 Berkeley Technology Law Journal 385.

[134] See Royal Society, 'Science as an Open Enterprise', available at <https://royalsociety.org/topics-policy/projects/science-public-enterprise/report/> accessed 13 January 2023.

- *Collaborative approach*: a final novel approach—and one which brings us back to the idea of patient empowerment and mutually beneficial ends—is illustrated by the case of PXE International, a patient and family support group for those affected by the genetic disorder pseudoxanthoma elasticum. The group announced in 2004 that one of its leading members had been named as a co-inventor of the gene associated with the condition together with the scientists responsible for its isolation. All rights have been assigned to PXE International, which considers itself the 'steward of the gene'. The Group entered various agreements to pursue further research and develop a diagnostic kit.[135]

We suggest that it is not so much the *existence* of IP rights that is the problem with an efficient incentive and reward system, but rather the ways in which they are *exercised*. Many developments to date have failed to see or address this distinction. So long as patents endure—and they will endure—then patent offices and courts should work together to limit the effects of overly broad patents by restricting protection to the precise contribution that an invention makes to human knowledge and no further.

14.8 CONCLUSION

This chapter examined the key aspects of past and current debates arising from the property approach to the human body, including its parts and tissue. It highlighted the complex inter-relationship of ethical, social, and legal issues at stake, as well as critically engaging with a range of stakeholder and judicial positions on the issue in the UK and internationally. It seems that whether we are dealing with living or dead bodies and related human tissue, whether we are looking at humanity at the structured or the molecular level, or whether we are considering ethical conundrums or legislation in the area, we are faced with a confounding approach to property rights in human tissue. On the one hand, there is an innate antipathy to the concept; on the other, we accept the inexorable march of science knowing that, if something is there to be discovered, someone will discover it—and with little concern for the consequences—and some will want to benefit, commercially or otherwise, from that discovery. Governments may set up regulatory authorities as the significance of each scientific advance becomes apparent, but they are relatively powerless in the face of global pressures. What does seem clear is that, so far as the UK context is concerned, our courts must appreciate that this is a field in which technology and societal attitudes are advancing and being fashioned rapidly—and the common law must keep pace and accelerate as is necessary.

FURTHER READING

1. Margaret Davies, 'Ownership: Persons, Property and Community' in Mariana Valverde et al. (eds.), *Routledge Handbook of Law and Society* (Routledge 2021).

2. Donna Dickenson, *Property in the Body: Feminist Perspectives* (CUP 2007).

---

[135] See PXE International, 'Welcome to PXE International', available at <https://www.pxe.org/> accessed 13 January 2023.

3. Imogen Goold et al. (eds.), *Persons Parts and Property: How Should We Regulate Tissue in the 21st Century* (Hart 2014).

4. Rohan Hardcastle, *Law and the Human Body: Property Rights, Ownership and Control* (Hart 2007).

5. Remigius Nwabeuze, *Biotechnology and the Challenge of Property: Property Rights in Dead Bodies, Body Parts and Genetic Information* (Routledge 2016).

6. Justine Pila, 'Property in Human Genetic Material: An Old Legal Question for a New Technological Age' in Tamara Hervey and David Orentlicher (eds.), *The Oxford Handbook of Comparative Health Law* (OUP 2020).

7. Muireann Quigley, *Self-Ownership, Property Rights, and the Human Body* (CUP 2018).

8. Jesse Wall, *Being and Owning: The Body, Bodily Materials and the Law* (OUP 2015).

15

CONTRACEPTION AND ABORTION

15.1 INTRODUCTION

This chapter covers an exceptionally wide spectrum of medical law and ethics. It can range in social significance from being a purely personal matter—as in the extreme example of abstinence from sexual intercourse—through contraception in its many guises, to termination of pregnancy. Attitudes to fertility control will vary with effect. At one end of the scale, there are those who perceive sexual intercourse and procreation as a unitary function and will, accordingly, object to barrier methods of contraception; somewhere in the middle are the purists who see any interference with the human body as unethical unless it be for therapeutic purposes; and, at the other end, are those who are committed to the concept that a woman's[1] body is hers to control as she pleases, and who advocate abortion on demand. Across the whole spectrum we must also accept that modern fertility control involves more than numerical limitation of the family; it also includes control of the timing and nature of the family, the latter of which may encompass anything from selection of the sex of one's children to manipulation of genetics, and it is in this field that the seeds of ethical conflict are sown.[2]

Here, we concentrate on the control of fertility as an aspect of what is, essentially, family planning, and discussion in this area is dominated by two overarching precepts. On the one hand, we have the fundamental bioethical and legal principle of respect for autonomy (see Chapter 2) which has now established itself as the cornerstone of modern medical jurisprudence. It is possible to regard *any* restriction of an adult's lifestyle as an affront to that autonomy, and reproductive choice is certainly one of its major components. On the other hand, given that quantitative and qualitative choice of one's offspring must involve rejection of some forms of future life, fertility control confronts personal autonomy with the essentially communitarian ideas that human life should be preserved whenever possible, and that we have duties toward future persons, and, perhaps more arguably, communities as well.

Both ethics and the law must, therefore, find a balance, and this chapter discusses how this is navigated in the face of varying levels of ethical controversy, which we consider in turn. There being no actual human life in isolated gametes, contraception stands as the most accepted form of fertility control,[3] and a form of 'quality' control that depends on

---

[1] We recognise that people who do not identify as women also use the contraceptives discussed here and require abortion services. In this chapter we predominantly use the term 'woman' to reflect the vocabulary used in law, for example in the Abortion Act 1967.

[2] For a full consideration of modern reproductive rights from the international perspective, see Rebecca Cooke and Bernard Dickens, 'Reproductive Health and the Law' in Pamela Ferguson and Graeme Laurie (eds.), *Inspiring a Medico-legal Revolution: Essays in Honour of Sheila AM McLean* (Routledge 2015), ch 1.

[3] Subject to the possible rejoinder 'abstinence excepted'.

gamete selection will attract less criticism than will one that depends on destruction of embryos. Sterilisation, on the other hand, while it involves prevention rather than loss of life, raises issues of both harm and consent and has, at least in the past, been the subject of intense debate. Embryocide resulting from contragestation, which involves the use of methods designed to prevent pregnancy after the formation of an embryo, is clearly more open to questioning than is contraception per se, but at the same time, it is less subject to moral objection than is feticide in the form of abortion.[4] Termination of pregnancy itself becomes progressively less acceptable, for most, as foetal maturity increases, and here the law steps in to provide some measure of protection for the foetus; finally, that protection becomes complete at birth where, subject to the vagaries of legal and medical necessity (for which, see Chapter 9), neonaticide remains unlawful irrespective of any opposing philosophical attractions.

What we can derive from the foregoing is that any distinction between contraception, contragestation, termination of pregnancy, and neonaticide, whether it be morally, legally, or even, in a slightly different context, medically based, depends upon the answer to the age-old question which arises at each point in the sequence, 'When does life begin?'

15.2 THE CONCEPT OF PERSONHOOD

The value that we place on human life is intimately linked with respect for personhood, but what constitutes personhood is certainly not a matter of scientific fact. Rather, it is an amalgam of legal expedience, cultural variation, and moral supposition; as such, it is likely to be subject to wide and varied interpretation.[5] For example, the view exemplified by the Roman Catholic Church lies at one extreme; this holds that personhood, and its consequent right to protection, exists from the moment of conception. There are relatively few who would support this extreme view as a matter of legal policy; there are, in fact, relatively good reasons, based, inter alia, on the totipotential[6] capacity of the early embryonic cells, for regarding the pre-implantation blastocyst[7] as being, also, pre-embryonic. We will see, however, that personhood may be one thing but that human life is another; hence, it is possible to argue that, while the zygote may not be a person, there is no logical alternative to regarding it as the first stage in human life.[8] At the other end of the scale, there are those who would equate personhood with consciousness, intellect, and with the power to make decisions.[9] There are also relatively few who would support this view,

[4] Though it is, perhaps, surprising how seldom the former is used. In one Scottish study, only 12% of women coming for abortion had used contragestative means to avoid their unwanted pregnancy, and this is the widespread experience: Fatim Lakha and Anna Glazier, 'Unintended Pregnancy and the use of Emergency Contraception' (2006) 368(9549) Lancet 1782.

[5] All of which is exemplified in the European Convention on Human Rights (ECHR), Art 2—'everyone's right to life shall be protected by law'. At what point in life is 'one' a 'person'? Barbara Hewson, 'Dancing on the Head of a Pin? Fetal Life and the European Convention' (2005) 13 Feminist Legal Studies 363.

[6] A cell capable of dividing into any kind of cell.

[7] The structure in early development that develops around day 5.

[8] Although recent advances in in vitro gametogenesis make this claim more complex, see César Palacious-González, John Harris, and Giuseppe Testa, 'Multiplex Parenting: IVG and the Generations to Come' (2014) 40(11) Journal of Medical Ethics 752.

[9] Michael Tooley, 'A Defense of Abortion and Infanticide' in Joel Feinberg (ed.), The Problem of Abortion (Wadsworth 1973); Helga Kuhse and Peter Singer, Should the Baby Live? (OUP 1985); in particular, ch 6. Another valuable discussion of 'personhood' from a rather different aspect is to be found in Mary Ford, 'The Personhood Paradox and the "Right to Die"' (2005) 13(1) Medical Law Review 80.

either, if for no reason other than an intuitive distaste for its natural consequence, which would be to deprive even relatively mature infants, or those in a coma, of a right to be valued as persons.

So, how is the dilemma to be resolved? Many attempts are made to define the point at which the embryo or foetus is morally entitled to, at least, consideration. Within these brackets, for example, the Jewish rabbinical law sets the time as when pregnancy is recognisable externally;[10] the early Christian moralists were attracted to the evidence of life exhibited by quickening[11]—or perceptible foetal movement;[12] and, in more modern terms, there is a widely accepted tendency to accord full protection to the foetus when it is capable of being born alive. The definitional complications of 'viability' are discussed later in this chapter.[13] At this point, we would only remark on the well-appreciated fact that the limits of viability in terms of gestation periods will be steadily lowered as improved neonatal medicine becomes more widely available. Perhaps as an indirect consequence of this, the law, in its search for certainty, draws a bright line at birth.[14] There is no legal personhood in a foetus, but a neonate has all the legal attributes and rights to protection of a 'reasonable creature in being'—and this distinction leads to some anomalous conclusions insofar as it excludes a moral dimension.[15] This was confirmed as a matter of legal principle in *CP (A Child) v Criminal Injuries Compensation Authority*,[16] in which the Court of Appeal held that because a foetus did not constitute a separate legal person, it could not be the victim of the criminal offence of grievous bodily harm. There, a pregnant woman excessively consumed alcohol in the knowledge that it could harm her unborn child. Notwithstanding, on the aforementioned reasoning, a subsequent claim to compensation by the seven-year-old daughter was unsuccessful. In *Criminal Injuries Compensation Authority v Y and Others*,[17] the Court of Appeal reaffirmed that the Criminal Injuries Compensation Act 1995 could not apply to Y, the infant, who was conceived as a result of rape (for which his mother, M, could be compensated), the Court holding that to suggest that Y, who had not been conceived at the time of the crime, was himself a victim of crime, or that it is possible to assess compensation on the postulate that Y would otherwise have been born without disability and so should be compensated for the genetic disorder from which he suffers, is to go beyond that which the Scheme was seeking to cover. An alternative approach can be couched in terms of potential—a human 'organism'[18] acquires humanity when it has the potential to become a human being.

[10] Avraham Steinberg, 'Induced Abortion in Jewish Law' (1980) 1(2) International Journal of Medicine and Law 187. Contrast: Mohammed Ghaly, 'Human Personhood in Contemporary Islamic Bioethical Discourse' [2014] (4) QScience Proceedings Online available at <https://www.qscience.com/content/papers/10.5339/qproc.2014.islamicbioethics.4> accessed on 18 December 2022.

[11] For a discussion of the history of quickening in law, see Catriona McMillan, *The Human Embryo: Breaking the Legal Stalemate* (CUP 2021) Ch 1.

[12] See George Dunstan, 'The Moral Status of the Human Embryo: A Tradition Recalled' (1984) 10(1) Journal of Medical Ethics 38 for a comprehensive review.

[13] Agota Peterfy, 'Fetal Viability as a Threshold to Personhood' (1995) 16(4) Journal of Legal Medicine 607 provides a most interesting overview.

[14] Achas Burin, 'Beyond Pragmatism: Defending the "Bright Line" of Birth' (2014) 22(4) Medical Law Review 494; although this line may be challenged by future technologies, see Elizabeth C Romanis, 'Challenging the Born Alive Threshold: Fetal Surgery, Artificial Wombs, and the English Approach to Legal Personhood' (2020) 28(1) Medical Law Review 93.

[15] But even this provides no absolute certainty—a foetus in the process of being born is not legally 'born' and requires the specific statutory protection of the Infant Life (Preservation) Act 1929—which does not apply in Scotland.

[16] [2014] EWCA Civ 1554.   [17] [2017] EWCA Civ 139.

[18] In *Attorney-General's Reference (No 3 of 1994)* [1998] AC 245 (HL) [256], Lord Mustill was unable to define the status of the foetus and referred to it as 'a unique organism'.

On this basis, the pre-implantation embryo has no potential, and implantation itself represents the critical moral watershed in human development.[19]

This discussion has already shown us that, whatever point we may choose as the marker for the acquisition of personhood, it represents no more than a convenient fare-stage in the continuum of early human development; an embryo in the process of implantation is the same embryo once it has become embedded, and a foetus in utero is the same foetus whether or not it could survive after birth.[20] The only absolute in the saga is that 'human life' as it is generally understood begins with the formation of the human zygote; on this view, the conservative Roman Catholic view represents the only tenable option—the difficulty being that it is also the least practical solution, and calls for the greatest degree of intervention by the law and removal of personal choice from the woman. It is, therefore, appropriate to begin our discussion of the control of fertility with discussion of this fundamental procedure—prevention of the formation of the zygote.

15.3 CONTRACEPTION

15.3.1 CONTRACEPTION AND RISK

There are few moral objections that can be levelled against contraception. While contraception may inhibit the production of a life that might otherwise materialise—an effect which, as we have already noted, is regarded as morally unacceptable by some—it does not involve the *destruction* of human *life* in any of its forms. Problems of a physical nature, however, arise with many forms of contraception which, therefore, should not be undertaken—and, certainly, not imposed—lightly. For these reasons, a brief consideration of the complications is essential.

Common side effects include headaches, nausea, mood swings, breast tenderness, and changes in sex drive.[21] Although oral hormone-based contraception has been refined over the years, there is little doubt that compounds with a high oestrogen content will predispose to intravascular thrombosis (blood clots),[22] and the risks of any form of hormonal contraceptive are increased when their use is combined with smoking (itself a potent cause of cardiovascular disease). A possible association between oral contraceptives and various forms of cancer is still debated; it is being increasingly agreed that there is no unacceptable added risk.[23] The very effective and widely used interceptive methods are also suspect in that, although any such association is certainly not a simple one, they may cause pelvic inflammation and permanent infertility. The formulation of intra-uterine devices (IUDs) has, however, undergone profound change and, in general, IUDs offer rather better protection against pregnancy than do depot hormonal contraceptives.[24] These are, however,

[19] This comes very close to the comparable theological position based on 'ensoulment': Norman Ford, *When Did I Begin?* (CUP 1988).

[20] Sally Sheldon, 'The Regulatory Cliff Between Contraception and Abortion: The Legal and Moral Significance of Implantation' (2015) 41(9) Journal of Medical Ethics 762.

[21] NHS, 'Combined Pill: Your Contraception Guide' (2022) available at <https://www.nhs.uk/conditions/contraception/combined-contraceptive-pill/> accessed 19 December 2022.

[22] Jacques Conard, 'Hormonal Treatments and Thrombosis' in Hau Kwaan and Meyer Samama (eds.), *Clinical Thrombosis* (CRC Press 1989).

[23] For a succinct analysis of the field, see Olav Meirik and Timothy Farley, 'Risk of Cancer and the Oral Contraceptive Pill' (2007) 335(7621) BMJ 621, 622. The US National Cancer Institute, *Oral Contraceptives and Cancer Risk* (2018) is a useful factsheet. The simple answer is that, where there is any increased risk, it is at best slight.

[24] Note that in *Re S (adult patient: sterilisation)* [2001] 3 Fam 15 (CA), the Court preferred the use of the Mirena coil to sterilisation.

mainly aspects of clinical medicine; they are introduced here only to emphasise that non-surgical contraception also has its pitfalls and cannot be *imposed* without forethought.[25]

Amidst the range of effective contraceptives available, we believe it is worth mentioning, in brief, a digital form has emerged in response to the risks discussed: 'femtech'. Femtech is a category of personal health tracking software, primarily used via a smartphone, that is specifically marketed at helping women to manage their reproductive processes. Unlike its contraceptive counterparts, this form of contraception requires no medical intervention or hormone-based medicine. Digital contraception uses an algorithm to calculate when women are in their 'fertile window' (sometimes with the aid of a device, such as a thermometer),[26] and produces a recommendation as to whether the user is likely to get pregnant if they have sex that day or week, on that basis. While popular, particularly among young women, this type of contraceptive has been critiqued for being not only relatively less effective than other forms of contraceptive[27] but also limited in scope in terms of the range of women, in their diversity, that can use it.[28] Digital contraceptives are caught by the medical devices regime[29] under certain circumstances,[30] yet this has been criticised as not going far enough to protect users considering the vulnerable position unwanted pregnancy can leave women in.[31]

Indeed, against this general background of 'risk', it must be remembered that, on a worldwide scale, the risk of death associated with pregnancy is several hundred times that of death associated with contraception.

15.3.2 CONTRACEPTION AND MINORS

The provision of contraceptives to minors was once a burning issue.[32] However, the evolution of educational policy has now stripped it of its urgency. Nevertheless, the dilemma confronting the doctor who is consulted by a female minor requesting contraceptive advice and treatment still merits consideration.[33] The practical problem lies in deciding whether the physician should do anything which might facilitate her engaging in sexual activity.

---

[25] *A Local Authority* v *A (capacity: contraception)* [2011] 3 All ER 706, points also to the practical near-impossibility of enforcing long-term contraception.

[26] Fertile women can typically only get pregnant for six days of their menstrual cycle: see Allen Wilcox, David Dunson, and Donald Baird, 'The Timing of the "Fertile Window" in the Menstrual Cycle: Day Specific Estimates from a Prospective Study' (2000) 321(7271) BMJ 1259.

[27] See, for example, Maryam Mehrnezhad, and Teresa Almeida, 'Caring for Intimate Data in Fertility Technologies' (2021) 409 Proceedings of the 2021 CHI Conference on Human Factors in Computing Systems 1; Marguerite Duane et al., 'The Performance of Fertility Awareness-Based Method Apps Marketed to Avoid Pregnancy' (2016) 29(4) Journal of the American Board of Family Medicine 508; Alexander Freis et al., 'Plausibility of Menstrual Cycle Apps Claiming to Support Conception' (2018) 6 Frontiers in Public Health 98.

[28] See Bethany Corbin, 'Digital Micro-Aggressions and Discrimination: Femtech and the "Othering" of Women' (2019) 44 Nova Law Review 337.

[29] Medical Devices Regulations 2002 (SI 2002/618), as amended. However, any changes to the scheme post-Brexit will be brought through the Medicines and Medical Devices Act 2021.

[30] See MHRA, 'Guidance: Medical Device Stand-Alone Software Including Apps (Including IVDMDs)' (2022) 25, available at <https://www.gov.uk/government/publications/medical-devices-software-applications-apps> accessed 19 December 2022.

[31] For a full discussion of the legal and regulatory issues in the UK, see Catriona McMillan, 'Monitoring Female Fertility Through "Femtech": The Need for a Whole-System Approach to Regulation' (2022) 30(3) Medical Law Review 410.

[32] See National Institute for Health and Care Excellence (NICE), 'Guidelines: Contraceptive services for Under 25s: Public Health Guideline [PH51]' (2014) available at <https://www.nice.org.uk/Guidance/PH51> accessed 19 December 2022.

[33] For interesting insights from Ireland, see Hilary Cronin et al., 'Attitudes of General Practitioners to Prescribing Contraception to Minors—A Medico-Legal Review' (2013) 19 Medico-Legal Journal of Ireland 28.

If the patient is, say, aged 14 or 15, the physician may well view the patient as being too young for sexual intercourse. This disapproval may be based on the view that sexual activity at such an age may lead to emotional trauma and, more obviously, a risk of disease. On the other hand, a refusal to prescribe contraceptives may ultimately be more damaging to the patient in that sexual activity may result in pregnancy—and giving birth to a child, or securing an abortion, at such an age is likely to be severely disruptive of the patient's life.[34] Aside from such 'social' considerations, a decision to provide contraception to a minor poses a number of ethical and legal dilemmas, including whether the physician can proceed without the consent of the parents, the nature and extent of their obligation of confidence to the minor (both explored in Chapter 9), and whether they attract any criminal liability as being a party to an offence of sexual intercourse with a minor.

All these issues were considered in *Gillick v West Norfolk and Wisbech Area Health Authority*,[35] a controversial case (explored in-depth in Chapter 9) that resulted from the publication of a circular by the Department of Health stating that practitioners could, in strictly limited circumstances, discuss and apply family planning measures to minors without the express consent of their parents; Gillick sought, inter alia, to have the instruction declared unlawful. In the absence of any binding authority, the trial judge relied heavily on the common law, and on the Canadian case of *Johnston v Wellesley Hospital*,[36] and concluded that a person below the age of 16 was capable of consent to contraceptive therapy provided she was of sufficient mental maturity to understand the implications. The Court of Appeal, however, concentrated on the duties and rights of parents, which it considered to be inseparable. The trial judge's decision was overturned unanimously. The Authority then appealed to the House of Lords which reverted to what might be loosely termed the 'mature minor' principle—and has come to be known as '*Gillick* competence'—and decided against Gillick by a majority of 3:2. For present purposes, we need only recall the overall tenor of the judgment as expressed by Lord Scarman:

> If the law should impose upon the process of growing up fixed limits where nature knew only a continuous process, the price would be artificiality and a lack of realism in an area where the law must be sensitive to human development and social change.[37]

This interpretation has materialised—social mores have altered and *Gillick* represents the law now even more firmly than it did 25 years ago.

At the same time, Lord Fraser laid down his Delphic 'five points' in which he said that the doctor would be justified in proceeding with contraceptive advice without the parents' consent or even knowledge provided that she was satisfied that the girl:[38]

    (i)   would, although under 16, understand the advice;

    (ii)   could not be persuaded to inform her parents or to allow the doctor to inform the parents that she was seeking contraceptive advice;

---

[34] The under-18 conception rate in 2020 was 13.1 conceptions per 1,000 women, continuing a trend of decreasing conception rates and record lows seen since 2007: Official for National Statistics, 'Conceptions in England and Wales: 2020' (2021) available at <https://www.ons.gov.uk/peoplepopulationandcommunity/birthsdeathsandmarriages/conceptionandfertilityrates/bulletins/conceptionstatistics/2020> accessed 19 December 2022.

[35] [1985] 3 All ER 402 (HL).   [36] (1970) 17 DLR (3d) 139 (ONSC).

[37] *Gillick* (n 35) [421].   [38] ibid. [413].

(iii) was very likely to have sexual intercourse with or without contraceptive treatment;

(iv) was likely to suffer physical or mental health issues unless she received contraceptive advice or treatment; and

(v) should receive, in her best interests, contraceptive advice, treatment, or both without parental consent.

Lord Fraser emphasised that the judgment was not to be regarded as a licence for doctors to disregard the wishes of parents whenever they found it convenient to do so, and he pointed out that any doctor who behaved in such a way would be failing to discharge their professional responsibilities and would be expected to be disciplined by their professional body accordingly.[39] The medical response to the decision was generally one of relief, and the guidelines of the General Medical Council (GMC) now state that the doctor who considers that the patient lacks capacity to give consent to treatment or disclosure, and who has failed to persuade the patient to allow the involvement of an appropriate third party, may disclose relevant information to an appropriate person or authority if it is essential to do so in the patient's medical interests. This, however, is subject to the person without capacity having been told of the intention.[40] It is fair to say, then, that Lord Fraser's guidance is still the template for good medical practice.[41]

The narrowness of the decision in *Gillick* cannot be overlooked—it is noteworthy that, on a simple head count, more judges supported the complainer than opposed her throughout the legal process. But, then, neither can the fact that a new generation has matured since *Gillick* was decided. One has only got to compare the lengthy arguments in *Gillick* with the almost summary dismissal in *R (on the application of Axon) v Secretary of State for Health*,[42] to appreciate the effects of time and custom. It is now fair to say that the sexual connotations of *Gillick* can be relegated to history, and the lasting importance of the case is its transformation of adolescent medical treatment generally, in which contraception plays but a minor role.

15.3.3 CONTRAGESTATION

Certain types of contraception are designed to—or, in practice, do—work after the embryo has formed. They are commonly referred to as interceptive methods, or as emergency contraception, although this is false nomenclature as conception has already occurred,[43] the prime examples being the so-called 'morning after' pill,[44] and the IUD (when it is used for this specific purpose rather than as a barrier). Such methods are designed to prevent the implantation and subsequent development of the embryo, and the question arises as

---

[39] The collateral question of the doctor's criminal liability for giving advice on sexual matters to young girls is now settled. The Sexual Offences Act 2003, s 73, states that a person is not guilty of aiding or abetting childhood sexual activity if, inter alia, the advice given is for the purpose of preventing the girl becoming pregnant.

[40] GMC, '0–18 years: Guidance for all Doctors' (2007) para 48a, available at <https://www.gmc-uk.org/ethical-guidance/ethical-guidance-for-doctors/0-18-years> accessed 19 December 2022.

[41] See Rachel Taylor, 'Reversing the Retreat from *Gillick*? *R (Axon) v Secretary of State for Health*' (2007) 19(1) Child and Family Law Quarterly 81.

[42] [2006] QB 539 (Admin).

[43] Nevertheless, the terminology is in general use and will be well understood.

[44] It has been pointed out that the term 'morning after' implies a spurious sense of urgency; in fact, emergency hormonal contraception need only be instituted within 72 hours of sexual intercourse and there is evidence that this is an over-cautious estimate: Anne Webb, 'Emergency contraception' (2003) 326(7393) BMJ 775.

to whether they offend against the Offences Against the Person Act 1861 which, as we will see, criminalises the procurement of a miscarriage of a woman.[45]

The greater part of the discussion turns on the interpretation of the word 'miscarriage' and whether this relates only to the *displacement* of the already implanted embryo. We find it illogical to suggest that there can be miscarriage in the absence of true carriage. In any event, the issue has now been put beyond doubt. It is currently legal for a pharmacist to dispense 'emergency contraception' without a doctor's prescription,[46] and an application for judicial review of the relevant order has been dismissed on the grounds that we have outlined earlier—interceptive methods of control of pregnancy are plainly excluded from the operation of the 1861 Act.[47]

A clear legal—and, possibly, moral[48]—distinction is, however, to be made between interception and the use of displacing methods that are specifically designed to displace the implanted embryo—the technique that is euphemistically termed 'menstrual extraction' is a common example of the latter while an IUD may also be used for this purpose; its intended function is, essentially, a matter of timing—was the embryo implanted at the time? These techniques are clearly on the same level as 'medical' methods of termination of pregnancy and we return to them later.

15.4 STERILISATION

The aim of sterilisation is to end the patient's reproductive capability. A number of surgical procedures may be used to achieve this. In males, the most common method is vasectomy, in which the vas deferens is cut and tied.[49] Sterilisation in women is usually achieved by division or clipping of the fallopian tubes, which carry the ova between the ovary and the womb.[50] An important feature of both operations from the legal and ethical standpoint is that they are generally intended to be irreversible; although it may be possible to repair the effects of the operation, prospective attempts to allow for reversibility are likely to result in procedures which fail in their primary purpose. Even so, it is generally assumed that a 'sterilisation operation' will bring a basic human function to an end.[51]

Ethical objections to sterilisation usually focus on this irreversibility. Those who object on this ground would argue that the individual may later change their mind and wish to

---

[45] Notably this Act applies to England and Wales only.

[46] The Prescription Only Medicine (Human Use) Amendment (No 3) Order 2000 (SI 2000/3231).

[47] *R (on the application of Smeaton)* v *Secretary of State for Health and Others* (2002) 66 BMLR 59, provides an exhaustive review of the relevant literature at the time. It has, however, been severely criticised by John Keown, '"Morning After" Pills, "Miscarriage" and Muddle' (2005) 25(2) Legal Studies 296. And see Jonathan Montgomery et al., 'Hidden law-making in the province of medical jurisprudence' (2014) 77(2) Modern Law Review 343.

[48] For which, see Valerie Satkoske and Lisa Parker, 'Emergency Contraception Policy: How Moral Commitments Affect Risk Evaluation' (2010) 9(3–4) Law, Probability and Risk 187.

[49] For discussion of the associated issues, Renu Barton-Hanson, 'Sterilization of Men with Intellectual Disabilities: Whose Best Interests is it Anyway?' (2015) 15(1) Medical Law International 49.

[50] Modern techniques rely on the body's self-defences against foreign bodies to seal the tubes: NICE, 'Hysteroscopic Sterilisation by Tubal Cannulation and Placement of Intrafallopian Implants: Interventional Procedures Guidance [IPG315]' (2009) available at <https://www.nice.org.uk/Guidance/IPG315> accessed 19 December 2022.

[51] Current methods, however, allow for reversal of vasectomy—a success rate of up to 40% successful pregnancies is claimed.

return to a reproductive potential which is probably now closed. They would also stress that the decision to sterilise is one which is taken in the midst of subtle social and personal pressures; the likelihood of the decision being entirely free is thereby diminished—yet it is one that cannot easily be retracted.[52] The objection of the Catholic Church is more direct: sterilisation is a mutilation of the body which leads to the deprivation of a natural function and which must, therefore, be rejected unless it is carried out for strictly therapeutic purposes—that is, where it is necessary for the physical health of the patient; the performance of a hysterectomy in the treatment of excessive menstrual bleeding, for example, is admissible.[53]

Insofar as it is possible to identify a lay consensus on the matter, sterilisation is an acceptable method of contraception provided the person undergoing the operation is adequately informed of the implications.[54] The legality of contraceptive sterilisation in the UK is now beyond doubt and would be governed by the general rules of consent (see Chapter 8).[55] It is also clear that the decision is personal to the individual, and the physician owes a duty of care to the patient, not to her spouse or partner, meaning the courts would never grant an injunction to stop a sterilisation or vasectomy.[56] As to the medical attitude to consent, there is no reason to suppose other than that the BMA still regards the routine search for a partner's agreement as being inappropriate—the decision to be sterilised is one for the individual patient.[57] Very strong objections may be voiced, however, when there is any question as to the validity of the patient's consent.

15.4.1 NON-CONSENSUAL STERILISATION AND THE RIGHT TO REPRODUCE

If consensual sterilisation raises ethical misgivings, then non-consensual sterilisation can be seen as a minefield of powerful objection. Neither legislatures nor courts can totally disregard the ghost of the eugenic movement which flourished in the first half of the twentieth century and led to legislative measures in several jurisdictions that provided for the sterilisation of 'mentally handicapped' persons, those suffering from certain forms of genetically transmissible diseases, and even criminal reoffenders. While eugenics on a national scale can now be relegated to history, there remain cases where the non-consensual sterilisation of adults and children with mental disabilities is permissible. We turn to discuss these going forward.

The root problem of non-consensual sterilisation lies in that it sits at odds with what is known as the basic human right to reproduce. The phrase seems to have originated in the US case *Skinner* v *Oklahoma*[58]—which, in fact, concerned the punitive sterilisation of a man—and has, since, come into common usage throughout the English-speaking world. In the UK, the concept was first articulated in the very significant case *Re D (a minor)*,[59] concerning an 11-year-old girl who suffered from a rare condition known as

---

[52] Edward Tuddenham, 'Sterilise in Haste: Repent at Leisure and at Great Expense' (2000) 321 BMJ 962.

[53] The attitude of orthodox Islam is just as rigid: Douwe Verkuyl, 'Two World Religions and Family Planning' (1993) 342(8869) The Lancet 473.

[54] For more on voluntary sterilisation, see Paddy McQueen, 'A Defence of Voluntary Sterilization' (2020) 26 Res Publica 237; and Seljka Buturovic, 'Voluntary Sterilisation of Young Childless Women: Not So Fast' (2019) 48(1) BMJ Journal of Medical Ethics.

[55] Many jurisdictions impose a legal age limit.

[56] *Paton* v *British Pregnancy Advisory Service Trustees* [1978] 2 All ER 987 at 990.

[57] BMA Ethics Department, *Medical Ethics Today* (3rd edn, John Wiley & Sons 2012) p 278.

[58] 316 US 535 (1942).   [59] [1976] 1 All ER 326.

Sotos syndrome, and who had an IQ of roughly 80. Heilbron J summarised her judgment as follows:

> A review of the whole of the evidence leads me to the conclusion that in a case of a child of 11 years of age, where the evidence shows that her mental and physical condition and attainments have already improved, and where her future prospects are as yet unpredictable, where the evidence also shows that she is unable as yet to understand and appreciate the implications of this operation and could not give valid or informed consent, that the likelihood is that in later years she will be able to make her own choice, where, I believe, the frustration and resentment of realising (as she would one day) what happened could be devastating, an operation of this nature is, in my view contra-indicated.[60]

She assumed that there was a 'basic human right of a woman to reproduce' and concluded that it would be a violation of that right if a girl were sterilised for non-therapeutic reasons without her consent.

Re B (a minor) (wardship: sterilisation) was the first of its kind to reach the house of Lords. It is unfortunate from the comparative perspective that *Re B* concerned a girl aged 17—she would shortly have passed out of the wardship jurisdiction and it was agreed that the *parens patriae* authority no longer applied in England to an adult.[61] A speedy decision was, thus, dictated, and there is no doubt that Lord Hailsham LC, on it being suggested that the girl's progress could well be observed for a year, laid open his defences when he said, 'We shall be no wiser in twelve months than we are now.'[62] B had a diagnosis of epilepsy and was said to have a mental age of five to six years. She had never conceived and was not pregnant but, absent being fully institutionalised, those caring for her considered she was in danger of becoming so. Medical opinion—which, in contrast to that given in *Re D*, was scarcely challenged—was that either she would have to be maintained on hormonal contraceptives for the rest of her reproductive life or her fallopian tubes could be occluded—and the court accepted this as being an irreversible procedure. It was common ground between the parties that any pregnancy that occurred would have to be terminated.

In authorising sterilisation, the House of Lords upheld the decisions of the court of first instance and the Court of Appeal. Lord Oliver emphasised that there was no question of a eugenic motive, no consideration was paid to the convenience of those caring for the ward, and no general principle of public policy was involved; the basic principle involved was the welfare of the girl.

Re B was widely criticised in the British academic literature, in particular for its failure to recognise the reproductive rights of individuals with mental disabilities.[63] Lord Hailsham, in addressing the question of rights,[64] stated:

> The right [of a woman to reproduce] is only such when reproduction is the result of informed choice of which the ward in the present case is incapable.[65]

---

[60] ibid. [335].

[61] Graeme Laurie, '*Parens Patriae* Jurisdiction in the Medico-Legal Context: The Vagaries of Judicial Activism' (1999) 3 Edinburgh Law Review 96.

[62] *Paton* (n 56) [212].

[63] Robert Lee and Derek Morgan, 'Sterilisation and Mental Handicap: Sapping the Strength of the State?' (1988) 15(3) Journal of Law & Society 229; Jonathan Montgomery, 'Rhetoric and "Welfare"' (1989) 9(3) Oxford Journal of Legal Studies 395.

[64] The problem of rights under the Human Rights Act 1998, Sch 1 may yet arise: see Emily Jackson, *Regulating Reproduction: Law, Technology and Autonomy* (Hart Publishing 2001) p 57.

[65] *Paton* (n 56) [213].

And:

> To talk of the 'basic right' to reproduce of an individual who is not capable of knowing the causal connection between intercourse and childbirth . . . [or who] is unable to form any maternal instincts or to care for a child, appears to me wholly to part company with reality.[66]

The concept of a right to reproduce is one which deserves discussion in depth but which we cannot provide in the space available. Put simplistically, it is not easy to envisage a right that requires the cooperation of another person who is under no obligation to provide it; moreover, an absolute right to reproduce would entail access by right to all means of assisted reproduction, including surrogate motherhood by way of womb-leasing—and this is clearly untenable.[67] Grubb and Pearl argued convincingly that the only such right currently recognised in English law is the right to choose whether or not to reproduce—this being grounded in the principle of individual autonomy.[68]

An alternative approach is to regard the 'right' as one to retain the capacity to reproduce. Such a right could well be subsumed within Article 8 (right to respect for private and family life) and Article 12 (right to marry and found a family) of the European Convention on Human Rights (ECHR). Indeed, the European Court of Human Rights (ECtHR) has recognised violations of Article 8 and Article 3 for failures to obtain informed consent for a sterilisation operation, especially where the operation was undertaken on an individual within a minoritised group.[69] Any court interference with that right would, then, have to be justified under Article 8(2) as a proportionate means to pursue a legitimate aim. This suggests some form of recognition of the right to reproduce, even if not couched in those terms.

Non-consensual Sterilisation of Women

Thus far, we have only discussed cases regarding minors where there was no doubt, at the time, of the courts' authority to make decisions about them under the wardship jurisdiction. The sterilisation of an adult considered to lack capacity to consent to treatment was first addressed in *T v T*,[70] a case which involved a 19-year-old woman said to born with a 'severe mental handicap' and who had significant daily care needs. Medical opinion was consistent that the pregnancy should be terminated under the terms of the Abortion Act 1967, and there was an additional application from her mother for her to be sterilised at the time of the termination. In the course of a wide-ranging determination, which had to be made in the absence of precedent, Wood J fell back on the expedient of an anticipatory declaration that the performance of the two operations would not be unlawful[71]—a solution which was later approved in House of Lords case *Re F (mental patient: sterilisation)*.[72]

Re F was concerned largely with court procedure. Nevertheless, it forms the basis for the 'best interests' test which is now an integral part of British medical jurisprudence; even if only for this reason, it still merits attention. The conditions of *Re B* were, effectively, replicated save that F, aged 36 at the time, was beyond the protection of wardship.

---

[66] ibid. [213]. For an opposing opinion, albeit at first instance, see *A Local Authority v K* [2013] EWHC 242 (COP).

[67] *Briody v St Helens and Knowsley Area Health Authority* [2002] 2 WLR 394 [404]–[405] (Hale LJ).

[68] Andrew Grubb and David Pearl, 'Sterilisation and the Courts' (1987) 46(3) Cambridge Law Journal 439. See also Nicholson CJ in the Australian case *Re Jane* (1989) FLC 92–007, who reasoned very similarly to that in *Re B*. Reproductive autonomy has been re-examined extensively by Emily Jackson (n 64), Ch 1.

[69] See e.g. *VC v Slovakia* [2011] WLUK 208, concerning non-consensual sterilisation of a Roma woman; see also *YP v Russia* (43399/13).

[70] [1988] 1 All ER 613.   [71] RSC Ord 15, r 16.   [72] [1990] 2 AC 1.

The lower courts tended to justify the operation on somewhat negative grounds—for instance:

- that treatments provided in a patient's best interests lay within the exceptions to the law of battery;[73]

- that there was nothing incongruous in doctors and others who had a caring responsibility being required to act in the interests of an adult who was unable to exercise a right of choice,[74] or;

- that the performance of a necessary, albeit serious, operation, including an operation for sterilisation, on a patient who could not consent would not be a trespass to the person or otherwise unlawful.[75]

The correctness of the decision to sterilise F was not challenged in the House of Lords, which was concerned primarily with the resolution of questions of law and of legal procedure. The most important aspect of the decision for our purposes was to establish that the common law provides that a doctor can lawfully give surgical or medical treatment to adult patients who are judged to lack capacity to consent, provided that the operation or treatment is in their best interests. The House of Lords held that it would be in their best interests if, but only if, it was carried out in order to save their lives or to ensure improvement, or prevent deterioration, in their physical or mental health.[76] Logically, this authority would also apply to sterilisation but six reasons were given for requiring special conditions for that operation—including its general irreversibility which would almost certainly deprive the woman of 'what was widely, and rightly, regarded as one of the fundamental rights of a woman, the right to bear a child'.[77]

At the same time, however, the House of Lords held that, whether the 'best interests' test had been met would be judged on *Bolam* principles,[78] and it seemed at the time that, having made a bid for judicial supervision, the Court, in so stating, effectively handed back control of the decisions to the doctors. The matter has, however, now been resolved and, the current Practice Direction makes it clear that sterilisation of a person who cannot consent to the operation is one of those special types of case that will require the prior sanction of a judge in virtually every instance.[79]

The precedent set by *Re F* is that, because the details of each case differ, decisions of this nature will continue to be made on a case-to-case basis. With that in mind, it is

[73] Per Scott Baker J, citing Goff LJ in *Collins v Wilcock* [1984] 3 All ER 374. These were devised, in the main, to cover the exigencies of everyday life, but Lord Donaldson MR found this a step too far.

[74] ibid. [18] (Lord Donaldson MR).

[75] ibid. [32] (Neill LJ).

[76] ibid. [55] (Lord Brandon). Note that this definition would now be too narrow to satisfy the terms of the Mental Capacity Act 2005, s 4(2) (see also Chapter 10).

[77] These historic cases now do little more than emphasise how they effectively implanted the 'best interests' or 'welfare' principle as the legal control of non-consensual treatment in adults. It has now been accepted as the cornerstone of the Mental Capacity Act 2005, ss 1(5) and 4, which would include therapeutic sterilisation.

[78] *Bolam v Friern Hospital Management Committee* [1957] 2 All ER 118 (HL).

[79] *Practice Note (Official Solicitor: Declaratory Proceedings: Medical and Welfare Decisions for Adults who Lack Capacity)* [2006] 2 FLR 373; it is to be emphasised that this note deals only with adults. The other situation is the discontinuation of nutrition and hydration of a person in a vegetative state (see Chapter 17). For Scotland, see Adults with Incapacity (Specified Medical Treatments) (Scotland) Regulations 2002, Sch 1 (SSI 2002/275). Note that the Code of Practice on the Mental Capacity Act 2005 repeats advice that a court order is to be obtained in all cases of non-therapeutic sterilisation.

useful to follow the fate of some of the cases that have subsequently been decided. *Re HG*[80] concerned a 17-year-old girl who was epileptic and suffered from an unspecified chromosomal abnormality. There was no dispute that pregnancy would be disastrous for her, and the contraceptive pill was unsuitable due to her epilepsy. In making the order, the Deputy Judge held:

> [My conclusion is that] a sufficiently overwhelming case has been established to justify interference with the fundamental right of a woman to bear a child. I am certainly satisfied that it would be cruel to expose [her] to an unacceptable risk of pregnancy and that that should be obviated by sterilisation in her interests.[81]

The adult patient in *Re W*[82] was also an epileptic who, again, was at small risk of becoming pregnant. Nevertheless, sterilisation was held to be in her best interests and a declaration was granted. A feature of the case was the reliance on *Bolam* as a measure of 'best interests'—an aspect that came in for some criticism.[83]

The Practice Note relevant at the time, however, specifically advised that a declaration in favour of non-consensual sterilisation should be granted only if there was a real danger rather than a mere chance of pregnancy resulting[84]—and this was reflected in *Re LC (medical treatment: sterilisation)*,[85] which seems to have been the first case since *Re D* in which sterilisation was refused in the face of medical opinion. The danger to the woman was, however, not so much that of pregnancy as of sexual assault—and the latter risk was present irrespective of her fertility. One notable feature was that the care afforded her was exceptional, and this, of itself, was thought to provide a good ground for not imposing the risks of a surgical intervention.

In 1998, two further cases were heard. In the first of these,[86] Johnson J found the circumstances to be indistinguishable from those in *Re LC* in that the risk of pregnancy was speculative rather than real. This aspect of the case was independent of any 'right to reproduce' which, it was agreed, was irrelevant in *Re B* terms.[87] The freedom from risk, however, was again due to the care expended by the woman's parents; it is probably this factor which mainly caused the judge to reach his conclusion and to follow *Re LC* 'with reluctance'. Thus, it seemed that a group of cases were being separated which depended on the immediacy of the risk of pregnancy. This was confirmed from the other side of the coin in *Re X (adult: sterilisation)*,[88] in which the woman concerned actually wanted to have a baby—sterilisation was authorised when it was agreed that she would have been incapable of looking after it.

All the cases thus far have been related to the person without capacity's way of life or best (social) interests, although it is arguable that the potential interests of the child where the woman is considered incapable of looking after them also play a role. At the same time, however, a line of cases was developing which referred to the subject's medical interests. The solution of some such cases will be obvious—clearly, for example, it would not

---

[80] *Re HG (specific issue order: sterilisation)* [1993] 1 FLR 587. The case is interesting in that, for financial reasons, the parents sought a specific issue order under the Children Act 1989, s 8. It was held that this was an appropriate, albeit not ideal, way of proceeding.

[81] ibid. [592].   [82] *Re W (mental patient: sterilisation)* [1993] 1 FLR 381.

[83] See Ian Kennedy, 'Commentary' (1993) 1(3) Medical Law Review 234.

[84] Practice Note (Official Solicitor: Sterilisation) [1993] 3 All ER 222.

[85] [1997] 2 FLR 258 (judgment in the case was given in October 1993).

[86] *Re S (medical treatment: adult sterilisation)* [1998] 1 FLR 944.

[87] See dicta of Lord Oliver and Lord Hailsham in that case. Johnson J did not feel the same way about the House of Lords' somewhat cavalier attitude to the risks of surgical operation.

[88] [1998] 2 FLR 1124.

be essential to obtain court approval before undertaking a hysterectomy in the treatment of carcinoma of the uterus despite the fact that the patient would be rendered infertile as a secondary effect.[89] Difficulty arises when the issue in question relates to menstruation, which could range from heavy and painful periods to the individual being caused distress by what would be considered a normal period. Sterilisation is a high price to pay for treating what may well have been, in ordinary circumstances, a comparatively simple menstrual disorder or, even, no more than a 'phobia'.

In the first such case, *Re E (a minor) (medical treatment)*,[90] concerning a 17-year-old, Sir Stephen Brown held that no formal consent of the court was necessary and that the parents were in a position to give a valid consent: 'A clear distinction is to be made between an operation to be performed for a genuine therapeutic reason and one to achieve sterilisation.'[91] This easy assurance in face of a significant operation is a little hard to accept. The matter came before the Court of Appeal once again in *Re S (adult patient: sterilisation)*.[92] Here, alternative methods of treatment were available and had been advocated. Wall J, at first instance, regarded S's menstrual problems as the most important issue and followed Bennett J in *Re Z*[93] in concluding that S's best interests lay in a subtotal hysterectomy rather than in the insertion of a coil—a procedure which, of itself, did not require court approval. Having declared the hysterectomy to be lawful, he then adopted the rather innovative strategy of leaving the choice of treatments to S's mother and her medical advisers in consultation.

The Court of Appeal was highly, and perhaps unfairly, critical of Wall J's decision, pointing out that the judge had run contrary to unanimous medical opinion. The declaration in favour of hysterectomy was reversed in favour of the insertion of a coil, with the option of a further hearing should this not prove an effective remedy. The Court of Appeal was unanimous in holding that any interpretation of Sir Stephen Brown's ruling on the need for involvement of the courts in cases such as these 'should incline towards the strict and avoid the liberal'[94]—a form of words which carries a ring of euphemism.

Contraception and sterilisation sit on the same spectrum of interference with reproductive capacity, albeit with one self-evidently far closer to an extreme than the other. Often, however, both options can be in play and sometimes favoured differently by different parties for different reasons. This was the case in *A Local Authority* v *K*,[95] which involved a 21-year-old woman with Down's syndrome and learning difficulties (and, unlike the cases discussed, was decided under the Mental Capacity Act 2005). K's parents sought medical advice to support their wish that she be sterilised in her own best interests. Her case came to the attention of a Matron for Safeguarding Vulnerable Adults, who sought further medical advice that contraception through the fitting of a coil was the preferable, least restrictive, course of action and so more in line with the woman's best interests. A best interest meeting took place with the local authority and all of the parties, and the conclusion was that non-therapeutic sterilisation was not in K's best interests; the parents then threatened to take K abroad and the action was raised by the local authority for a declaration once the parents gave an undertaking not to remove their daughter from the jurisdiction.

---

[89] But circumstances may make it highly desirable to do so. For an illustrative decision, see *DH NHS Foundation Trust* v *PS* (2010) 116 BMLR 142 (carcinoma of the uterus—the special condition being the potential use of force). Also see *University Hospital Coventry and Warwickshire NHS Trust v K & Anor* [2020] EWCOP 31, where a young woman (K) without capacity required urgent cancer treatment that would trigger menopause (in effect, sterilising her). Notwithstanding the consensus that existed between clinicians and K's mother, Haydn J endorsed a pre-emptive application to the court by the Trust.

[90] (1992) 7 BMLR 117.   [91] ibid. [119].   [92] [2000] 3 WLR 1288.

[93] (2000) 53 BMLR 53.   [94] *Re S* (n 92).   [95] [2013] EWHC 242 (COP).

To begin, the court determined the criteria for assessing the question of K's capacity to take contraception decisions by herself,[96] and concluded, based on those criteria, that she did not have capacity and therefore best interests fell to be considered. The court then took the opportunity to reiterate its role and the appropriate approach in such difficult cases. In stressing the serious nature of non-therapeutic sterilisation, the court reminded the parties of the need for court approval in all such applications (through the Court of Protection, as discussed in Chapter 10), and for the importance of prior consultation with the Official Solicitor's department. In addition to further procedural safeguards, the court stressed the importance of least restrictive approach as a matter of human right: was sterilisation a necessary and proportionate interference? As to best interests, the court tried to strike a balance between protection and empowerment, and after considering the nature, risks and consequences of both procedures, concluded that sterilisation in this case would be a disproportionate step at the time to achieve contraception for K. It would be lawful to attempt less restrictive methods of contraception than sterilisation.

We can contrast the *K* case with *Mental Health Trust & Ors* v *DD*,[97] in which sterilisation was considered to be in D's best interests in preference to other forms of contraception. D was a 36-year-old woman with Autistic Spectrum Disorder and an IQ of 70. She had six children, aged between six months and 12 years, none of whom had any continuing contact with their mother. D was in a long-term loving and sexual relationship with BC, who had an IQ of 62. This ruling was the culmination of a series of hearing about D's circumstances relating to her sixth pregnancy, and involving questions of her capacity for the use of short-term contraception before, at, and post-delivery of her child. Matters had clearly reached a head, and the court here was concerned, primarily, with D's capacity to take decisions on long-term contraception/non-therapeutic sterilisation, and the nature of best interests if capacity was found to be lacking. On this very point, the court followed unanimous medical opinion that D lacked capacity both with respect to contraception, and the more serious intervention of sterilisation.

As to best interests in *DD*, the court acknowledged that any proposed intervention would interfere with D's Article 8(1) ECHR rights, and so could only be justified in terms of Article 8(2) as necessary and proportionate. Thus—as a matter of broad legal approach—this perfectly mirrors *K*. On the facts, however, the conclusion was radically different. A central concern was the risk of future pregnancies in two senses: first, that D would have yet more children for whom she could not care, but more importantly, that further pregnancies would themselves pose serious risks, including uterine rupture, placenta previa, and a thrombotic event, all of which led the Official Solicitor to suggest a risk of about 70% of a life-threatening event. Against this, the court was cognisant of its statutory duty (under section 1(6) of the 2005 Act) to have 'regard' to the less restrictive intervention with respect to impact on a person's rights and freedoms. In doing so, Mr Justice Cobb acknowledged that sterilisation was by no means the least restrictive medical measure, but that best interests admit a wider set of considerations. In particular, he opined that sterilisation would free D from repeated examinations and interventions that would necessarily accompany the use of a contraceptive coil. And, in a thorough execution of

---

[96] Relying on *A (Capacity: Refusal of Contraception)* [2010] EWHC 1549 (Fam), it identified the criteria as the ability to weigh up the following factors: (i) the reason for contraception and what it did; (ii) the types of contraception available and their uses; (iii) the advantages and disadvantages of each type; (iv) possible side effects; (v) how easily each type could be changed; and (vi) the generally accepted effectiveness of each type.

[97] [2015] EWCOP 4. This was the culmination of a series of cases relating to D's pregnancy, the others being *Mental Health Trust & Ors* v *DD* [2014] EWCOP 8, [2014] EWCOP 11, [2014] EWCOP 13, and [2014] EWCOP 44.

the balance sheet approach[98] that listed the pros and cons of each possible intervention, the ultimate conclusion was that sterilisation was in D's best interests, assisted by 'two factors of "magnetic" importance':

(i) Future pregnancy poses such a high risk to DD's life that the option which most effectively reduces the prospects of this should be preferred; this is one of those exceptional cases where medical necessity justifies the considerable interference.

(ii) Sterilisation is the treatment which most closely coincides with DD's dominant wishes and feelings to be left alone to enjoy a 'normal' life free from intrusion by health and social services.

These two cases represent extreme opposite ends of the contraception/sterilisation spectrum, but they confirm the same points of fundamental legal principle: the outcome of the best interests test will turn on the particular facts of a case. Nonetheless, whether one agrees that the final step of authorising non-therapeutic sterilisation can *ever* by justified will remain a point of central concern.

Non-consensual Sterilisation of Men

Our final case concerns something that we once thought would never happen—the non-consensual, non-therapeutic sterilisation of a *male* adult without capacity. In *An NHS Trust* v *DE*,[99] declarations were sought on the lawfulness of non-therapeutic sterilisation in relation to D, a man who had learning difficulties, lived with his parents, but had a child with a woman in 2009, leading to concerns about his ability to consent to sex. This resulted in him being under constant supervision, and this in turn severely restricted his freedoms. D was very clear that he did not want any more children, and it was accepted that he lacked capacity with respect to decisions about contraceptives. His parents were of the view that it was in his best interests to have a vasectomy, and the case turned on (i) his capacity to consent to such a procedure, and (ii) whether this would be in his best interests in the absence of capacity. Having held that there was no capacity, the court's view on best interests was—once again—entirely driven by the particular facts. Relevant considerations here were that: D was in a loving relationship with a woman and it was important for him that this continue; there was a sexual element that would be supported by this course of action; the birth of another child (and its removal) would distress his partner and jeopardise the relationship; D himself had been clear that he did not want another child; and D wished to remain with his parents while enjoying his previously hard-won independence. All of this led to the view that the only way to preserve this situation was by way of a vasectomy, with the court stating: 'it is both the entitlement and in the best interests of any person with significant disabilities (whether learning or physical), that they be given such support as will enable them to be as much an integral part of society as can reasonably be achieved'.[100]

From this discussion, it is evident that the non-consensual sterilisation of individuals (both adults and minors) with mental disabilities is legally permissible as long as it is sanctioned as being in their best interests. Despite the run of cases discussed, in recent years their appearance has been less frequent, with cases in the Court of Protection often focusing on capacity to engage in sexual relations themselves, rather than a need for sterilisation to prevent the consequences of such relations. Equally, the range of protections

[98] For discussion see Camilia Kong et al., 'An Aide Memoire for a Balancing Act? Critiquing The "Balance Sheet" Approach to Best Interests Decision-Making' (2020) 28(4) Medical Law Review 753.
[99] (2013) 133 BMLR 123.   [100] ibid. [94].

and safeguards is extensive, and none of these cases depart from the central legal principle of the paramountcy of best interests and its all-encompassing nature. Still, we confess to a residual degree of disquiet when the ever-expanding nature of this test seems to know no limits as to which considerations can be added to the mix to (potentially) justify not only diametrically opposing outcomes but significant interferences with the reproductive liberty of individuals with disabilities.[101]

15.5 TERMINATION OF PREGNANCY

The abortion debate is one that is centred on morality and ethics. Any legal argument is confined to how, and to what extent, the ethics should be constrained by the law. The passing of the Abortion Act 1967 did, however, exercise a profound and direct influence on the medical ethos. Once the Act was accepted by doctors, the profession abrogated a main tenet of its Hippocratic conscience. The Declaration of Geneva 1948 was amended in 1994 to state, 'I will maintain the utmost respect for human life' (replacing the old provision, which stated, 'I will maintain the utmost respect for human life from its beginning'). This shift is also evident in the Declaration of Oslo 1970, as amended, which now adds: 'Diversity of response to this situation [circumstances which bring the vital interests of a mother into conflict with the vital interests of her unborn child] results from the diversity of attitudes towards the life of the unborn child. This is a matter of individual conviction and conscience.' This ethical watershed has spilled over to influence the attitudes of doctors towards all aspects of life and death; as discussed in Chapter 17, modern medicine now clearly accommodates the concept of death as a therapeutic option.

In the wider context, however, attitudes to abortion depend almost entirely on where the holder stands in respect of, on the one hand, the foetal interest in life and, on the other, a woman's right to control her own body, and it is this which perpetuates a near intractable moral conflict with which the law must come to terms—and, until recently, it has singularly failed to do so. An opportunity to define the moral status of the foetus arose in *Attorney-General's Reference (No 3 of 1994),*[102] a case of fatal foetal injury resulting from an attack on its mother. However, the House of Lords' only concession to recognition of foetal interests was to accept (overriding the Court of Appeal) that the foetus was more than an adjunct of its mother; it then, however, declined to elaborate on what its status was.[103] It is true to say that harm to the foetus *before* birth can be actionable *after* birth; even so, the subsequent live birth is an essential prerequisite.[104] This means that any protection provided by the common law is, essentially, protection of the neonate. An antenatal foetal right to life is recognised in the criminalisation of child destruction. Again, however, any recognition of foetal interests under this head is indirect, as the relevant legislation was enacted primarily to close a gap in the law of infanticide. Nowhere is there any mention of feticide as an offence per se, and it is against this background that we must consider the development of abortion law in the UK and Ireland.

---

[101] Renu Barton-Hanson (n 49); Sam Rowlands and Jean-Jacques Amy, 'Involuntary Sterilisation: We Still Need to Guard Against it' (2018) 44 BMJ Sexual & Reproductive Health 233.

[102] [1998] AC 245 (HL).

[103] For discussion of the case, see Mary Seneviratne, 'Pre-Natal Injury and Transferred Malice: The Invented Other' (1996) 59(6) Modern Law Review 884, and John K Mason, '"A Lords" Eye View of Fetal Status' (1999) 3 Edinburgh Law Review 246.

[104] *Burton* v *Islington Health Authority, de Martell* v *Merton and Sutton Health Authority* [1993] QB 204; *Hamilton* v *Fife Health Board* 1993 SLT 624. See Adrian Whitfield, 'Common Law Duties to Unborn Children' (1993) 1(1) Medical Law Review 28.

15.5.1 THE EVOLUTION AND STATE OF BRITISH ABORTION LAW

Offences Against the Person Act 1861

The fundamental law in England and Wales lies in sections 58 and 59 of the Offences Against the Person Act 1861. The Act proscribes procuring the miscarriage of a woman by a third party, self-induced miscarriage, attempted procurement of miscarriage, and supplying the means to do so.[105] It is to be noted that the word 'abortion' appears only in the marginal note to the sections,[106] and the offences can also apply to the late insertion of an IUD, although challenges arise as to the certainty of the pregnancy in such situations.[107] This was demonstrated in an unreported case which involved a charge under section 58 of the 1861 Act against a doctor who fitted a contraceptive coil to his secretary some 11 days after they had had intercourse.[108] The judge, having heard gynaecological evidence that implantation would not have occurred, withdrew the case from the jury on the ground that the woman could not have been pregnant 'in the true sense of the word'. He is also reported as saying, 'Only at the completion of implantation does the embryo become a foetus. At this stage, she can be regarded as pregnant'.[109]

The question of what would be the result if an IUD were to be fitted after the 11th day post-intercourse remains open, but it seems unlikely that a prosecution would succeed—the difficulty of proving intent would be almost insurmountable. Whatever may be the true situation in England and Wales, it is apparent that a prosecution in these circumstances for the common law crime of procuring an abortion could not succeed in Scotland, where proof of pregnancy is essential to a successful prosecution for that offence.

The Act makes no distinction between criminal and therapeutic activity and, despite frequent scrutiny, these sections have not been repealed. It is, however, important to note that there is still no engagement of foetal interests. Criminalisation of procuring the miscarriage of a woman was undoubtedly intended for the protection of *women's* health—once again, no direct concern for the foetus was shown.

The first statutory variation is to be found in the Infant Life (Preservation) Act 1929, which introduced the offence of child destruction or causing the death of a child capable of being born alive before it has an existence independent of its mother. There is no offence, however, if the act was done in good faith for the purpose only of preserving the mother's life. This meagre concession, in the main, served only to decriminalise killing the infant in the event of an impacted labour. It was left to *R v Bourne*[110] to temper the legal influence on medical practice in the field. Bourne performed an abortion, with no attempt at secrecy, on a 15-year-old girl who was pregnant following a rape. Although

---

[105] But limited to some 'thing'—e.g. not by coercion or fraud: *R v Ahmed* [2011] QB 512, CCA.

[106] The distinction, if any, between 'miscarriage' and 'abortion' is of academic interest in relation to pre-implantation methods of contraception. Some writers believe the terms to be interchangeable: John Keown, '"Miscarriage": A Medico-Legal Analysis' (1984) Criminal Law Review 604. We believe that 'abortion' implies interference, whereas miscarriage is a natural misfortune.

[107] *R v Price* [1968] 2 All ER 282. The conviction was quashed on the ground of a misdirection.

[108] *R v Dhingra* (Daily Telegraph, 25 January 1991) p 5. The case was quoted with approval in *R (on the application of Smeaton) v Secretary of State for Health and Others* (2002) 66 BMLR 59, but that case was not concerned with mechanical displanting methods.

[109] He may have been attentive to the terms of the Human Fertilisation and Embryology Act 1990, s 2(3) which states that '*For the purposes of this Act*, a woman is not to be treated as carrying a child until the embryo has become implanted.' The emphasis is added but the wording could be persuasive in other branches of the law.

[110] [1938] 3 All ER 615.

Bourne was indicted under the Offences Against the Person Act 1861, Macnaghten J took the opportunity to link the 1861 and 1929 statutes and ruled that, in a case brought under the 1861 Act, the burden rested on the Crown to satisfy the jury that the defendant did not procure the miscarriage of the girl in good faith for the purpose only of preserving her life: the word 'unlawful' in the 1861 Act 'imports the meaning expressed by the proviso in section 1(1) of the Infant Life (Preservation) Act 1929'.[111] The summing-up essentially recognised that a woman's life depended upon her physical and mental health, and that an abortion was not unlawful if it was performed because these were in jeopardy. Bourne was acquitted and the law and the medical profession then lived in harmony for many years; the *Bourne* decision was undoubtedly stretched to the limits of interpretation by many doctors, but the authorities turned a sympathetic eye.[112]

The Abortion Act 1967

But it is never a good thing for any section of the public to flirt with illegality; moreover, there was still no authority for termination of the pregnancy in the event of a serious disability of the child. The situation was resolved with the adoption of the Abortion Act 1967 (which, despite repeated attacks, remained unchanged until amended by section 37 of the Human Fertilisation and Embryology Act 1990). In summary, section 1(1) of the 1967 Act states that a person shall not be guilty of an offence when a pregnancy is terminated by a registered medical practitioner, and two registered medical practitioners have formed the opinion in good faith that:

(a) the continuance of the pregnancy would involve risk, greater than if the pregnancy were terminated, of injury to the physical or mental health of the pregnant woman or any existing children of her family;[113]

(b) there is a risk of grave permanent injury to the physical or mental health of the pregnant woman;

(c) the continuance of the pregnancy would involve risk to the life of the pregnant woman greater than if the pregnancy were terminated; or

(d) there is a substantial risk that, if the child were born, it would suffer from such physical or mental abnormalities as to be severely handicapped.

Though the therapeutic and social grounds articulated in section 1(1)(a) are subject to the pregnancy not having exceeded its 24th week, the justifications in sections 1(1)(b), (c) and (d) are now free of such temporal restriction. Subsections (b) and (c) are, additionally, not restricted by requiring the opinion of two registered medical practitioners; single practitioners may operate on their own initiative in such circumstances.[114]

[111] ibid. [617], [619].

[112] It is interesting to compare the historical attitudes in England with those prevailing in Scotland, where procuring a woman's miscarriage has always been a common law offence. The difference in concern lies in the emphasis laid in Scots law on 'evil intent' as a measure of criminality; there is little doubt that *Bourne* would have been unlikely to provoke a test case in Scotland. Indeed, it is arguable that there was no need to extend the Act to Scotland, but its inclusion was justified in that it removed any doubt as to the limits of therapeutic abortion in that country where, in effect, a policy similar to that recognised in *Bourne* had been openly followed for decades.

[113] These therapeutic and social grounds account for the vast majority of all abortions performed: UK Government, 'Abortion statistics, England and Wales: 2021' (2022) available at <https://www.gov.uk/government/statistics/abortion-statistics-for-england-and-wales-2021/abortion-statistics-england-and-wales-2021> accessed 19 December 2022.

[114] It is to be noted that s 1(1)(b) contains no comparative element—there simply has to be a risk and it is arguable that pregnancy always carries such a risk, even though it is minimal.

Termination under the 1967 Act may be carried out in National Health Service (NHS) hospitals or in places approved for the purpose by the Minister or the Secretary of State (section 1(3)). The advent of termination of pregnancies via 'medical methods' has dictated a change in the location rules, which are now relaxed for this purpose.[115] While it was held in *British Pregnancy Advisory Service* v *Secretary of State for Health*[116] that the courts will not sanction any further extension on the basis of semantic wrangling, it should be noted that legislators have now—in recognition of the realities of women's lives, the difficulty of securing multiple surgery visits, and the immediacy of the effects of these abortifacient drugs—decided to change the rules on abortion by legalising the home-use of early medical abortion pills; in essence allowing women to take the second of the two pills in the clinic or in their own home.[117] During the Covid-19 pandemic, telemedical abortion (where the patient takes both pills at home, normally received by post after a telephone or virtual consultation) was available due to the severe restriction in access to services. While this was originally introduced as a temporary measure, in 2022 both the Scottish Government and Westminster[118] made this permanently available for those where the pregnancy has not exceeded ten weeks.[119]

As noted, the vast majority of legal terminations are performed under section 1(1)(a) of the 1967 Act for minor therapeutic or social reasons. It is arguable that the risks of an abortion to the health of a woman are always less than those of a full-term pregnancy—particularly if the termination is carried out in the first trimester,[120] and that now at least half the terminations carried out in the UK are 'medical' in nature. Equally, it is obvious that the mental health of a woman who is carrying an unwanted pregnancy must suffer more damage if she is forced to carry her foetus than it would if she were relieved of her burden. Simple economics dictate that a *risk* to the well-being of any existing members of the family is occasioned by the advent of another mouth to feed. The indications are, therefore, that it is impossible for a doctor to perform an abortion in Great Britain[121] that can be shown to have been unlawful, provided that all the administrative conditions are met.[122]

As a corollary, the doctor who applies the letter of the law must always be acting in good faith—indeed, possibly the only way in which a termination can be carried out in *bad* faith is when it is done without the woman's consent.[123]

---

[115] Section 1(3A).   [116] [2011] 3 All ER 1012.

[117] In October 2017, the Scottish Government recognised that it could be safely taken outside of a clinical setting, and claimed that a legislative change did not need to occur because it came within its power under the Abortion Act 1967. The Welsh Government followed suit in June 2018. See Jonathan Lord et al., 'Early Medical Abortion: Best Practice now Lawful in Scotland and Wales but not Available to Women in England' (2018) 44(3) BMJ Sexual & Reproductive Health 153; Allie Nawrat, 'Abortion in England: Legalising Home Medical Abortion pills' (Pharmaceutical Technology, 28 August 2018) available at <https://www.pharmaceutical-technology.com/analysis/abortion-in-england-home-use-pills/> accessed 19 December 2022. See generally Jordan Parsons and Elizabeth Chloe Romanis, *Early Medical Abortion, Equality of Access, and the Telemedical Imperative* (OUP 2021).

[118] Health and Care Act 2022, s 178 amends s 1 of the Abortion Act 1967.

[119] See Health and Care Act 2022, s 178(4), which inserts subss (3B)–(3D) into s 1 of the 1967 Act.

[120] Abortion methods are becoming increasingly safe but complication rates still increase with the period of gestation.

[121] The Abortion Act 1967 does not extend to Northern Ireland, discussed further. The Channel Islands have adopted legislation which is similar to, although rather stricter than, that of Great Britain. See e.g. Termination of Pregnancy (Jersey) Law 1997.

[122] One could, in fact, apply much the same reasoning to s 1(1)(c), though this sub-section is plainly intended to cover terminations in late pregnancy when the dangerous toxaemias of pregnancy most commonly arise.

[123] Even then, the charge would be under the Offences Against the Person Act 1861 rather than under the 1967 Act.

Apparently paradoxically, this also applies when considering terminations under section 1(1)(d)—the 'foetal abnormality' ground—which one might have thought was there for the benefit of the foetus that may, otherwise, lead to a child born with a significant disability. Apart from anything else, the prospect of a disabled child is likely to affect a woman's mental health more than if she terminated the pregnancy; from the woman's aspect, there is, therefore, no absolute need for section 1(1)(d)—other than, if necessary, to take advantage of the concession as to the length of gestation. More specifically, the sub-section is, again, open-ended in its phraseology. What is a substantial risk? What is a serious handicap? Neither is defined and each can be interpreted on a wholly subjective basis. As a result, it will be difficult, if not impossible, to demonstrate that a decision to terminate the pregnancy was not taken in good faith. Ms Jepson, who succeeded in obtaining access to judicial review of a termination performed because the foetus had a cleft palate, received no sympathy from either the police or the medical profession, and the Crown Prosecution Service refused to take action, on the ground that the decision had been taken in good faith.[124]

It is hardly surprising that we have been able to find only one conviction under the Act[125] and this appears to have arisen mainly because of the way the operation was performed. It should be noted, however, that dozens of police investigations into women who have been suspected of having 'illegal abortions' have taken place over the past ten years or so.[126]

The medical profession tends to look on the Act as a success and resists any attempt to stiffen its conditions.[127] Circumstances must, however, arise when the proportionality between termination of pregnancy and the severity of the mischief it avoids is so balanced as to make one wonder if the law should not intervene—abortion on the basis of foetal sex selection provides such an example. Most people, we imagine, would instinctively regard it as an abuse of medical skills. Moreover, the clear restrictions on gender-based embryocide[128] must surely imply parliamentary disapproval of the practice. Nevertheless, it cannot necessarily be illegal. Section 1(2) of the 1967 Act specifically states that, in making a determination as to the risk of injury to the woman's or her existing children's health, 'account may be taken of the pregnant woman's actual or reasonably foreseeable environment'. For some who hold particular beliefs, or simply have several children of the same sex, the birth of a child of a particular sex could affect a woman's mental health and, possibly, her physical well-being; there is nothing in the Act which limits such risks to those directly associated with the condition of pregnancy. A positive argument for sex selection can be based on the concept of procreative autonomy,[129] and it has even been suggested that, once one accepts termination on the grounds of foetal disability, one is logically bound to accept abortion on the basis of sex.[130] While the latter may not constitute a

---

[124] *Jepson* v *Chief Constable of West Mercia* [2003] EWHC 3318.

[125] *R* v *Smith (John)* [1974] 1 All ER 376 (CA).

[126] Shanti Das, 'Women Accused of Illegal Abortions in England and Wales after Miscarriages and Stillbirths' (The Observer, 2 July 2022) available at <https://www.theguardian.com/world/2022/jul/02/women-accused-of-abortions-in-england-and-wales-after-miscarriages-and-stillbirths> accessed 19 December 2022.

[127] Studies have found that the majority of UK medical students support the availability of abortion and it being included in their education. See Pollyana Cohen et al., 'What Should Medical Students be Taught About Abortion? An Evaluation of Student Attitudes Towards their Abortion Teaching and their Future Involvement in Abortion Care' (2021) 21(1) BMC Medical Education 4.

[128] See Human Fertilisation and Embryology Act 1990, Sch 2, para 1ZA(1)(b)–(c).

[129] Julian Savulescu, 'Sex Selection: The Case For' (1999) 171(7) Medical Journal of Australia 373.

[130] Jeremy Williams, 'Sex Selective Abortion: A Matter of Choice' (2012) 31(2) Law and Philosophy 125. This depends upon one also accepting that s 1(1)(d) is there for the benefit of the mother.

major problem in the UK,[131] it illustrates how wide is the facility for termination within the wording of the 1967 Act.

Those who support the interests of the foetus have always been concerned to prevent the abortion, or feticide, of those capable of a free existence by lowering the foetal age beyond which termination is impermissible so as to keep in step with the increasing medical capacity to lower the age of 'viability'. They can be said to have succeeded to an extent by having this set at 24 weeks for the relatively slight medical and social reasons described in section 1(1)(a) of the 1967 Act. There have been repeated attempts to lower the age at which a 'social' abortion can be performed still further. The UK Government has not, however, supported this to date.[132]

The offset of the 24-week timescale is that it may be difficult, particularly in the face of human error, to make a prognosis of serious neonatal handicap within that timescale. Accordingly, the 1990 Act removed the prevailing 28 weeks' legal limit and imposed no other time restrictions on abortions performed by reason of foetal abnormality. Similar de-restriction applies in the event of risk or grave injury to the pregnant woman—and such conditions are likely to arise particularly in late gestation. The *need* for late abortion thus remains, and to avoid any risk of a live aborted foetus, the Royal College of Obstetricians and Gynaecologists now recommends feticide as a preliminary to all terminations beyond a gestational age of 22 weeks.[133] Feticide has become a routine part of late termination of pregnancy—and this is not only to ensure no live birth results but also to ensure that the foetus suffers no pain in the process.

The availability of lawful termination has been further extended by section 37(4) of the 1990 Act, which amends section 5(1) of the 1967 Act so as to read: 'No offence under the Infant Life (Preservation) Act 1929 shall be committed by a registered medical practitioner who terminates a pregnancy in accordance with the provisions of this Act.' This means the criminal associations with 'viability' of the foetus[134] are therefore now almost, although not quite, entirely dispelled.

15.5.2 ABORTION AND PERSONS HELD TO LACK CAPACITY

We have no reason to believe that termination of pregnancy in persons judged to lack capacity or minors is to be regarded differently from any other aspect of medical treatment. In respect of minors, the courts will, in the event of conflict, always put the interests of a young mother above those of her foetus—indeed, they *must* do so.[135]

Specific problems as to confidentiality—and particularly in respect of parental rights and duties—are, however, likely to arise in the unique context of under-age pregnancy. At one time, these caused particular concern in the US; the matter has now probably been

---

[131] For a global gender justice perspective on this, see Agomoni Ganguli-Mitra, 'Sex Selection and Global Gender Justice' (2021) 52(2) Journal of Social Philosophy 217.

[132] Adrian O'Dowd, 'No Evidence Backs Reduction in Abortion Time Limit, Minister Says' (2007) 335 BMJ 903. It is arguable that the discussion is misplaced—viability has little fundamental importance in the abortion debate in that abortion destroys human life at any stage of fetal development.

[133] Royal College of Obstetricians and Gynaecologists, 'Termination of Pregnancy for Fetal Abnormality' (ROCG, 2010) at 29, available at <https://rcog.org.uk/guidance/browse-all-guidance/other-guidelines-and-reports/termination-of-pregnancy-for-fetal-abnormality-in-england-scotland-and-wales/> accessed 19 December 2022.

[134] For a review of attitudes to late terminations, see Julian Savulescu, 'Is Current Practice Around Late Termination of Pregnancy Eugenic and Discriminatory?' (2001) 27(3) Journal of Medical Ethics 165.

[135] Children Act 1989, s 1(1). See the criticism of an expert witness in *Re B (wardship: abortion)* [1991] 2 FLR 426 [431].

settled in *Planned Parenthood of Southeastern Pennsylvania* v *Casey*,[136] where the need for parental consent was confirmed. In Britain, the concept of the 'understanding child' has gone unchallenged since it was first mooted by Butler-Sloss J in 1982.[137] There can be no doubt, however, that to perform an operation without parental permission on a child too young to understand the issues—and, hence, to give a valid consent—would constitute an assault. In practice, absent strongly held religious views, it must be very rare for the parents of an unmarried girl below the age of 16 not to consent to termination of pregnancy,[138] but the question remains—*must* the parents be informed prior to legal termination of a minor's pregnancy? The 1967 Act makes no distinctions as to age. One might suppose that the majority of children who are old enough to *become* pregnant are also old enough to understand the consequences, but there are bound to be exceptions. A case in point is *Re X (A Child) (Capacity to Consent to Termination)*,[139] where a 13-year-old girl was assessed to be non-*Gillick*-competent on account of her failure to appreciate the consequence of continued pregnancy and childbirth. Notwithstanding, it was deemed to be in her best interests for a termination to proceed, though her supportive wish for this outcome was heavily influential. One wonders what would have happened had she objected.

The other issue that arises in the case of minors relates to the confidentiality conditions laid down in *Gillick*.[140] The circumstances surrounding pregnancy—including termination of pregnancy—and childcare are, however, so unique that, until recently, there have been lingering doubts. These have now been put to rest in *R (Axon)* v *Secretary of State for Health*.[141] In that case, the claimant, Axon, a divorced mother of five who had herself undergone a termination, sought a declaration to the effect that, since a doctor owed no duty of confidentiality to a minor in respect of advice and proposed treatment related to contraception, sexual health, and abortion, she could not provide such advice or treatment without the consent of the minor's parents; Axon also sought a declaration that guidelines issued by the Department of Health, which failed to acknowledge this exception to the general rule, were unlawful. It is hard to see that these claims were anything other than doomed from the start, and they were rejected essentially on the ground that, to accept them would involve overturning *Gillick*. In anticipation of this, the claim was amended to apply to abortion only.

Silber J recognised the distinctive aspects of abortion to which we have already alluded, and accepted that about one-third of terminations in England and Wales involving girls under the age of 16 were carried out without at least one parent being informed. In the end, however, he fell back on Lord Fraser in *Gillick*, who pointed out that the medical professional was only justified in proceeding without parental consent or knowledge if they are satisfied that 'the girl will understand his advice', and on Lord Scarman, who opined that it is not enough that she should understand the nature of the advice which is being given; she must also have a sufficient maturity to understand what is involved. In other words, the *Gillick* test is a pliable test that can be adjusted so as to apply to the precise circumstances—the benchmark being that the more intricate or significant in the long term the treatment to be given, the more mature must be the minor before she can be entrusted with her own destiny. There was nothing in *Gillick* to suggest that it depended

---

[136] *Planned Parenthood of Southeastern Pennsylvania* v *Casey* 112 S Ct 2791 (1992).

[137] *Re P (a minor)* [1986] 1 FLR 272.

[138] But see *Re B (wardship: abortion)* [1991] 2 FLR 426, where a mother opposed a termination for her 12-year-old daughter.

[139] [2014] EWHC 1871 (Fam).

[140] The position in Scotland is covered by the Age of Legal Capacity (Scotland) Act 1991, s 2(4). See Chapter 9 for a full discussion.

[141] (2006) 88 BMLR 96 (HC).

on the nature of the treatment under review.[142] Which does not allay one's misgivings as to the unique nature of abortion, but which nevertheless makes perfect logic so long as *Gillick* represents the relevant law.[143]

Thus, although the knowledge and agreement of the parents are clearly desirable, a doctor who has made reasonable efforts to induce their patient to confide in her parents and is still faced with an adamant refusal of consent to disclosure, and who goes on to terminate a minor's pregnancy, would be secure from action in the courts or before the GMC. The trend in medical, legal, and societal attitudes towards children's rights over the last three decades gives added support to this view.[144]

Concerning adults judged to lack capacity, abortions may be carried out under the Mental Capacity Act 2005 if the procedure is considered to be in their best interests and meets the requirements of the Abortion Act 1967. As Hilder J stated in *S v Birmingham Women's and Children's NHS Trust*:

> Consent, either by the pregnant woman capacitously or by the Court of Protection in the best interest of a non-capacitous pregnant woman, is fundamental to the lawfulness of abortion, as it is to any medical procedure. It is not, however, sufficient. Ultimately, lawful termination of a pregnancy depends on their being two medical practitioners who are satisfied that the conditions of the Abortion Act are met and one who is willing to perform it. Ethical considerations arise. The Court of Protection cannot require a clinician to perform this (or any) procedure if s/he is unwilling to do so.[145]

The courts have also confirmed that the proposition-specific nature of any capacity assessment equally applies to termination of pregnancy. Thus, in *Re SB (A Patient) (Capacity to Consent to Termination)*,[146] a 37-year-old woman with bipolar disorder who was detained under the Mental Health Act 1983 was assessed to have sufficient capacity under the Mental Capacity Act 2005 to decide to have an abortion at almost 24 weeks' gestation, despite psychiatric assessment to the contrary. While she suffered from paranoia and delusional thoughts, she had given additional sound reasons for desiring a termination that demonstrated her ability to make her own decision *on this matter*. Similarly, in *S*, which also concerned a woman with bipolar disorder detained under the Mental Health Act 1983, Hilder J considered her capacity to decide to terminate her pregnancy and whether a change of view was indicative of a loss of capacity to decide:

> The clinicians note that S's wish for a termination is a marked change of position to her wish to become pregnant in the first place; and that this change of position coincides with a deterioration in her mental health. They conclude that the wish for termination is a reflection of the negative cognitions of S's mental health condition and therefore S lacks capacity to make the decision. In my judgment this reasoning is not sufficient. A person can change their mind. I do not agree that S's consideration of termination is 'new and

---

[142] Perhaps the most determinant effect of *Axon* is to quash any attempt to say that *Gillick* was concerned with contraceptive advice alone.

[143] *Axon* also claimed that her Art 8 ECHR rights were violated by the guidelines, but this claim was dismissed in a lengthy judgment which is not directly relevant to this chapter, but which merits acknowledgement. In brief, *Axon* had no Art 8(1) rights because these only accrued if her daughter was found to be without *Gillick* competence.

[144] Jordi Ribot, 'Underage Abortion and Beyond: Developments of Spanish Law in Competent Minor's Autonomy' (2012) 20(1) Medical Law Review 48.

[145] [2022] EWCOP 10, [33].   [146] [2013] EWHC 1417 (COP).

impulsive'. It has been maintained at least since the point of detention. A month is a long time in the context of abortion time limits. Moreover S has articulated reasons for her current stance, consistently, and Dr. Jancevic 'completely agree[d]' that those reasons are not irrational. The clinicians may not agree with the S's reasons for seeking termination. They are free to disagree but their disagreement does not justify a conclusion that S's decision-making is incapacitous.[147]

15.5.3 REDUCTION OF MULTIPLE PREGNANCIES

Original doubts as to the legality of the reduction of multiple pregnancies were based mainly on terminological grounds—first on whether the phrase 'termination of pregnancy' in the 1967 Act relates to the pregnancy as a whole, and, if this strict interpretation is inappropriate, whether individualised feticide in situ can be regarded as an abortion.[148] Whatever the solution of this academic argument may be, the situation has been resolved in practice—both selective reduction and reduction of multiple pregnancy in utero are legal when the requirements of section 5(2) of the 1967 Act are fulfilled in relation to the individual foetus.

Given that account may be taken of the woman's actual or reasonably foreseeable environment, there is no legal difficulty in justifying pregnancy reduction on the grounds that continuance of a multiple pregnancy would involve a risk of injury to the mental health of the pregnant woman greater than if it was reduced.[149] It might be equally appropriate to plead risk to the physical or mental health of the existing family—particularly if the intended remaining foetus or foetuses were regarded as 'existing children of the family'. Selective destruction of an abnormal foetus is, of course, justified under the serious handicap clause of the 1967 Act. Whether there is tort liability in the event of damage to a surviving foetus is arguable; the probability is that the doctor would not be liable in the absence of negligence in the operation.[150]

It scarcely needs emphasising that all the foregoing relates to legal justification—the morality of the procedure is open to question. There is, clearly, a difference between reducing a twin pregnancy and reducing one involving sextuplets. To say that both are wrong in that they offend against the principle of respect for human life is to ignore the equally valid argument that ensuring the death of all six foetuses by inaction is equally disrespectful; the death of all octuplets following refusal of foetal reduction in an, at the time, *cause célèbre* provides an extreme example. The subject opens up the age-old question of whether it is permissible to use unacceptable means to achieve a desirable end—at which point, multiple perspectives come into play (see earlier discussion of the concept of personhood, and Chapter 2).

Some regard abortion in Great Britain as being unreasonably restricted as compared with other jurisdictions, and indeed much of the public are supportive of access to abortion.[151] The number of terminations carried out in England and Wales in 2021 was the

---

[147] [2022] EWCOP 10 [57].

[148] For somewhat opposing views, see John Keown, 'Selective Reduction of Multiple Pregnancy' (1987) 137(6335) New Law Journal 1165; and David Price, 'Selective Reduction and Feticide: The Parameters of Abortion' (1988) Criminal Law Review 199.

[149] Richard Berkowitz, 'From Twin to Singleton' (1996) 313 BMJ 373.

[150] Margaret Brazier, 'Unfinished Feticide: A Legal Commentary' (1990) 16(2) Journal of Medical Ethics 68, discussing of Robert Jansen, 'Unfinished feticide' (1990) 16(2) Journal of Medical Ethics 61.

[151] It has been suggested that some 42% of the British public would support the availability of abortion without any reason other than the woman's choice: Jacqui Wise, 'British Public Supports Legal Abortion For All' (1997) 314 BMJ 627.

highest since records began, at 214,256.[152] The figures for Scotland show that 13,896 abortions took place in 2021.[153] The number of terminations provided for non-resident women in England and Wales in 2021 was 613,[154] a significant decrease from 4,908 in 2017 which, at the time was the lowest figure since 1969. Clearly, there have been policy changes in other countries in the intervening years and it is worth considering some of these briefly.

15.5.4 NORTHERN IRELAND

The position in Northern Ireland differs from the rest of the UK and has undergone significant transformation via the Abortion (Northern Ireland) Regulations 2020.

The Abortion Act 1967 has never applied to Northern Ireland, and until recently the Offences Against the Person Act 1861, subject to modification by jurisprudence, continued to hold sway. In *Re K (a minor)*,[155] it was held that the 1861 Act was modified by the charge to the jury in *R v Bourne*,[156] and termination of a 13-week pregnancy in a severely handicapped ward of court was authorised. In *Re A (Northern Health and Social Services Board)*,[157] the court used the reasoning in *Bourne* to apply section 25 of the Criminal Justice Act (Northern Ireland) 1945 to the 1861 Act, and a termination was held to be in the handicapped woman's best interests. The application of the law was summarised by the Northern Ireland Court of Appeal in *Family Planning Association of Northern Ireland v Minister for Health and Social Services and Public Safety*:

> A termination will . . . be lawful where the continuance of the pregnancy threatens the life of the mother, or would adversely affect her mental or physical health; The adverse effect on her mental or physical health must be a 'real and serious' one, and must also be 'permanent or long term'; In most cases the risk of the adverse effect occurring would need to be a probability, but a possibility might be regarded as sufficient if the imminent death of the mother was the potentially adverse effect; It will always be a question of fact and degree whether the perceived effect of a non-termination is sufficiently grave to warrant terminating the pregnancy in a particular case.[158]

The real-world effect of this was there was no automatic entitlement to services, even in cases of rape or incest, and no account was taken of foetal abnormality as a basis for termination. The extent of the unequal treatment of Northern Irish women under the previous law can be seen by the stark difference in the numbers of terminations in Northern Ireland in any given year as compared with the mainland figures.[159] In the first half of 2018, some 342 women and girls were reported to have travelled to England for a termination through the British Pregnancy Advisory Service.[160] In the past, such women's

---

[152] Office for Health Improvement and Disparities, 'Abortion Statistics, England and Wales: 2021' (GOV. UK, 21 June 2022) available at <https://www.gov.uk/government/statistics/abortion-statistics-for-england-and-wales-2021/abortion-statistics-england-and-wales-2021> accessed 19 December 2022.

[153] Public Health Scotland, 'Termination of Pregnancy Statistics' (31 May 2022) available at <https://www.publichealthscotland.scot/publications/termination-of-pregnancy-statistics/termination-of-pregnancy-statistics-year-ending-december-2021/> accessed 19 December 2022.

[154] Office for Health Improvement and Disparities (n 152).

[155] (1991) 2 Med LR 371.   [156] [1938] 3 All ER 615.   [157] (1991) 2 Med L Rev 274.

[158] [2004] NICA 37 [12].

[159] For current figures, see Office for Health Improvement and Disparities (n 152). See also Department of Health, *NI Termination of Pregnancy Statistics, 2015/16* (2017), which indicates that 16 terminations of pregnancy were carried out on women normally resident in Northern Ireland in 2015/16.

[160] James Tapper, 'Rise in Women Travelling from Northern Ireland to England for Abortions' *The Guardian* (21 July 2018) available at <https://www.theguardian.com/world/2018/jul/21/women-travelling-from-northern-ireland-to-england-for-abortions> accessed 19 December 2022.

situation would be complicated by the refusal of the Secretary of State in England to pay for their treatment, a refusal which was upheld as reasonable in judicial review.

In the wake of the *Family Planning Association* case, social pressure increased to change the law. A consultation was later held, which emphasised the appetite for change.[161] The desire for fundamental law reform continued to rise,[162] and the Northern Ireland Human Rights Commission (NIHRC) challenged the law as incompatible with Articles 3, 8, and 14 ECHR insofar as it failed to provide for abortions in cases of rape, incest, or serious foetal abnormality; it sought a declaration of incompatibility under section 4(2) of the Human Rights Act 1998. The matter reached the UK Supreme Court in *Re Northern Ireland Human Rights Commission's Application for Judicial Review*,[163] which offered a rather unsatisfactory (non-)resolution.

In a lengthy judgment,[164] a narrow majority (Lords Mance, Reed, Lloyd-Jones, and Lady Black) held that the NIHRC did not have standing because it had not identified any unlawful act with any victim or potential victim.[165] However, a majority, in obiter, would have made a declaration of incompatibility with Article 8 (Ladies Hale and Black, and Lords Mance, Kerr, and Wilson), and with Article 3 (Lords Kerr and Wilson). Lord Mance concluded as follows:

> I am . . . satisfied that the present legislative position in Northern Ireland is untenable and intrinsically disproportionate in excluding from any possibility of abortion pregnancies involving fatal fetal abnormality or due to rape or incest. My conclusions about the Commission's lack of competence to bring these proceedings means that there is however no question of making any declaration of incompatibility. But the present law clearly needs radical reconsideration. Those responsible for ensuring the compatibility of Northern Ireland law with the Convention rights will no doubt recognise and take account of these conclusions, at as early a time as possible, by considering whether and how to amend the law, in the light of the ongoing suffering being caused by it as well as the likelihood that a victim of the existing law would have standing to pursue similar proceedings to reach similar conclusions and to obtain a declaration of incompatibility in relation to the 1861 Act.[166]

---

[161] Department of Health, Social Services and Public Safety, *Summary of Consultation Responses Received* (2013).

[162] Stephen Cragg, 'Abortion, Northern Ireland and the NHS in England: Can Respect for Devolved Governments Be a Justification for Discrimination' (2017) 4 Journal of International and Comparative Law 377; Jennifer Thomson, 'Free Abortions in England will not Remove the Fundamental Injustice Northern Irish Women Suffer' (LSE British Politics and Policy, 07 July 2017) available at <https://blogs.lse.ac.uk/politicsandpolicy/free-abortions-in-england-will-not-remove-the-fundamental-injustice-northern-irish-women-suffer/> accessed 19 December 2022; Angel Li, 'From Ireland to Northern Ireland: Campaigns for Abortion Law' (2018) 391(10138) Lancet 2403; Abigail Aiken et al., 'The Impact of Northern Ireland's Abortion Laws on Women's Abortion Decision-Making and Experiences' (2018) BMJ Sexual Reproduction & Health, available at <https://pubmed.ncbi.nlm.nih.gov/30341065/> accessed 19 December 2022.

[163] [2018] UKSC 27.

[164] For more on which, see Sandy Goldbeck-Wood et al., 'Criminalised Abortion in UK Obstructs Reflective Choice and Best Care' (2018) 362 BMJ k2928, and Tom Frost, 'Abortion in Northern Ireland: Has the Rubicon Been Crossed?' (2018) 39 Liverpool Law Review 1.

[165] Under s 69(5)(b) of the Northern Ireland Act 1998, as amended by the Justice and Security (Northern Ireland) Act 2007, the NIHRC has the power to bring human rights proceedings without itself being a victim, but s 71(2B)(c) of the 1998 Act states that actual or potential victims of an unlawful act should be identified. For more on why the minority's view on standing was more tenable, see Shona Wilson Stark, 'In Re Northern Ireland Human Rights Commission's Application for Judicial Review [2018] UKSC 27: A Declaration in All but Name?' (UK Constitutional Law Association, 12 June 2018) available at <https://ukconstitutionallaw.org/2018/06/12/shona-wilson-stark-in-re-northern-ireland-human-rights-commissions-application-for-judicial-review-2018-uksc-27-a-declaration-in-all-but-name/> accessed 19 December 2022.

[166] [2018] UKSC 27, [135].

He went on to state that if a specific individual were to challenge the compatibility of the legislation, it is 'inevitable' that a declaration would be made.

Appetite for change continued to gather; the same year, the United Nations Committee on the Elimination of Discrimination Against Women (UN CEDAW) released a report stating that the existing law of Northern Ireland is a 'grave and systematic' breach of women's rights',[167] and Sarah Ewart successfully brought a case to the High Court in Belfast, which declared that the law breached the UK's human rights commitments.[168] In 2019, the law on abortion in Northern Ireland began to change dramatically when the UK Government introduced section 9 of the Northern Ireland (Executive Formation etc) Act 2019, which repealed sections 58 and 59 of the Offences Against the Person Act 1861, introduced a moratorium on abortion-related criminal prosecutions, and placed a duty on the UK Government to introduce a new framework for abortion in Northern Ireland which ensured the recommendations of the UN CEDAW report were implemented.[169] Following this, a new legal framework for abortion services was introduced on 25 March 2020, the Abortion (Northern Ireland) Regulations 2020.[170] Abortion in Northern Ireland is now permitted at up to 12 weeks' gestation in all circumstances, provided it is certified by one medical professional.[171] Termination of pregnancy is also allowed up to 24 weeks where there is risk of injury to the physical or mental health of the woman.[172] The Regulations also include grounds for termination where there is no gestational limit, namely immediate necessity, risk to life or grave permanent injury, and severe foetal impairment or fatal foetal abnormality.[173]

Despite the progress that has been made, it is reported that in practice, access to abortion services in Northern Ireland remains difficult,[174] and concerns were raised after the implementation of the 2020 Regulations that full commissioning of services had not yet taken place.[175] This eventually led to the Abortion (Northern Ireland) Regulations 2022, which came into force on 20 May 2022 and place an obligation on the Northern Ireland Department of Health to commission and fund abortion services. At time of writing, it remains to be seen whether this will in fact happen and thereby ease patient access to these services.

15.5.5 REPUBLIC OF IRELAND

Historically, the Republic of Ireland conferred constitutional rights to life on the foetus, sometimes privileging that right over the rights of the mother.[176] Previous to the enactment of the Health (Regulation of Termination of Pregnancy) Act 2018, the Irish law on

---

[167] United Nations Human Rights Treaty Bodies, 'Inquiry Concerning the United Kingdom of Great Britain and Northern Ireland under Article 8 of the Optional Protocol to the Convention on the Elimination of All Forms of Discrimination Against Women' (2019) available at <https://tbinternet.ohchr.org/_layouts/15/treatybodyexternal/TBSearch.aspx?Lang=en&TreatyID=3&DocTypeCategoryID=7> accessed 19 December 2022.

[168] Re NIHRC Application for Judicial Review [2019] NIQB 88.

[169] At the time the Northern Irish Executive was suspended, and it set out that if the Executive was not in place by 21 October 2019, s 9 would come into force on 22 October 2019. This ended up being the case.

[170] Subsequently re-made as the Abortion (Northern Ireland) (No. 2) Regulations 2020 (SI 2020/503), which corrects drafting errors.

[171] 2020 regulations, reg 3.

[172] This must be certified by two medical professionals; see reg 4.   [173] Regs 5–7.

[174] See Sydney Calkin and Ella Berny, 'Legal and Non-Legal Barriers to Abortion in Ireland and the United Kingdom' (2021) 5 The Journal of Medicine Access.

[175] Re NIHRC Application for Judicial Review (n 168).

[176] For example, see A-G v X (1994) 15 BMLR 104; and A and B v Eastern Health Board [1998] 4 IR 464.

abortion was derived from the UK Offences Against the Person Act 1861, when Ireland was subject to British rule. Subsequently to Irish independence, this was incorporated into the Health (Family Planning) Act 1979, and then displaced by the Protection of Life During Pregnancy Act 2013, which was adopted after the tragic death of a woman who was miscarrying but left on a wait-and-see policy by hospital staff.[177] The 2013 Act did not make provision for cases of incest, rape, or foetal abnormality, permitting abortions only where there is a 'real and substantial risk' to a woman's life, but not necessarily to her health. Moreover, its access provisions required the input of three medical practitioners to certify that a woman qualifies, and in the case of a suicide risk, two of the practitioners needed to be psychiatrists.

Against this legislative background, the history of access to safe abortions in Ireland has been a study in conflict, with many cases working their way to Europe.[178] In *Society for the Protection of Unborn Children Ireland Ltd v Grogan*,[179] which concerned the Republic of Ireland's prohibition on the distribution of information relating to UK abortion facilities, the European Court of Justice (ECJ) held that, as a matter of morality, the Irish Government was entitled to follow its own public policy. The problems of providing information and arranging travel to another jurisdiction were then considered by the ECtHR,[180] when an injunction of the Supreme Court restraining such counselling was challenged. While agreeing that the purpose of the injunction was to protect the national morality, the ECtHR held that the degree of restraint imposed was disproportionate to the aim pursued. Accordingly, Article 10 (freedom of expression) ECHR was infringed. Two national referenda supported this conclusion, and the Regulation of Information Act 1995 was thereafter passed, resulting in the lifting of the injunctions against the provision of information concerning the availability of abortion in Great Britain, subject to there being no advocacy of termination. A third referendum in 2002 was confined to an attempt to exclude potential suicide as a legal justification for termination of pregnancy.

A further case was *D v Ireland*, which involved the carriage of a foetus with trisomy-18—a lethal chromosomal anomaly but one which did not involve danger to the life of the mother.[181] D was advised that she was not medically eligible for an abortion in Ireland, so she underwent a termination in the UK. On her return, she lodged a complaint with the ECtHR to the effect that existing Irish law as applied to a fatal foetal diagnosis was incompatible with her rights under Articles 3, 8, 10, and 14 ECHR. The ECtHR deemed the application inadmissible on the ground that the full range of domestic resources had not been exhausted.[182] The legislative inertia resulted in another ECtHR case, this one brought by three women who claimed that their Article 8 rights were infringed due to their

[177] Radhika Sanghani, 'Ireland's Abortion Problem: New Report Lays Bare the Horrifying Truth' *The Telegraph* (9 June 2015) available at <https://www.telegraph.co.uk/women/womens-life/11660028/Irelands-abortion-problem-New-report-lays-bare-the-horrifying-truth.html> accessed 19 December 2022.
[178] Brenda Daly, 'Braxton Hicks or the Birth of a New Era? Tracing the Development of Ireland's Abortion Laws in Respect of the ECHR Jurisprudence' (2011) 18(4) European Journal of Health Law 375.
[179] (1992) 9 BMLR 100 (ECJ).
[180] *Open Door Counselling and Dublin Well Woman v Ireland* (1993) 15 EHRR 244.
[181] ECtHR (App No 26499/02), 28 June 2006. The transcript contains a very detailed analysis of abortion law in Ireland. The case is not to be confused with that involving another 'Ms D' who was carrying an anencephalic foetus. The High Court overruled a decision by the District Court not to authorise her travel for a termination: Clare Dyer, 'Girl Carrying Anencephalic Foetus is Granted Right to Travel' (2007) 334(7602) BMJ 1026.
[182] Its significance lies in the government's complaints about courts. It claimed that the courts would be unlikely to interpret the law with remorseless logic particularly when the facts were exceptional, and that the tenor of the submissions demonstrated an almost palpable anxiety for the courts, rather than the politicians, to be given the opportunity to acknowledge the viability of D's case.

being unable to obtain terminations in Ireland despite the grounds for permissibility being expanded to include a real and substantial risk to their lives.[183] In the event, the ECtHR found that the rights of C, who had cancer, were infringed, but not those of A and B.

In sum, Irish law on abortion remained one of the most draconian in Europe, and the situation remained highly contested until a 2018 referendum resulted in a landslide vote (66.4% in favour) to rescind the 8th Amendment of the Irish Constitution, which acknowledged the right to life of the unborn child.[184] The government subsequently adopted the Thirty-Sixth Amendment of the Constitution Act 2018, which stipulates that Article 40 of the Constitution is to be amended by adding the following words: 'Provision may be made by law for the regulation of termination of pregnancy. As such, abortion in Ireland is now regulated by the Health (Regulation of Termination of Pregnancy) Act 2018, under which abortion is permitted in all circumstances during the first 12 weeks of pregnancy.'[185] Thereafter, abortion is only permitted where there is serious risk to the life or health of the mother[186] or where there is a fatal foetal abnormality.[187] It has been reported that significant barriers exist within this framework for those seeking abortions, however, including rigid cut-off times for seeking an abortion under sections 11 and 12.[188]

15.5.6 TERMINATION OF PREGNANCY AND THE NON-GESTATIONAL PARENT

The anomalous position of the father, or non-gestational parent, in the right to life debate also falls to be considered. It is clear that, insofar as abortion is concerned, they have for practical purposes, *no* rights. It seems incongruous that this should be so, irrespective of the reason for the abortion, and that it should apply even in cases which do not relate to the health of the mother; a non-gestational parent could not, for example, save the existence of a potentially haemophiliac child. Some may argue that the non-gestational parent should be entitled to a hearing, but this would surely be as far as one could go—it would not be possible to support any legal right to the unacceptable consequences that might attend acceptance of their wishes.

The English position was established in *Paton v British Pregnancy Advisory Service Trustees*,[189] where it was held that a husband cannot by injunction prevent his wife from undergoing a lawful abortion. The decision was upheld by the European Commission of Human Rights; the Commission was, however, clearly worried by the possible complication of foetal 'viability'—the matter was not decided and it remains an area of potential doubt.[190] It was clarified no further in *C v S*,[191] in which the unmarried father's *locus standi* was firmly rejected—and the decision was not appealed—but in which the main thrust of the hearing was to establish that the foetus in question was *not* viable.[192] Any possibility

---

[183] *A v Ireland* (2011) 53 EHRR 13. See Stephanie Palmer, 'Abortion and Human Rights' (2014) 6 EHRLR 596.

[184] Henry McDonald, et al., 'Ireland Votes by Landslide to Legalise Abortion' *The Guardian* (26 May 2018) available at <https://www.theguardian.com/world/2018/may/26/ireland-votes-by-landslide-to-legalise-abortion> accessed 19 December 2022.

[185] Health (Regulation of Termination of Pregnancy) Act 2018, s 12.

[186] ibid., ss 9–10.   [187] ibid., s 11.

[188] For discussion, see Sydney Calkin and Ella Berny (n 174).

[189] *Paton v British Pregnancy Advisory Service Trustees* [1979] QB 276. And see Sheila McLean, 'Abortion Law: Is Consensual Reform Possible?' (1990) 17(1) Journal of Law & Society 106.

[190] [1978] 2 All ER 987; *Paton v United Kingdom* (1980) 3 EHRR 408.

[191] [1987] 1 All ER 1230.

[192] Nor can a father recover for distress on hearing diagnosis of miscarriage: *Wild v Southend University Hospital NHS Foundation Trust* [2014] EWHC 4053 (QB).

that a Scottish foetus might be able to petition through its tutor—that is, its father—for interdict of any threatened harm has now also been excluded; in *Kelly* v *Kelly*,[193] the Inner House of the Court of Session agreed that a review of the extensive Commonwealth decisions supported the view that the foetus had no rights for the protection of which the remedy of interdict might be invoked. It followed, therefore, that the father, as the guardian of the foetus, had no standing by which to prevent his wife's abortion.[194]

There is every reason to suppose that this attitude to paternal and foetal rights will persist. Nothing can alter the fact that it is the woman who carries the foetus and whose health is mainly at risk, and it is this factor which explains the difference in legal attitudes to the father's or non-gestational parent's interest in the foetus (and in their in vitro embryo, discussed in Chapter 16). An objecting father may well deserve sympathy but, in the final analysis, a woman's right to control her body must take precedence.

15.5.7 THE CARER'S ROLE AND CONSCIENTIOUS OBJECTION

The rights of those who, of necessity, participate in terminations of pregnancy receive comparatively little attention in the abortion debate. Yet, they are of considerable communitarian importance.[195] In addition to physicians, who obviously hold a central role, nurses are significant in treatment and care, exemplified in the abortion context by the widespread use of prostaglandin infusions for induction of premature labour. Indeed, nurses have so great a part to play that some doubt was raised as to whether they were, in fact, guilty of performing illegal abortions insofar as they were not 'registered medical practitioners', as required by the 1967 Act. In 1980, the Royal College of Nursing thus sought a declaration to the effect that the advice in a Departmental Circular was wrong in law, stating that irrespective of the precise action taken, an abortion was legal provided that it was initiated by and was the responsibility of a registered medical practitioner. The complexities were such that the Royal College lost its case in the High Court, won in the Court of Appeal, and lost in the House of Lords, which held, by a 5–4 margin, that abortion, no matter how it is performed, is accomplished by way of a team effort and is no different in this respect from any other form of treatment.[196]

But of course, as all of the this should make clear, abortion is not like any other form of treatment, a fact recognised by the inclusion in the 1967 Act of section 4, which excuses the conscientious objector from participating in termination treatments unless that treatment is directed towards saving the life or preventing grave permanent injury to the health of the mother.[197] The exercise of this 'out'—which is not found in relation to most other lawful treatments—deserves careful consideration, not least because of the history of discrimination against reproductive health. It is important to recall that equitable access to adequate health care, including reproductive health care, is a universally accepted human

---

[193] 1997 SCLR 749.

[194] *X* v *United Kingdom* (App No 8416/79) 1980. By contrast, paternal rights as to the neonate have been confirmed by the ECtHR. An unmarried father can veto the adoption of his child: *Keegan* v *Ireland* (App No 16969/90) (1994) 18 EHRR 342.

[195] See the (failed) attempt before the European Committee of Social Rights to challenge Sweden's absence of conscientious objection laws for health workers with respect to induced abortion: *Federation of Catholic Families in Europe (Fafce)* v *Sweden* (2015) 61 EHRR SE12.

[196] *Royal College of Nursing* v *Department of Health and Social Security* [1981] AC 800 (HL).

[197] Whereas the 'conscience clause' in the 1967 Act refers to participation in 'any treatment' authorised by the Act, s 38 of the Human Fertilisation and Embryology Act 1990, which 'governs' abortion by way of s 37, refers to participation in 'any activity' governed by the Act. The latter is, arguably, open to wider interpretation.

right; that women's health, which has long been marginalised around the world, has special status and demands special protection;[198] that abortion is a critical element of reproductive health care with relevance to respecting women's dignity, autonomy, equality, and citizenship;[199] and that political and legal efforts have been undertaken to include abortion in the public health system.

Of course, a result of section 4 is that some discrimination must be levelled against doctors, especially those seeking to become gynaecologists, who, regardless of their objection, remain under an obligation to (1) advise the patient of their objection and of her right to see another doctor, provide information, and refer the patient to another carer in a timely manner, or (2) treat a woman when the continuation of the pregnancy is life-threatening. Providing information is subject to the normal rules of medical negligence, and in doing so, a physician should not express disapproval of a patient's lifestyle, choices, or beliefs. Further, the referral must be made in a timely manner, since it will inevitably delay the termination.[200] And these considerations apply equally to other carers, including the nursing staff.[201]

In the result, the GMC published supplementary guidance on the issue which attempts to balance physician and patients' rights.[202] The BMA stated that physicians should have a right to object to participation in certain treatments, including abortion, but that they should not allow their religious or cultural beliefs to impact negatively on the doctor-patient relationship; the right is not absolute and must not impact on the patient's right to care, and it cautions against discriminatory practices.[203] The Royal College of General Practitioners allows for wide-ranging opt-outs,[204] and it has been argued that there now exists a lack of clarity about which treatments health carers may validly opt out of using conscientious objection.[205]

---

[198] Committee on Economic, Social and Cultural Rights, *General Comment 14 on the Right to Health* (2000), UN CEDSCR 22nd Sess. UN Doc E/C.12/2000/4.

[199] See Rebecca Cook and Bernard Dickens, 'Human Rights Dynamics of Abortion Law Reform' (2003) 25(1) Human Rights Quarterly 1.

[200] For a critical review, see Julian Savulescu, 'Conscientious Objection in Medicine' (2006) 332(7536) BMJ 294.

[201] In general, the sensibilities of the nursing staff are inadequately recognised. The damage that conscientious objection causes to their career prospects may well be greater than that confronted by doctors—a doctor does not have to practise gynaecology but, as Lord Denning emphasised in *Royal College of Nursing*, nurses are expected to be mobile throughout the hospital system. Moreover, current methods of termination beyond week 12 of pregnancy involve the nursing staff in an uncompromising way—whether it be in the delivery of what is comparable to a premature birth or in counting the fragmented parts of a formed foetus. The seminal work—Jonathan Glover, *Causing Death and Saving Lives* (Penguin 1986) p 142—points to the effects on the health carers as providing a major moral distinction between, say, contraception and abortion.

[202] GMC, *Personal Beliefs and Medical Practice* (2013), which refers to objection to 'a particular procedure', not just to an intervention for which there is statutory relief, an open-endedness which was criticised by the BMA, which suggested that the guidance should be limited to a shortlist of clearly defined procedures. See *Barr v Matthews* (2000) 52 BMLR 217, wherein Alliott J approved an arrangement whereby a conscientious objector referred a termination case to a colleague, and Jean McHale, 'Faith, Belief, Fundamental Rights and Delivering Health Care in a Modern NHS: An Unrealistic Aspiration?' (2013) 21(3) Health Care Analysis 224.

[203] BMA, 'Expression of Doctors' Beliefs' (2018). And see *Eweida and Others v UK* [2013] ECHR 37, and Daniel Hill and Daniel Whistler, *The Right to Wear Religious Symbols* (Springer 2013).

[204] Royal College of General Practitioners, 'Good Medical Practice for General Practitioners' (2008).

[205] Sara Fovargue and Mary Neal, 'In Good Conscience: Conscience-Based Exemptions and Proper Medical Treatment' (2015) 23(2) Medical Law Review 221.

Difficulties arise, predictably, in practice. McHale has noted a slow growth of 'opt out' across healthcare provision.[206] It has been reported that some 20% of British GPs are against abortion on the basis of their religious beliefs, and that some of them actively work to delay or prevent women from securing abortion services.[207] In at least one case, this has led to a claim of medical negligence against the physician.[208] Further, there have been efforts to expand the use of conscientious objection to more health carers and to more peripheral elements of abortion treatment.

The first British case is that of *R v Salford Health Authority, ex parte Janaway*,[209] wherein the applicant regarded herself as having been unfairly dismissed following her refusal to type a letter referring a patient for termination of pregnancy. Ultimately, Janaway failed on the grounds that the right in section 4 was predicated on actual participation in treatment administered in a hospital or other approved place. Janaway was clearly well distanced from the actual treatment.[210] This reliance on a proximity test was revisited in *Doogan v Greater Glasgow and Clyde Health Board*,[211] a largely unsatisfactory decision[212] wherein the Supreme Court rejected a claim to section 4 conscientious objection by two midwives whose primary duties consisted of coordinating the work of the labour ward. It reiterated that section 4 only extends to those professionals taking part in the medical treatment itself, not to those who carry out ancillary, administrative, and managerial tasks which are necessarily, but indirectly, associated with the provision of termination services.[213]

The advent of medical termination also raises the unusual position of the conscientiously objecting pharmacist who is asked to fill the necessary prescriptions. Almost certainly, the proximity test would be satisfied (depending on one's view of the professional relationship between pharmacists and physicians), but *Doogan's* adoption of a narrow approach to those 'actually performing the tasks involved in the course of treatment' throws this into some question.[214] Guidance from the General Pharmaceutical Council emphasises that pharmacy professionals must provide person-centred care, which means, among other things, that they 'recognise their own values and beliefs but do not

---

[206] Jean McHale, 'Conscientious Objection and the Nurse: A Right or a Privilege?' (2009) 18(20) British Journal of Nursing 1262. A finding in keeping with warnings about 'conscience creep' in the US: Julie Cantor, 'Conscientious Objection Gone Awry: Restoring Selfless Professionalism in Medicine' (2009) 360(15) New England Journal of Medicine 1484.

[207] Ellie Lee et al, *A Matter of Choice? Explaining National Variations in Teenage Abortion and Motherhood* (Joseph Rowntree Foundation 2004).

[208] In *Enright v Kwun* [2003] EWHC 1000 (QB), the High Court found a physician negligent for failing to counsel a patient on genetic screening, a failure that was, on the evidence, partially driven by his religious beliefs.

[209] [1989] AC 537 (CA); aff'd as *Janaway v Salford Area Health Authority* [1989] AC 537 (HL).

[210] But see Charles Foster, 'When Two Freedoms Collide' (2005) 155 New Law Journal 1624.

[211] [2015] UKSC 68.

[212] See Shaun Harmon, 'Abortion and Conscientious Objection: Doogan – A Missed Opportunity for an Instructive Rights-Based Analysis' (2016) 16 Medical Law International 143.

[213] For comment, see Harmon, ibid.; Valerie Fleming, Beate Ramsayer, and Teja Škodič Zakšek, 'Freedom of Conscience in Europe? An Analysis of Three Cases of Midwives with Conscientious Objection to Abortion' (2018) 44(3) Journal of Medical Ethics 104.

[214] The philosophical arguments have been aired by Deborah Flynn, 'Pharmacist Conscience Clauses and Access to Oral Contraceptives' (2008) 34(7) Journal of Medical Ethics 517. This is from the US view, where the impression is gained that the woman's right to treatment would trump the pharmacist's moral stance in the US courts. Even so, it is reported that four US states have passed legislation to allow pharmacists to refuse to fill prescriptions for emergency contraception and similar draft legislation is in preparation in nearly half the states. By contrast, nine states have 'must fill' policies: Veronica English et al., 'Ethics Briefings' (2006) 32(12) Journal of Medical Ethics 743, 744. More recently, Zuzana Deans, 'Conscientious Objections in Pharmacy Practice in Great Britain' (2013) 27(1) Bioethics 48.

impose them on other people' and 'take responsibility for ensuring that person-centred care is not compromised because of personal values and beliefs'.[215] The Council's guidance allows for conscientious objection, though it indicates that pharmacy professionals must still act in accordance with equalities and human rights law and make sure that person-centred care is not compromised. To this end, the guidance suggests its members consider in advance the areas of their practice which may be affected and make the necessary arrangements, so they do not find themselves in the position where a person's care could be compromised. The guidance also suggests that if a pharmacy professional is unwilling to provide a certain service, they should take steps to make sure the person asking for care is at the centre of their decision-making, so they can access the service they need in a timely manner and without hindrance. As it states, 'this might include considering any time limits or other barriers to accessing medicines or other services, as well as any adverse impact on the person'.[216] With respect to referrals, the guidance states that referral to another health professional may be an appropriate option, including handover to another pharmacist at the same or another pharmacy or service provider. However, it cautions that a referral 'may not be appropriate in every situation: for example, if a service is not accessible or readily available elsewhere for the person, or if, due to the person's vulnerability, a referral would effectively obstruct timely access to the service'.[217]

One should also note the case of *Pichon & Sajous* v *France*,[218] wherein two French pharmacists were convicted for refusing to sell contraceptives on a doctor's prescription to three women. The pharmacists claimed that the freedom to manifest one's religion under Article 9 ECHR implied that a pharmacist was entitled not to stock contraceptives whose use amounted to an interference with their religious beliefs, and in consequence, their human right had been violated as a result of their conviction. However, the ECtHR concluded that Article 9 ECHR does not always guarantee the right to behave in public in a manner governed by that belief. As the sale of contraceptives was legal and could only occur by way of medical prescription at a pharmacy, the pharmacists could not give precedence to their religious beliefs and impose them on others as justification for their refusal to sell the contraceptives, since they could manifest those beliefs in many ways outside the professional sphere. Thus, their refusal to sell contraceptives did not fall within the scope of Article 9 ECHR.

We have certainly not heard the final word on conscientious objection; the Conscientious Objection (Medical Activities) Bill 2017–2019 was introduced in the House of Lords. This was intended to clarify the extent to which a medical practitioner with a conscientious objection may refrain from participating in certain medical activities. It clearly establishes the right for doctors, nurses, pharmacists, and those registered with the Health and Care Professions Council to object and refrain from treating certain conditions. This is, in no uncertain terms, attempted to extend of the previsions already in place. It would have forbidden an employer from discriminating against someone who lawfully invokes the right, and would lay the burden of proving the conscientious objection on the claimer, who may do so by a sworn statement. However, after entering committee stage in the House of Lords, the Parliamentary prorogation of 2019 occurred, and its progress was halted. This of course does not preclude a similar bill from being proposed in the future.

---

[215] General Pharmaceutical Council, 'In Practice: Guidance on Religion, Personal Values and Beliefs' (2017). See also, General Pharmaceutical Council, 'GPhC Council approves guidance on religion, personal values and beliefs' (22 June 2017), available at <https://www.pharmacyregulation.org/news/gphc-council-approves-guidance-religion-personal-values-and-beliefs> accessed 25 January 2023.
[216] ibid.   [217] ibid.   [218] [2001] ECHR 898 (ECtHR).

15.6 FOETAL RESEARCH AND EXPERIMENTATION

While several of the legal and moral attitudes to foetal life have already been discussed, the possibilities of foetal research and experimentation extend the area of debate and merit further discussion.[219] Research on the foetus is of considerable importance given that a major proportion of morbidity of infancy is congenital in origin. Major areas of disease will never be properly understood in the absence of research on the foetus and the uterine environment.[220] Nor will the outstanding dilemma of drug therapy during pregnancy be fully resolved. Recent renewed interest in foetal cells holds some promise for wider therapeutic application.[221]

15.6.1 SOURCES OF FOETAL MATERIAL AND THE PROBLEMS OF CONSENT

Other than those that are born alive prematurely and with which we are not currently concerned, fetuses become available for research either through spontaneous miscarriage or as a result of therapeutic abortion. It is axiomatic that any necessary consent to their use can only be given by the mother, and both her attitude and that of her physicians may be different in the two scenarios.[222]

The position seems clear in the case of miscarriage. It seems unlikely in the circumstances that a research project will be contemplated but, were it so, the informed consent of the mother would be required. The therapeutic abortion situation is rather different. Historically, the mother will have requested termination and it could be held that, in so doing, she has effectively 'abandoned' her foetus. The Peel Committee, as the first body to conduct an in-depth examination of the issues, in 1972, made the following recommendation:

> There is no legal requirement to obtain the patient's consent for research but, equally, there is no statutory right to ignore the parent's wishes—the parent must be offered the opportunity to declare any special directions about the foetus.[223]

This recommendation would now be considered inadequate. The very strict rules as to consent to research on the abandoned embryo should, in theory, be extrapolated to the abandoned foetus.[224] Moreover, the Peel Report was overtaken by that of the Polkinghorne Committee,[225] which detected no material distinction between the results of therapeutic

---

[219] See Amel Alghrani and Margaret Brazier, 'What is it? Whose is it? Re-Positioning the Foetus in the Context of Research?' (2011) 70(1) Cambridge Law Journal 51.

[220] See e.g. Sandra Rees, Richard Harding, and David Walker, 'An Adverse Intrauterine Environment: Implications for Injury and Altered Development of the Brain' (2008) 26(1) International Journal of Developmental Neuroscience 3.

[221] Constance Holden, 'Fetal Cells Again?' (2009) 326(5951) Science 358; Julie Steenhuysen, 'Fetal Tissue Research Declining, Still Important' (Reuters, 4 August 2015) available at <https://www.reuters.com/article/us-usa-plannedparenthood-research-insigh-idUKKCN0Q63BX20150803> accessed 19 December 2022; Sally Temple and Lawrence Goldstein, 'Why We Need Fetal Tissue Research' (2019) 363(6424) Science 207.

[222] Simon Woods and Ken Taylor, 'Ethical and Governance Challenges in Human Fetal Tissue Research' (2008) 3(1) Clinical Ethics 14.

[223] The Peel Committee listed 53 ways in which fetal research could be valuable at the time of its report in the early 1970s: Report of the Committee on the Use of Fetuses and Fetal Material for Research (1972). This quote is at para 42.

[224] Human Fertilisation and Embryology Act 1990 as amended, Sch 3.

[225] Review of the Guidance on the Research Use of Fetuses and Fetal Material (Cmnd 762).

or spontaneous miscarriage.[226] It was firmly recommended that positive consent be obtained from the mother before foetal tissue is used for research or treatment in either circumstance[227]—for it was thought to be too harsh a judgement to infer that she has no special relationship with her foetus that has been aborted under the terms of the Abortion Act 1967;[228] the mother was entitled, at least, to counselling on the point. The Committee also recommended that her consent should include the relinquishing of any property rights. The Committee rejected the notion of any control by 'the father' over the disposal of 'his child'—this being on the grounds that paternal consent was not required for an abortion and that his relationship to the foetus is less intimate than that of the mother.[229] This view is reflected in the Human Tissue Authority's Code of Practice, which states that 'the needs of the woman are of paramount importance in the development of a disposal policy' following pregnancy loss.[230]

The Polkinghorne Committee was established mainly in response to concerns over foetal brain implants, and, as a consequence, one of its main concerns was that the research worker seeking consent should be wholly independent of the caring gynaecologist—every moral and public policy principle dictates that it be made absolutely clear that abortions are not being performed in order to provide research or therapeutic material; the timing of a therapeutic abortion should be subject only to considerations of care for the pregnant woman.[231]

The Human Tissue Act 2004 now governs this area;[232] it is an ambitious piece of legislation that tries to juggle many balls in the air at once. There are no specific provisions relating to foetal material, although undoubtedly the provisions extend to such matter since the exclusions of 'relevant material' relate only to embryos outside the human body and hair and nails from the body of a living person. The Human Tissue Authority (HTA) has the responsibility to produce Codes of Practice in respect of the Act.

The HTA deals with issues of research separately, and primarily as a matter of consent, the legal position is confirmed that foetal tissue—which is defined for the purposes of the Code as being derived from pregnancy loss before 24 weeks' gestation—is regarded as the 'mother's tissue'.[233] This brings foetal tissue firmly within the provisions of the Human Tissue Act 2004, requiring appropriate consent of the mother—and, assuming her to be still alive, only of the mother—for all of the relevant scheduled purposes in the legislation.[234] By contrast, the Code does not apply to stillbirths,[235] nor to neonatal deaths, whose disposal is governed by the same provisions as apply to the deceased under the 2004 Act. The Code notes that, in the absence of dedicated legal provisions with respect

---

[226] ibid., para 2.09.   [227] ibid., para 3.10.   [228] ibid., para 2.08.

[229] At para 6.07. For this and several other criticisms of the recommendations, see John Keown, 'The Polkinghorne Report on Fetal Research: Nice Recommendations, Shame About the Reasoning' (1993) 19(2) Journal of Medical Ethics 114.

[230] Human Tissue Authority, 'Guidance on the Disposal of Pregnancy Remains Following Pregnancy Loss or Termination' (2015), para 15. The guidance refers throughout to 'the woman', but takes into account that a woman may choose to delegate the decision to her partner, a family member, or a friend.

[231] For comment on the potential impact on women of allowing fetal research, see Naomi Pfeffer, 'How Work Reconfigures an "Unwanted" Pregnancy into "the Right Tool for the Job" in Stem Cell Research' (2009) 31(1) Sociology of Health & Illness 98.

[232] A helpful FAQs site is available at Human Tissue Authority, 'Disposal of Pregnancy Remains FAQs' (HTA, 26 October 2018) available at <https://www.hta.gov.uk/guidance-professionals/regulated-sectors/post-mortem/guidance-sensitive-handling-pregnancy-0> accessed 19 December 2022.

[233] HTA, 'Code A: Guiding Principles and the Fundamental Principle of Consent' (2020) paras 141–143.

[234] Human Tissue Act 2004, s 3.

[235] A stillbirth is defined as a child born after the 24th week of gestation which did not breathe or show other form of life: Still-birth (Definition) Act 1992.

to foetal material, the relevant guidance for research on such tissue is derived from the Polkinghorne Guidelines, but with one important difference. Whereas Polkinghorne recommended that women should not be told what the foetal tissue would be used for, or indeed whether it would be used at all, this is no longer lawful under the Human Tissue Act 2004. The guidance is clear that women must be given sufficient information to make an informed decision about the storage, use, and disposal of 'their' tissue.[236]

15.6.2 THE DEAD FOETUS AND FOETAL MATERIALS

Much useful research can be done on foetuses which are clearly dead or are incomplete; the major debate as to the morality of such research depends on how the foetus came to be dead—any objection on principle to the use of tissue from dead foetuses is almost certainly grounded on an overall objection to abortion. Disposal of the dead foetus—as opposed to the stillbirth—is, effectively a matter of societal rather than lawful practice. We have seen that foetal tissue, whether alive or dead, is now considered to be the mother's tissue; it follows that the dead foetus of less than 24 weeks' gestation, itself, must be 'maternal tissue'.[237] The question remains: how far does this give control to the woman over her 'own' tissue? In particular, does she own it? We discuss the complexities of this in Chapter 14. Suffice it to say, the Polkinghorne Committee condemned out of hand the sale of foetal tissues and materials for commercial purposes; this sentiment certainly persists in Article 21 of the European Convention on Human Rights and Biomedicine (Oviedo Convention), which prohibits commerce in 'the human body and its parts, as such',[238] although this makes no specific mention of the placenta, in which, there *is* a recognised commercial value.

Closer to home, the Human Tissue Act 2004 imposes a prohibition on commercial dealings in human material for transplantation purposes. This is particularly pertinent given the suggested value of foetal material for a growing range of therapeutic possibilities. Only the permission of the HTA can elide the possibility of prosecution in such cases. Note, however, material that has become property because of the application of human skill—for example, through suitable preservation techniques—is excepted from this.[239] This raises the prospect that researchers, rather than the mother, might ultimately claim property rights in foetal material, albeit that failure to obtain her consent to the 'work' to be done at all would serve as a complete veto.

15.7 CONCLUSION

The control of fertility and pregnancy continues to be a central feature of political and legal landscapes worldwide. Access to contraception and termination of pregnancy is a matter of profound importance. We imagine that the landscape in this field will continue to change (for better in some places, for worse in others) in the coming years, as we have

[236] HTA (n 231), paras 141 and 108–112.
[237] Leaving aside the difficulty of equating this with the House of Lords' decision in *A-G's Reference (No 3 of 1994)* (1998) AC 245.
[238] Council of Europe, Convention for the Protection of Human Rights and Dignity of the Human Being with regard to the Application of Biology and Medicine (1997), Art 21. See also, Department of Health, 'Human Bodies, Human Choices' (2002), which raised the possibility of legislation specifically excluding property rights in the body of a foetus or fetal tissue.
[239] Human Tissue Act 2004, s 32(9)(c).

seen recently, for example, in the *Dobbs* case in the US Supreme Court.[240] At the time of writing, MPs have backed proposals to enforce buffer zones in England and Wales under the Public Order Bill[241] and momentum is gathering for the provision of safe access zones (also known as buffer zones) around all abortion clinics in Scotland to prevent would-be patients from intimidation or harassment from so-called 'pro-life' protesters.[242] In early 2022, the Northern Ireland Assembly passed a similar Bill, only for it to be referred to the UK Supreme Court by the Office of the Attorney General for Northern Ireland before it could come into effect.[243] The result of this case and the Scottish Bill remain to be seen, or indeed whether England and Wales will follow in their footsteps.

FURTHER READING

1. Sally Sheldon, *Beyond Control: Medical Power and Abortion Law* (Pluto Press 1997).

2. Sally Sheldon et al., *The Abortion Act 1967: A Biography of A UK Law* (CUP 2022).

3. Elizabeth Romanis, Alexandra Mullock, and Jordan Parsons, 'The Excessive Regulation of Early Abortion Medication in the UK: The Case for Reform' (2022) 30 Medical Law Review 4.

4. Zoe Tongue, '*Crowter* v *Secretary of State for Health and Social Care* [2021] EWHC 2536: Discrimination, Disability, and Access to Abortion' (2022) 30(1) Medical Law Review 177.

5. Sheelagh McGuinness and Michael Thomson, 'Conscience, Abortion and Jurisdiction' (2020) 40(4) Oxford Journal of Legal Studies 819.

6. Sally Sheldon, 'The Regulatory Cliff Between Contraception and Abortion: The Legal and Moral Significance of Implantation' (2015) 41(9) Journal of Medical Ethics 762.

7. Kate Greasley, *Arguments About Abortion: Personhood, Morality, and Law* (OUP 2017).

8. Emily Ottley, 'Fixed Buffer Zone Legislation: A Proportionate Response to Demonstrations Outside Abortion Clinics in England and Wales?' (2022) 30(3) Medical Law Review 509.

---

[240] *Dobbs* v *Jackson Women's Health Organization*, No 19-1392, 597 US (2022).
[241] UK Parliament, 'Public Order Bill' (2022) available at <https://bills.parliament.uk/bills/3153> accessed 19 December 2022.
[242] Proposed Abortion Services Safe Access Zones (Scotland) Bill.
[243] Reference by the Attorney General for Northern Ireland (AG for NI)—Abortion Services (Safe Access Zones) (Northern Ireland) Bill [2022/0077].

16

ASSISTED REPRODUCTION

16.1 INTRODUCTION

Assisted reproduction is an umbrella term for a range of treatments that help people[1] to address fertility issues with a view to starting a family. Such treatments may be required where a woman and/or her male partner suffers from issues with fertility, or where a same-sex couple or single person wish to start a family. There may be individuals who may not wish to conceive 'naturally' for genetic reasons, either because one carries a dominant deleterious gene (for example, Huntingdon's disease) or because both are known to bear adverse recessive characteristics (for example, Tay-Sachs disease). While adoption remains an option, for many years, attention has focused on the elaboration of methods designed either to substitute the gametes (i.e. eggs or sperm) of one or other persons or to bypass the natural process in other ways. Assisted reproduction will therefore continue to shape individuals' lives and family formation practices for years to come, particularly with recent expansions in capabilities in this field on the scientific, ethical, and legal horizon for human use, including gene therapy and artificial wombs.

Many reproductive techniques currently involve the fertilisation of the egg in laboratory—or in-vitro—conditions, and which will also involve the subsequent transfer of the embryo from the petri dish to the uterus. Strictly speaking, therefore, in-vitro fertilisation (IVF) and embryo transfer (ET) are technical terms applicable to a number of specific treatment regimes. Standard IVF treatment involves collection of eggs from a biological female, fertilisation of these eggs with sperm in the laboratory, and then the transfer of the resulting embryo to her uterus. An IVF cycle does, however, involve complex hormonal priming to ensure superovulation.[2] This is important to the process, as an excess of subsequent embryos is needed so that a choice can be made so as to ensure that those inserted are normal. A significant collateral advantage is that unused eggs can be made available for egg donation, a process also known as 'egg sharing'—to which we return going forward. For approximately half of all individuals who experience fertility issues, the cause is sperm-related.[3] The most common treatment for this is intracytoplasmic sperm injection (ICSI), which is a very similar process to IVF. The only difference is that sperm are injected into the egg in vitro, rather than mixed and left to fertilise on their own.

---

[1] We wish to recognise that while the majority of those who can get pregnant identify as women, trans men and people who identify otherwise can also get pregnant. For that reason, in this chapter, we use gender-neutral language where possible, except for where the law discussed specifically refers to gendered terms, e.g. 'woman', 'mother', 'father'.

[2] HFEA, 'IVF' (2022) available at <https://www.hfea.gov.uk/treatments/explore-all-treatments/in-vitro-fertilisation-ivf/> accessed 30 November 2022.

[3] Manon Oud et al., 'A De Novo Paradigm for Male Infertility' (2022) 13 Nature Communications 154.

The legal and moral issues involved have been considered since the inception of IVF. In general, the major differences of opinion with regard to such issues in and across jurisdictions are determined by attitudes toward the respect to be paid to the embryo in vitro. This has led to what has been described as procreative 'shopping around', as individuals wishing to avail of IVF seek a jurisdiction that permits their preferences with regards to family formation.[4] The UK is in some ways atypical in that, while the creation and management of embryos outside the body is tightly regulated, the status of those embryos is, at best, left in a legal limbo.[5] This is largely due to the position of the UK Parliament and regulatory oversight bodies in the area, which have consistently leant towards the philosophy that medical research—and medical advancement—should not be restrained unless it can be shown to be positively harmful.[6] Positive harm to an embryo that is destined to die is difficult to establish, and we will see later that embryonic research in the UK has extended significantly beyond the limits recommended in other jurisdictions,[7] as well as by international bodies.[8] In its way, this leads to a paradox. It is easy to see why a government should be concerned to protect the embryo—for some view it as the most vulnerable form of human life. But it is also difficult to justify the control of assisted reproduction: why, it may be asked, should we do so in this particular instance, when any attempt to control natural reproduction would probably be condemned out of hand?[9] There is no simple answer, yet that is the way that has been chosen.

16.2 REGULATING ASSISTED REPRODUCTION IN THE UK

The Human Fertilisation and Embryology Act 1990, as amended by the Human Fertilisation and Embryology Act 2008 (hereinafter referred to as 'the 1990 Act') provides the UK's legal framework for regulating assisted reproduction. For present purposes, it is important to note that the 2008 Act makes extensive amendments to the 1990 Act,[10] with Part I now representing the substantive law in this field. Part 2 is freestanding and now regulates parenthood in cases involving assisted reproduction.[11] Part 3 amends, inter alia, the Surrogacy Arrangements Act 1985. All such matters will be considered in this chapter.

[4] Margaret Brazier, 'Regulating the Reproduction Business?' (1999) 7(2) Medical Law Review 166.
[5] Catriona McMillan, *The Human Embryo In Vitro: Breaking the Legal Stalemate* (CUP 2021).
[6] House of Commons Science and Technology Committee, *Fifth Report: Human Reproductive Technologies and the Law* (HC 7–1, 2005). The report itself was controversial: see Sheila McLean, 'De-Regulating Assisted Reproduction: Some Reflections' (2006) 7(3) Medical Law International 233.
[7] For comparison see Rosario Isasi and Bartha Knoppers, 'Mind the Gap: Policy Approaches to Embryonic Stem Cell and Cloning Research in 50 Countries' (2006) 13(1) European Journal of Health Law 9.
[8] See e.g. Art 18(2) of the Council of Europe Convention on Human Rights and Biomedicine (1997).
[9] There is a mass of literature on the subject. See e.g. Amel Alghrani and John Harris, 'Reproductive Liberty: Should the Foundation of Families be Regulated?' (2006) 18(2) Child and Family Law Quarterly 191; Sandra Samardžić, 'Saviour Siblings – Current Overview, Dilemmas and Possible Solutions?' (2019) 12(2) Medicine, Law & Society 89; and, for an alternative approach, Roger Brownsword, 'Happy Families, Consenting Couples, and Children with Dignity: Sex Selection and Savour Siblings' (2005) 17(4) Child and Family Law Quarterly 435.
[10] For a full analysis, see Rachel Fenton, Susan Heenan, and Jane Rees, 'Finally Fit for Purpose? The Human Fertilization and Embryology Act 2008' (2010) 32(3) Journal of Social Welfare and Family Law 275.
[11] 2008 Act, s 57.

16.2.1 THE HUMAN FERTILISATION AND EMBRYOLOGY AUTHORITY

The main thrust of the 1990 Act was to establish a Human Fertilisation and Embryology Authority (HFEA),[12] which is mandated to supervise, and to provide information and advice to the Secretary of State about embryos and about treatment services governed by the Act.[13] Perhaps the most important specific function of the HFEA in the present context is to maintain a Licence Committee through which four basic types of licence can be issued to clinics approved for the purposes of the 1990 Act. These authorise activities in the course of providing:

- treatment services;[14]

- non-medical fertility services;[15]

- the storage of gametes and/or embryos;[16] and

- research.[17]

In respect of assisted reproductive treatment, the 1990 Act, in broad practical terms, prohibits the use or storage of gametes and the creation of embryos outside the body unless the clinic is in possession of a licence to do so.[18] Thus, it allows for a flexible development of reproductive technologies under the control of peer and lay review.[19] Yet the HFEA's regulatory powers are not limitless; for example, it cannot have a say in the nature and extent of any fertility treatment sought abroad, which is an increasingly popular practice.[20]

The HFEA must also prepare and maintain a Code of Practice outlining the proper conduct of activities carried on under licence.[21] As with all such mandated codes, the Code is not legally binding per se—though it may, of course, include provisions that *are* legally binding. The fact that it had been disregarded would, however, count heavily in any criminal or civil actions brought against the offending IVF clinic. Of greater practical importance, the Licence Committee is empowered to vary, revoke, or refuse to renew a licence in light of any deviations from the provisions of the Code,[22] operating on more routine matters through its Executive Licensing Panel.[23]

---

[12] 1990 Act, s 5.

[13] For details, see Lynn Hagger, 'The Role of the Human Fertilisation and Embryology Authority' (1997) 3(1) Medical Law International 1. An interesting appraisal from the lay aspect is given by Thérèse Callus, 'Patient Perception of the Human Fertilisation and Embryology Authority' (2007) 15(1) Medical Law Review 62.

[14] 1990 Act, s 13, Sch 2, s 1.   [15] 1990 Act, s 13A, Sch 2, s 1AS.   [16] 1990 Act, s 14, Sch 2, s 2.

[17] 1990 Act, s 15, Sch 2, s 3. Treatment can also be provided under a 'third-party agreement' which, effectively, covers the use of non-medical—i.e. commercial—fertility services provided by persons licensed to do so. The purpose of this is to allow cooperation with, say, internet suppliers of sperm (1990 Act, s 2A inserted by 2007 Regulations, reg 7).

[18] Interestingly, the licence-holder, or person responsible for the clinic, is not necessarily responsible for criminal activity under the Act by a senior member of the staff: *Attorney-General's Reference (No 2 of 2003)* [2005] 3 All ER 149.

[19] The Chair of the Authority may not be a registered medical practitioner or directly associated with the provision of treatment services; such persons must, however, constitute at least one-third but not more than one-half of the total membership (Sch 1, para 4).

[20] See Ilke Turkmendag, 'When Sperm Cannot Travel: Experiences of UK Would-Be Parents Seeking Treatment Abroad' (2013) in Mark Flear et al. (eds.), *European Health Law and New Health Opportunities* (OUP 2013).

[21] 1990 Act, s 25.   [22] 1990 Act s 25(6).   [23] HFEA, *Code of Practice* (9th edn, 2018).

16.2.2 ACCESS TO ASSISTED REPRODUCTIVE TECHNOLOGIES

While the 1990 Act does not contain formal restrictions on access to fertility treatment per se, there are three crucial ways in which access to fertility treatment is constrained in the UK: funding, screening, conscientious objection, and the requirement that the welfare of any child born as a result must be considered before providing treatment services. In addition to these restrictions, inequalities in access to access to assisted reproduction have only heightened due to the Covid-19 pandemic, which resulted in treatments decreasing by 20% between 2019 and 2020.[24]

Funding

Those who are seeking fertility treatment[25] have two options: they can self-fund or receive treatment on the NHS if they are 'eligible'.[26] Private clinics are free to set their own costs, and these can vary greatly; one cycle can cost around £5,000.[27] More than one cycle is required more often than not.[28] Whether one has to resort to these costs (unless doing so by pure choice) depends largely on where one lives in the UK. Each nation in the UK has different regimes with respect to funding fertility treatment. Currently, all prospective patients in Scotland may receive up to three cycles of IVF/ICSI where there is a 'reasonable expectation of live birth', as long as they meet an extensive list of eligibility criteria.[29] In England, decisions regarding eligibility for treatment are guided by the National Institute for Clinical Excellence (NICE), but direct decisions for particular areas made by local Integrated Care Boards (ICBs, previously Clinical Commissioning Groups), this has been widely criticised for causing a 'postcode lottery'.[30] In Northern Ireland, the Department of Health is responsible for commissioning fertility services, and presently only one fresh and one frozen embryo transfer is NHS funded for patients.[31] And in Wales, where two cycles of fertility treatment are funded, access criteria are standardised nationwide.[32] Unfortunately, funding is not the only limit to access to fertility treatment; age, sexuality, and marital status all play a factor too, which we turn to next.

[24] HEFA, 'HEFA Regulatory Response to the COVID-19 Pandemic' (2022) available at <https://www.hfea.gov.uk/about-us/publications/research-and-data/impact-of-covid-19-on-fertility-treatment-2020/#section-2> accessed 30 November 2022.

[25] For a discussion of national policies on fertility preservation, e.g. for cancer patients, see Sania Latif et al., 'Fertility Preservation Provision in the NHS: A National Assessment of Care Policies' (2022) Human Fertility 1.

[26] For various eligibility criteria for England, Northern Ireland, Scotland and Wales see Fertility Network UK, 'NHS Funding' (2022) available at <https://fertilitynetworkuk.org/access-support/nhs-funding/> accessed 30 November 2022.

[27] HEFA, 'In Vitro Fertilisation (IVF)' (2022) available at <https://www.hfea.gov.uk/treatments/explore-all-treatments/in-vitro-fertilisation-ivf/> accessed 30 November 2022.

[28] HFEA, 'National Patient Survey 2021' (2022) available at <https://www.hfea.gov.uk/about-us/publications/research-and-data/national-patient-survey-2021/> accessed 30 November 2022.

[29] Fertility Network UK, 'NHS Funding in Scotland' (2017) available at <https://fertilitynetworkuk.org/access-support/nhs-funding/scotland/> accessed 30 November 2022.

[30] See Jacqui Wise, 'NICE Calls for End to "Postcode Lottery" of Fertility Treatment' (2014) g6383 BMJ 349; BPAS, 'BPAS Investigation into the IVF Postcode Lottery: An Examination of CCG Policy for the Provision of Fertility Services' (2021) available at <https://www.bpas.org/media/3369/bpas-fertility-ivf-postcode-lottery-report.pdf> accessed 30 November 2022.

[31] Belfast HSCB, 'Eligibility for HSC Funded IVF and Related Treatments Effective From 1st June 2019' (2020) available at <https://belfasttrust.hscni.net/wpfd_file/eligibility-for-hsc-funded-ivf-and-related-treatments-effective-from-1st-june-2019/> accessed 30 November 2022. Previously, this was managed by the Health and Social Care Board (HSCB), which closed in March 2022; responsibility for its functions transferred to the Department of Health.

[32] Welsh Health Specialised Services Committee, 'Specialised Services Commissioning Policy: CP38' (2017) available at <https://whssc.nhs.wales/commissioning/whssc-policies/fertility/specialist-fertility-services-commissioning-policy-cp38-july-2018/> accessed 30 November 2022.

Screening

Age is a limiting factor when it comes to access to fertility treatment. NICE recommends that three free cycles of IVF are provided by the NHS to women under 40.[33] The access considerations are different (and more onerous) for women between 40 and 42, for whom only one cycle is recommended. Given that we would not consider depriving 42-year-old women of pregnancy without technological assistance, it seems paternalistic in the extreme to deny assisted reproductive services on the grounds of age alone; however, the policy reason behind the age limit is deemed to be the scarcity of NHS resources and evidence surrounding age-associated fertility decline.[34] It is for this reason that the courts, which are traditionally reluctant to interfere with clinical judgement, have supported at least one health authority's decision not to fund infertility services for women above the age of 35.[35] It is important to note that these are only guidelines and there is room for discretion. The HFEA therefore recommends that those seeking treatment check the criteria for their local area.[36] While IVF may well be the optional treatment for fertility issues stemming from other underlying reasons, the success rates (i.e. a live birth) are around 32% for women under 35 and drop as the woman's age increases, to 4% for women over the age of 44.[37]

Access to treatment services is also limited by sexual orientation and marital status; access is notably unequal across the UK for LGBTQ+ and single people in general. In Scotland, England, and Wales, same-sex couples, single women, and single men have to go through six non-stimulated cycles of artificial insemination (AI) to prove infertility before being deemed eligible for NHS funded services.[38] More justification may be required when it comes to ICBs commissioning services. For example, at the time of writing, a test case has launched against a Clinical Commissioning Group (CCG) by a female same-sex couple on the grounds of direct and indirect discrimination under the Equality Act 2010, and Articles 8 and 14 of the European Convention on Human Rights (ECHR) for this very reason.[39] The CCG in question reportedly required single women and people with wombs, as well as female same-sex couples, to pay for twelve rounds of AI to demonstrate their infertility before they are eligible for treatment. A similar action for unlawful discrimination was brought by a female same-sex couple in 2017 against their CCG, though this was settled out of court. Promising developments have happened on this

---

[33] National Institute for Health and Care Excellence, 'Fertility Problems: Assessment and Treatment' (2017) available at <https://www.nice.org.uk/guidance/CG156> accessed 30 November 2022. Notably, the NICE guidelines apply to England only, but very similar limits with regards to age are followed across the four nations.

[34] For general discussion, see Giulia Cavaliere and James Fletcher 'Age-Discriminated IVF Access and Evidence-Based Ageism: Is There a Better Way?' (2022) 47(5) Science, Technology, and Human Values 986.

[35] *R v Sheffield Health Authority, ex parte Seale* (1994) 25 BMLR 1. Note also that the HFEA imposes age limits for gamete donors. In respect of treatment, gametes should not be taken from women over 36 and men over 41, and gametes must not be taken for treatment (other than the patient's own treatment or treatment of his/her partner), storage, or research from persons below the age of 18: HFEA (n 23) ch 11 Guidance.

[36] HEFA, 'Women Over 38' (2022) available at <https://www.hfea.gov.uk/i-am/women-over-38/> accessed 30 November 2022.

[37] NHS, 'Overview: IVF' (2022) available at <https://www.nhs.uk/conditions/ivf/> accessed 30 November 2022.

[38] National Institute for Health and Care Excellence (2017) (n 33) (similar guidance is used in Scotland); WHSSC, Specialised Services Commissioning Policy: Welsh Health Specialised Services Committee (n 32), p 9.

[39] Abi Rimmer, 'Same Sex Couple take Commissioners to Court over "Discriminatory" IVF Policy' (2021) n2769 BMJ 375.

matter recently, however. In 2022 as part of its 'Women's Health Strategy for England', the UK Government announced that it planned to remove 'additional barriers' to IVF for female same-sex couples in England by no longer requiring them to pay for AI to prove their fertility status, and committed to providing six rounds of AI on the NHS before giving access to IVF services.[40]

Conscientious Objection

It is also worth noting here that, similar to the Abortion Act 1967 (see Chapter 15), a 'conscience clause' embedded in section 38(1) of the 1990 Act provides that health-care professionals can refuse to participate in treatment services where they have a conscientious objection to the activity. This has limits, however.[41] The doctor who is morally opposed to extramarital procreation of any sort, or to these 'non-traditional' family forms, could attempt to plead the 'conscience clause', but the chances of that happening seem increasingly remote. Additionally, Parliament has limited the objections to providing treatment for such women insofar as ss 43–53 of the 2008 Act allow not only for the application of the terms of the Civil Partnership Act 2004 but also for a homosexual woman to consent to being, and to be accepted as, a second parent.[42] The implication is that there is no objection in principle to same-sex parenting, an inevitable and logical conclusion once it is appreciated that there is no suggestion that single and lesbian women should be prevented from having children by natural means.[43] There remain some concerns, however, as to whether equality is being enjoyed in practice, or indeed whether lesbian prospective mothers require their own treatment pathways.[44]

The Welfare of the Child

For all potential patients, the decision whether to make IVF available to any person or couple involves a consideration of the motives behind the request—and these are many and varied. The well-being of the resultant child is to be taken into consideration before IVF treatment is provided. Here, medical involvement in the procedure is essential; it follows that the doctor cannot opt out of making moral judgements, despite the fact that they may involve purely social values. No legally enforceable principles have been established, but the Code of Practice contains a number of conditions, some of which are markedly intrusive, not only as to the welfare of the child but also in relation to each patient and their partner. The clinic may make widespread inquiries and, while the patients should be given the opportunity to respond to adverse information, ultimately, treatment may be refused.[45] Of note, under section 13(6), all patients and any partner(s) must be given suitable opportunity for counselling, but this must be private and discussions should not be

[40] Department of Health and Social Care, 'Women's Health Strategy for England' (2022) available at <https://www.gov.uk/government/publications/womens-health-strategy-for-england/womens-health-strategy-for-england> accessed 30 November 2022.

[41] See s 38(2).

[42] Here, the Marriage (Same Sex Couples) Act 2013 is relevant, and in such circumstances, no man is to be regarded as the father (2008 Act, s 45(1)).

[43] Although the 'logic' depends on whether the word 'parent' is interpreted in procreative or social terms. It also leaves open the underlying question of whether NHS resources should be used for non-medical purposes.

[44] Helen Priddle, 'How Well are Lesbians Treated in UK Fertility Clinics?' (2015) 18(3) Human Fertility 194.

[45] The full list of conditions is to be found in the HFEA, 'Code of Practice' (n 23), ch 8 Guidance.

taken into consideration when considering whether the conditions of licencing treatment are met (including the welfare of the child).

Section 13(5) of the 1990 Act states that 'A woman shall not be provided with treatment services unless account has been taken of the welfare of any child who may be born as a result of the treatment (including the need of that child for supportive parenting), and of any other child who may be affected by the birth.'[46] All prospective parents should be presumed to be supportive as a starting point.[47] However, the HFEA Code of Practice also expands on the factors to be considered in the assessment of the welfare of any future child, which it frames as an assessment of 'risk of significant harm or neglect'.[48] These factors include (but are not limited to): previous convictions relating to harming children, mental or physical conditions, and medical history. While this provision is named the 'welfare of the child principle', it has been noted that it is commonly used to scrutinise the adequacy of patients as prospective parents.[49] This provision has been subject to rigorous criticism for various reasons,[50] perhaps most significantly the unfair burden and scrutiny it places on infertile couples relative to those who are able to conceive naturally. And as to their actual interpretation, it is a matter of considerable conjecture as to what the 'supportive parenting' provision is actually designed to achieve, how this can be policed, whether (and how) it is invoked, and whether it does little more than provide subjective licence to discriminate against those seeking fertility services.[51]

16.3 ARTIFICIAL INSEMINATION

As previously mentioned, artificial insemination (AI) is a procedure where a doctor (but not always a doctor, as we will see) injects sperm into the uterus; this may be done using partner sperm, or the sperm of a donor. This process is thus distinct from much of the discussion elsewhere in this chapter first, because it occurs in vivo, and secondly, it may be done privately in the confines of one's home without any medical intervention.

In general terms, both artificial insemination by the husband (AIH) and partner (AIP) are affected by the 1990 Act only tangentially. It is important to note that section 4(1)(b) states that no person shall use the sperm of any man *other than partner donated sperm which has been neither processed nor stored* (our emphasis) in the course of providing treatment services for a woman except in pursuance of a licence. Both, however, come within the scope of the Act if technical expertise has been involved, in which case the clinic is providing 'basic partner treatment services'. Even then, however, the regulations

---

[46] It is of note that s 13(5) formerly required consideration of 'the need of that child for a father', yet this was replaced with 'supportive' parenting in the 2008 amendments to align the Act with reforms in equality legislation and family law.

[47] Para 8.15.   [48] HFEA, 'Code of Practice' (n 23), 8.14.

[49] See Emily Jackson, 'Conception and the Irrelevance of the Welfare Principle' (2008) 65(2) The Modern Law Review 176.

[50] See Julie McCandless, 'Cinderella and her Cruel Sisters: Parenthood, Welfare and Gender in the Human Fertilisation and Embryology Act 2008' (2013) 32(3) New Genetics and Society 135; Julie McCandless and Sally Sheldon, '"No Father Required"? The Welfare Assessment in the Human Fertilisation and Embryology Act 2008' (2010) 18(3) Feminist Legal Studies 201.

[51] For discussion, see Sally Sheldon, Ellie Lee, and Jan Macvarish, '"Supportive Parenting", Responsibility and Regulation: The Welfare Assessment Under the Reformed Human Fertilisation and Embryology Act (1990)' (2015) 78(3) The Modern Law Review 461; Samuel Walker, 'Potential Persons and the Welfare of the (Potential) Child Test' (2014) 14(3) Medical Law International 157.

are less strict: for example, basic partner treatment services do not have to be recorded in the clinic's 'register of information'.[52]

Much of the difficulty previously experienced as to the definition of 'partner' is now negated by section 1(5), which states that, for the purposes of the Act, sperm is to be treated as partner-donated sperm if the donor and the recipient declare that they have an intimate physical relationship. This, however, still begs several questions; in particular, it ignores the duration of that relationship in both prospective and retrospective senses. It is, perhaps, inevitable that much still depends on the good sense of those called upon to interpret the 1990 Act and its associated Code. In this connection, it is to be noted that the problem, such as it is, is a matter of providing treatment, and is distinct from the legal determination of fatherhood.[53] Leaving aside any aspects of family law which depend upon marital status, it is tempting to conclude that uncomplicated AI gives rise to no major legal problems. This, however, is something of a simplistic view because a major issue raised by AI lies in the possibility of 'sperm banking', either as an insurance against later sterility due to treatment—for example, radiotherapy for malignant disease—or for use after the death of a partner. These possibilities can, obviously, arise in combination.

AI may also be carried out using donor sperm. While IVF is more often used as a solution for female infertility (among other reasons), donor insemination (DI) may provide a solution to male infertility (for example, where ICSI is not a viable option). It is also used as a solution where a woman (or person who can get pregnant) does not have a (male) partner. In this procedure, semen obtained from a donor is injected into the neck of the womb; this results in conception in a surprisingly low proportion of cases.[54] The partner's semen may similarly be introduced by artificial means—a need which might arise from impotence, from inadequate formation of spermatozoa, or from a vaginal reaction to constituents of the semen; treated semen would be used in the last two instances[55] which would, accordingly, require a licence from the HFEA.

DI introduces two legal complexities. First, in some cases the procedure involves a second (in the case of a single prospective parent) or third (in the case of a couple) party whose contribution lies at the heart of the enterprise. Second, sperm donation in a clinical setting inevitably results in the production of an excess of gametes and, consequently, to the creation of options for their storage and later use. We have seen already that the wording of section 4(1)(b) of the 1990 Act excludes the need for a licence when carrying out AI without recourse to storage or processing of the sperm; whether privatised DI is also excluded is, however, less obvious. The same section equally makes it an offence to use any sperm other than as limited 'in the course of providing any treatment services for a woman except in the pursuance of a licence'. Because the meaning of treatment services which are defined in section 2(1) as 'services provided to the public or a section of the public', it is widely agreed that, taken together, sections 2(1) and 4(1)(b) combine to exclude 'do-it-yourself' inseminations from coverage under the Act and that this is irrespective of whether the sperm used is that of a partner or an altruistic donor. Control of a public insemination programme is, however, both desirable and

---

[52] A register kept by the HFEA containing donors, persons seeking treatment services, etc. See 1990 Act, s 31(2).

[53] The definition of a 'partner' here is to be compared with that given in the Human Tissue Act 2004, s 54(8) as one of two persons, of either sex, living as partners in 'an enduring family relationship'.

[54] The live birth rate was over 45% in 2016 for the age range 18–34, and success diminishes rapidly with increasing age: HEFA, 'HEFA Regulatory Response to the COVID-19 Pandemic' (2022) (n 24) 27.

[55] Intra cytoplasmic sperm injection would then be the ideal treatment and its increasing use must contribute to the recent fall in the number of DI cycles provided.

possible and, to this end, the use of the sperm of a man other than a partner—and, conversely, the use of any other woman's eggs—in providing treatment services is permitted only in pursuance of a licence.[56] Ultimately, the legality and morality of DI (and egg donation) depend on the consent of the donors to their use; as we discuss in the next section, consent provides the foundation on which control is based and its form is detailed in Schedule 3 to the 1990 Act.

16.4 THE REGULATION OF GAMETES AND EMBRYOS FOR REPRODUCTION

In this section we explore the regulation of the creation, use, and disposal of gametes and embryos for reproductive purposes under the 1990 Act. A clear distinction is made between embryos to be used for therapy and research (the latter of which we discuss further). In this respect, sections 3–4A of the 1990 Act define activities which *cannot* and *will not* be licensed. These include: placing in a woman any live gametes or embryos other than those designated as permitted—a permitted gamete being one which is produced by or extracted from a man or woman and whose nuclear or mitochondrial DNA has not been altered, and a permitted embryo being one produced by the fertilisation of a permitted egg by permitted sperm; there must have been no alteration of the DNA of any cell and no cell may be added to it other than by division of the embryo's own cells.[57]

Probably the most significant development introduced in the 2008 Act lies in the acceptance of the production of embryos containing admixed human and animal DNA—currently for the purposes of research only. This has more recently been extended to research involving mitochondrial donation.[58] In practical terms, the 2008 Act recognises four main categories of 'admixed human embryos':[59]

- **Cytoplasmic hybrids**, in which a human nucleus is inserted and replaces the nucleus of an animal oocyte which is then stimulated to form an embryo. The scientific need for this procedure is stimulated by the lack of human ova from which to develop human stem cells. It is to be noted that embryos are being created here rather than being destroyed.

- **Human–animal hybrid embryos** created using human eggs and the sperm of an animal or vice versa.[60]

- **Human transgenic embryos** created by introducing animal DNA into cells of the embryo.

- **Human–animal chimeras**, which are human embryos altered by the addition of one or more animal cells.

The therapeutic use of admixed embryos of any sort is not allowed, and a licence to do so cannot be issued. Precisely the same restrictions are now placed on any egg or embryo developed with respect to mitochondrial research.[61]

---

[56] 1990 Act, s 4(1)(b).   [57] 1990 Act, s 3ZA.

[58] Human Fertilisation and Embryology (Mitochondrial Donation) Regulations (SI 2015/572).

[59] Inserted into the 1990 Act as s 4A(6).

[60] The same hybrid could be created by combining an animal pronucleus with that of a human pronucleus—the pronucleus being that part of the germ cell which is normally discarded in the formation of the gamete. Generally speaking, the Act governs the use of the pronucleus in the same way as it does that of the nucleus.

[61] 1990 Act (n 14) reg 10.

Of equal, if not greater, significance is the ban on keeping or using an embryo after the appearance of the primitive streak (we return to this)—defined in the Act as equating with not later than 14 days from the day on which the process of creating the embryo began, but excluding any time for which the embryo was stored.[62] After the commotion caused by the *Quintavalle* case,[63] an embryo is now defined, except where otherwise stated, as a live human embryo other than an admixed human embryo, including an egg that is in the process of fertilisation or is undergoing any other process capable of resulting in an embryo.[64] Insofar as the 1990 Act governs the creation of an embryo, the definition applies only to the creation of an embryo *outside* the human body and to those where fertilisation or any other process by which the embryo was created began *outside* the human body.[65] We now turn to the legal complexities associated with each stage of the reproductive process governed by the Act from the sourcing of gametes, through to the disposal of 'spare' gametes and embryos.

16.4.1 GAMETE DONATION

Egg Donation

Most IVF cycles use patient eggs and partner sperm,[66] but an alternative therapeutic scenario is that eggs are donated by one woman for use by another who is experiencing fertility issues. For example, the need might arise as being the only way in which a woman with, say, abdominal adhesions or genetic disease could have children. The procedure is, then, that the donated egg is fertilised by the partner's semen and the embryo then transferred to the woman's uterus.[67]

The obvious practical difference between harvesting eggs and sperm is that, whereas sperm is plentiful and easily harvested, eggs are relatively scarce and their recovery involves some discomfort and inconvenience to the donor. They must be stimulated hormonally in order to coincide with the recipient's optimal menstrual state and, in many cases, a laparoscopy will be required. As such, the difficulties associated with egg donation lie not only in the technique, but also in finding egg donors; altruism generally provides no more than a fraction of the overall requirement. Eggs may also be obtained from women in the course of other surgery—in particular, during sterilisation. The process is not without risk for the donor,[68] but clinics in the UK may still pursue such arrangements

---

[62] Section 3(4) as amended.

[63] For discussion see Catriona McMillan, *The Human Embryo In Vitro: Breaking the Legal Stalemate* (CUP 2021) chapter 2.

[64] 1990 Act, s 1(1). This covers the fact that it has been agreed in the House of Lords that an organism produced as a result of cell nuclear replacement is an embryo. But, the restriction on the use of such an embryo imposed by the Human Reproductive Cloning Act 2001 (now repealed) is continued under ss 3(2) and 3ZA(4), which prohibit the placing in a woman of an embryo other than a permitted embryo.

[65] For example, gamete intra-fallopian transfer, i.e. the introduction of the sperm to the egg in their natural habitat (the fallopian tube, not a Petri dish), is not subject to licensing unless either the sperm or eggs are donated. Even so, the HFEA maintains a watchful eye on the process, now used relatively rarely. By contrast, in zygote intra-fallopian transfer, the preformed zygote is placed in the tube; fertilisation is, therefore, in vitro.

[66] 89% of IVF cycles in the UK use patient eggs and partner sperm. See HEFA, 'Fertility Treatment 2019: Trends and Figures' (2019) available at <https://www.hfea.gov.uk/about-us/publications/research-and-data/fertility-treatment-2019-trends-and-figures/#Section5> accessed 1 December 2022.

[67] The HFEA established a National Donation Strategy Group in 2011. In addition to a wide advisory function, it launched the 'Lifecycle' initiative to improve sperm and egg donation in the UK.

[68] See Susan Bewley, Lin Foo, and Peter Braude, 'Adverse Outcomes from IVF' (2011) d436 BMJ 342.

provided that very strict criteria as to counselling, management, and consent are met.[69] The HFEA has also accepted the practice of 'egg sharing'—in which women who are, themselves, undergoing fertility treatment involving ovarian stimulation donate a proportion of their surplus eggs or others to use in treatment, almost always in return for an adjustment in the costs of treatment.[70] Very stringent requirements as to consent are imposed, including a double consent by the women providing the eggs both as an IVF patient and a donor and consent by her partner; there is no relaxation of the assessment of donors' suitability for parenthood because one or both are receiving payment in kind.[71] Currently, the demand for eggs greatly outstrips their availability and egg sharing is a near-essential component of satisfactory treatment services.[72]

Around 40% of donated eggs in the UK come from egg sharing.[73] As an increasingly popular practice, it is worth considering the benefits and drawbacks for sharers and recipients in brief.[74] The main advantage for donors is of course that taking part can substantially alleviate the costs of treatment services. It has been reported that many donors feel rewarded by taking part in these schemes,[75] and further egg sharing helps reduce wastage of eggs,[76] which can inevitably occur in some people's IVF and/or ICSI cycles. The disadvantages of egg sharing are fundamentally associated with the emotional impact this procedure can have, primarily that those who choose to become egg sharers may feel they are giving their 'future children' up for adoption, and/or they may end up regretting it, especially if they are unsuccessful with their own treatment. Yet empirical evidence suggests only rarely do donors express regret, even when their own treatment has not succeeded.[77] For all parties involved—donor, prospective parent(s), and future child—a further issue is the matter of genetic and donor identity, discussed next.

Donor Information

When the 1990 Act was drafted and for many years thereafter, anonymity of the donor was ensured. This was only subject to the HFEA being obliged to keep a register of identifiable individuals who had been treated, whose gametes had been stored or used, and who

---

[69]   Egg donors may be compensated a fixed sum of £750 per cycle of donation plus expenses, and sperm donors a fixed sum of £35 per visit: HEFA (n 23) ch 13. For discussion of the regime, see Stephen Wilkinson, 'Is the HFEA's Policy on Compensating Egg Donors and Egg Sharers Defensible?' (2013) 21(2) Medical Law Review 173.

[70]   A range of benefits in kind is encouraged. The HFEA also accepts the practice in respect of donating ova for research. The evidence is that egg sharing does not affect the success rate in donors.

[71]   HEFA, 'Code of Practice' (n 23) ch 12.

[72]   See Timothy Bracewell-Milnes et al., 'Exploring the Knowledge and Attitudes of Women of Reproductive Age From the General Public Towards Egg Donation and Egg Sharing: A UK-Based Study' (2021) 36(8) Human Reproduction 2189. In particular there is a shortage of donors from BAME backgrounds. See HFEA, 'Ethnic Diversity in Fertility Treatment 2018' (2021) available at <https://www.hfea.gov.uk/about-us/publications/research-and-data/ethnic-diversity-in-fertility-treatment-2018/?utm_source=Twitter&utm_medium=Tweet&utm_campaign=EDIFT_report_23/03/2021> accessed 01 December 2022.

[73]   Kamal Ajuka, 'The Case for Egg-Sharing' (New Scientist 2012) available at <https://www.newscientist.com/article/dn21379-the-case-for-egg-sharing/> accessed 21 September 2022.

[74]   For more detailed discussion, see Eleanor Blyth, 'Subsidized IVF: The Development of "Egg Sharing" in the UK' (2012) 17(12) Human Reproduction 3254; Boon Chin Heng, 'Egg Sharing in Return for Subsidized Fertility Treatment – Ethical Challenges and Pitfalls' (2008) 25(4) Journal of Assisted Reproduction and Genetics 159; Timothy Bracewell-Milnes et al., 'Investigating Knowledge and Perceptions of Egg Sharing Among Healthcare Professionals in the United Kingdom' (2019) 236 European Journal of Obstetrics and Gynaecology and Reproductive Biology 98.

[75]   See Eleanor Blyth (n 74).

[76]   During IVF treatment, usually one or two embryos are transferred to the recipient's uterus, but egg donors usually produce around 10–12 eggs.

[77]   Kamal Ajuka (n 73).

were, or may have been, born as a result of treatment services.[78] However, after a successful human rights challenge,[79] new regulations came into force in April 2005 which allow a person over the age of 18 access to the name, date and place of birth, appearance, and last known address of a donor parent.[80] However, since a change in the regulations cannot be retrospective,[81] the new facility cannot be invoked until 2023 at the earliest. This position is in contrast to other countries in Europe where the right to discover the identity of the donor has been recognised, although there is far from consensus on the matter. For example, in Italy anonymity is absolute, whereas in Sweden, a child has a right to identify the father on reaching maturity. In Germany, a need for knowledge of the truth of one's heredity is so much ingrained in the national psyche that laws provide for compulsory examinations in order to obtain the evidence from reluctant parties.[82] Elsewhere in the world, for example in Victoria, Australia, retrospective access to anonymous donors has been introduced.[83]

The recognition of such a right is based not only on the supposition that knowledge of one's genetic parentage is a fundamental right but also that children have a strong psychological urge to acquire this knowledge,[84] which may be related to developing a sense of their personal identity.[85]

On this matter, analogies with adoption are frequently drawn, where, in the UK, there is a statutory right for the child in question to discover a true genetic relationship.[86] Yet for some it is doubtful if the statutory creation of the right of children to question their genetic parentage can be to the overall benefit of family relationships;[87] some authors have raised concern about its effects on the cultural significance of kinship[88] and single motherhood.[89] Moreover, such a right may challenge parent–child relationships

[78] 1990 Act, s 31(2).

[79] For the balance between parental anonymity and the child's desire to know, see the ECtHR opinion (particularly the minority's) in *Odièvre v France* (2004) 38 EHRR 871, an adoption case peculiar to French law. And see Thérèse Callus, 'Tempered Hope? A Qualified Right to Know One's Genetic Origin: *Odièvre v France*' (2004) 67(4) The Modern Law Review 658.

[80] Human Fertilisation and Embryology Authority (Disclosure of Donor Information) Regulations 2004 (SI 2004/1511). The change in the law was heavily influenced by the concept of 'the child's right to personal identity': Ilke Turkmendag, 'The Donor Conceived Child's "Right to Personal Identity"' (2012) 39(1) Journal of Law and Society 58.

[81] 1990 Act, s 31(5).

[82] §372a of the German Civil Procedure Code (ZPO). For discussion of legal frameworks on donor anonymity in Europe, see Rafal Lukasiewicz, 'The Scope of Donor-Conceived Person's Right to Access Information about the Gamete Donor in Europe: A Comparative Review' (2020) 13(4) Journal of Politics and Law 88.

[83] See Fiona Kelly et al., 'From Stranger to Family or Something in Between: Donor Linking in an Era of Retrospective Access to Anonymous Sperm Donor Records in Victoria, Australia' (2019) 33(3) International Journal of Law, Policy and the Family 277.

[84] For recent empirical evidence, see Elena Canzi, Monica Accordini, and Federica Facchin, '"Is Blood Thicker than Water?" Donor Conceived Offspring's Subjective Experiences of the Donor: A Systematic Narrative Review' (2019) 38(5) Reproductive Biomedicine Online 797; Lucy Frith et al., 'Secrets and Disclosure in Donor Conception' (2018) 40(1) Sociology of Health and Illness 188.

[85] For discussion of identity and bioinformation, see Emily Postan, *Embodied Narratives: Protecting Identity Interests Through Ethical Governance of Bioinformation* (CUP 2022) ch 5.

[86] Adoption and Children Act 2002, s 60; Adoption and Children (Scotland) Act 2007, s 55(4).

[87] Much the same concerns were expressed by John Harris, 'Assisted Reproductive Technological Blunders' (2003) 29(4) Journal of Medical Ethics 205. An interesting, alternative perspective is given in I Glenn Cohen, 'Response: Rethinking Sperm-Donor Anonymity: Of Changed Selves, Non-Identity, and One-Night Stands' (2012) 100 Georgetown Law Journal 431.

[88] Carol Smart, 'Law and the Regulation of Family Secrets' (2010) 24(3) International Journal of Law, Policy and The Family 397.

[89] Fiona Kelly, 'Autonomous Motherhood in the Era of Donor Linking: New Challenges and Constraints' (2021) 32(2) Canadian Journal of Family Law 387.

and family functioning,[90] and there is some evidence that hurtful psychological consequences can result from the receipt of such information.[91]

Even so, it must be acknowledged that much of modern opinion is strongly in favour of early disclosure of genetic parentage,[92] and there is longitudinal evidence that other factors (including absence of a gestational connection, and maternal distress in childhood) are more likely to negatively affect children born from donation than knowledge of a lack of genetic connectedness.[93] Counselling and family environment are clearly a large part of the picture,[94] and current HFEA policy on the subject is unequivocal on this matter: 'The centre should encourage and prepare patients to be open with their children from an early age about the circumstances of their conception' and further '[t]he centre should tell people who seek treatment with donated gametes or embryos that it is best for any resulting child to be told about their origin early in childhood'.[95]

Finally, there is always the possibility that the supply of suitable semen specimens will be compromised even further than is currently the case if donor anonymity continues, or is removed entirely—and the recognition of 'nonmedical fertility services' indicates official recognition of the problem. As is to be expected, reports of the effect of the radical policy reversal are conflicting, but may not be as negative as was feared.[96]

Future reform notwithstanding, revisions of the 1990 Act have included extensive provisions for exchange of far-reaching information between the HFEA, the donor, and the recipient. Among the more interesting are the right of the resultant young adult (the 'relevant individual') to know how many and the nature of any half-siblings they may have,[97] and to know if they are related to the person whom they intend marry, form a civil partnership with, or establish an intimate relationship with.[98] The donor, on the other hand, is entitled to know, anonymously, that such inquiries are afoot[99] and, should they wish to know, they must be informed as to the number, sex, and age—but not the identity—of any children born as a result of their donation.[100] Significantly, a father is specifically prevented from knowing the identity of his children, meaning the information available may not be given if it appears to the provider doing so may lead to identifying the children.[101] There are also provisions for inter-sibling disclosure of a relationship[102] and, throughout the section, disclosure can only be legal if counselling has been offered.

[90] Susan Imrie et al., 'Families Created by Egg Donation: Parent-Child Relationship Quality in Infancy' (2018) 90(4) Child Development 1333; Claudia Lampic, Agneta Skoog Svanberg, and Gunilla Sysjö, 'Attitudes Towards Disclosure and Relationship to Donor Offspring Among a National Cohort of Identity-Release Oocyte and Sperm Donors' (2014) 29(9) Human Reproduction 1978.

[91] Sophie Zadeh et al., 'The Perspectives of Adolescents Conceived Using Surrogacy, Egg or Sperm Donation' (2018) 33(6) Human Reproduction 1099.

[92] For discussion, see I Glenn Cohen, 'Sperm and Egg Donor Anonymity: Legal and Ethical Issues' in Leslie Francis (ed.), Oxford Handbook of Reproductive Ethics (OUP 2015).

[93] Susan Golombok et al., 'Children Born Through Reproductive Donation: A Longitudinal Study of Psychological Adjustment' (2013) 54(6) Journal of Child Psychology and Psychiatry 653.

[94] Tetsuua Ishii and Iñigo de Miguel Beriain, 'Shifting to a Model of Donor Conception that Entails a Communication Agreement Among the Parents, Donor, and Offspring' (2022) 23(18) BMC Medical Ethics.

[95] HEFA, 'Code of Practice' (n 23) D20.8 and D20.7. It would seem that individual clinics could refuse to provide treatment if the patients were adamant in rejecting such advice.

[96] Ranging from 'a national crisis' in the more sensational press (John Ely, 'Nationwide Sperm Shortage Means 75% of Donated Swimmers Used by British Women Trying to Conceive Come from Abroad' (Daily Mail, 2022) available at <https://www.dailymail.co.uk/health/article-10940975/Nationwide-sperm-shortage-means-75-donated-swimmers-come-abroad.html> accessed 07 December 2022) to the HFEA's estimate that the number of donors rose by 6% in the year following the enforcement of the new legislation: Michael Day, 'Number of Sperm Donors in UK Rises Despite Removal of Anonymity' (2007) 334 BMJ 971.

[97] 1990 Act, s 31ZA(2)(b).   [98] 1990 Act, s 31ZB(2).   [99] s 31ZC.   [100] s 31ZD(3).
[101] s 31ZD(5).   [102] s 31ZE.

16.4.2 CONSENT TO USE OF GAMETES AND EMBRYOS

Following the case of *Evans* (as discussed further), amendments were made to the conditions governing modification and withdrawal of consent to the use of gametes and embryos. So-called 'effective consent' must be in writing and signed, and can apply to the use, storage, and/or disposal of gametes or of embryos resulting from their use.[103] The obligation to sign can be waived if the person lacks capacity, provided that it is signed at their direction. But this concession does nothing for those in a position where direction cannot be given. Consent to the use or storage of gametes implies consent to the use of any resulting embryo or admixed embryo.[104] Conversely, gametes cannot be used or received other than in accordance with the terms of an effective consent[105] and this extends to the use of any embryo created from those gametes, in which case the consent must be by each 'relevant person'.[106] A consent to storage of gametes—which is, itself, governed by the clinic's possession of a 'storage licence'[107]—can be subject to conditions and, again, this applies to any embryo so formed.[108] The 1990 Act makes provision for storage without consent of the gametes of children below the age of 18 and of adults above the age of 16 considered to lack capacity to consent to the storage. For the latter group, gametes may be stored only if the person is to undergo treatment that is likely to result in significant impairment of their fertility, and is subject to stringent medical conditions as to the need for so doing.[109] Lastly, the person giving consent to storage must specify what is to be done with the gametes or created embryos in the event that they die or lost capacity and must specify the maximum period of storage if this is less than the statutory storage period.[110] In addition, the donor must be given adequate information and must be counselled before consenting to procedures under the Act and particular aspects of counselling are now detailed.[111]

It goes without saying that the conditions surrounding effective consent have been modified throughout the 1990 Act so as to accommodate the creation and use of admixed embryo, with the requirements as follows:

- the terms of any consent can be varied or withdrawn by the person giving consent by giving notice to the person keeping the relevant gametes or embryos;

- the terms of any consent to the use of any embryo or admixed embryo cannot be varied or withdrawn once the embryo has been used;

- where the embryo in storage was created for treatment purposes and one of its progenitors gives notice of withdrawal of consent before the embryo is used, the person keeping the embryo must, so far as is reasonably possible, notify each interested person—including a person who was to be treated by the use of the embryo—of that notice;

- then, storage of the embryo remains lawful for 12 months from the day on which notice of withdrawal was received or until each interested person consents to the destruction of the embryo within that time.[112]

---

[103] It is now open to gamete donors to specify extra conditions for their storage or use, subject to compatibility with the Equality Act 2010, which prohibits clinics from discriminating by treating people less favourably because of various protected characteristics.
[104] 1990 Act, Sch 3, para 2(4).   [105] ibid., Sch 3, para 5.   [106] ibid., Sch 3, para 6(3A).
[107] ibid., s 11(b).   [108] ibid., Sch 3, para 8(2).
[109] ibid., Sch 3, paras 9 and 10. Including that the person is not only incapacitated at the time but is also likely to regain capacity to consent to storage. Non-consensual storage is subject to a 'best interests' test and the gametes may not be stored after the patient's death.
[110] ibid., Sch 3, para 2(2).   [111] ibid., Sch 3, paras 3, 4, and 4A and Sch 3ZA.
[112] ibid., Sch 3, paras 4 and 4A.

The matter of consent, of course, becomes more complex when it comes to using gametes or embryos posthumously, which we turn to next.

Posthumous use of Gametes and Embryos

In the UK, posthumous use of gametes and embryos for assisted reproduction per se is governed by the common law and is not unlawful.[113] Indeed, Schedule 3 paragraph 2(2) to the original 1990 Act allows for the relevant consent prior to his death as long as it is written. Nevertheless, as we saw previously, section 13(5) of the 1990 Act and its associated Code of Practice allow the clinics considerable leeway as to the use of available techniques; the indications are that a significant proportion disapprove of at least some aspects of the process, including perhaps those that infringe the dignity of a dying person or a corpse.[114]

The problem of consent and posthumous use of gametes was at the heart of the *Blood* case.[115] Despite the fact that it has been largely overtaken by the events it catalysed, the case still merits discussion for its wider implications. Mr Blood was in a terminal coma due to contracting meningitis, and his wife Diane Blood requested and obtained a specimen of semen, which she hoped to use for insemination after his death. If it could have been established clearly that he was alive, removal of the specimen could have been seen as treatment for a husband and wife together and, since it was arguably in his 'best interests',[116] there would have been little to stop his wife's immediate AI.[117] However, the clinical team was reluctant to proceed along this road without authority. The legality of storage of gametes under licence depends on the written consent and counselling of the donor, and since neither condition could be satisfied, the HFEA held that storage of the specimen and its future use would be unlawful. It also declined to exercise its discretion to allow the gametes to be exported to another country where treatment could be given in the absence of the donor's written consent.

Mrs Blood applied for judicial review of this decision. Her application was dismissed. The Court of Appeal agreed with the High Court decision, finding the HFEA was, effectively, following the will of Parliament. It did, however, conclude that in failing to exercise its discretion to facilitate treatment abroad, the HFEA had not been properly advised as to the importance of EU law in relation to access to cross-border reproductive services and had been over-concerned with the creation of an undesirable precedent. The case was, therefore, remitted to the HFEA, which exercised its discretion in the light of the further evidence adduced in the Court of Appeal. In the end, then,

[113] See *L v Human Fertilisation and Embryology Authority* (2008) 104 BMLR 200.

[114] For criticism of this last practice, see Robert Orr and Mark Siegler, 'Is Posthumous Semen Retrieval Ethically Permissible?' (2002) 28(5) Journal of Medical Ethics 299. In an unusual case, which is also of interest as to the meaning of 'undue pressure', a clinic put pressure on a man to withdraw his consent to posthumous use of his sperm, and the court found that he had done so: *Centre for Reproductive Medicine v U* [2002] EWHC 36 (Fam), aff'd [2002] Lloyd's Rep Med 259. More recently, the widow of a man who had clearly given consent to ongoing storage of his sperm after his death was allowed extended storage for use even though the statutory time period had expired. The reasoning was that to do otherwise would be a disproportionate burden on human rights considerations, and also in recognition of the fact that the clinic had failed to inform the husband of changed regulations for storage and to seek his written consent thereto: *Warren v Care Fertility (Northampton) Ltd* [2015] Fam 1.

[115] *R v Human Fertilisation and Embryology Authority, ex parte Blood* [1997] 2 All ER 687 (CA).

[116] It is an assault to touch a person who is incapable of consenting unless, among other possibilities, it is in her best interests to do so: *Re F (mental patient: sterilisation)* [1990] 2 AC 1.

[117] Accepted by Lord Woolf in the Court of Appeal [1997] 2 All ER 687 [696].

Blood's main contribution to the jurisprudence was to accelerate the changes to UK law that were so clearly desirable.[118]

Since the 2008 Act, the necessity of written consent has been further tested. *R (M) v Human Fertilisation and Embryology Authority*[119] concerned a deceased woman's frozen unfertilised eggs. The parents sought to export the eggs to the US for use with a surrogate, and presented evidence of conversations to this effect with their daughter. At first instance, the Court held that the HFEA was entitled to refuse to surrender the eggs for want of clear, effective, written, and informed consent.[120] On appeal, however, the decision was overturned and the case remitted to the HFEA for further consideration.[121] In finding that the HFEA's decision was flawed, the Court of Appeal held that:

- The HFEA had misstated the facts when it suggested that the daughter had not expressed an explicit wish for her mother to carry a child after her death, and that she did not consent to the use of her eggs after death; this disregarded the evidence presented by the parents.[122] Moreover, the HFEA's conclusion that there was no evidence the daughter would consent to the use of anonymous donor sperm 'would be perverse' if this was what the mother proposed, or was the only way of achieving the daughter's wishes.[123]

- The HFEA failed to explain why the daughter would need to receive information about the likely steps which would be required in order for her to give effective consent, given it was her mother who would likely undergo the treatment.[124]

- The HFEA failed to decide what information would need to be disclosed to the daughter in accordance with the circumstances of the case.[125]

The requirement for written consent has also been thrown into question by the recent high-profile judgment in *Jennings v Human Fertilisation and Embryology Authority*,[126] concerning the posthumous use of embryos. Mr Jennings sought a declaration that it was lawful to use an embryo created from his sperm and the eggs of his late wife, Ms Choya, in treatment with a surrogate. In this case, Ms Choya had died from complications of pregnancy and had not provided written consent to posthumous use of the embryos she and her husband had created. Mr Jennings submitted that his wife had not been given the sufficient opportunity or information required to provide consent in writing as none of the forms Ms Choya had been directed to concerned posthumous use of their embryos, and further that the court can infer from evidence that Ms Choya would have consented, had she had the opportunity.

In consideration of the Schedule 3 consent requirements of the 1990 Act (i.e. that consent must be in writing and signed by the relevant person(s)), Theis J noted that '[t]he reference to written consent is an evidential rule with the obvious benefits of certainty but it is not inviolable where the circumstances may require the Court to intervene.'[127] It was held that because refusal to grant this declaration would be a disproportionate interference with Mr Jennings' right to family life under Article 8 ECHR,[128] the three

---

[118] The generally uncertain nature of the law, even since *Blood*, is demonstrated by the length of the judgment in *L v Human Fertilisation and Embryology Authority* (2008) 104 BMLR 200.

[119] [2015] EWHC 1706 (Admin).

[120] Noting at the time that, given that the store of sperm exists, the HFEA has the authority to allow its export under s 24(4) of the 1990 Act and, as a prerequisite to this, to modify the conditions for storage.

[121] [2016] EWCA Civ 611.   [122] ibid. [70]–[72].   [123] ibid. [71].   [124] ibid. [74]–[76].

[125] ibid. [22]–[83].   [126] [2022] EWHC 1619 (Fam).   [127] ibid. [101].

[128] Specifically 'respect for the decision to become a parent in the genetic sense', see ibid. [102].

requirements for written consent 'can and should be read down . . . to dispense with the requirement for written and signed consent in this limited situation'.[129] Interestingly, at present, neither the HFEA Code of Practice nor their Guidance for Clinics provides information on how a woman may formally consent to posthumous use of an embryo created with her partner.[130] Theis J suggested that the HFEA consider clarifying their forms.[131]

It is important to note that emphasis was made in this judgment that this was a case that turned on particular facts. Indeed, Theis J specifically noted that 'it will not open any floodgates'.[132] The extent to which this sets a precedent for posthumous use of embryos without written consent is therefore doubtful, especially if the aforementioned forms are 'clarified'. At the time of writing, it remains to be seen whether this case will be appealed. It is of note that cases like this highlight flaws in the consent system for posthumous use of the product of the body (for more on this, see Chapters 13 and 14).

16.4.3 SELECTING EMBRYOS

Preimplantation Genetic Diagnosis

Preimplantation genetic diagnosis (PGD) raises a number of moral difficulties, in particular, the obvious proposition that, in deliberately selecting for destruction embryos that are likely to result in disabled infants, we are open to the charge of denigrating the disabled population in general. The argument runs from, on the one hand, that the procedure should be outlawed on that ground alone to, on the other, that persons carrying defective genes have a duty to ensure that, so far as is possible, they are eliminated from the overall gene pool—a version of so-called intergenerational justice—all of which, in turn, drive us into the wider reaches of reproductive freedom and its legitimate extent.[133] There is now a wealth of literature on the subject, the agreement with which is very much a matter of personal morality. Essentially, a balance must be reached between the importance of reproductive autonomy and the moral value of any human embryo,[134] and the justification for 'risk-taking' in the context of the 'do no harm' principle.[135] But there remain legitimate spaces for disagreement as to what constitutes 'doing harm' in this context.

The 2008 Act clarifies ambiguity insofar as it added new sections to Schedule 2 to the 1990 Act. Thus, an embryo may now be tested for genetic abnormality where there is a particular risk that the embryo may have that abnormality.[136] In addition, an embryo may be tested to establish the sex if there is a corresponding risk of a gender-related abnormality.[137] It is to be noted, however, that an abnormality must carry with it a significant risk of serious disability, illness, or condition in the person affected,[138] and embryo sex testing for any gender-related abnormality, illness, or condition must affect

---

[129] ibid. [104].   [130] ibid. [90].   [131] ibid. [105].   [132] ibid. [104].

[133] A helpful analysis is to be found in Amel Algharani and John Harris, 'Reproductive Liberty: Should the Foundation of Families be Regulated?' (2006) 18(2) Child and Family Law Quarterly 191. See also Reuven Brandt, 'Mandatory Sex Selection and Mitochondrial Transfer' (2018) 32(7) Bioethics Online 437.

[134] Rosamund Scott, 'Choosing Between Possible Lives: Legal and Ethical Issues in Preimplantation Genetic Diagnosis' (2006) 26(1) Oxford Journal of Legal Studies 153.

[135] Much depends, of course, on the definition of 'disability': John Harris, 'Is There a Coherent Social Conception of Disability?' (2000) 27(2) Journal of Medical Ethics 95; John Harris, 'One Principle and Three Fallacies of Disability Studies' (2001) 27(6) Journal of Medical Ethics 383; Solveig Rendal, 'Disability, Gene Therapy and Eugenics—A Challenge to John Harris' (2000) 26(2) Journal of Medical Ethics 89.

[136] 1990 Act, Sch 2 s 1ZA(1)(b).   [137] ibid., Sch 2 s 1ZA(1)(c). See also ibid., Sch 2 s 1ZA(3).

[138] For a particularly useful analysis of this criterion, see Timothy Krahn, 'Preimplantation Genetic Diagnosis; Does Age of Onset Matter (Anymore)?' (2009) 12(2) Medical Healthcare Philosophy 187. See also 1990 Act, Sch 2 s 1ZA(2).

only one sex or one sex significantly more than the other. The lawfulness of 'negative selection' of embryos is therefore acknowledged, but considerable difficulty still lies in the interpretation of 'serious' in this context.[139] This is, perhaps, particularly so in the case of chromosomal disease where the clinical and social effect is variable—as in Down's syndrome.[140] In the end, we must depend on the virtue ethics which govern good medical practice, and on the guidance provided by the HFEA.[141]

Even greater moral uncertainty surrounds the extension of PGD into the realm of therapy—currently into therapy for an existing sibling who suffers from genetic disability; this involves the production of an embryo that is not only genetically but also tissue-type compatible with the elder child so that, following its birth, its umbilical stem cells can be used to supply a normal gene for its affected sibling (i.e. a 'saviour sibling'). The HFEA's policy of agreeing to license such activity was challenged by way of judicial review—the 'Hashmi case'—and the application was successful.[142] The finding was, however, reversed on appeal.[143] The basis for the unanimous decision can be summed up in the words of Lord Phillips who said, in respect of PGD:

> [I]f the impediment to bearing a child is concern that it may be born with a hereditary defect, treatment which enables women to become pregnant and to bear children in the confidence that they will not be suffering from such defects can properly be described as 'for the purpose of assisting women to carry children'.[144]

This precipitated the inclusions in the 1990 Act outlined earlier. As to tissue typing, he added:

> No evidence suggests that the wish of a woman to bear a child in order to provide a source of stem cells for a sick or dying sibling was anticipated at [the time the Act was passed]. Such a wish is now the reality, and the only difference between activities that were already regularly licensed and tissue typing was the nature of the 'desired characteristics' of the embryo.[145]

Lord Phillips concluded that IVF treatment that includes PGD constituted 'treatment for the purpose of assisting women to bear children', irrespective of the purpose of the PGD. Once more, this is now incorporated in the 1990 Act.[146] The Hashmi ruling survived examination in the House of Lords[147] and the great majority of the misgivings discussed earlier are now covered in the HFEA's Code of Practice.[148]

---

[139] For a very full discussion, see Rosamund Scott et al., 'The Appropriate Extent of Pre-Implantation Genetic Diagnosis: Health Professionals' and Scientists' Views on the Requirement for a "Significant Risk of a Serious Genetic Condition"' (2007) 15(3) Medical Law Review 320.

[140] The example is analysed in depth by Timothy Krahn, 'Regulating Preimplantation Genetic Diagnosis: The Case of Down's Syndrome' (2011) 19(2) Medical Law Review 157.

[141] HFEA, 'Code of Practice' (n 23) ch 10 Guidance.

[142] R (Quintavalle on behalf of Comment on Reproductive Ethics) v Human Fertilisation and Embryology Authority [2003] 2 All ER 105.

[143] R (Quintavalle) v Human Fertilisation and Embryology Authority [2003] 3 All ER 257.

[144] ibid. [43].   [145] ibid. [47].   [146] At Sch 2, s 1ZA(1)(d).

[147] R (Quintavalle) v Human Fertilisation and Embryology Authority [2005] 2 AC 561—largely on an extended definition of the breadth of the Authority's discretion.

[148] HFEA, 'Code of Practice' (n 23) ch 10 Guidance. The whole topic is well summarised in Amel Alghrani, '"Suitable" to be a "Saviour"' (2006) 18 Child and Family Law Quarterly 407.

'Non-medical' Selection of Embryos

A rather more unusual form of procreative planning takes the form of requests for 'positive selection' of embryos *with known* genetic defects, an example of which arose were a lesbian couple suffering from congenital deafness sought IVF in order to create a child with a similar condition.[149] It is possible to construct a justification for this on the grounds of procreative autonomy, and adoption of a social or affirmative model of disability, although on the other side are considerations of intergenerational justice.[150] In the revised 1990 Act it states, in effect, that embryos which are known to have a genetic or a chromosomal abnormality that involves a significant risk that the child will develop a serious physical or mental disability must not be preferred to those that are not known to have such an abnormality. The same goes for gender-related disabilities.[151] Again, of course, this begs the questions of what constitutes 'significant' or 'serious', and it has been suggested that the law is disproportionate and little more than symbolic.[152]

Non-medical reasons for using IVF are of several types, the extreme being, perhaps, that of sex selection as a matter of parental choice for social reasons.[153] An example of this could arise where a couple might wish to ensure the birth of a girl, having lost their only daughter in tragic circumstances.[154] The HFEA was, at the time, ambivalent on the subject and, in this particular instance, no clinic could be found which was willing to undertake the case. The Authority is now, however, firmly opposed—'The law requires that the centre should not, for social reasons: a) select embryos of a particular sex, b) separate sperm samples, or use sperm samples that have been separated, for the purpose of sex selection, or c) participate in any other practices designed to ensure that a resulting child will be of a particular sex.'[155] Yet, it will be seen that the case demonstrates the difficulties of categorisation. If the parents can show that they are suffering from, say, a demonstrable reactive depression as a result of their loss, selective replacement of their child *becomes* a medical treatment. In such circumstances, the moral high ground may shift, though perhaps not far enough to justify disregard for the interests of the resulting child. Even so, there is a tenable case for holding that we should not pass judgement in respect of a personal dilemma which affects no other person.[156]

Public concern has been aroused by the entry into the marketplace of preconception sex selection of children. Most methods claiming scientific respectability depend upon

---

[149] Julian Savulescu, 'Deaf Lesbians, "Designer Disability", and the Future of Medicine' (2002) 325 BMJ 771.

[150] For more on this topic see Alicia Ouellette 'Selection Against Disability: Abortion, ART, and Access' (2015) 43(2) Journal of Law, Medicine & Ethics 211; Adrienne Asch and David Wasserman, 'Reproductive Testing for Disability' in *The Routledge Companion to Bioethics* (Routledge, 2014); Isabel Karpin and Roxanne Mykitiuk, 'Reimagining Disability: The Screening of Donor Gametes and Embryos in IVF' (2020) 8(2) Journal of Law and the Biosciences.

[151] Section 13(9) and (10) inserted by s 14(4) of the 2008 Act:

[152] Jackie Leah Scully, '"Choosing Disability", Symbolic Law and the Media' (2011) 11(3) Medical Law International 197.

[153] Purely preferential reasons are criticised, inter alia, on sexist grounds. John Robertson, 'Extending Pre-Implantation Diagnosis: Medical and Non-Medical Uses' (2003) 29(4) Journal of Medical Ethics 213, has pointed out that this applies only to the selection of the sex of a first child. See also Olya Kudina, 'Accounting for the Moral Significance of Technology: Revisiting the Case of Non-Medical Sex Selection' (2019) 16(1) Journal of Bioethical Inquiry 75.

[154] See e.g. Kirsty Scott, 'IVF Selection Still Off Limits' *The Guardian* (19 October 2000) available at < https://www.theguardian.com/science/2000/oct/19/genetics.uknews> accessed 07 December 2022.

[155] HFEA, 'Code of Practice' (n 23) ch 10D Guidance.

[156] It is, of course, equally possible to argue that the deontological problem involved is a matter for public decision.

altering the proportion of male- and female-bearing sperm, followed by AI with the processed specimen. Opinions differ as to whether such methods are efficient and to what
extent they can be relied upon, but the HFEA is clearly concerned as to their effect on the
gametes. It states that a licensed clinic should not use sperm samples which have been
separated for the purpose of sex selection for medical reasons.[157]

16.4.4 STORING GAMETES AND EMBRYOS

Other 'non-medical' reasons for IVF treatment include the early removal of eggs and their
impregnation for use in later life (i.e. embryo freezing). Women are now also increasingly
freezing their eggs unfertilised,[158] although this is sometimes done for medical reasons
such as undergoing a hysterectomy. Under the original iteration of the 1990 Act, there
was a ten-year limit on storage of gametes and embryos. This limit was set to alleviate
practical difficulties in estate planning for example that are inherent within a permitted
policy of indefinite preservation of embryos.[159] However, in 2009 the maximum time
was extended to 55 years, provided the storage was for 'treatment purposes', and certain
conditions were met, namely there being genuine cases of premature infertility (or being
likely to become prematurely infertile), with the person's written consent, and with a (ten
years renewable) medical confirmation from a medical practitioner.[160]

While renewable ten-year extensions have worked for those storing sperm and
embryos, this has been critiqued on behalf of those who wish to freeze their eggs for
'social' reasons (and thus are not prematurely infertile).[161] To explain, if a woman
freezes her eggs in advance, at the recommended age (i.e. around 25),[162] she is unlikely
to be prematurely infertile in her mid-30s and thus her eggs would be destroyed. This
critique has gained momentum in recent years, and in 2020, in the wake of the Covid-19
pandemic and the resultant suspension of fertility services during lockdown, the UK
Government enacted regulations to automatically extend the storage time limit by two
years.[163] In 2021, it announced plans to change the time-limit for storage of gametes
and embryos, so they may be stored for up to 55 years (with a review every ten years,
as before) regardless of whether the patient is prematurely infertile.[164] This has clear
benefits for individuals and society with respect to the clear trend toward postponement of childbearing, with some workplaces even offering its staff stipends for assisted

---

[157] HFEA, 'Code of Practice' (n 23) ch 10.

[158] Known as 'social egg freezing', where women choose to delay starting a family, for various reasons.
It is less common that women do this for career reasons; it is more often that they have not yet found a
partner they wish to have children with. See Kylie Baldwin et al., 'Running out of Time: Exploring Women's
Motivations for Social Egg Freezing' (2018) 40(2) Journal of Psychosomatic Obstetrics & Gynaecology 166.

[159] The relatively academic problems of succession of 'twin embryos' that are implanted at different times
are settled by the elimination of 'storage time' from the age of an embryo (1990 Act, s 3(4)).

[160] Human Fertilisation and Embryology (Statutory Storage Period for Embryos and Gametes)
Regulations (SI 2009/1582).

[161] From 2019–2021 the Progress Educational Trust successfully campaigned for a change to this rule,
see PET, 'Our Campaigns' (2022) available at <https://www.progress.org.uk/get-involved/our-campaigns/>
accessed 21 August 2022.

[162] Bana Borovecki et al., 'Social Egg Freezing Under Public Health Perspective: Just a Medical Reality or
a Women's Right? An Ethical Case Analysis' (2018) 7(3) Journal of Public Health Research 1484.

[163] The Human Fertilisation and Embryology (Statutory Storage Period for Embryos and Gametes)
(Coronavirus) Regulations 2020 (SI 2020/566).

[164] This was implemented Health and Care Act 2022 Sch 17(2), which amended s 14 of the 1990 Act.

reproductive technologies;[165] some concerns have been raised about its cost-effectiveness.[166] Notably, HFEA cautions women over the age of 40 against freezing their eggs as a 'sensible option'.[167]

While this technique is increasingly being used in the UK as a method of preserving fertility,[168] it is reported that a low number of people end up using their 'thawed' eggs.[169] Whether this changes as a result of the recent change to the storage limit of course remains to be seen, but where individuals or couples opt not to use their eggs, they will be allowed to perish, a matter which we turn to next.

16.4.5 DISPOSAL OF GAMETES AND EMBRYOS

It is inevitable that surplus embryos will be produced, whether IVF or egg donation is being attempted. The status and disposal of such embryos have significance which is independent of the problems of successful implantation. Insofar as the embryo has no legal status, the problem can be characterised as purely ethical, and one which turns on the *nature* of the embryo.

The Surplus Embryo

It is clear that 'over-production' of embryos is inherent in the treatment of infertility by IVF. It follows that any legislation that attempted to criminalise the necessary destruction of embryos would, at the same time, effectively shut the door on this form of treatment. It is arguable that, so long as we accept that such treatments are morally acceptable, it is logical to accept the production and destruction of embryos for *any* reputable purposes, such as embryo research, for example. However this argument may be difficult to accept without some qualification.[170]

Under the terms of the 1990 Act, the disposal of gametes and embryos depends almost entirely on the consent and, hence, the decision of those donating the gametes. It follows that whether or not an embryo can be used for treatment or research or whether it is to be destroyed at a certain time or in certain circumstances—for example, on the death of the

---

[165] Suzanne Moore, 'It's Not a Perk When Big Employers Offer Egg-Freezing – It's a Bogus Bribe' *The Guardian* (2017) available at <https://www.theguardian.com/society/commentisfree/2017/apr/26/its-not-a-perk-when-big-employers-offer-egg-freezing-its-a-bogus-bribe> accessed 22 September 2022.

[166] See Alex Polyakov and Genia Rozen, 'Social Egg Freezing and Donation: Waste Not, Want Not' (2020) 47(12) BMJ Journals.

[167] HFEA, 'Press Release: Age is the Key Factor for Egg Freezing Success Says New HFEA Report, as Overall Treatment Numbers Remain Low' (2022) available at <https://www.hfea.gov.uk/about-us/news-and-press-releases/2018-news-and-press-releases/press-release-age-is-the-key-factor-for-egg-freezing-success-says-new-hfea-report-as-overall-treatment-numbers-remain-low/> accessed 07 December 2022.

[168] According to the HFEA, in 2019 'there were 7,027 frozen eggs donated for treatment, an 80% increase on 2015. The number of frozen embryos donated during this period increased by 44%'. See HFEA, 'Health and Care Bill: Changing the Storage Limits for Human Eggs, Sperm, and Embryos' (2022) available at <https://www.hfea.gov.uk/about-us/news-and-press-releases/2022-news-and-press-releases/hfea-briefing-health-and-care-bill-changing-the-storage-limits-for-human-eggs-sperm-and-embryos/> accessed 07 December 2022.

[169] Angela Leung et al., 'Clinical Outcomes and Utilization From Over a Decade of Planned Oocyte Cryopreservation' (2021) 43(4) Reproductive BioMedicine Online 671.

[170] For discussion, see Sarah Chan and John Harris, 'Consequentialism Without Consequences: Ethics and Embryo Research' (2010) 19(1) Cambridge Quarterly of Healthcare Ethics 61.

donor—depends upon the agreed consent of the two progenitors and any other 'relevant persons'.[171] Even after amendment, however, the Act provides no permanent alternative resolution for the condition most likely to cause difficulty: that is, when there is disagreement between the two parties concerned, as was highlighted in the joined cases of *Evans and Hadley*, which we turn to examine in the next section.

Disputes over Frozen Embryos

Evans and Hadley concerned two couples who had stored embryos which they had not used successfully before they parted.[172] The women wished to become pregnant, but both male gamete donors withdrew their consent to storage and subsequent use of the embryos, which meant that they should be allowed to die. Ms Evans and Mrs Hadley argued their case along two main lines. First, they sought injunctions requiring restoration of their partners' consent and declarations that they could be lawfully treated during an extended period of storage, and, second, they applied for a declaration that the restrictions imposed by the 1990 Act were incompatible with their rights under the ECHR (Articles 8, 12, and 14). Additionally, Articles 2 and 8 were pleaded in respect of the embryos themselves. This case eventually reached the Grand Chamber of the European Court of Human Rights (ECtHR).[173] In the end, the issue was essentially a matter of statute law, the ethical component being aired, in the main, in the accompanying public debate. It seemed that the primary actions were bound to fail in the light of the very clear provisions as to consent embodied in Schedule 3 to the 1990 Act and, indeed, this proved to be the case.

The court of first instance, backed by the English Court of Appeal,[174] disposed of the first and second pleas on the ground of the clear statutory requirements as to consent. Consent had been given to the use of the embryos for treatment of the donors 'together'; treatment together was provided when the embryos were transferred into the woman[175] and, by this time, the couples were no longer together. Thus, there was no effective consent either to storage or use of the embryos by either of the women on their own and, accordingly, the clinic could not store or use the embryos lawfully.[176] Wall J found the human rights aspects of the case to be far more demanding, particularly those governed by Article 8 ECHR. In the end, he decided that the provisions of Schedule 3 to the 1990 Act

---

[171] 1990 Act, Sch 3, para 6. Relevant persons include not only those whose gametes were used to create an embryo (embryo A) but also any persons whose gametes were used in the creation of an embryo that was later used to create embryo A (1990 Act, Sch 3, para 6(3E) inserted by 2008 Act, Sch 3, para 9(5)). The paragraph also makes provision for consent by minors.

[172] *Evans* v *Amicus Healthcare Ltd, Hadley* v *Midland Fertility Services Ltd* [2003] 4 All ER 903 (Fam).

[173] An extensive literature developed around the case: John K Mason, 'Discord and Disposal of Embryos' (2004) 8(1) Edinburgh Law Review 84; Anne Scully-Hill, 'Consent, Frozen Embryos, Procreative Choice and the Ideal Family' (2004) 63(1) Cambridge Law Journal 47; Sally Sheldon, '*Evans* v *Amicus Healthcare, Hadley* v *Midland Health Services*—Revealing Cracks in the "Twin Pillars"' (2004) 16(4) Child and Family Law Quarterly 437; Sally Sheldon, 'Gender Equality and Reproductive Decision Making' (2004) 12(3) Feminist Legal Studies 303; Amel Alghrani, 'Deciding the Fate of Human Embryos' (2005) 13(2) Medical Law Review 244; Craig Lind, '*Evans* v *United Kingdom*—Judgments of Solomon: Power, Gender and Procreation' (2006) 18(4) Child and Family Law Quarterly 576; Lorenzo Zuca and Jacco Bomhoff, 'The Tragedy of Ms Evans: Conflicts and Incommensurability of Rights, *Evans* v *the United Kingdom*, Fourth Section Judgment of 7 March 2006, Application No 6339/05' (2006) 2(2) European Constitutional Law Review 424; Tim Annett, 'Balancing Competing Interests Over Frozen Embryos: The Judgment of Solomon?' (2006) 14(3) Medical Law Review 425.

[174] [2005] Fam 1 (CA).

[175] See also *Re R (IVF: paternity of child)* [2005] UKHL 33, which disposes of the argument that insertion of the embryo is merely consequential to the mixing of the sperm and eggs.

[176] 1990 Act, Sch 3, para 6(3).

do interfere with the right to respect for a person's private life but that the infringement applies equally to each gamete donor. Moreover, the court considered that the provisions of the 1990 Act, based as they were on consent of the parties and the interests of the unborn child, were proportionate to the restrictions they imposed. A possible infringement of the rights of the embryo to life was dismissed fairly peremptorily, largely on the ground that it is illogical to attribute a right to life to the embryo when no such right attaches to the foetus.

An appeal by Evans was subsequently dismissed.[177] Thorpe LJ summed up:

> To dilute [the requirement for bilateral consent to implantation] in the interests of proportionality, in order to meet Ms Evans's otherwise intractable biological handicap, by making the withdrawal of the man's consent relevant but inconclusive, would create new and even more intractable difficulties of arbitrariness and inconsistency . . . The sympathy and concern which anyone felt for Ms Evans was not enough to render the legislative scheme of Schedule 3 disproportionate.

The issue was, apparently, so clear-cut that permission to appeal to the House of Lords was refused, and Ms Evans therefore applied the ECtHR.[178] This further appeal proved unsuccessful, mainly on the grounds that the UK's 'bright line' policy lay within a national jurisdiction's margin of appreciation when determining the balance between the conflicting rights of Ms Evans—not to be prevented from having a family—and those of her partner—not to be forced into unwanted parentage.[179]

Our main concern with *Evans* lies in the fact that, in this particular area, UK law is founded on the principle of equality between the gamete donors. It is, indeed, to be noted that the powerful dissenting opinion in *Evans* in the Grand Chamber was based largely on the fact that the interests of and effects on Ms Evans and on her partner were so disproportionate that the decision could not be compatible with Article 8 or with the Convention's general purposes of protecting human dignity and autonomy. In the event of disagreement between the parties in question, it is suggested that legislation should allow for 'a right of management' (akin to a quasi-property claim) to be vested in the person for whom the embryos were intended—that is, the proposed woman recipient.[180] This solution, admittedly, ignores the man's interest in his own genetic survival (or extinction) and it opens the door to imposing unwanted financial obligations on him in the future.[181] The former seems a relatively small price to pay for the advantage to women, many of whom, like Evans, will have no more gametes to provide.[182] The latter can be dealt with by legislation—there is little reason why a man who wishes to opt out of an arrangement should not be granted the same legal immunity as that accorded the sperm donor.[183]

The government's response to *Evans* was to propose that it will be legal to store embryos for a further period of 12 months after a gamete provider has notified his or her withdrawal of consent to their being used for treatment services.[184] This was clearly

---

[177] *Evans* v *Amicus Healthcare Ltd* [2004] 3 All ER 1025.

[178] *Evans* v *United Kingdom* (2006) 43 EHRR 21.

[179] ibid. [65].

[180] We discuss this further in Chapter 14. A similar—and seemingly unique—attitude has been adopted in the Israeli Supreme Court: *Nachmani* v *Nachmani* (1996) 5(4) PD 661.

[181] E.g. by way of the Child Support Act 1991.

[182] A Mrs Grant of Inverness was in the same position and her embryos were destroyed on the instructions of her former husband. Frances Gibb, 'Woman Who Lost IVF Embryos Wins Change in the Law' *The Times* (20 May 2003). Other interested parties will, in future, have to be informed whenever possible before unilateral action can be taken: 1990 Act, Sch 3, para 4A(2) inserted by 2008 Act, Sch 3, para 7.

[183] 1990 Act, s 28(6).   [184] 1990 Act, Sch 3, para 4A(4).

a well-intentioned effort to introduce a 'cooling-off period' during which disagreement might be resolved between the parties in question. However, this issue has continued to create dilemmas for the law post-Evans.[185] As noted, the power of each gamete donor to decide the fate of the embryo is limited by statute even when they are in accord, but in the unusual case of *ARB* v *Hammersmith Ltd*,[186] consent requirements were evaded by a forgery. Here, a couple ('R' and 'ARB') underwent IVF treatment and froze five embryos. The couple later separated, yet it transpired that the clinic later allowed R to thaw and implant the embryos without ARB's knowledge or consent, and as a result a child was born. While a breach of contract was found, the court refused to award ARB damages for the cost of financial upkeep of the child.[187] It would appear therefore, that the issue is yet to be satisfactorily resolved.

16.5 SURROGACY

Surrogacy introduces another third party into the reproductive process. At its simplest, and as the term is most commonly used, a couple (the intended parents, or IPs) arrange with a woman that she will carry a child conceived by donor insemination using the husband's semen and will surrender it to its genetic father after birth ('partial surrogacy'). The alternative, which also concludes with the return of the infant to the IPs, is that an embryo which is created in vitro from the gametes of a couple is then implanted in the uterus of a 'surrogate' ('full surrogacy', 'complete surrogacy', 'womb-leasing', or 'IVF surrogacy').

When considered as part of the emerging 'reproductive revolution', the great majority of early commentators shied away from accepting it as a means of satisfying an urge to parenthood. The reason was summarised many years ago in the classic words of Winslade: 'The practice has a potential for economic exploitation, moral confusion and psychological harm to the surrogate mothers, the prospective adoptive parents and the children.'[188] This view crystallises the debate which surrounded surrogacy when it first came to the attention of British courts years ago; it is only fair to say, however, that the evolution of society's sexual and reproductive mores has served to restrict controversy to relatively case specific issues. Indeed, the issues have exploded on the global stage, particularly in countries like the US, where commercial surrogacy is increasingly seen as the norm and attracts considerable numbers of interested parties from around the world, as well as academic commentary.[189] Here, we concentrate on the UK position.

16.5.1 SURROGACY REGULATED UNDER THE 1985 ACT

The practice of surrogacy is now regulated by the Surrogacy Arrangements Act 1985 and related case law, the recent evolution of which has been described as demonstrating

---

[185] See Amel Alghrani, *Regulating Assisted Reproductive Technologies: New Horizons* (CUP 2018) p 82.

[186] [2017] EWCH 2438 (HC).　　　[187] See Chapter 12.

[188] William J Winslade, 'Surrogate Mothers: Private Right or Public Wrong?' (1981) 7(3) Journal of Medical Ethics 153.

[189] Anne Donchin, 'Reproductive Tourism and the Quest of Global Gender Justice' (2010) 24(7) Bioethics 323; Jyotsna Gupta, 'Reproductive Biocrossings: Indian Egg Donors and Surrogates in the Globalized Fertility Market' (2012) 5(1) International Journal of Feminist Approaches to Bioethics 25; John Tobin, 'To Prohibit or Permit: What is the (Human) Rights Response to the Practice of International Surrogacy?' (2014) 63(2) International and Comparative Law Quarterly 317.

the insufficiency of law and practice in this area.[190] We outline its key elements in the following section.

Permissible but not Enforceable

While surrogacy arrangements are permissible under certain conditions, the principals involved are expressly excused from criminal liability.[191] A key aspect of the regime created is that such arrangements (or contracts) are not enforceable by or against any of the persons making it.[192] A surrogate arrangement is clearly a difficult contract to draw up[193]—it must allow for changes of heart on either side, illness in the surrogate, abnormalities in the resultant child, and other imponderables, some of which can be seen as basic rights. Several cases are illustrative of the difficulties associated with surrogacy contracts and enforcement.[194]

Nonetheless, to retain the uncertainties of a breakable agreement which is not against public policy seems to do little more than reflect a persistent ambivalence in a Parliament which, while unable to follow the German model in outlawing the practice,[195] seems determined to avoid any signs of approval. Surrogacy is to be seen as a form of legal liberty, although an increasingly tolerant approach in the courts has been evident for some time. Even so, a system which depends upon the vagaries of the courts cannot be satisfactory, and some formula must be evolved if the IPs are to have a legal right to receive the child, especially considering at present they are not automatically its parents (discussed further going forward).

The fundamental problem lies in the nature of the current regulation—it is currently negative and would be improved if it were to provide some positive statutory conditions under which a surrogacy contract can be legally binding. The difficulty with this, of course, is the problem of enforcement. Florida is one of the few US states that have addressed the question of parenthood independent of a paternity/adoption process, by way of Pre-Planned Adoption Agreements.[196] These include comprehensive requirements of both a positive and negative type, two of which are particularly significant in the present context: (1) the agreement is not binding until seven days after the birth of the child; and (2) it can be terminated at any time by any party. It is difficult to see how such agreements are anything other than dependent on the goodwill of the parties—and this is the position as it stands at present in the UK.

No Commercialisation

A key ambition of the 1985 Act is to prohibit the making of surrogacy arrangements on a profit-making basis. Indeed, outside the US, there appears to be a consensus which condemns, not the making of private arrangements, but rather the manifest commercialisation

---

[190] See Kirsty Horsey, 'Fraying at the Edges: UK Surrogacy Law in 2015' (2016) 24(4) Medical Law Review 608; Emily Jackson, 'UK Law and International Commercial Surrogacy: The Very Antithesis of Sensible' (2016) 4(3) Journal of Medical Law and Ethics 197.

[191] 1985 Act, s 2(2). This also excludes any suggestion of a criminal ancestry for the resulting children.

[192] ibid. s 1A. For the practical implications of this, see *Re TT (Surrogacy)* [2011] EWHC 33 (Fam).

[193] Nevertheless, it can be done; the judicial decision at first instance in the celebrated US case of *Re Baby M* 525 A 2d 1128 (NJ, 1987) was largely based on the law of contract.

[194] See *Re P (minors) (wardship: surrogacy)* [1987] 2 FLR 421; *Johnson v Calvert* 851 P 2d 776 (Cal, 1993); *W and B v H (child abduction: surrogacy)* [2002] 1 FLR 1009. Also see Andrew Grubb, 'Surrogate Contract: Parentage' (1994) 2(2) Medical Law Review 239.

[195] *Embryonenschutzgesetz* [Embryo Protection Act] 1990, s 1(1)(vii). Surrogacy is also banned in France (*Code Civil*, art 16–7, 1994) although the courts will sometimes confer civil status on 'surrogate children' when it is to the child's advantage.

[196] Florida Statutes § 63.212.

of childbearing by way of intermediate, profit-making agencies.[197] Thus, under the 1985 Act, payments made to or for the benefit of the surrogate are not regarded as being made on a commercial basis,[198] but a range of systematised and commercialised practices are prohibited. For example, it is a criminal offence to advertise that one is looking for a surrogate or willing to act as a surrogate, and for third parties to advertise that they facilitate surrogacy, or to negotiate the terms of a surrogacy agreement for any payment (i.e. a solicitor cannot represent IPs or surrogates in agreeing the terms).[199] However, there are some exemptions for not-for-profit organisations, known as altruistic organisations, which now lawfully assist potential surrogates and IPs in navigating their surrogacy (e.g. Surrogacy UK, Brilliant Beginnings, and Childlessness Overcome Through Surrogacy).[200] Again, all of this is meant to de-commercialise the process and remove the financially motivated entrepreneur from the scene.

What remains is to determine what constitutes commercial activity as opposed to reasonable expenses. In *J* v *G (Parental Orders)*,[201] the court exercised its discretion when granting a parental order to authorise payment in excess of reasonable expenses with respect to a professional surrogate who had been engaged in the US.[202] The surrogate was paid $56,750 to cover an allowance for unspecified 'incidental expenses', an inconvenience fee for the IVF transfer, and a pregnancy compensation fee. The court justified its action on the basis that the payment was not so disproportionate as to be an abuse of public policy, and because the parties had acted at all times in good faith and with every attempt to comply with parenting laws in the UK.[203]

This can be contrasted with the comparable Scottish case of *C* v *S*,[204] wherein the (unemployed) surrogate received £8,000 in expenses but then regretted her decision to give up the child. A parental order was, therefore, unavailable on the grounds of lack of consent by the legal mother and the IPs sought to adopt the child a year after its birth. The sheriff, while holding that consent to adoption was being withheld unreasonably, nonetheless refused an adoption order because he considered that the monetary transaction breached the terms of the statute;[205] a custody order was granted in lieu. On appeal to the Court of Session, however, it was held that the money had been paid in the expectation of a parental order rather than of adoption; the Act had, accordingly, not been contravened and an adoption order was substituted. While it is unclear to us why a provision for unreasonable withdrawal of consent should be available in respect of an adoption order but not of a parental order, *C* v *S* serves, at least, to harmonise policy as to the authorisation of 'reasonable' payments in respect of surrogacy on both sides of the border.

The cases indicate that the public, as represented by its judiciary, are sympathetic to surrogate motherhood—an attitude which probably derives more from the fait accompli nature of the proceedings than from any basic empathy with the practice. Accordingly, it

---

[197] For a critical discussion, see Jason Hanna, 'Revisiting Child-Based Objections to Commercial Surrogacy' (2010) 24(7) Bioethics 341.

[198] 1985 Act s 2(3).   [199] ibid. s 3.

[200] Their operation, permitted by s 2(8A) of the 1985 Act as amended by the Human Fertilisation and Embryology Act 2008, acknowledges that amateur action in such a delicate field is beset with pitfalls.

[201] [2013] Fam Law 972.

[202] Such discretion is granted under s 54(8) of the Human Fertilisation and Embryology Act 2008.

[203] For a discussion of 'reasonable expenses' with respect to payments made to an Indian surrogate (being the equivalent of £6,875), see *Re X (A Child) (Surrogacy: Time Limit)* [2015] Fam 186.

[204] 1996 SLT 1387, sub nom *C and C* v *GS* 1996 SCLR 837. For practical guidance and commentary on further cases, see Alan Inglis, 'Hagar's Baby: Surrogacy Arrangements' (2014) 25 Scots Law Times 105.

[205] Adoption (Scotland) Act 1978, ss 24(2) and 51 then in force.

is very unlikely that a parental order will be withheld in the event of an application by the IPs and consent on the part of the surrogate and the legal father—if there is one. While it would always be possible for the court to override agreement by the parties, it is difficult to see how the motivation of the couple and their almost inevitable superior material status could be irrelevant to the child's 'best interests'—which is not to say that economic advantage will always take precedence.[206]

Insofar as it is possible to apply pre-1990 standards to the present-day conditions, the indications are that the prime factor in the court's thinking in the event of disagreement between the parties would be the extent of family bonding—much would depend on where, and for how long, the child was living at the time of adjudication. It is, however, impossible to generalise. The paramount feature lies in the child's best interests. The published cases provide no indication of what would result if the IPs were to refuse to accept the infant; the precise details of each case would be all-important, but it is difficult to see an alternative to intervention by the local authority by way of care proceedings.

While there is no firm evidence on the point, and despite the contrary evidence from the US, we suspect that British judges would take much the same approach whether the surrogate had incubated her own egg, that of the commissioning woman, or one donated—concern for the welfare of the child would trump any other arguments. This has, perhaps, been demonstrated in *N (a child)*,[207] where there was a deliberate deception on the part of a surrogate mother, as a result of which she had managed to retain care of the child for 18 months before the commissioning father became aware of its existence. The court held that the case represented a classic discretionary balancing exercise by which to determine the best interests of the child.[208] In the end, it was decided that the child would thrive best in the care of his biological father and his wife. Nevertheless, the decision might easily have gone the other way and still have been acceptable.[209]

16.5.2 LAW REFORM AND SURROGACY

The law relating to surrogacy is still in an uncertain state and, as suggested, is likely to be further confused with the clear growth in travelling abroad (as most of the recent legal cases demonstrate).[210] Many would say that it is right that customs so private as reproductive choice should be allowed to evolve by way of public opinion as represented by the common law. Others, however, would feel that the implications of surrogacy are such that it ought to be controlled by statute, and that as things stand, regulation in the UK is unsatisfactory because it is largely both indirect and inconsistent.

---

[206] See e.g. *Re P (minors) (wardship: surrogacy)* [1987] 2 FLR 421.

[207] *N (a child), In the matter of* [2007] EWCA Civ 1053; [2008] 1 FLR 198. It is interesting that, even in 2007, there was some conflict in the Court of Appeal as to the legal fatherhood of the child—see Lloyd LJ at [19].

[208] As regulated by the Children Act 1989, s 1.

[209] Assistance in this field is now available in Department of Health and Social Care, 'Care in Surrogacy: Guidance for the care of surrogates and intended parents in surrogate births in England and Wales' (2021) available at <https://www.gov.uk/government/publications/having-a-child-through-surrogacy/care-in-surrogacy-guidance-for-the-care-of-surrogates-and-intended-parents-in-surrogate-births-in-england-and-wales> accessed 21 August 2022, and 'The Surrogacy Pathway: Surrogacy and the legal process for intended parents and surrogates in England and Wales' (2021) available at <https://www.gov.uk/government/publications/having-a-child-through-surrogacy/the-surrogacy-pathway-surrogacy-and-the-legal-process-for-intended-parents-and-surrogates-in-england-and-wales> accessed 21 August 2021.

[210] See e.g. *A, Re* [2021] EWFC 103 (08 February 2021); *X, Re* [2020] EWFC 39 (20 May 2020); *A-B, Re* [2020] EWFC 81 (13 August 2020); *A & B (Children) (Surrogacy: Parental orders: time limits)* [2015] EWHC 911 (Fam) (01 April 2015).

At present, while IVF associated surrogacy clearly lies within the framework of the 1990 Act, standard surrogacy does not, unless it involves donor insemination with manipulation of the sperm,[211] and this leaves an unsatisfactory dichotomy. While very few would now wish to criminalise what is an accepted form of treatment, most would also agree that it must be regulated, and uniformly.[212] The recent cases suggest that the formula for successful regulation remains extremely elusive. If well-intentioned and economically empowered IPs are able to obtain receipt of a child and bring the child to the UK, the odds are now very much stacked in their favour. And yet, this does not remove the legal precariousness of the strategy. To paraphrase one judge: surrogacy is probably the least satisfactory way to become a parent.

It was against this background that the Brazier Review Team was set up in 1997, intending to ensure that the law continued to meet public concerns.[213] It recommended that:

- Payments to surrogate mothers should cover only genuine expenses associated with the pregnancy and that additional payments should be prohibited in order to prevent surrogacy arrangements being entered into for financial benefit; reasonable expenses should be defined by the Ministers.

- Agencies to oversee surrogacy arrangements should be established and registered by Health Departments which would be required to operate within a Code of Practice; an advisory code would be drawn up to provide guidance for the registered agencies and also for those acting in a private capacity.

- Current legislation dealing with surrogacy should be repealed and replaced by a consolidated Surrogacy Act which would address the whole subject rather than specific aspects. It was further recommended that surrogacy arrangements should remain unenforceable, that the ban on commercial agencies and advertising should remain in force, and that the prohibition should include the operation of unregistered agencies.

There is much to commend in these proposals, and it is a matter of concern that none has as yet been incorporated into statute.[214] Nevertheless, some are open to question. The question of payment remains, the rejection of which is central to the Brazier position. The concepts of provision of a service and recompense for that service are so closely linked that, save in unusual circumstances, the majority of persons would expect them to go hand in hand. Given that the demand for surrogates has not abated, and given that private surrogacy arrangements are not prohibited, it is possible the effect of prohibiting paid arrangements in the registered field will force the process onto the 'back streets',[215] which would overturn the whole purpose of regulation.

---

[211] HFEA, 'Code of Practice' (n 23) ch 14, the Code of Practice states that the HFEA does not regulate surrogacy but gives advice to clinics on counselling as to the law and on the mandatory requirements as to gamete donation. The impression gained is that, while clinics are not barred from taking part in surrogacy, they are certainly not encouraged to do so.

[212] With respect to that which falls within the ambit of the HFEA, note the Human Fertilisation and Embryology (Amendment) Regulations 2018 (SI 2018/334), which address the movement and traceability of gametes and embryos across borders. The possibility that regulation offends against the Human Rights Act 1998 is discussed by Joanne Ramsey, 'Regulating Surrogacy—A Contravention of Human Rights?' (2000) 5(1) Medical Law International 45.

[213] Margaret Brazier (Chair), 'Surrogacy: Review for Health Ministers of Current Arrangements for Payment and Regulation' (Cm 4068, 1998).

[214] Kirsty Horsey and Sally Sheldon, 'Still Hazy After all These Years: The Law Regulating Surrogacy' (2012) 20(1) Medical Law Review 67; Kirsty Horsey (ed.), *Revisiting the Regulation of Human Fertilisation and Embryology* (Routledge 2015) ch 8.

[215] Michael Freeman, 'Does Surrogacy Have a Future After Brazier?' (1999) 7 Medical Law Review 1.

Of note, in 2018 the Scottish and English Law Commissions began a joint review of surrogacy law, including a consultation, and published their final report along with a draft Bill in 2023.[216] The Commissions' consultation paper listed a series of proposals on a range of issues, many relating to those discussed, including payment and the way in which parenthood is transferred. It is not clear from the consultation whether and how the payment regime will change, if at all, but it was clear that surrogacy agreements should remain legally unenforceable. Despite the overwhelming consensus that law reform is urgently needed in this field,[217] the extent to which there will be uptake of the Commissions' recommendations remains to be seen.

16.6 ASSISTED REPRODUCTION AND PARENTAGE

The question of who, in law, is or are the parent(s) of a child is a question of fundamental importance—what can be more emotionally, psychologically, socially, and legally important than the answer to the questions: Who is my parent? Is this my child? The parentage of children born as a result of treatment carried out under this legislation is therefore a major ethical and legal question, and it is dealt with in Part 2 of the 2008 Act. While it is fair to say that the major ethical problems associated with DI have been eliminated from the standard husband/wife or heterosexual partnership setting, issues can arise in light of the more diverse family structures and configurations that are entered into today, including same-sex couples, polyamorous relationships with a desire for the recognition of more than two parents, and so on.[218]

The statutory definitions of parenthood are covered by sections 27–29 of the amended 1990 Act and sections 33–47 of the 2008 Act.[219] Which is applicable is simply a matter of timing; the provisions of the 1990 Act do not have effect in relation to children born after the commencement of sections 33–48 of the 2008 Act.[220] Accordingly, we use the 2008 statute as our template, noting not only that much new law is introduced but also that a number of anomalies which previously existed between England and Wales and Scotland are eliminated.[221]

16.6.1 'THE MOTHER'

Legal motherhood is fairly straightforward, unless transfer of parenthood is required where a child has been born in treatment of a surrogate. Section 33 of the 2008 Act holds that a woman who carries a child as a result of the placing in her of an embryo or of sperm and eggs—and no other woman—is to be treated as the mother of the child. This is the

---

[216] Law Commission, 'Surrogacy' (2023) available at <https://www.lawcom.gov.uk/project/surrogacy/> accessed 30 May 2023.

[217] ibid.

[218] Although note that these new forms are not always accepted as meeting the demands of statutory support schemes. For example, in *T v B* [2011] 1 All ER 77 (Fam), the biological mother of a child born to a lesbian couple failed in a claim for financial relief from her partner after they separated.

[219] Sch 6, para 35(3) of the 2008 Act states that both remain 'relevant statutory provisions'. See also Child Support Act 1991, s 26, Case B1, where the sections are regarded as alternatives.

[220] 2008 Act, s 57.

[221] Note that the original 1990 Act is also subject to considerable amendment by way of the European Directives.

case regardless of whether a donated egg or embryo has been used.[222] Where a woman is in a same-sex relationship, the non-gestational partner is not treated as 'the mother' of the child, but rather as a 'parent'.[223]

16.6.2 'THE FATHER'

According to section 35, where a woman has been inseminated with the sperm of a person other than her husband or civil partner, and provided that her husband has consented, her husband will be 'treated as the father of the child'; the donor is covered against withdrawal of consent by the husband.[224] The section 35 rule is voided if the husband can show that he did not, in fact, consent to the procedure. The somewhat confusing terms of sections 38(2) and 38(3) do, however, retain the common law principle of *pater est quem nuptiae demonstrant*: the husband who does not consent to DI will still have to rebut that presumption in an acceptable way. The statutory provisions will prevail in the event of disagreement between the partners.[225]

Section 36 extends the responsibilities and privileges of fatherhood to a man other than a woman's husband subject, first, to the insemination being carried out in a licensed clinic, and, second, to satisfaction of the 'agreed fatherhood' provisions laid down in section 37. These are that both the man and the woman concerned have given the person responsible for the treatment notice in writing that they consent to the man's fatherhood, and that neither has withdrawn their consent or otherwise altered the agreed conditions of parenthood.[226] Reciprocal protection of the donor when such an agreement is reached is provided by section 38(1) in respect of both married and unmarried couples. Section 37 makes no mention of the quality of the relationship or its duration—all that matters is bilateral consent between a man and a woman. Sections 42-47 contain analogous provisions where there is no father but a 'second parent' who will be a woman.

16.6.3 POSTHUMOUS PARENTHOOD

Where posthumous use of gametes or embryos is deemed lawful (as discussed), it could lead to complex problems in relation to probate and succession.[227] However, absent specific regulations, a child born as a result of posthumous insemination or embryo donation could be, in legal terms, 'fatherless'—a situation which would be, at best, undesirable (for some) and, at worst, incompatible with their ECHR rights. Under the 2008 Act, if a child has been carried by a woman as a result of the placing in her of an embryo, or of sperm and eggs, or her artificial insemination involving the use of a man's sperm after his death,

---

[222] 2008 Act ss 35–36.   [223] 2008 Act, s 44(1).

[224] ibid., s 41(1). There is nothing to prevent a man claiming paternity under the common law: *X v Y* 2002 SLT 161, Glasgow Sheriff Court. The potential advantages of this to the child were expressed in the Australian case *Re Patrick* (2002) 28 Fam LR 579.

[225] *Re CH (contact: parentage)* [1996] 1 FLR 569.

[226] The mischief of the concepts of 'agreed fatherhood' and 'treatment together' are well illustrated in *U v W* (1997) 38 BMLR 54. For a more recent consideration, see *ARB v IVF Hammersmith* [2018] EWCA Civ 2803, wherein the woman forged the partner's consent, who then sued for a wide range of consequent expenses, and which were refused on policy and other grounds.

[227] Although these do not seem insuperable in the US: *Woodward v Commissioner of Social Security* 435 Mass 536 (2002). The 1990 Act left open the related questions of the man who is reported missing but is, in fact, dead and of the woman who reasonably believes her dead partner to be alive—we think it is likely that legal paternity could be established in either case.

then, subject to a number of conditions, that man's particulars can be entered as the particulars of that child's father in a register of live or still births.[228]

No special relationship is demanded by section 39—the essential element is the man's written consent. Section 40 also provides for the posthumous transfer of an embryo that was created during a man's life by way of consensual sperm donation. Here, however, a distinction persists as to the married or unmarried status of the woman in that, if she is unmarried, the embryo must be formed during the course of treatment in the UK by a person to whom a licence applies.[229] In either case, however, the conditions as to posthumous fatherhood apply whether the actual impregnation took place in the UK or elsewhere.[230] It is to be noted that the law as to succession is unaltered—the child will not inherit from its 'father's' estate—and that the purpose of these concessions is strictly limited to providing the resulting child with a traditional birth certificate. The conditions validating the grant of the birth certificate are strict. In particular, the woman must elect in writing that the man be treated as the father of the child within 42 days of the child's birth.[231] Most importantly, either party must have given their written consent to posthumous parenthood before their death, although as we saw in *Jennings* there may be exceptions in particular circumstances.

16.6.4 PARENTAGE AND SURROGACY

In cases of surrogacy, in accordance with section 33 of the 2008 Act, the surrogate is clearly the child's legal mother irrespective of whether or not it is the product of her own egg and, if she is married and conception was via consensual donor insemination, her husband is its father.[232] Neither can simply surrender their parental duties.[233] Thus, after the child is born, a legal process is required to transfer legal parenthood from the surrogate to the IP(s): the parental order process. In some cases an adoption order is required.

Parental Orders and Conditions

Under the 2008 Act,[234] a child carried by a woman who is not one of the IPs as a result of placing in her an embryo or sperm and eggs, or her artificial insemination, is to be treated as the child of the applicants, provided that the gametes of at least one of the applicants were used to bring about the creation of the embryo.[235] To qualify for an order, the applicants must be either husband and wife (the original requirement), or (now also) civil partners or two persons who are living as partners in an enduring family relationship. This is the same criterion as applies to the provision of treatment as opposed to agreed fatherhood, which is simply a matter of consent. Presumably, this is to allow some discretion to the clinics and the courts. This condition has led to significant difficulty in the past for would-be single parents, although this has now changed following *Re Z (A Child)*

---

[228] 2008 Act, s 39.

[229] 2008 Act, s 40(2)(b). There is now no reference to 'treatment together'. But since, in either situation, an embryo must be created in vitro, it is a little difficult to see the distinction as being other than one without a difference.

[230] 2008 Act, ss 39(2) and 40(3).

[231] The period is 21 days in Scotland (s 28(5E)). The period can be extended in both jurisdictions with the consent of the Registrar General provided he is satisfied that there are compelling reasons why he should do so (s 28(5F) and (5G)).

[232] 1990 Act, ss 27 and 28.   [233] Children Act 1989, s 2(9).   [234] Section 54.

[235] In an unusual case, the biological father died between the application and the hearing; it was held that 'the applicants' involved were those who made the application: *A v P* [2012] 1 FCR 408.

(Human Fertilisation and Embryology Act: Parental Order)[236] and the subsequent insertion of section 54A.

Applications are heard in private, and a guardian ad litem is appointed to watch over the child's interests.[237] Further conditions for granting a parental order include the following:

- both IPs must be over 18 years old;

- the application must be made within six months of the birth of the child whose home must be with the applicants (i.e. the IPs);

- the surrogate and, where applicable, any other parent of the child[238] if they can be found, must give their free consent with full understanding;

- the agreement of the woman who carried the child is ineffective if made less than six weeks after the child's birth; and

- the court is satisfied that no money other than reasonable expenses has been given or received by the applicants in relation to the surrogacy arrangement other than as authorised by the court.

On the whole, when the aforementioned conditions are fulfilled, it will be exceptional for a parental order to be refused. Most British cases now confirm the paramountcy of the child's welfare in surrogacy cases in general and the granting of parental orders in particular. For example, in *Re L (A child) (Parental order: foreign surrogacy)*,[239] although he had some misgivings on the facts, Hedley J held that, 'it will be only in the clearest case of the abuse of public policy that the court will be able to withhold an order if otherwise welfare considerations support its making'. Similarly, in *J v G*,[240] Theis J opined that 'the court is only likely to refuse parental orders in the clearest case of the abuse of public policy where otherwise the child's welfare requires the order to be made'.[241] As such, retrospective payments, clearly beyond 'expenses', to surrogates in the US and India have been authorised on 'welfare' grounds.[242]

The last suggests that, even when the conditions are not strictly met, parental orders might follow. Indeed, in *JP v LP (Surrogacy Arrangement: Wardship)*,[243] where the solicitors had drawn up an illegal agreement, leading to considerable complications surrounding any parental order including non-compliance with the parental order time limit, the Court held, first, that it should be within the competence of a legal family practitioner to know the particularities of the law on surrogacy and to advise accordingly, and, second, as to the time limits, a purposive approach is warranted, especially when set against the

---

[236] [2016] EWFC 42; Human Fertilisation and Embryology Act 1990 (as amended), s 54A.

[237] Parental Orders (Human Fertilisation and Embryology) Regulations 1994 (SI 1994/2767); Parental Orders (Human Fertilisation and Embryology) (Scotland) Regulations 1994 (SI 1994/2804), both repealed by the Human Fertilisation and Embryology (Parental Orders) (Consequential, Transitional and Saving Provisions) Order (SI 2010/986). Also, see 2008 Act, s 54(8). The first 'order' was, in fact, made pre-emptively: *Re W (minors) (surrogacy)* [1991] 1 FLR 385.

[238] Including a man who is the father by virtue of ss 35 or 36 of the 2008 Act and a woman who is a parent according to ss 42 or 43.

[239] [2011] Fam 106.   [240] [2014] 1 FLR 297.

[241] The great advantages of the parental order system were illustrated in the US cases: *Doe v Doe* 710 A 2d 1297 (Conn, 1998) and *Doe v Roe* 717 A 2d 706 (Conn, 1998), the gist of which was to apply parental rights in the best interests of a child who had been accepted into a family.

[242] See *Re S (Parental order)* [2010] 1 FLR 1156; *Re X and Y (Children: foreign surrogacy)* [2012] Fam Law 286.

[243] [2015] 1 All ER 266.

welfare of the child. As such, failure to meet the six-month limit was not seen to be as hard and fast as the wording of the law suggests.

Other developments have included guidance coming from clearly frustrated courts when parties have not sufficiently considered the implications of their actions in producing the child. In *AB v CT*,[244] civil partners who had paid £16,000 to an Indian agency (with £2,250 to the surrogate) sought a UK parental order some three years after the birth of twins. In allowing the order, the court highlighted the need for prospective parents undertaking surrogacy abroad to seek specialist advice; they were urged to establish the necessary legal steps involved in all relevant jurisdictions, and to make any parental order promptly after birth in whichever jurisdiction they might wish to move to (the present couple had been living in Australia and moved to the UK). The court also stressed the importance of maintaining clear lines of communication with the surrogate mother, which had been lost in this case, with the resulting order being granted in her absence. It finally recommended the maintenance of honest and accurate records of sums paid, and the purposes for same.

This case—and many others like it[245]—suggests that the law and the courts are in an intractable bind. The trumping principle of the welfare of the child is sweeping away all legislative efforts toward specificity and detail in regulating these practices. This having been said, this 'welfare of the child' line of authority[246] is probably to be preferred over cases like *AB v CD and The Z Fertility Clinic*,[247] which, though not a surrogacy case, involved a same-sex couple seeking a declaration of parenthood with respect to children born through reproductive services. The formalities of the 2008 reforms that recognise same-sex partners as parents had not been complied with, and the judge took a firm, literal line in interpreting the rule. The justification for denying the partner's recognition of parentage was the importance of certainty in the law. The judge was not persuaded by the argument that public policy required a more accommodating approach, nor by the claim that the decision might otherwise be discriminatory to same-sex couples. This case is probably an outlier in light of recent decisions, with even here the judge warning against behaviours clearly not in the interests of the children.

The Adoption Regime

Harmony between the statutory provisions of the Adoption Acts[248] and the practicalities of surrogacy has been virtually achieved with the introduction of the parental order, but where intended parents cannot apply for or obtain a parental order, the only way through which they can acquire legal parenthood is through the adoption regime.[249] This may also be required where neither the surrogate nor the IPs can take care of the child after their birth.[250]

---

[244] [2015] EWFC 12.
[245] See *Re A* [2015] EWHC 1756 (Fam) (child born in South Africa—first case to consider this), and *D v ED (Parental Order: Time Limit)* [2015] EWHC 911 (Fam); [2015] Fam Law 1052 (couple commissioned surrogacy in the US and were legally advised they would be parents).
[246] For just one example, see *H v S (Surrogacy Arrangement)* [2015] EWFC 36.
[247] [2013] EWHC 1418 (Fam).
[248] See the Adoption and Children Act 2002; the Adoption and Children (Scotland) Act 2007.
[249] For example, single people, before they became eligible to apply for parental orders: see *X v Z* [2018] EWFC 86.
[250] See *Re A (A Child)* [2014] EWFC 55.

16.7 EMBRYO RESEARCH

Research into human fertility issues and an understanding of embryonic development and implantation are inseparable. Embryonic research is also essential to the study of genetic disease. Systematic study in both these fields depends upon a supply of human embryos, for there always comes a time when animal models are inadequate for human research purposes. Essentially, there are at least two potential positions that could be adopted: either one can be totally opposed to research and experimentation on what are considered to be living human beings who cannot refuse consent to manipulation; or one can hold that the benefits to humanity are likely to be so great that the opportunity for study must be grasped if it is presented. Given that the case for human research is agreed—and we consider it must be—the problem then arises as to how the necessary material is to be obtained, generated, and used within an acceptable legal framework. We discuss each in turn in the next section.

16.7.1 THE MORAL STATUS OF THE HUMAN EMBRYO

Arguments against a policy that prohibits embryo research rely, ultimately, on the view that, although the embryo may have human properties, it is not a human being invested with the same moral rights to respect as are due to other living members of the human community (see Chapter 2). This approach has a familiar ring to it; indeed, it introduces the same concepts of personhood that have been so much a part of the abortion debate (see Chapter 15). There is, however, a crucial distinction to be made between lethal embryo research and abortion. The life of the aborted foetus is extinguished because its interests are outweighed by a more powerful and tangible set of interests—namely, by those who are pregnant. The embryo subjected to research, by contrast, in the pursuit of medical knowledge.

The Warnock Committee, whose recommendations formed the basis of the 1990 Act (see previous section), recommended that human embryos should be afforded *some* protection in law.[251] What this means and whether this is even possible has been the subject of much discussion,[252] and is perhaps indicative of the measure of the moral difficulties involved. However, in practice, it is commonly accepted that by affording some protection (or 'respect')[253] to in vitro embryos in the 1990 Act, a 'compromise' between two extreme positions has been reached.[254]

The extreme positions can be summarised as holding either that the embryo is a full human being—in accordance with rigid Christian theological doctrine—or, as the pure scientist might claim, it is simply a product of the laboratory, comparable to a culture of human tissue. It has been argued that there may be acceptable reasons for suggesting that morally relevant 'humanity' is not established until implantation—this being largely on

---

[251] The Report of the Committee of Inquiry into Human Fertilisation and Embryology (1984) para 11.17.

[252] See for example, Natasha Hammond-Browning, 'Ethics, Embryos, And Evidence: A Look Back at Warnock' (2015) 23(4) Medical Law Review 588; Mary Ford, 'Nothing and Not-Nothing: Law's Ambivalent Response to Transformation and Transgression at the Beginning of Life' in Stephen Smith and Ronan Deazley (eds.), *The Legal, Medical and Cultural Regulation of the Body* (Routledge 2016).

[253] Warnock later stated she regretted the use of the word 'respect' in the report, as you cannot 'respect something you pour down the sink'. She suggested 'non-frivolity' would be more accurate. See Emily Jackson, 'Fraudulent Stem Cell Research and Respect for the Embryo' (2006) 1(3) BioSocieties 349.

[254] See Hammond-Browning (n 252).

the grounds that it is only at implantation that the embryo achieves a capacity for meaningful development.[255] The acceptance of a 'specific moment' theory as to the acquisition of humanity is, however, by no means universal; an alternative approach is to regard the process of becoming a human person as 'a progression through a series of linked developmental stages' and to attribute rights to the embryo because it represents a phase in the whole human form.[256]

Importantly, even after implantation, much is required for viability and birth to take place; it is entirely dependent on further processes in utero to become a person. Acceptance of this premise may help to address some moral conundrums arising from embryonic research which, when done well, could be argued to be of value to the community as a whole. Nevertheless, this conclusion cannot be accepted without qualification—at the very least, the embryo must be accorded the respect due to any living human tissue. It could be replied that, in logic, there is no need to control laboratory interference with a research object that one believes has no human status. However, there is a degree of public disquiet over scientific involvement in the reproductive process and, on this ground alone, it must be contained within a controlling framework.[257] Most importantly, the moral argument rests upon the limitations of current technology. It is clear that this formula would be inadequate should technology advance to the state of being able to 'grow' foetuses to full term in vitro.[258]

If one accepts the undeveloped in vitro embryo merits a certain, albeit unspecified, respect based on its moral status, its management presents a dilemma of which there are three major elements. The first is closely related and concerns the pre-implantation selection of embryos which we have discussed. The second relates to the practical problems surrounding the disposal of those that are surplus to immediate therapeutic needs, and third is that of the use of and, indeed, the production of embryos for research purposes, and it is to this that we now turn.

16.7.2 SOURCES OF EMBRYOS FOR RESEARCH

In order to obtain embryos for research purposes, there are two possibilities (which are not mutually exclusive):

- use the inevitable surplus of embryos that are produced through fertility treatment; or
- create embryos in vitro for the explicit purpose of using them for research.

Matters have been complicated further by the prospect of, and legal acceptance of, the creation of 'admixed embryos' for research. It is first necessary to look at the general proposition.

If we consider, first, the surplus embryo, we have to ask: 'What is the alternative to embryocide?' The techniques used in IVF and the welfare of the patient demand that

[255] John K Mason, *Medico-Legal Aspects of Reproduction and Parenthood* (2nd edn, Routledge 1998) p 234. For the argument based on 'ensoulment', see Norman Ford, *When Did I Begin? Conception of the Human Individual in History, Philosophy and Science* (CUP 1988) pp 56, 171. Perhaps 'humanity' and 'ensoulment' are different expressions of the same thing.

[256] Nikodem Poplawski and Grant Gillett, 'Ethics and Embryos' (1991) 17(2) Journal of Medical Ethics 62; Catriona McMillan, *The Human Embryo In Vitro: Breaking the Legal Stalemate* (CUP 2021).

[257] Michael Mulkay, 'Frankenstein and the Debate Over Embryo Research' (1996) 21(2) Science, Technology, & Human Values 157; Michael Mulkay, *The Embryo Research Debate: Science and the Politics of Reproduction* (CUP 1997).

[258] Partial ectogenesis via artificial wombs is on the horizon, yet full ectogenesis is not yet possible.

more embryos are created than are strictly necessary; to say that all must be implanted would be to fly in the face of the reality and what is now clear HFEA policy on point.[259] The alternatives then lie between embryocide and the reduction of multiple pregnancy, of which the former is clearly the less objectionable insofar as it involves the destruction of organisms which, left to themselves, have no future. It is now the policy in many jurisdictions that the use of so-called 'surplus embryos' is an ethically acceptable approach in the conduct of embryo research.[260] Indeed, for any jurisdiction that accepts and permits an active IVF programme, the dilemma of outright destruction of these human organisms or their use for wider social benefit cannot be avoided.

Between the two 'extreme' positions discussed lies the middle view that, whereas research on surplus embryos is acceptable, the creation of embryos for that purpose is not. This latter is, in fact, expressly prohibited by Article 18 of the Council of Europe Convention on Biomedicine and Human Rights (Oviedo Convention). While this may be considered an acceptable position to hold, it is not easy to establish a valid ethical basis for the position. This is because, insofar as the ultimate outcome destruction, the harm done to surplus embryos is the same in each case. A possible ethical solution depends on distinguishing harm from wrong. No *wrong* is done to the embryo at the time it is formed with a view to implantation; a later failure to achieve that goal is due to circumstances which are, to a large extent, beyond the control of the person who has brought it into being. By contrast, the embryo which is developed with the express intention of harming is clearly *wronged* at the moment of its formation. While the ultimate harm done to each is the same, the wrong done is of a different quality. But do those who take the middle road adopt such reasoning in reality? It seems more probable that they accept instinctively that a utilitarian argument which holds that the benefit to mankind exceeds the harm done to what are the unfortunate rejects of a legitimate therapeutic activity cannot be substantiated in the case of specially created research subjects (see Chapter 2). This problem has raised what has been, perhaps, the most difficult hurdle in legislative terms in a range of jurisdictions. The UK Parliament is a world 'leader', if that is not an inappropriate use of the term, in having opted in favour of the similar moral status of in vitro embryos, whether they be surplus or purposeful creations. In this regard, the UK stands in stark contrast to a range of other countries in allowing the creation of embryos for the specific purpose of performing research on them.[261]

There may, of course, be tenable scientific reasons for creating embryos for research purposes, if these new entities possess qualities not found in their foregone counterparts. Arguments in favour of embryo creation include the role that embryo research can play in providing autologous transplants, in which the embryonic material must have the same genetic profile as the future recipient of the transplant. Other examples include specific disease modelling, whereby the embryonic material is manipulated to maximise its utility for investigations into particular diseases. Arguments in favour of 'admixed embryos' are far-ranging and were sufficiently influential in relation to the 2008 reforms to the 1990 Act, allowing the creation of, and research on, human admixed embryos subject to an HFEA licence. We now turn to discuss the parameters of UK legislation on the matter.

[259] HFEA, 'Code of Practice' (n 23).
[260] Kirstin Matthews and Daniel Moralí, 'National Human Embryo and Embryoid Research Policies: A Survey of 22 Top Research-Intensive Countries' (2020) 15(7) Regenerative Medicine 1905.
[261] Countries which prohibit the creation of embryos for research include: Australia, Canada, Japan, the Netherlands, Spain, South Korea, Switzerland, and Turkey.

16.7.3 THE LEGAL RESPONSE

The entire legal framework regulating embryo research in the UK is contained within the 1990 Act (as amended). Under its terms, it is illegal to conduct any research on human or admixed embryos except under licence from the HFEA.[262] The HFEA can only issue such a licence if the project is thought to be desirable for specific 'principal purposes'.[263] This includes increasing knowledge or developing treatments about serious disease or other serious medical conditions; promoting advances in the treatment of infertility; increasing knowledge about the causes of miscarriage; developing more effective techniques of contraception; developing methods for detecting the presence of gene, chromosome, or mitochondrion abnormalities in embryos before implantation; or increasing knowledge about the development of embryos.

It is a criminal offence, punishable by up to ten years' imprisonment, to keep or use an embryo in vitro, however created, that is more than 14 days old (the time around which the primitive streak appears)—excluding any time spent in suspended animation while frozen.[264] Even so, this specific time limit can be attacked, mainly on the grounds that a 13-day embryo is no less alive than is one of 15 days' gestation and that it is entitled to the same respect—as is the embryo formed at fertilisation.[265] The counter-argument is that *some* controlled embryonic research is essential if the attack on genetic disease—which may well be the most important single factor dictating morbidity in humans—is to be carried on in a scientifically acceptable way.[266] It was not until 2016, however, that arguments such as this had any practical force as until then an embryo had not been maintained alive in vitro to the 13-day point.[267] This advancement reignited debates about extending the 14-day limit, and whether we are missing out on valuable scientific and therapeutic benefits by not doing so.[268]

Importantly, the UK has placed no restrictions on the source of the embryos used; the HFEA has no mandate to impose an overall embargo on the creation of embryos for that specific purpose. In 2004, the HFEA granted its first licence to create human embryonic stem cells using cell nuclear transfer. Since that time, there has been an explosion of interest in this branch of science and its associated ethical concerns.

16.7.4 EMBRYONIC STEM CELL RESEARCH

The framers of the 1990 legislation may have imagined that the issue of embryo research would no longer be controversial once Parliament had answered the fundamental moral question and a system of tight regulation was in place. If so, they were proved wrong and the decisions of the HFEA have been subject to a wide array of judicial review proceedings

---

[262] 1990 Act, s 4A(2).   [263] 1990 Act, Sch 2.   [264] Sections 3(3)(a) and 41(1)(b) of the 1990 Act.

[265] For a recapitulation of the issues and arguments, see Giulia Cavaliere, 'A 14-Day Limit for Bioethics: The Debate over Human Embryo Research' (2017) 28 BMC Medical Ethics 18.

[266] See Nicholas Rivron et al., 'Debate Ethics of Embryo Models from Stem Cells' (Nature, 2018) available at <https://www.nature.com/articles/d41586-018-07663-9> accessed 07 December 2022.

[267] Alessia Deglincerti et al., 'Self-Organization of the In Vitro Attached Human Embryo' (2016) 533(7602) Nature 251; Marta Shahbazi et al., 'Self-Organization of the Human Embryo in the Absence of Maternal Tissues' (2016) 18 Nature Cell Biology 700.

[268] Giulia Cavaliere (n 265); John Appleby and Annelien Bredenoord, 'Should the 14-Day Rule for Embryo Research Become the 28-Day Rule?' (2018) 10 EMBO Molecular Medicine e9437; Catriona McMillan, 'When is Human? Rethinking the Fourteen-Day Rule' in Graeme Laurie et al. (eds.), *The Cambridge Handbook of Health Research Regulation* (CUP 2021) pp 365–372.

ever since its inception.[269] It was partly for this reason that the 2008 reforms sought to clarify and confirm the role of the HFEA in this realm. It was perhaps with the successful production of stable cell lines from human embryonic stem cells in 1998 that the controversy moved up to yet another level.[270]

Before considering the contours of the debate, it is valuable to cover some of the scientific ground. The adult human body is composed of 50 trillion cells of around 200 different kinds, each with a particular function, be it an eye cell, a muscle cell, a blood cell, etc. In the beginning, however, it is not so complicated. Over a matter of hours from the initial creation of the zygote, this entity divides again and again but the cells that are created at this stage have no dedicated function—they are said to be *undifferentiated*. Indeed, within this initial period of division—which lasts no more than three to four days—these undifferentiated stem cells are *totipotent*—that is, each has the capacity to become a complete and separate embryo. This quality is soon lost, however, and by days five to seven the organism has become a *blastocyst*, a ball of around 100 cells each of which is now *pluripotent*—that is, each has the capacity to develop into any of the 200 cell types that make up the human body, but it is no longer possible for them to develop into separate embryos. As time passes, the organism—which we might now wish to call an *embryo*—will continue to grow so long as it is furnished with an appropriate environment and nutrition. These are provided by implantation in the lining of the womb from which a blood supply can be drawn (occurring around day eight of development). It is arguable that it is not until this point that the organism achieves the potential for 'human life'—a distinction which is very important when considering the status of the embryo in the Petri dish.

Thereafter, the embryo will continue to develop, with the first signs of a nervous system appearing at days 14 to 15 (the primitive streak). As the embryo grows, its cells slowly become more task-orientated (*differentiated*) and begin to assume their eventual role within the body. While there is no hard and fast rule, an embryo is generally referred to as a *foetus* from week eight of its development onwards. Clearly, one would be holding an immensely powerful research and therapeutic resource if one could produce a pluripotent cell line— that is, a self-perpetuating line of cells that can be replicated indefinitely in the laboratory.

Stem cells can also be derived from aborted fetal germ cells—that is, the cells that would have become the sperm or egg cells. These germ cells can be cultivated into stem cells in the same way as can occur naturally in the case of embryos. They were first developed in 1998 and they can now be differentiated into an increasingly broad range of dedicated cells. A final and further source of stem cells can be found in adults, but in the main these tend to be *multipotent*—that is, they can only evolve into particular kinds of cell, or *progenitor cells*, which, although they are clearly destined for a particular end, are as yet undifferentiated. Even so, it now appears that adult stem cells can differentiate into a far broader range of cells than was originally thought and many advances are being made towards the production of clinical grade cell lines.

Most promise with embryonic stem cells lies with those extracted from the blastocyst when they have pluripotent qualities. It is important to re-emphasise that no embryo can be derived from such cells. Equally important, however, is the fact that the blastocyst is destroyed in this process. If one views this organism at this stage as embryonic life we have, then, the makings of a classic ethical controversy. Notwithstanding, embryonic stem cell therapies are already here, at least in trial form.

---

[269] See for example *Quintavalle* v *HFEA* [2005] UKHL 28.

[270] James Thomson et al., 'Embryonic Stem Cell Lines Derived from Human Blastocysts' (1998) 282 Science 1145.

The ethical and legal issues surrounding human stem cell research of this nature differ from those addressed in the earlier debate on embryo research in that, whereas other forms of embryo research may be intended to assist reproductive medicine and future embryos, this type involves using embryos for the benefit of society in general. This has invigorated the opposition of those who have a principled objection to any form of embryo research. At the same time, arguments in favour of such research have been forcefully advanced, often on the grounds that the benefit to humanity of the resulting therapies outweighs the interests of the embryos, particularly if use is made of cells derived from embryos which were rendered surplus within the accepted IVF treatment programme. A major milestone in addressing the ethical concerns is the recent announcement that Nature journals have formalised a policy encouraging scientists to conform to uniform guidelines on human-embryo and stem cell research.[271] As an added incentive, certain types of manuscript are required to be accompanied by ethics statements and/or show ethics expert consultation.

The phenomenon of induced pluripotent stem cells (iPSCs) has been heralded by some as a sufficiently scientifically robust and ethically preferable route to follow in this field of research.[272] In brief, iPSCs can be created from human somatic cells, such as skin cells, without the need to use embryos. Ethically speaking, it is self-evident that many of our moral concerns disappear if it is the case that we do not need to use and destroy embryos in research; unfortunately, other ethical concerns may surface to take their place, for example, the concern that viral vectors are often used in iPSCs techniques raising the prospect of transmission of carcinogenic retroviruses to mammals. Such objections, which are based on concerns about technical limitations or scientific risks, are being overtaken quickly by developments in the field. Accordingly, a strong consensus remains, in the scientific community at least, that for now all avenues of stem cell research should be followed.

The value of stem cells of whatever origin is twofold. First, they can divide and multiply more or less indefinitely without differentiation and, second, they can be manipulated so as to differentiate into particular specialised cells. These qualities mean that scientists have both a potentially endless supply of raw research material and also the means to develop a number of therapeutic applications. These range from gene therapy to developments in regenerative medicine whereby diseased or damaged cells can be replaced in conditions such as diabetes, Parkinson's disease, chronic heart failure, and injuries to, or degenerative disease of, the spinal cord. As we discuss in Chapter 13, one of the main drawbacks in transplantation therapy is the rejection by the body of the implanted foreign tissue. Embryonic stem cell biology has developed its own way round this problem whereby the nucleus of an embryonic cell is replaced with a nucleus taken from the cell of the prospective patient. Stem cells are then taken from the resulting embryo and tissue is grown from them, which can be transplanted back to the patient without risk of rejection. The process of creating such an embryo is known as therapeutic cloning. This is quite distinct from reproductive cloning because the embryo is not allowed to develop beyond an early point and is not implanted in a uterus.

Embryonic stem cell research for therapeutic purposes is now legal, and encouraged, in the UK, provided a licence is obtained from the HFEA, the first of which, as

---

[271] Nature, 'Announcement: Stem-Cell Policy' (2018) available at <https://www.nature.com/articles/d41586-018-05030-2> accessed 07 December 2022.

[272] For discussion of this topic, see John Harris, Murieann Quigley, and Sarah Chan, *Stem Cells: New Frontiers in Science and Ethics* (World Scientific Publishing 2012).

we have seen, was granted in 2004. The UK Stem Cell Bank—the world's first—was established in 2003 in order to provide quality research materials under optimal governance restrictions in this field. In part, it was also established to minimise the moral impact of embryonic stem cell research on the philosophy that more sharing would lead to less destruction of early stage human life. All stem cell and tissue collections are now subject to the provisions of the EU Tissue and Cells Directive,[273] adopted in April 2004, and currently incorporated into domestic law. While this instrument is largely concerned with matters of storage and safety, it is important to point out that earlier versions were subject to intense lobbying in the European Parliament in an attempt to use the Directive to outlaw embryo and stem cell research entirely. These attempts did not succeed—there is, in fact, probably no legal authority for the Union to so legislate—but the attempt demonstrates well the continuing controversial nature of the research. As with so many other issues detailed in this book, the advent of Brexit leaves these standards in a considerable state of flux. Even if the UK begins down the road of 'regulatory alignment', it is by no means guaranteed that these robust measures of safety and quality will be maintained over time.

While the UK has proved ready to facilitate stem cell research, other countries have been either more cautious or, in some cases, frankly hostile to the process.[274] It seems to us to be rather difficult—if not impossible—to maintain a consistent ethical stance in these circumstances. It cannot be the case that the ethics of embryonic stem cell research can fundamentally change depending on who funds the work or which colour of political party is in power. In the final analysis, however, we cannot divorce the ethical debate from the socio-economic imperatives that are also at stake. The realities are that many people suffering from degenerative and other conditions could stand to benefit considerably if stem cell technologies can deliver on the hype that has accompanied them. The commercial benefits for countries that take the lead in such research are not far behind. Whatever one might think of the ethical issues, it is undeniable that other pressures are mounting in favour of these technologies, including the development of embryonic stem cell lines. The resultant attitudes with respect to controversial technologies such as embryonic stem cell research—at present, seems decidedly equivocal. Thus, the EU regulation establishing the parameters for funding within the Horizon Europe Programme prohibits the financing of: '[research] activities intended to create human embryos solely for the purpose of research or for the purpose of stem cell procurement, including by means of somatic cell nuclear transfer'.[275] Nevertheless, research on human stem cells both adult and embryonic may be financed, depending both on the contents of the scientific proposal and the legal framework of the Member States involved. This compromise position has been welcomed by many, but it will contribute little towards a more harmonised approach to stem cell research in the future.

---

[273] 2004/23/EC.

[274] Rosario Isasi et al., 'Legal and Ethical Approaches to Stem Cell and Cloning Research: A Comparative Analysis of Policies in Latin America, Asia, and Africa' (2004) 32(4) Journal of Law, Medicine & Ethics 626; Timothy Caulfield et al., 'International Stem Cell Environments: A World of Difference' (2009) Nature Reports Stem Cells, available at <https://www.nature.com/articles/stemcells.2009.61#citeas> accessed 07 December 2022.

[275] Regulation EU 2021/695 of the European Parliament and of the Council of 28 April 2021 establishing Horizon Europe—the Framework Programme for Research and Innovation, laying down its rules for participation and dissemination, and repealing Regulations (EU) No 1290/2013 and (EU) No 1291/2013, Art 18.

16.8 THE FUTURE OF ASSISTED REPRODUCTION

As a fast-paced field of medicine, new forms of assisted reproduction have continued to crop up over the past 30 years, in some senses far beyond the imaginings of the Warnock Committee, whose ground-breaking considerations recommendations formed the basis of the 1990 Act.[276] To consider all possible new technologies[277] would venture into the realms of legal prophecy, but there are several new technologies that, while not yet in common usage, have engaged the attention of law and regulation. We discuss a select few of these current and emerging technologies here.

16.8.1 MITOCHONDRIAL REPLACEMENT THERAPY (MRT)

An emerging possibility for the prevention of particular inheritable disorders is that of MRT. Mitochondria are cytoplasmic organelles with their own genome that have a major role in energy generation. Transmission of germline mtDNA mutations—currently thought to be inherited exclusively from the egg (i.e. maternally)—can cause disease in the next generation. The two current techniques are pronuclear transfer (PNT), which involves the transfer of two pronuclei from a zygote with disease-linked mitochondria into an enucleated zygote with healthy mitochondria, and maternal spindle transfer (MST), which involves the transfer of the spindle of chromosomes from an unfertilised egg with disease-linked mitochondria into an enucleated egg with healthy mitochondria. Ultimately, it is germline gene therapy resulting in a permanent genetic alteration of the germ cells, and it is not unanimously agreed that mtDNA does not encode components that are prime determinants of genetic identity or kinship.[278]

The primary ethical concerns are that (1) it is a form of germline therapy, which could create a 'slippery slope' towards alterations of the nuclear germline; (2) the safety of interventions is uncertain and will remain so until several generations of people have been born from the procedure, implicating intergenerational justice; and (3) a person born with three genetic contributors might have a conflicted or confused self-image or perceptions of the social roles of others in relation to themselves.[279] This in turn gives rise to questions as to whether mitochondrial donors should be treated anonymously or not.[280] With respect to the latter concern, we have already noted that there exist

---

[276] See Secretary of State for Education and Science, the Secretary of State for Scotland, and the Secretary of State for Wales, 'The Warnock Report (1978): Special Educational Needs' (1978) available at <http://www.educationengland.org.uk/documents/warnock/warnock1978.html> accessed 20 August 2022.

[277] For in-depth discussions of technologies on the horizon, see Amel Alghrani, 'The Legal and Ethical Ramifications of Ectogenesis' (2007) 2(1) Asian Journal of WTO & International Health Law and Policy 18; Elizabeth Chloe Romanis, 'Partial Ectogenesis: Freedom, Equality and Political Perspective' (2020) 46(2) Journal of Medical Ethics 89; Elizabeth Chloe Romanis, 'Artificial Womb Technology and the Choice to Gestate Ex Utero: Is Partial Ectogenesis the Business of the Criminal Law?' (2020) 28(2) Medical Law Review 342; and Sonia Suter, 'In Vitro Gametogenesis: Just Another Way to Have a Baby?' (2016) 3(1) Journal of Law and the Biosciences 87.

[278] Don Wolf, Nargiz Mitalipov, and Shoukhrat Mitlipov, 'Mitochondrial Replacement Therapy in Reproductive Medicine' (2015) 21(2) Trends in Molecular Medicine 68.

[279] For a useful discussion, see Nuffield Council on Bioethics, 'Novel Techniques for the Prevention of Mitochondrial DNA Disorders' (2012); Françoise Baylis, 'The Ethics of Creating Children with Three Genetic Parents' (2013) 26(6) Reproductive Biomedicine 531; Julie McCandless and Sally Sheldon, 'Genetically Challenged: The Determination of Legal Parenthood in Assisted Reproduction' in Tabatha Freeman et al. (eds.), *Relatedness in Assisted Reproduction: Families, Origins and Identities* (OUP 2014);

[280] See e.g. John Appleby, 'Should Mitochondrial Donation be Anonymous?' (2017) 43(2) Journal of Medicine and Philosophy 261; Ilke Turkmendag, 'It Is Just a "Battery": Right to Know in Mitochondrial Replacement' (2018) 43(1) Science, Technology, & Human Values 56.

many different kinds of family arrangements where more than two people take on the role of caring for a child and serving as parents, including fostering, (open) adoption, step-parenting and informal arrangements within families. Moreover, in *A v B and Another*,[281] the Court of Appeal observed that, although the lesbian couple desired to bring up the child as a two-parent nuclear family, and it is generally accepted that a child gains by having two parents, it does not follow from that that the addition of a third is necessarily disadvantageous.[282]

Under the 1990 Act, an embryo is a 'permitted embryo' for transfer to a woman only if no nuclear or mtDNA of any cell of the embryo has been altered (i.e., the egg produced by or extracted from the ovaries of a woman must have unaltered nuclear or mtDNA).[283] But the 2008 Act grants the Secretary of State for Health the power to create regulations specifically for the prevention of inherited mitochondrial disorders that would permit the alteration of eggs or embryos as part of treatment, expanding the definition of a permitted egg. Thus, the Human Fertilisation and Embryology (Mitochondrial Donation) Regulations 2015 were adopted. Part 2 of the Regulations enable eggs and embryos created following PNT or MST to be 'permitted' for use in treatment subject to certain conditions, including the HFEA having given a determination that there is a particular risk that the eggs or embryos of the woman seeking treatment may have mitochondrial abnormalities caused by mtDNA, and that there is a significant risk that the potential child will have or develop serious mitochondrial disease.[284]

16.8.2 UTERUS TRANSPLANTATION

In the past few decades advances in the realms of transplantation of reproductive organs has come forward in leaps and bounds.[285] More recently, in 2014, a child was born as a result of the first human uterine transplant in Sweden.[286] Now, uterine transplantation (UTx) is the established treatment for absolute uterine factor infertility (AUFI) (where a uterus does not function correctly, or is missing), which before now was deemed as an untreatable condition.[287] UTx thus provides an alternative to surrogacy and adoption for those with AUFI.

The crossover between assisted reproduction and organ donation has caused significant moral dilemma.[288] A 2021 review estimated that at least 80 procedures have been

---

[281] [2012] EWCA Civ 285.

[282] Similarly, in *AA v BB & CC* (2007) ONCA 2, the Ontario Court of Appeal made a declaration of parentage in favour of a lesbian co-mother as the child's third legal parent.

[283] Section 3ZA of the 1990 Act, as amended. And this is largely in keeping with international views that germ line genetic therapy should not be permitted: UNESCO Universal Declaration on the Human Genome and Human Rights (1997), Arts 1 and 24; Council of Europe's Convention on Human Rights and Biomedicine (1997), Art 13.

[284] Regulations 4, 5, 7, and 8.   [285] For example, ovaries and testes.

[286] Rose Buchanan, 'Womb Transplant Baby: First Picture Emerges of Child After Pioneering Womb Transplant Operation' *Independent* (2014) available at <https://www.independent.co.uk/life-style/health-and-families/first-picture-of-baby-born-after-pioneering-womb-transplant-operation-9774497.html> accessed 21 August 2021.

[287] See Mats Brännström et al., 'Livebirth After Uterus Transplantation' (2015) 385(9968) The Lancet 607.

[288] For discussion, see Katvita Shah and Valarie Blake, 'Uterus Transplantation: Ethical and Regulatory challenges' (2014) 40(6) Journal of Medical Ethics 396; Elizabeth Romanis et al., 'Re-Viewing the Womb' (2020) 47(12) Journal of Medical Ethics 820.

performed, with around 50 live births following.[289] UTx is currently being carried out through clinical trials in the UK. IVF and cryo-preservation of embryos is required for UTx to take place, and the procedure therefore engages not only the Human Tissue Act 2004 as a form of organ donation but also the Human Fertilisation and Embryology Act 1990, as amended. This gives rise to legal complexities, which vary, for example, depending on whether the donor is living or deceased.[290] What is clear, however, is that this form of assisted reproduction[291] bypasses the complexities of parenthood discussed when it comes to surrogacy. Section 33 of the 2008 Act is clear that the woman who carries a child born as a result of placing an embryo in her is the legal 'mother'.[292]

16.9 CONCLUSION

Baroness Warnock and her committee could scarcely have imagined the multiple dimensions to regulation that would spring from their recommendations for more active legal intervention in the field. The complexities arise at numerous points, from the fact that, in many respects, the law in this area is caught in a double bind. The idea of the 'right to reproduce'—in the negative sense of not placing obstacles in people's way—is incredibly powerful; there are few arguments or actions that can stand up to it. However, ethical dilemmas continue to arise surrounding the use of the embryo within and beyond the reproductive context. The traditional understandings of parenthood appear to be in need of continual update to meet our evolving technological capabilities, and our understanding of the nature of families. It would also appear, therefore, that legislative evolution will continue to be required to make sense of these competing interests and keep up with the new questions posed by technological advancement and social change.

FURTHER READING

1. Emily Jackson, 'The Legacy of the Warnock Report', in Edward Dove and Niamh Nic Shuibhne (eds.), *Law and Legacy in Medical Jurisprudence: Essays in Honour of Graeme Laurie* (CUP 2022).

2. Amel Alghrani, *Regulating Assisted Reproductive Technologies* (CUP 2018).

3. Catriona McMillan, *The Human Embryo In Vitro, Breaking the Legal Stalemate* (CUP 2021).

4. Isabel Karpin and Roxanne Mykitiuk, 'Reimagining Disability: The Screening of Donor Gametes and Embryos in IVF' (2021) 8(2) Journal of Law and the Biosciences lsaa067.

---

[289] Mats Brännström et al., Uterus Transplantation Worldwide: Clinical Activities and Outcomes 2021 26(6) Current Opinion in Organ Transplantation 616–626.

[290] For discussion see Saaliha Vali et al., 'Uterine Transplantation and Regulatory Implications in England' (2021) 129(4) Obstetrics and Gynaecology 590.

[291] If not 'assisted gestation'. For discussion, see Elizabeth Chloe Romanis, 'Assisted Gestative Technologies' (2022) 48(7) Journal of Medical Ethics 439.

[292] Note this technology has potential to offer reproductive options for transgender women. For discussion, see Benjamin Jones et al., 'Uterine Transplantation in Transgender Women' (2018) 126(2) Obstetrics and Gynaecology 153; and for further discussion, see Natasha Hammond-Browning, 'Uterine Transplantation in Transgender Women: Medical, Legal and Ethical Considerations' (2018) 126(2) Obstetrics and Gynaecology 157.

5. Giulia Cavaliere, 'A 14-day Limit for Bioethics: The Debate Over Human Embryo Research' (2017) 18(1) BMC Medical Ethics 1.

6. Annelien Bredenoord and John Appleby, 'Mitochondrial Replacement Techniques: Remaining Ethical Challenges' (2017) 21(3) Cell Stem Cell 301.

7. Zaina Mahmoud and Elizabeth Chloe Romanis, 'On Gestation and Motherhood', (2022) 31(1) Medical Law Review, available at <https://pubmed.ncbi.nlm.nih.gov/35980020/> accessed 07 December 2022.

17

WITHHOLDING AND WITHDRAWING MEDICAL TREATMENT FROM ADULTS

17.1 INTRODUCTION

There may come a time in life where the opposite status quo is considered preferable, by virtue of a person being in a permanently vegetative (or minimally conscious) state, and treatment being futile. This status raises questions of both law and ethics that surround the decision-making process, the identities of the decision-makers, and the interests of the patient.

In this chapter, we are concerned with the judicial sanction of the ending of life in the medical treatment environment. We consider cases in which patients suffer from degenerative diseases, or find themselves in situations in which treatment would be futile, and where the best interests test is judicially applied. The application of that test determines whether a patient should be allowed to die. That could be because they are in a minimally conscious state, and active treatment such as artificial nutrition and hydration is withdrawn; that is justified by collapsing the distinction between the act of withdrawing treatment and the omission to treat, where the latter allows physicians to escape allegations of active killing.

We consider those situations first, before going on to look at cases which are not so much about breaking down the act/omission distinction, but applying the related doctrine of 'double effect'. This refers to a different class of cases and the physician's intent with respect to terminally ill patients. Here an analgesic may be prescribed for the treatment of symptoms, which will also have the justifiable effect of shortening that person's life. Returning to cases of patients in a prolonged disorder of consciousness allows us to consider cases in which life-sustaining treatment is withdrawn, and medication restricted to that which would allow a peaceful death. We reflect on the fact that much of the debate centres on the importance of accuracy in diagnosis, given the consequences of treatment withdrawal.

Through each of these cases we consider the human rights implications, as well as what is known or understood of the patient's prior wishes—whether or not these were formally expressed by way of an advance decision to refuse treatment, which we discuss in closing.

As we will see, courts have struggled for objectivity in their end-of-life determinations. While there is great normative appeal—and judicial refuge—in the use of legal constructs such as 'futility' and 'best interests', that process is very much a value-laden one. At the same time, a trend has emerged that shows a greater judicial willingness to state clearly which values have informed their decisions.[1] This is most obviously illustrated in *R (on the application of Burke) v General Medical Council*,[2] which we discuss in the next section. Consideration of this case serves as a bridge between our discussions of futility at the beginning of life, and

---

[1] See Richard Huxtable, 'Autonomy, Best Interests and the Public Interest: Treatment, Non-Treatment and the Values of Medical Law' (2014) 22(4) Medical Law Review 459.
[2] [2004] 2 FLR 1121.

then at its end. *Burke* is also the starting point of our discussion of the case law on withdrawal of treatment in a vegetative patient's 'best interests'. Withdrawal of treatment in these circumstances has an alarming similarity to permitting active euthanasia.

17.2 THE ENDING OF MR BURKE'S LIFE

Mr Burke suffered from cerebellar ataxia, a degenerative disease which would eventually leave him unable to communicate, while still retaining his mind. He did not want artificial nutrition and hydration (ANH) to be removed in any circumstances, no matter his state of health. He challenged the General Medical Council (GMC) guidance that it would be within the bounds of good medical practice to withhold or withdraw ANH when the conditions were considered so severe and the prognosis so poor that providing ANH would be too burdensome for the patient in relation to the possible benefits. For Mr Burke, ANH would never be futile; it would be in his own best interests to continue to receive such care even when nothing else could be done for him medically, and when the sole function of that care would be to keep his body alive.

In a controversial ruling, the court of first instance held: (i) the GMC guidance concentrated too much on the right of the competent patient to refuse treatment rather than to require treatment; (ii) the guidance did not stipulate that a doctor who did not wish to follow the patient's wishes must continue to treat until a doctor who was willing to do so was found; (iii) the guidance failed to acknowledge a very strong presumption in favour of prolonging life; and (iv) the standard of best interests was that of intolerability as judged from the patient's own perspective. Article 8 of the European Convention on Human Rights (ECHR) implied that it was for the competent patient, not the doctor, to decide what treatment should be given to achieve what the patient thought conducive to their dignity. However, there would be no breach of Articles 2, 3, or 8 ECHR if ANH was withdrawn when it was serving absolutely no purpose, but this would not be the case in Mr Burke's envisaged circumstances.

Munby J's analysis was based on ethical principles for which he found support in human rights law: prominence was given to *sanctity of life* (protected by Article 2 ECHR), *dignity* (which underpins the entire Convention but is most clearly seen in Article 3), and *autonomy* or *self-determination* (inherent in the interpretation of Article 8). Munby J rated dignity highly[3] as a fundamental recognition of our humanity, particularly a person's interest in the manner of their death. It is therefore surprising how little attention was paid to its meaning by both the Court of Appeal and the European Court of Human Rights (ECtHR).

Dignity is a concept that is widely embraced but not easily defined. It can be seen from subjective or objective perspectives, and both feature in Munby J's analysis. On the one hand, the decisions divide along the categories of competency. At first instance it was held that it is for the patient to *determine*—and we should note with care the use of this expression—what treatment *should* or *should not* be given in order to achieve what the patient believes conducive to their dignity and in order to avoid dying in what the patient would find to be 'distressing circumstances'.[4] Where the patient is incompetent, best interests applies, and the dignity test is what 'right-thinking persons'

---

[3] Quoting his judgment in *R (on the application of A, B, X and Y) v East Sussex County Council and the Disability Rights Commission (No 2)* [2003] EWHC 167 (Admin), [57] et seq.

[4] *R (on the application of Burke) v General Medical Council* [2004] EWHC 1879 (Admin) [130].

would consider undignified in such circumstances. This statement lacks definition and it is not straightforward to express what is meant by the term 'protection of human dignity'. Dupré has suggested two approaches.[5] First, that dignity can be conflated with personality—or, respect for dignity is, in effect, respect for the uniqueness, or the moral integrity, of the individual person. Second, she suggests that the 'right to life' can be seen as more than a conflict between life and death and, rather, as a right to a dignified or a 'good' life. The difficulty is that, in either case, the ethical principle of respect for dignity can conflict with those of the sanctity of life and of self-determination, and it is this which led to the rejection of Munby J's analysis by the superior courts.[6]

The Court of Appeal[7] overruled Munby J on the basis that he had ruled beyond the bounds of the facts of the case. The Court of Appeal did, however, endorse the position that to remove ANH from a patient with capacity who wished to keep it would be a breach of their ECHR rights (Articles 2, 3, and 8), and an affront to their dignity, and that specific parts of the GMC guidelines were unlawful.[8] By far the more interesting feature of the court's ruling is its attitude towards the management of patients who lack capacity. Once again, in *Burke*, we find it falling back on the best interests test: it can be lawful to withdraw ANH if its provision is not in the patient's best interests. Any doctor in doubt should seek a court declaration, but they are not obliged by law to do so. Finally, on the scope of rights of the competent patient, the Court of Appeal stated in obiter that their views will not be *determinative* in the last stages of life if the continuation of ANH might hasten death, because no patient can require a doctor to treat against their best clinical judgement.[9]

17.3 FUTILITY: DIFFERENT FOR ADULTS

As we discussed Chapter 9, non-treatment in infancy has been, at least in part, about the management of physical disability. This has been considered morally permissible only because treatment itself would result in an intolerable life which it would be inhumane to enforce on the child who would, at the same time, die naturally if they were not treated. Such conditions are uncommon in adult life and, when they do occur—as, for example, in accidental quadriplegia—their management is more allied to euthanasia or assisted suicide[10] than to selective non-treatment.

Disability due to brain damage is common to both infancy and adulthood and while the courts will not tolerate the deliberate shortening of life, they are fully prepared to accede to non-treatment of associated lethal disease in the severely brain damaged child—and to base this on a 'quality of life' standard as measured by a 'best interests' test. It is interesting to speculate on why this has been easily accepted in the case of children, while the legal attitude to the management of the brain-damaged adult has taken so long to mature and has done so amid so much controversy. Do we give greater weight to life

---

[5] Catherine Dupré, 'Human Dignity and the Withdrawal of Medical Treatment: A Missed Opportunity?' (2006) 6 European Human Rights Law Review 678.

[6] This conflict with autonomy is considered in Conor O'Mahony, 'There is No Such Thing as a Right to Dignity' (2012) 10(2) International Journal of Constitutional Law 551.

[7] *R (Burke)* v *General Medical Council and Others* [2005] EWCA Civ 1003.   [8] ibid. [81].

[9] For critical reflection on this ruling, see Hazel Biggs, 'Taking Account of the Views of the Patient, but Only if the Clinician (and the Court) Agrees' (2007) 19(2) Child and Family Law Quarterly 225.

[10] See also the case of Daniel James which did not come to trial but was discussed in *R (on the application of Purdy)* v *DPP* [2009] UKHL 45. Euthanasia and assisted suicide are discussed in Chapter 18 of this book.

that has 'been lived' than to life which has no past? Do we see a sustainable distinction between starting life with disability and continuing life in a disabled state? Whatever the possible distinctions, in all cases the courts are clear that they will not order a clinician to treat against their considered professional opinion. They will not allow argument about possible benefits to a patient to be used to pressure health professionals and authorities into continuing interventions that professionals consider to be futile. For example, in *AVS v An NHS Foundation Trust*,[11] the Court of Appeal made it clear that it would not entertain hypothetical arguments about possible benefits and future health carers' willingness to provide treatment in the case of a severely affected patient with Creutzfeldt Jakob's disease. The brother of the patient was unable to produce evidence refuting the unanimous opinion of his brother's carers that it would be futile to replace a failed pump delivering a compound which had failed to produce results over the previous two years. The Court therefore refused any declaration along the lines that *if* a willing professional could be found, the pump should be replaced. The Court of Protection has since further confirmed that:

> In determining whether treatment would be in a patient's best interests, the court ha[s] to consider whether it would be futile in the sense of being ineffective or of no benefit to the patient. The treatment [does] not have to be likely to cure or palliate the underlying condition or return the patient to full or reasonable health, rather it should be capable of allowing the resumption of a quality of life which the patient would regard as worthwhile.[12]

Another common feature of these cases is that we are constantly assured that we are *not* practising euthanasia in allowing such persons to die. As Hoffmann LJ put it:

> This is not a case about euthanasia because it does not involve any external agency of death. It is about whether, and how, the patient should be allowed to die.[13]

That is why we have detached the management of adults with brain damage—and, particularly, adults diagnosed as being in a permanent vegetative state—from our discussion of euthanasia. Legally—if less certainly logically—it sits more easily under the heading of 'futile treatment'; as Lord Goff put it in the House of Lords in *Bland*, 'it is the futility of the treatment [of Anthony Bland] which justifies its termination.'[14]

17.4 THE PATIENT IN THE PERMANENT VEGETATIVE STATE

It is common knowledge that the cells of the body depend upon oxygen to survive, and it is well understood that brain cells are the most sensitive to oxygen deprivation. That the brain itself is not uniformly sensitive to hypoxia[15] means that depriving the brain of oxygen can result in anything from mild intellectual deterioration to death. Whatever the cause, hypoxic *anatomic damage* to the brain is irreversible, since destroyed brain cells cannot be replaced. Yet further damage can be prevented if an efficient oxygen supply is

---

[11] [2011] EWCA Civ 7. For comment, see Gillian Douglas, 'Vulnerable Adult: Medical Treatment' (2011) 41 Family Law 363.

[12] *United Lincolnshire Hospitals NHS Trust v N* [2014] EWCOP 16.

[13] *Airedale NHS Trust v Bland* [1993] 1 All ER 821, [856].   [14] [1993] 1 All ER 821, [870].

[15] The relative term 'hypoxia' is used advisedly to emphasise that lack of oxygen need not be absolute—'anoxia'—in order to cause brain damage.

restored. One can therefore speak of *degrees* of brain damage and resultant coma but not of *stages* of coma, because the condition is static once oxygen supply is restored.

Even if all appropriate cases may properly be given intensive care for the purposes of diagnosis and assessment, it is all but impossible to justify initiating long-term treatment for a patient who is likely to retain no cortical and only minimal thalamic function. This presents a formidable technical dilemma because some *functional* or *physiological* damage may be recoverable while some 'dormant' brain cells may have survived to become activated later. This potential for evidence of clinical recovery underlies the distinction between a persistent and a permanent stage of cerebral dysfunction; it also partially accounts for the fact that recovery of brain function is more likely when it has been lost as a result of direct head injury than due to pure hypoxic damage.[16] It also helps to explain the more recent emergence of an additional (legal) category of patient: the minimally conscious, or patients with a 'prolonged disorder of consciousness' (as we discuss further).[17] Once again, medical science presents the law with a seemingly infinitely granular spectrum of human experiences and catastrophes that require responsible management.[18]

At one extreme end of such a spectrum sits the wholly decorticated patient who falls into the category originally defined by Jennett and Plum[19] as the persistent vegetative state (PVS). Such a person will have periods of wakefulness but still be permanently unconscious; a state of 'eyes-open unconsciousness'. A human who has lost all brain function might be considered to have lost their human personality, but as long as they are capable of oxygenating their tissues without mechanical support—that is, their cardiorespiratory system is intact and functional—they are equally certainly not dead. Nonetheless, the patient has no consciousness, a condition summed up in the phrase, 'Consciousness is the most critical moral, legal, and constitutional standard, not for human life itself, but for human personhood.'[20] The unconscious or comatose patient is incapable of fulfilling their human function in a way which transcends the loss of any other capacity; it follows that the whole status of the person in a position of persistent unconsciousness is in doubt.

It is notoriously difficult to identify a satisfactory definition of PVS. The distinguishing features include cycles of sleeping and waking, without any detectable expressions of self-awareness, specific recognition of external stimuli, or consistent evidence of responsiveness.[21] Despite common perception, patients in this state are not immobile and, to varying extents, are able to respond to certain forms of stimuli, reflecting the degree of their brain damage. As we see later, the law is now responding to these shades of grey

---

[16] Robert Howard and David Miller, 'The Persistent Vegetative State' (1995) 310(6976) BMJ 341.

[17] See *An NHS Trust* v *Y* [2018] UKSC 46.

[18] *Cf.* Joseph Giacino et al., 'Disorders of Consciousness After Acquired Brain Injury: the State of the Science' (2014) 10(2) Nature Reviews Neurology 99; Sarah Nettleton, Jenny Kitzinger, and Celia Kitzinger, 'A Diagnostic Illusory? The Case of Distinguishing Between "Vegetative" and "Minimally Conscious" States' (2014) 116(100) Social Science and Medicine 134. See generally Aurore Thibault et al., 'Therapeutic Interventions in Patients with Prolonged Disorders of Consciousness' (2019) 18(6) The Lancet 600.

[19] Bryan Jennett, *The Vegetative State: Medical Facts, Ethical and Legal Dilemmas* (CUP 2002). For a revisitation of Jennett's contribution, see Klaus von Wild et al., 'The Vegetative State—a Syndrome in Search of a Name' (2012) 5(1) Journal of Medical Life 3. For the legal vagaries of diagnosis, see Clare Dyer, 'Court Case Adjourned After Diagnosis of Persistent Vegetative State Changes' (2012) 345 BMJ e5803.

[20] Ronald Cranford and David Smith, 'Consciousness: The Most Critical Moral (Constitutional) Standard for Human Personhood' (1987) 13(2–3) American Journal of Law & Medicine 233.

[21] Multi-Society Task Force on PVS, 'Medical Aspects of the Persistent Vegetative State' (1994) 300(22) New England Journal of Medicine 1499 (Pt 1); 1572 (Pt 2). See more recently Frederica Pisa et al., 'The Prevalence of Vegetative and Minimally Conscious States: A Systematic Review and Methodological Appraisal' (2014) 29(4) Journal of Head Trauma Rehabilitation e23.

matter in recognising patients who are 'near PVS' or 'minimally conscious',[22] under the umbrella term of patients 'with a prolonged disorder of consciousness', suggesting a gamut of possible experiences and diagnoses.

The concept of PVS also has its built-in semantic difficulties, the most urgent of which lies in the word 'persistent'. A persistent state is one which persists until it is relieved—from which it follows that the diagnosis of PVS envisages a potential for recovery; this was the understanding of those who coined the term.[23] In our opinion it is essential that discussion—and any legislation based upon it—should be devoted to the management of the *permanent* vegetative state, even as 'permanent' has an evolving definition in respect of the number of years of unconsciousness.[24] Though the Royal College of Physicians recognised that for its purposes the definition is required more for medical than legal decision-making, it also noted that following *Aintree* (as we discuss further), 'the emphasis [is no longer] on the likelihood of regaining consciousness, but on whether a patient could ever recover a quality of life that they personally would value.'[25]

Permanence is a presumption rather than a certainty; whether or not that presumption is acceptable depends on empirical evidence, which must also bow to practicality. As such, the Multi-Society Task Force in America defined PVS as a vegetative state present one month after acute traumatic or non-traumatic brain injury; it concluded that a permanent state can be assumed if the patient has been vegetative for one year.[26] But to say that a state is permanent if it has been present for a year[27] involves a balancing act between reasonableness and certainty. No matter how high the degree of clinical certainty, the compromise is unlikely to satisfy everyone, and the possibility of exceptions to the rule cannot be denied. Nevertheless, the advantages of establishing a cut-off point outweigh the disadvantages of indefinitely prolonging the decision. Equally important is the fact that the word 'vegetative' fails to define the degree of brain damage involved. Therapeutic decisions in PVS therefore depend not only on its permanence but also on the definition

---

[22] See the minimally conscious state as involved in the case *W (by her litigation friend B)* v *M (by her litigation friend, the Official Solicitor) and Others* [2011] EWHC 2443 (Fam), described as being a state of awareness above that of the vegetative state, but for which diagnosis was a heavily specialised and problematic area, and one which had come to attention in the years since *Bland*. See also Justice Baker, 'A Matter of Life and Death' (2017) 43(7) Journal of Medical Ethics 427.

[23] Steven Laureys et al., 'Permanent Vegetative State and Persistent Vegetative State are not Interchangeable Terms' (2000) 321 BMJ 916.

[24] See especially Royal College of Physicians, *The Vegetative State: Guidance on Diagnosis and Management* (2003) available at <https://pubmed.ncbi.nlm.nih.gov/12848260/> accessed 02 November 2022. This is a restatement of the guidance originally provided in 1996, on the key requirements for the diagnosis: (i) no evidence of self or environment awareness at any time; (ii) no response to visual, auditory, tactile, or noxious stimuli of a kind suggesting volition or conscious purpose; and (iii) no evidence of language comprehension or meaningful expression.

[25] Royal College of Physicians, 'Prolonged Disorders of Consciousness Following Sudden Onset Brain Injury: National Clinical Guidelines' (2020) available at <https://www.rcplondon.ac.uk/guidelines-policy/prolonged-disorders-consciousness-following-sudden-onset-brain-injury-national-clinical-guidelines> accessed 25 October 2022, p 36.

[26] See Multi-Society Task Force on PVS (n 21).

[27] See Royal College of Physicians (n 25). See also GMC, BMA, and RCP, 'Decisions to Withdraw Clinically-Assisted Nutrition and Hydration (CANH) from Patients in Permanent Vegetative State (PVS) or Minimally Conscious State (MCS) Following Sudden-Onset Profound Brain Injury: Interim Guidance for Health Professionals in England and Wales' (2017) available at <https://www.rcplondon.ac.uk/file/8465/download?token=Uqr8eJgZ> accessed 25 October 2022.

of vegetativeness. This must, to some extent, involve a value judgement,[28] and disputes by experts over diagnosis can lead to adjournment and delay in legal proceedings.[29]

Emergent medical understanding also requires that guidelines be kept under constant review. The current Royal College of Physicians' guidelines from 2020 retain reference to 'prolonged disorders of consciousness', 'vegetative state', and 'minimally conscious state', finding that 'there are clear definitions for them and both the public and commissioners generally know what they mean'; it is also stated that '[i]f and when a more acceptable, internationally agreed term emerges, this will be adopted in future iterations of these guidelines'.[30] **Table 17.1** provides a brief taxonomy of varying degrees of disorders, as defined in the guidelines.

Having reached a diagnosis, we are then left with what may be regarded as the ultimate tragedy in human life—a human being who is alive in the cardiovascular sense, yet at the same time has no contact with the outside world and will never have such contact again. The law on killing is unaffected by the mental state of the victim; persons in a PVS still represent 'persons in being'. They present an additional jurisprudential difficulty in that, being unconscious, they are free from pain—or, at least, from treatable pain; the doctrine of 'double effect'[31] cannot, therefore, be applied within their management. In this respect it should be noted that, absent an intercurrent infection or similar complication, well-managed PVS patients have a life expectancy that is measurable in years.

We have spent some time on the definitional difficulties of the condition because without understanding them, it is impossible to appreciate the distinctions which have been made in the various cases that have come before the courts, and the reasons underlying those decisions. We now turn to these cases in detail.

17.5 THE ENGLISH CASES

The first and most important case in which the matter was addressed in the UK was *Airedale NHS Trust* v *Bland*.[32] Anthony Bland was crushed in a football stadium incident

Table 17.1 Prolonged disorders of consciousness[33]

Coma	A person is unresponsive and cannot be woken for longer than 6 hours. They do not respond to stimuli (pain, light, or sound) and do not initiate voluntary actions.
Vegetative state (VS)	A person is in a state of wakefulness without awareness. They exhibit a range of reflexive and spontaneous behaviours, but there is no behavioural evidence of self or environmental awareness
Minimally conscious state (MCS)	A person is in a state of severely altered consciousness, where there is evidence of self or environmental awareness, but this is minimal. Responses are inconsistent but are reproducible and suggest the person is able to interact to some degree with their surroundings.

---

[28] Adrian Owen, et al., 'Detecting Awareness in the Vegetative State' (2006) 313(5792) Science 1402.
[29] Clare Dyer (2012) (n 19).   [30] Royal College of Physicians (n 25), pp 23–24.
[31] This doctrine will be discussed further.   [32] [1993] 1 All ER 821.
[33] Table adapted from ibid., p 25.

in 1989 and sustained severe anoxic brain damage, from which he lapsed into a PVS. There was no improvement in his condition by 1992, at which point the hospital sought a declaration[34] that they could lawfully discontinue all life-sustaining treatment and medical support measures, including artificial ventilation, nutrition, and hydration; that any subsequent treatment given should be for the sole purpose of enabling him to end his life in dignity and free from pain and suffering; that, if death should then occur, its cause should be attributed to the natural and other causes of his present state; and that none of those concerned should, as a result, be subject to any civil or criminal liability.

This declaration—save for the final clause, which was considered inappropriate[35]—was granted in the Family Division essentially on the grounds that it was in Bland's best interests to do so; the Court considered there was overwhelming evidence that the provision of artificial feeding by means of a nasogastric tube was 'medical treatment' and that its discontinuance was in accord with good medical practice. An appeal was unanimously dismissed in the Court of Appeal. From three exceptionally well-considered opinions, we extract only that of Hoffmann LJ:

> This is not an area in which any difference can be allowed to exist between what is legal and what is morally right. The decision of the court should be able to carry conviction with the ordinary person as being based not merely on legal precedent but also upon acceptable ethical values.[36]

And, later:

> In my view the choice the law makes must reassure people that the courts do have full respect for life, but that they do not pursue the principle to the point at which it has become almost empty of any real content and when it involves the sacrifice of other important values such as human dignity and freedom of choice. I think that such reassurance can be provided by a decision, properly explained, to allow Anthony Bland to die.[37]

The inherent difficulty of the declarator procedure is that it is concerned only with the *lawfulness* of an action[38] and, when the *Bland* case came to the House of Lords, Lord Browne-Wilkinson and Lord Mustill were at particular pains to emphasise that the ethical issues should be considered and legislated for by Parliament.[39]

Although the Lords could not entirely avoid addressing the ethical and moral problems involved, it was therefore not surprising that they did so to a lesser extent than did the Court of Appeal. In this respect, the fundamental conflict lies in the inevitable distortion of the principle of the sanctity of life which would result from a decision to terminate

---

[34] The English courts were initially in a dilemma in such cases since their authority under the *parens patriae* jurisdiction was removed by way of the Mental Health Act 1959 and revocation of the last warrant under the Sign Manual. The courts could no longer give effective consent to medical treatment on behalf of an adult who lacked capacity unless that treatment is directed to the cause of the mental condition. Procedural matters were addressed by the establishment of the Court of Protection under the Mental Capacity Act 2005.

[35] This problem was considered in greater detail in the comparable Scottish case *Law Hospital NHS Trust v Lord Advocate* 1996 SLT 848; (1996) 39 BMLR 166, for which see discussion below on 'The Position in Scotland'.

[36] *Bland* (n 33) [850].   [37] ibid. [855].

[38] See Catherine Constable, 'Withdrawal of Artificial Nutrition and Hydration for Patients in a Permanent Vegetative State: Changing Tack' (2010) 26(3) Bioethics 157. For criticism, see Simon Halliday, Adam Formby, and Richard Cookson, 'An Assessment of the Court's Role in The Withdrawal of Clinically Assisted Nutrition and Hydration from Patients in the Permanent Vegetative State' (2015) 23(4) Medical Law Review 556.

[39] *Bland* (n 33) [878].

the care on which life depended.[40] The majority of the House was able to dispose of this on the ground that the principle was certainly not absolute. Moreover, since the right to refuse treatment—including life-sustaining treatment—is now firmly part of common law and medical ethics, the principle of the sanctity of life must yield to that of the right to self-determination. It is this which seems to us to bind all five Law Lords most closely. As Lord Goff put it,[41] the right to self-determination should not be eclipsed by the fact of incapacity—it must always be present. This also forms the basis of Lord Mustill's reasoning, which is summarised later and which justifies the withdrawal or withholding of treatment.

We are less happy with the alternative view taken, in particular by Lords Lowry and Browne-Wilkinson. In essence, this also started from the premise that non-voluntary treatment was lawful only if it was justified by necessity; but once necessity could no longer be claimed—by reason of the futility of treatment—further invasion of the patient's body constituted either the crime of battery or the tort of trespass. On this view, any potential medical offence lies not in *withholding* treatment but in *continuing* it to no purpose. This argument seems to us to be dangerously open-ended in relation to conditions less clear-cut than PVS. It was this situation which Lord Mustill was anxious to avoid. His concern was later borne out in guidance from the BMA, which proposed extending the PVS ruling to other incapacitated patients.[42]

The greater part of the opinions in *Bland* was concerned for the doctors' position vis-à-vis the criminal law. First, it was essential to eliminate the possibility of murder by classifying removal of support as an omission rather than as a positive act.[43] There was wide agreement that, while there was no moral or logical difference, a distinction was certainly to be made in law. The House came to a unanimous conclusion that discontinuance of nasogastric feeding was an omission; their Lordships achieved this in various ways, but it was generally considered impossible to distinguish between withdrawal of, and not starting, tube feeding—and the latter was clearly an omission.

Next, the problem of the duty of care had to be addressed. Lord Mustill's argument can be summarised as follows:

(i)   treatment of an adult who lacks capacity is governed by necessity and necessity is, in turn, defined in terms of the patient's best interests;

(ii)   once there is no hope of recovery, any interest in being kept alive disappears and, with it, any justification for invasive therapy; and

(iii)   in the absence of necessity, there can be no duty to act and, in the absence of a duty, there can be no criminality in an omission.

This argument leads to a major hurdle: can feeding be regarded as medical treatment and, therefore, a subject fit for medical decision-making, or is it always such a fundamental duty that it can never be wilfully withheld? The Lords in *Bland* had rather more trouble with

---

[40] For major discussion, see John Keown, 'Restoring Moral and Intellectual Shape to the Law After *Bland*' (1997) 113 Law Quarterly Review 481. Singer, at one extreme, saw the decision as an explicit rejection of the sanctity of life principle: Peter Singer, *Rethinking Life and Death: The Collapse of Our Traditional Ethics* (OUP 1994) 75.

[41] *Bland* (n 33) [866].

[42] BMA, 'Withholding and Withdrawing Life-Prolonging Medical Treatment: Guidance for Decision Makers' (3rd edn, 2007) para 30.2. This was expanded, though not updated, by the later guidance in BMA and RCP, 'Clinically-Assisted Nutrition and Hydration (CANH) and Adults Who Lack The Capacity to Consent: Guidance for Decision-Making In England and Wales' (2018).

[43] See discussion of the doctrine of double effect.

this than their counterparts in the United States.[44] Eventually a consensus was reached that nasogastric feeding at least formed part of the general medical management.[45] While it is certainly more difficult to see nasogastric feeding as medical treatment than it is to accept gastrostomy feeding as such, we do not share some of the academic distrust of the concept.[46]

The House of Lords was able to justify its unanimous decision on the basis of the patient's best interests—or non-interest in the case of futility, according to Lord Mustill's logical formulation. All the opinions stressed that it was not a matter of it being in the best interests of the patient to die but, rather, that it was not in his best interests to treat him so as to prolong his life in circumstances where 'no affirmative benefit' could be derived from the treatment.[47] We confess to some difficulty in accepting a 'best interests' test in these circumstances and we return to the matter later. For the present, we point out that its application dictates the concurrent acceptance of 'good medical practice' as the yard-stick of assessment. This led the House of Lords to conclude that the *Bolam* test[48]—that the doctor's decision should be judged against one which would be taken by a responsi-ble and competent body of relevant professional opinion—applied in the management of PVS. This gives considerable discretion to the medical profession to decide what amounts to the patient's best interests by reference to its own standards.[49]

In deciding that artificial feeding was, at least, an integral part of medical treatment, the House of Lords opened the door to the health carers to withdraw alimentation. Nevertheless, the requirement to seek court approval in every case was maintained[50]—subject to the hope that the restriction might be rescinded in the future—and there was, in fact, a strong undercurrent to the effect that the decision was specific to *Bland* rather than a general statement on the removal of alimentation from brain damaged persons. Indeed, as we see later with respect to *Briggs* and *Re Y*,[51] the law did move to a position of not requiring court permission to withdraw medical treatment.

17.5.1 THE PRINCIPLE OF 'DOUBLE EFFECT'

The law condemns active euthanasia on the ground of intent. The terminally or incurably ill are by definition beyond curative therapy, and their management is aimed at relief of suffering. Achieving this may inevitably involve some risk to life, but the patient's comfort, and not their premature death, is the intended therapeutic outcome. The principle of

---

[44] See e.g. *Bush v Schiavo* (Fla 2004) 885 So. 2d 321; *Schindler v Schiavo* (11th Cir. 2005) 403 F 3d 1289.

[45] The Australian courts have approached the question from a different and interesting angle. In *Gardner: re BWV* [2003] VSC 173, the central legal issue was whether the provision of ANH was 'medical treatment' (which can be refused under the Victorian Medical Treatment Act 1988, s 3) or 'palliative care' (which cannot be rejected by way of an advance statement). It was held that the provision of ANH was medi-cal treatment. Similarly, the Supreme Court of Canada confirmed in *Cuthbertson v Rasouli* [2013] SCC 53 that withdrawal and withholding of life support constitutes 'treatment' under the Ontario Health Care Consent Act 1996. This, in turn, required consent from the patient or their proxy decision-maker to be legal.

[46] See, e.g., John Finnis, '*Bland*: Crossing the Rubicon?' (1993) 109 Law Quarterly Review 329; John Keown, 'Restoring Moral and Intellectual Shape to the Law After *Bland*' (1997) 113 Law Quarterly Review 481.

[47] *Bland* (n 33) [883] (Lord Browne-Wilkinson), see also [865].

[48] *Bolam v Friern Hospital Management Committee* [1957] 1 WLR 582.

[49] See *Bland* (n 33) [883].

[50] Practice Note [1996] 4 All ER 766, and see now Practice Note (Official Solicitor: Declaratory Proceedings: Medical and Welfare Decisions for Adults who Lack Capacity) [2006] 2 FLR 373.

[51] *Director of Legal Aid Casework & Ors v Briggs* [2017] EWCA Civ 1169; *An NHS Trust v Y* [2018] UKSC 46.

double effect allows performing an action with a good objective, despite that positive effect being possible only at the expense of a coincident harmful effect.[52] This needs to be qualified: the action itself must be either good or morally indifferent, the good effect must not be produced by means of the ill-effect, and there must be a proportionate reason for allowing the expected ill to occur.[53] It might well be ethically right to administer pain-killing drugs in such dosage as simultaneously shortens the life of a terminally ill patient; it would not be justifiable to give the same dose to a young person with identical pain who stood a reasonable chance of recovery.

The seminal case in the UK is that of *R v Adams*,[54] and the dictum of Devlin J, that 'the doctor is entitled to relieve pain and suffering even if the measures he takes may incidentally shorten life'. Devlin J also noted that it was not universally approved. Twenty years after the *Adams* verdict, Lord Edmund Davies commented: 'Killing both pain and patient may be good morals but it is far from certain that it is good law.'[55] Nonetheless, Williams found the proposition easily justified by necessity.[56] The potential conflict has now been at least partially resolved. Devlin J's direction was followed in *R v Cox*,[57] and the charge to the jury in *Cox* was cited with approval by the House of Lords in *Bland*.

However, since *Bland*, the House of Lords has pronounced on the meaning of 'intention' in the non-medical case of *R v Woollin*.[58] It was directed that a consequence could be said to be intentional if the actor was 'virtually certain' that it would arise—in this case throwing a toddler onto a hard surface and to their death. In *Re A (children) (conjoined twins: surgical separation)*,[59] Ward LJ said that it could be difficult to reconcile the doctrine of double effect with *Woollin*, but he could 'readily see' how the doctrine would work in cases where painkillers are administered for acute pain.[60] Essentially, *Woollin* crystallises a major objection to the use of the 'doctrine' in courts of law—that is, the difficulties juries may face in applying the intention/foresight distinction, which is the 'core requirement' of double effect. It has been argued that clinicians 'have an unarticulated, intuitive grasp of the rule of double effect in almost all their therapeutic interventions';[61] the same can be said of the judiciary.[62] The UK Supreme Court has most recently and unquestioningly endorsed the role of the double effect in *Nicklinson v Ministry of Justice*,[63] citing Lord Goff in *Bland*.

---

[52] For a wide-ranging analysis of double effect see David Price, 'What Shape to Euthanasia After Bland? Historical, Contemporary and Futuristic Paradigms' (2009) 125 Law Quarterly Review 142. See also Joshua Stuchlik, *Intention and Wrongdoing: In Defense of Double Effect* (CUP 2021).

[53] It will be seen that Dr Cox (discussed in the next chapter) would have failed on at least two counts to justify his action as one of 'double effect'.

[54] Henry Palmer, 'Dr Adams' Trial for Murder' [1957] 365 Criminal Law Review 365.

[55] Herbert Edmund-Davies, 'On Dying and Dying Well—Legal Aspects' (1977) 70(2) Proceedings of the Royal Society of Medicine 73.

[56] Glanville Williams, *Textbook of Criminal Law* (2nd edn, 1983) p 416.   [57] (1992) 12 BMLR 38.

[58] [1999] 1 AC 82 (HL).   [59] [2000] 4 All ER 961 (CA).

[60] For a major analysis of the effect of *Woollin* on the management of terminal illness, and distinguishing foreseeability and intent, see Andrew McGee, 'Finding a Way Through the Ethical and Legal Maze: Withdrawal of Medical Treatment and Euthanasia' (2005) 13(3) Medical Law Review 357.

[61] Daniel Sulmasy and Edmund Pellagrino, 'The Rule Of Double Effect: Clearing Up The Double Talk' (1999) 159(6) Archives of Internal Medicine 545; cf, Charles Douglas, Ian Kerridge, and Rachel Ankeny, 'Double Meanings Will Not Save the Principle of Double Effect' (2014) 39(3) Journal of Medicine and Philosophy 304.

[62] David Price (n 52) [146]–[147] points out that to deny the legality of double effect in the present context is going a long way towards denying the legality of any medical procedure which may cause harm.

[63] *R (Nicklinson) v Ministry of Justice* [2014] UKSC 38.

17.5.2 TERMINAL SEDATION

'Deep continuous' or 'terminal' sedation is defined by Williams as 'the administration of a sedating drug for the purpose of relieving suffering by diminishing consciousness at the end of life'.[64] This is a reasonably innocuous goal that seems to be plausibly justified under a modified principle of double effect.[65] McStay, however, speaks of the 'induction of an unconscious state' and adds 'which is frequently accompanied by the withdrawal of any life-sustaining intervention, such as hydration and nutrition'.[66] Insofar as it implies an intention to hasten death, McStay's interpretation introduces a far less easily acceptable motive, but one which is becoming acceptable under the guise of 'early' terminal sedation.[67]

Such interventions provide a vivid example of the application of the 'slippery slope' philosophy to the management of the terminally ill patient. Seen as palliative treatment for those whose death is imminent and whose dying is painful, terminal sedation could be accommodated within the acceptable processes of good medical practice—as defined by double effect.[68] 'Early terminal sedation', however, involves patients whose death is not imminent and even those who are able to take part in decision-making.[69] In such cases we have clearly moved into the fields of assisted suicide and euthanasia hiding under emollient terminology,[70] and further confusing the taxonomy of assisted dying.[71]

To the best of our knowledge, the legality of early terminal sedation has not been addressed directly in the UK courts,[72] at least with respect to adults. It was announced in 2007 that a Mrs Taylor was bringing an action to test the legality of the procedure but the case never came to fruition.[73] And yet the role for sedation at the end of life appears to have found a legal foothold in the ruling in *King's College Hospital NHS Foundation Trust v Y (By Her Children's Guardian), MH*.[74] The judgment concerned a child, yet is applicable here because the application of the legal principles of best interests are now largely the same for neonates, children, and adults. In that case the judge ruled, with respect to a seven-year-old child with spinal muscular atrophy, that in the case of their severe discomfort and pain it would be lawful in her best interests to receive pain or sedation medication, even if it would shorten her life.

---

[64] Glanville Williams, 'The Principle of Double Effect and Terminal Sedation' (2001) 9(1) Medical Law Review 41.

[65] See Ruth Horn, 'The "French Exception": the Right to Continuous Deep Sedation at the End of Life' (2018) 44(3) Journal of Medical Ethics 204.

[66] Rob McStay, 'Terminal Sedation: Palliative Care for Intractable Pain, Post *Glucksberg* and *Quill*' (2003) 29(1) American Journal of Law & Medicine 45. See also Yale Kamisar, 'Are the Distinctions Drawn in the Debate About End-Of-Life Decision Making "Principled"? If Not, How Much Does it Matter?' (2012) 40(1) Journal of Law, Medicine & Ethics 66.

[67] For intuitive concern, see Victor Cellarius, 'Terminal Sedation and the "Imminence Condition"' (2008) 34(2) Journal of Medical Ethics 69.

[68] See John Lombard, 'Sedation of the Terminally Ill Patient: The Role of the Doctrine of Double Effect' (2015) 21(1) Medico-Legal Journal of Ireland 22.

[69] See Adrian Serey et al., 'Deep Continuous Patient-Requested Sedation Until Death: A Multicentric Study' (in press) BMJ Supportive & Palliative Care, available at <https://pubmed.ncbi.nlm.nih.gov/31005881/> accessed 02 November 2022.

[70] Consider, however, Victor Cellarius, '"Early Terminal Sedation" is a Distinct Entity' (2011) 25(1) Bioethics 46, and the proposal of a new legal category.

[71] Nevertheless, the US Supreme Court appears to have approved the practice in *Washington v Glucksberg* 521 US 702 (1997) and *Vacco v Quill* 521 US 793 (1997).

[72] See, however, *Fleming v Ireland & Ors* [2013] IEHC 2.

[73] Clare Dyer, 'Dying Woman Seeks Backing Dose of Morphine to Hasten Death' (2007) 334(7589) BMJ 329.

[74] [2015] EWHC 1966 (Fam), to be read in conjunction with the earlier ruling at [2015] EWHC 1920 (Fam).

17.5.3 ENGLISH PVS CASES AFTER *BLAND*

Consideration of cases subsequent to *Bland* suggests that the previous note of caution on diagnostic precision may not have been misplaced; neither is the threat of a slippery slope entirely countered.

Almost exactly a year later, we had *Frenchay Healthcare NHS Trust* v S.[75] This concerned a young man who had been in apparent PVS for two-and-a-half years as a result of a drug overdose. When it was discovered that his gastrostomy tube had become detached, a declaration was sought that the hospital could lawfully refrain from renewing or continuing alimentary and other life-sustaining measures and could restrict any medical treatment to that which would allow him to die peacefully and with the greatest dignity. The declaration was granted and the decision was upheld on appeal.

Frenchay differed fundamentally from *Bland* in that the actual decision to discontinue treatment was not a considered one but was one forced by events. As a corollary, the judicial inquiry was certainly hurried and this was the factor which most concerned Waite LJ in the Court of Appeal. The decision has also been subject to academic criticism on these grounds.[76] More importantly, Sir Thomas Bingham MR considered it plain that the evidence in *Frenchay* was neither as emphatic nor as unanimous as that in *Bland*.[77] We must also consider the potential results of failing to make, or countermanding, the declaration sought—either the doctors would have been forced into an operation which was, in the opinion of the consultant in charge, of no benefit to the patient and which possibly verged on criminal intervention, or they would have had to do nothing and take their chance with the law.

Sir Thomas accepted the medical opinion that was provided but he was conscious of a qualitative difference between the two cases. The question arises as to whether *Frenchay* represents a 'slippery slope' on which we could descend from PVS to little more than physical or mental disability when assuming that the patient's 'best interests' lie in non-treatment. Alternatively, is it a judicial effort to homogenise non-treatment decisions—during which process, PVS becomes merely the end-point for decision-making, rather than a condition to be considered on its own? We discuss in due course the difficulties in harmonising the 'specific-case' stance adopted in *Bland* with the relatively open-ended direction in *Re J*[78] on withholding 'futile' treatment. Perhaps the main inference to be drawn is that each case is special and must be judged on its own facts.[79]

Later English cases have been reported only spasmodically. We comment briefly on some of these mainly to indicate the quality of the evidence that was available.

Re C[80] concerned a 27-year-old man who had been in PVS for four years following an anaesthetic disaster. Clinically, the case was of great severity and the judge appears to

---

[75] [1994] 2 All ER 403.

[76] See e.g. Andrew Grubb, 'Commentary' (1994) 2 Medical Law Review 206.

[77] [1994] 2 All ER 403 [411]. [78] *Re J (a minor) (wardship: medical treatment)* [1990] 3 All ER 930.

[79] A point which was emphasised in *Bland* and also in the even more doubtful Irish case of *In the matter of a Ward* (1995) 2 ILRM 401. The same result was achieved in this case although the reasoning was complicated by considerations of Irish constitutional law. For discussion, see John K Mason and Graeme Laurie, 'The Management of the Persistent Vegetative State in the British Isles' [1996] 4 Juridical Review 263; John Keown, 'Life and Death in Dublin' (1996) 55(1) Cambridge Law Journal 6.

[80] The importance of continued post-mortem anonymity was considered in *Re C (adult patient: restriction of publicity after death)* [1996] 2 FLR 251 and see *Practice Direction* [2002] 1 WLR 325. For professional guidance to this effect, see GMC, 'Confidentiality: Good Practice in Handling Patient Information' (2018) available at <https://www.gmc-uk.org/ethical-guidance/ethical-guidance-for-doctors/confidentiality> accessed 25 October 2022.

have accepted without demur the evidence provided by the relatives as to the likely wishes of the patient.

Re G[81] related to a young man whose brain damage, sustained in a motorcycle accident, was intensified by a later anoxic episode. Of particular interest was a dispute among the relatives as to the course to be adopted. Sir Stephen Brown P concluded that the dissenting views of the patient's mother should not be allowed to operate as a veto when his best interests—as defined by the surgeon in charge—favoured removal of nutrition. This reflected the comments of Lord Goff in *Bland*[82] that the views of relatives should be respected, but are not determinative in the event of conflict.

Swindon and Marlborough NHS Trust v *S*[83] was unique among reported cases in being concerned with a patient who was being nursed at home. Like *Frenchay*, the issue was forced by blockage of the gastrostomy tube; but in this case further treatment would have involved hospitalisation. Ward J held that, given the certain diagnosis of PVS, to discontinue life-sustaining measures would be in accordance with good medical practice as recognised and approved within the medical profession. Once again, as in *Re G*, the court firmly adopted *Bolam* as the benchmark. That gives rise to a strong suggestion that good medical practice is being seen as a test of lawfulness.[84]

There was no doubt as to the diagnosis in any of these three cases. Conversely, *Re D*[85] concerned a 28-year-old woman who had sustained very severe brain damage following a head injury some six years before. Again, an emergency arose following displacement of her gastrostomy tube. Medical opinion was united to the effect that D was totally unaware of anything or anyone, but she did not fully satisfy the conditions laid down by the Royal College of Physicians for the diagnosis of PVS. The President of the Family Division regarded her as suffering 'a living death' and was unable to accept that, because she did not fulfil one of the diagnostic criteria, she was not in a PVS. He did not believe he was extending the range of cases in which a declaration as to the removal of feeding and hydration might properly be considered. It was appropriate and in her best interests to make such a declaration.

Re H[86] involved a 43-year-old woman who had existed for three years in a severely brain-damaged state following a vehicular accident. She, too, was agreed to be wholly and unalterably unaware of herself or her environment, but it was agreed that she did not fit squarely within one of the Royal College of Physicians' diagnostic criteria. Sir Stephen Brown P thought that, in this instance, 'it may be that a precise label is not of significant importance'. Indeed, the whole area is prey to semantic juggling—one expert, while agreeing that the case did not fit the criteria for PVS, nevertheless thought that H was in a vegetative state which was permanent. The court reiterated that, while it was aware of the consequences that would follow the suspension of treatment, it did not in any sense sanction anything which is *aimed* at terminating life. H's best interests favoured suspension of treatment.[87]

While all these cases show distinctive variations, they also have common features on which the jurisprudence continues to be built. The precedents having been set, the

---

[81] (1995) 3 Med LR 80. In passing, it was held that the public interest in these cases determined that they should be heard in open court: *Re G (adult patient: publicity)* [1995] 2 FLR 528.

[82] *Bland* (n 33) [872].   [83] (1995) 3 Med LR 84.

[84] It does not follow that medical opinion in a case must be unanimous. As long as there is a high degree of probability that medical evidence supported withdrawal of treatment in the patient's best interests, then the court would be entitled to support it: see *An NHS Trust* v *X* [2005] EWCA Civ 1145.

[85] (1997) 38 BMLR 1.   [86] *Re H (adult: incompetent)* (1997) 38 BMLR 11.

[87] (1997) 38 BMLR 11 [16].

baseline lies in the confirmed diagnosis of PVS. Once made, the conclusion follows automatically that the patient's best interests dictate the termination of assisted feeding and, indeed, there may well be an obligation on the doctor to discontinue treatment.[88] Following from this, the Official Solicitor has been loath to oppose any applications for withdrawal once the diagnosis is confirmed. Complete medicalisation of treatment decisions in the condition may, then, still be accepted. This having been said, a Practice Direction makes it clear that court approval should be sought in almost all cases where removal of feeding and hydration is contemplated.[89] Despite the court being charged with weighing the advantages and disadvantages of treatment removal, it is difficult to see how any conclusion other than withdrawal could be reached when faced with a good faith assessment of medical futility by the care team. We say this in light of recent developments which demonstrate that the provisions of the Human Rights Act 1998 make little or no difference to the position of patients in PVS.

In *NHS Trust A v Mrs M, NHS Trust B v Mrs H*,[90] declarators of legality were sought on the proposed withdrawal of feeding and hydration from two patients in PVS. In authorising this the High Court endorsed and went further than the position under *Bland*, in testing that precedent against possible human rights objections under the 1998 Act, namely Article 2 (right to life), Article 3 (prohibition of cruel and inhuman treatment), and Article 8 (right to respect for private life). Rather than considering the particularised reasoning of Butler-Sloss P in respect of each of these provisions,[91] a few points of principle and policy should be noted.

The court clearly adopted a good faith approach to the issue, focusing on the fact that, because a 'responsible body of medical opinion' had reached a conclusion as to futility, there was little more to be said on the matter. This, however, makes professionalism rather than principle the measure of patient protection. We have already shown that medical professionals are qualified only to comment on the medical futility of any proposed course of action and that the court retains the ultimate role as arbiter of best interests.

Second, in examining the content of the human rights laid before it, the court fixed on the principle of respect for personal autonomy. It concluded that, because the PVS patient could not consent to continued intervention, to continue to intervene against their best interests—as determined by (medically qualified) others—would violate protection under Article 8. This, however, turns self-determination on its head. Its relevance is questionable for someone who cannot meaningfully experience or exercise this state. It is because the patient cannot do so that 'best interests' enters the equation. The error lies in the failure to appreciate that it is *respect* for the human being that is required, not only (or necessarily) respect for their 'right to choose'.

The court also relied upon the incapacity of these patients to justify restricting their rights in another respect. It held that, because PVS patients cannot appreciate their state of being, it is not cruel and degrading to subject them to the vagaries of withdrawal of feeding and hydration—adopting a narrow interpretation of Article 3, that a victim must be able to experience the inhuman treatment before a violation will occur.[92] This is a

[88] Following the argument put forward by Andrew Grubb in 'Commentary' (1995) 3 Medical Law Review 85. This seems to have been confirmed by Baker J in *W (by her litigation friend B)* (n 22) [35].

[89] *Practice Note (Official Solicitor: Declaratory Proceedings: Medical and Welfare Decisions for Adults Who Lack Capacity)* [2006] 2 FLR 373. See, however, discussion of *An NHS Trust & Ors v Y & Anor* on court involvement being unnecessary.

[90] [2001] 2 WLR 942; (2001) 58 BMLR 87.

[91] For such an analysis, see Alasdair MacLean, 'Crossing the Rubicon on the Human Rights Ferry' (2001) 64(5) Modern Law Review 775.

[92] Article 3 states: 'No one shall be subjected to torture or to inhuman or degrading treatment or punishment.'

distorted view of European jurisprudence, which has held that only a victim's own subjective reactions to treatment can impact on the question of whether violation has occurred.[93] It does not automatically follow that subjectivity is a prerequisite for violation.[94]

We see Lord Mustill's fears as to extending the precedent in *Bland* to other, non-PVS cases being realised in *Re G (adult incompetent: withdrawal of treatment)*.[95] The patient was a 45-year-old woman who had suffered serious anoxic brain damage after inhaling her own vomitus following surgery. She had been kept alive for nine months by means of ANH when the NHS Trust responsible for her care brought the matter to court for a declaration of legality as to the withdrawal of her means of artificial sustenance. G's family supported the application, stating that she would not have wished to remain in such a state. One expert witness was enough to convince the court that there was no reasonable prospect of her ever recovering and that she should be allowed to 'die with dignity'. Moreover, it was held to be not inconsistent with her human right to life that a decision be made to discontinue treatment, despite her inability to give a valid consent to its withdrawal. A declaration to this effect was granted.

We view this decision with a degree of concern. It comes very close to the controversial guidance of the BMA, already mentioned, which suggested that an assessment of futility leading to the withdrawal of feeding and hydration may be appropriate for patients with dementia or for those who have suffered serious stroke.[96] We consider it a positive step that references to dementia and stroke do not appear in the most recent update of that guidance.[97] It remains problematic, however, because it demonstrates the ongoing possibility of an expansionist development of clinical discretion,[98] if criteria can be easily altered.

A further ruling from the Court of Appeal reflects our views and concerns, but at the same time, it reveals the tragedy of so many of these cases which often feel like lose–lose scenarios. *W Healthcare NHS Trust v H and Another*[99] concerned KH, who had suffered from multiple sclerosis for 30 years. She had required artificial feeding for five years and needed 24-hour nursing care to survive. She could scarcely speak and recognised nobody; she was, however, conscious and sentient. Her feeding tube had fallen out and her health carers wished to replace it. The family was opposed to this and appealed the trial judge's opinion in favour of continued treatment. The Court of Appeal upheld the trial judge's ruling that KH should continue to be fed, while expressing the deepest sympathy for her and her family.

The Court stated that three tests have to be applied in cases such as this. First, is the patient capable of taking an informed decision herself? There was no doubt as to

[93] *Campbell and Cosans* v *United Kingdom* (1983) 7 EHRR 165 [28].

[94] Inability or awareness to feel pain in PVS or in a minimally conscious state has been challenged: Mélanie Boly et al., 'Perception of Pain in the Minimally Conscious State with PET Activation: An Observational Study' (2008) 7(11) The Lancet Neurology 1013.

[95] (2002) 65 BMLR 6.

[96] BMA (2007) (n 42). See also GMC, 'Treatment and Care Towards the End of Life: Good Practice in Decision Making (2010)' available at <https://www.gmc-uk.org/ethical-guidance/ethical-guidance-for-doctors/treatment-and-care-towards-the-end-of-life> accessed 02 November 2022, paras 119–122, though absent from the 2022 update, which somewhat allays our concerns.

[97] GMC, 'Treatment and Care Towards the End of life: Good Practice in Decision Making' (2022) available at <https://www.gmc-uk.org/ethical-guidance/ethical-guidance-for-doctors/treatment-and-care-towards-the-end-of-life> accessed 25 October 2022.

[98] On this problematic element, see Graeme Laurie and John K Mason, 'Negative Treatment of Vulnerable Patients: Euthanasia by Any Other Name?' (2000) 3 The Juridical Review 159.

[99] [2004] EWCA Civ 1324.

the negative response in the instant case. Second, is there a valid advance statement or directive which covers the present circumstances? In KH's case there was insufficient evidence of what she would have wanted, so as to justify relying on an advanced refusal. Finally, if neither test applies, what is in the patient's best interests? It is important to note, as the Court itself does, that the legal test in the UK is not substituted judgement: the Court could not rely on the strong evidence from the family that KH would not have wanted to continue living in this undignified state to refuse on her behalf. The onerous task for the Court was to ask, 'What is in the patient's best interests given that the decision not to feed would effectively mean that the patient would starve to death?' Unlike the PVS cases, KH would have some level of awareness of the process. Brooke LJ emphasised the high value that English law places on life and stated:

> The Court cannot in effect sanction the death by starvation of a patient who is not in a PVS state other than with their clear and informed consent or where their condition is so intolerable as to be beyond doubt.[100]

As to the process of establishing overall best interests, the Court of Appeal approved Thorpe LJ's suggested 'balance sheet' of pros and cons. *KH* appears to endorse intolerability as the touchstone for measuring best interests. As suggested earlier in this chapter, the decision in *KH* suggests a higher intolerability threshold for adults than for neonates such as was considered by the Court of Appeal in *Wyatt v Portsmouth Hospitals NHS Trust*, where it was merely a useful signpost on the route towards best interests. This might be an echo once again of the strains of the personhood argument, whereby a sentient adult with a lived life may be held in higher regard than a newborn with little or no experiential existence. Later cases adopt a more straightforward application of the best interests test, as conventionally understood.[101]

17.5.4 THE DIRECTION OF TRAVEL FOR PROLONGED DISORDERS OF CONSCIOUSNESS

Here we draw on four illustrative examples. In *An NHS Trust v L*,[102] patient L was, like Mrs M, initially determined to be in PVS following a cardiac arrest which resulted in 'devastating neurological injury', but was later reassessed as a minimally conscious state (MCS) at a very low level of the spectrum. Medical opinion suggested a less than 1 per cent chance of recovering capacity as defined by the Mental Capacity Act 2005 (MCA 2005). The medical team sought a declaration of lawfulness with respect to no further intervention in the event of further deterioration. The family objected, taking an essentially vitalist position by arguing that L would have wanted to be kept alive. In making the declaration on non-intervention, the court endorsed two important principles: (i) family and patient views are but one element in the balancing exercise required by law, and (ii) while a court is entitled to disagree with unanimous clinical evidence, it could not require professionals to treat against their better judgement.[103]

In *United Lincolnshire Hospitals NHS Trust v N*,[104] the legal question was the permissibility of withholding intravenous fluids from a patient in MCS. In declaring this lawful,

---

[100] [2004] EWCA Civ 1324.

[101] *Gloucestershire Clinical Commissioning Group v AB* [2014] EWCOP 49.

[102] [2013] EWHC 4313 (Fam).

[103] This fortifies the point made in *Re J (a minor) (wardship: medical treatment)* [1991] Fam 33 and followed *An NHS Trust v MB* [2006] EWHC 507 (Fam) [116].

[104] [2014] EWCOP 16.

the court reiterated the previous point about non-compunction of medical staff, now buoyed by confirmation of the point from the Supreme Court.[105] In determining whether treatment would be in a patient's best interests, the court had to consider whether it would be futile to continue in the sense of being ineffective, or of no benefit to the patient. The court clarified that the treatment did not have to be likely to cure or palliate the underlying condition or return the patient to full or reasonable health; rather, it should be capable of allowing the recovery of a quality of life 'which the patient would regard as worthwhile'. The evidence in the present case overwhelmingly supported non-intervention.

In *Sheffield Teaching Hospitals NHS Foundation Trust v TH*,[106] the court faced the detailed issue of the *management* of non-intervention, that is, even if it is lawful to withhold or withdraw treatment, is there nonetheless an enduring obligation to treat supervening conditions, such as infection? The court adjourned in this decision for a full assessment of the facts, reminding all parties that the law now requires a holistic evaluation and this had not been forthcoming. Tellingly, '"[w]ishes" and "best interests"' were never to be conflated, being 'separate matters which may ultimately weigh on dif-ferent sides of the balance sheet'.[107] Finally, whether treatment with antibiotics was in the patient's best interests was always case-dependent. In this case, evidence supported the view that relatively minor infections would be treated with a short course of antibiotics to maintain the patient's general comfort, but it was not in his interests to treat overwhelm-ing infections such as pneumonia or septicaemia with antibiotics. Whether an infection was mild or overwhelming was a matter of clinical judgement, dependent in turn on the invasiveness of any medical response.

Finally, in *St George's Healthcare NHS Trust v P*,[108] we find an example of an MCS patient in which the court held that it was in the patient's best interest for renal replacement therapy to continue. After an initial diagnosis of PVS, family video led to a reassessment of P's condition and re-diagnosis as MCS. Applying a strict level of scrutiny to the evidence as a whole and beginning with the presumption in favour of life, the court found almost no evidence to rebut the presumption that it was in P's best interests to be treated. Indeed, there was contrary evidence that it could extend life a further four years, that he gained benefit from his family's love and affection, that the treatment was not unduly burdensome and had a prospect of success, and he did not seem to be in pain. The court went to some lengths to emphasise the absolute necessity for a structured assessment in all such cases *before* any application to the court. As it said: '[w]ithout a rigorous evidential analysis, real mistakes could be made'.

Two streams of futile cases emerge in these catastrophic cases. It is important to recog-nise the role of the Official Solicitor's Practice Note of 2006 in all of this.[109] It was deemed that an application to court should always be sought before withdrawal of ANH from patients in PVS and a range of treatments from patients with MCS patients as well.[110] In most circumstances, for PVS this was little more than a confirmatory exercise in respect of the diagnosis from which a declarator of legality of withdrawal would follow,[111] and

---

[105] *Aintree University Hospitals NHS Foundation Trust v James* [2013] UKSC 67, discussed further.
[106] [2014] EWCOP 4.   [107] ibid. [31], [35]–[39], [53]–[56].   [108] [2015] EWCOP 42.
[109] *Practice Note (Official Solicitor: Declaratory Proceedings: Medical and Welfare Decisions for Adults who Lack Capacity)* [2006] 2 FLR 373.
[110] *W v M* [2012] 1 All ER 1313; (2011) 122 BMLR 67. The Court of Protection re-emphasised that all cases involving the PVS and now also MCS should be referred to the Court (COP Practice Direction 9E, para 5). The Court of Protection Rules 2007 (SI 2007/1744), along with COP Practice Direction 9E, were replaced by the Court of Protection Rules 2017 (SI 2017/1035) as amended, which came into force on 1 December 2017.
[111] *Practice Note (Official Solicitor: Declaratory Proceedings: Medical and Welfare Decisions for Adults who Lack Capacity)* [2006] 2 FLR 373, Appendix 2.

with respect to *An NHS Trust* v *Y*,[112] an application to the court is no longer deemed necessary.

The 'confirmatory exercise' prior to a declarator of legality of treatment withdrawal was not necessarily true in MCS cases. Indeed, the cases could often overlap in the sense that medical evidence can change circumstances, as a number of the aforementioned cases worryingly demonstrate. In *An NHS Trust* v *J*,[113] a challenge by the Official Solicitor was successful based on evidence in the literature of a possible beneficial effect of a drug called Zolpidem on the condition of some PVS patients. The request was to delay the declaration for three days to try this, albeit unproven, intervention. It was accepted that if there was no improvement within three days then withdrawal could proceed. The stay was granted by the court but there was no improvement. Still, the need for 'structured assessment' must clearly be the guiding parameter in all of these cases. From there the question arises as to whether it is helpful or defensible to continue to treat these kinds of cases as distinct in legal and ethical terms.

What began as a seemingly aberrational and tragic set of circumstances for the House of Lords in *Bland* 30 years ago has become a staple for many of the courts today: the consideration of what is futile treatment and how this is to be accommodated within the best interests test. The UK Supreme Court considered these questions in *Aintree University Hospitals NHS Foundation Trust* v *James*,[114] which was the first case to reach the Supreme Court on the meaning of 'best interests' under section 1(5) of the MCA 2005.

The patient had suffered a series of debilitating physical and mental onslaughts, leaving him in a decidedly grey area of the spectrum of mental capacity. While the trial judge had accepted him as being in MCS, the Supreme Court seemed to accept the view that 'Mr James's current level of awareness when not in a medical crisis "might more accurately be described [as] very limited rather than minimal"'.[115] This is important, because it suggests that the ruling that follows is not dependent on the attachment of such particular labels. The case came to the Supreme Court because the judges at first instance and the Court of Appeal had adopted different approaches in their assessment of best interests, and the patient's widow appealed. The legal question was by now the standard one: is it lawful to withhold treatment from a patient without capacity such that this might lead to their death? The unanimous medical view was one of futility, while the family took the opposite position—that he gained benefit from seeing family and friends, had overcome all infections to date, and had been determined to beat the cancer which was the instant cause of his ultimate condition. Although the patient had died by the time the case reached the Supreme Court, the ruling was considered and handed down for the important points of law and principle that it confirmed:

- When dealing with the incapacitated patient, the court has no more powers than the patient would have if he had capacity; therefore, the court cannot demand or require a particular form of treatment.[116]

- The correct formulation of the question is not whether it is lawful to withhold treatment, but rather whether it is lawful to give it in the patient's best interests. If the treatment is not in the patient's best interests, then the court cannot lawfully consent to it.[117]

---

[112] [2018] UKSC 46.　　[113] [2006] EWHC 3152 (Fam).　　[114] [2013] UKSC 67.
[115] ibid. [6].　　[116] ibid. [18].　　[117] ibid. [22].

- The case of *Bland* (and PVS in general) is particular because there is no benefit at all to be gained by intervention; in all other cases the approach should be: 'in considering the best interests of this particular patient at this particular time, decision-makers must look at his welfare in the widest sense, not just medical but social and psychological; they must consider the nature of the medical treatment in question, what it involves and its prospects of success; they must consider what the outcome of that treatment for the patient is likely to be; they must try and put themselves in the place of the individual patient and ask what his attitude to the treatment is or would be likely to be; and they must consult others who are looking after him or interested in his welfare, in particular for their view of what his attitude would be'.[118]

- Accordingly, 'futile' should be seen as meaning ineffective or of no benefit to the patient, and 'benefit' must be considered relative to the patient's welfare in the widest sense: 'recovery does not mean a return to full health, but the resumption of a quality of life which Mr James would regard as worthwhile'.[119]

The appeal was then dismissed. The case is important for a number of reasons. In precedent terms it drew liberally on the range of judgments we have already discussed with respect to patients with prolonged disorders of consciousness. The ruling applies across the board. Equally, it appears that PVS cases remain distinct as examples of patients for whom intervention represents no benefit whatsoever and therefore no balance exercise is required.[120] Such a conclusion is not restricted to that class of patient, but only to those for whom benefit cannot be found. In all other cases, the balance sheet must be deployed. Most tellingly, the assessment must be recognised for the moveable target that it is, and the bullseye must be seen determinedly from the patient's perspective and from the circumstances in which they now find themselves.[121]

The UK Supreme Court more recently settled another point of law that was unclear since *Bland*. In *Re Y*,[122] it considered whether a court order must *always* be obtained before 'clinically assisted nutrition and hydration' (CANH, which has come to replace the term ANH), which is keeping alive a person with a 'prolonged disorder of consciousness' can be withdrawn (PDOC encompasses *both* PVS and MCS). Case law was conflicted (as, it seemed, was the MCA 2005's Practice Direction 9E and Code of Practice) regarding whether legal proceedings were, in fact, necessary prior to withholding or withdrawing CANH, even when an incapacitated person's family and clinicians agreed that CANH was no longer in the person's best interests and the clinicians were acting in accordance with the MCA 2005 and with recognised medical standards.[123]

---

[118] ibid. [39].   [119] ibid. [40]–[45].

[120] The case against reliance on 'best interests' in the context of PVS is argued by Alan Fenwick, 'Applying Best Interests to Persistent Vegetative State—A Principled Distortion?' (1998) 24(2) Journal of Medical Ethics 86. An alternative view is given in the same issue: Raanan Gillon, 'Persistent Vegetative State, Withdrawal of Artificial Nutrition and Hydration, and the Patient's "Best Interests"' (1998) 24(2) Journal of Medical Ethics 75.

[121] For comment, see Ian Wise, 'Withdrawal and Withholding of Medical Treatment for Patients Lacking Capacity Who are in Critical Condition—Reflections on the Judgment of the Supreme Court in *Aintree University Hospitals NHS Foundation Trust v James*' (2014) 82(4) The Medico-Legal Journal 144.

[122] *An NHS Trust v Y* [2018] UKSC 46.

[123] *Re M (Adult Patient) (Minimally Conscious State: Withdrawal of Treatment)* [2011] EWHC 2443 (Fam) (with Baker J finding at paras 78, 82, 257 that reference to the court was necessary); *Re M (Incapacitated Person: Withdrawal of Treatment)* [2017] EWCOP 18 (with Peter Jackson J finding at paras 37 and 38 that reference to the court was not necessary).

This case concerned Mr Y, who suffered a cardiac arrest which resulted in severe cerebral hypoxia and extensive brain damage.[124] He never regained consciousness and required CANH to keep him alive. There was a clinical consensus that Mr Y was in a vegetative state and that there was no prospect of improvement. Mrs Y and their children believed that he would not wish to be kept alive, given the doctors' assessment of his prognosis. The clinical team and the family agreed that it would be in Mr Y's best interests for CANH to be withdrawn, which would result in his death within two to three weeks.

The NHS Trust sought a declaration in the High Court that it was not mandatory to seek court approval for the withdrawal of CANH from a patient with PDOC when the clinical team and the patient's family agreed that it was not in the patient's best interests to continue treatment, and that no civil or criminal liability would result if CANH were withdrawn. The High Court granted a declaration that court approval was not mandatory in such cases. Fraser J invited the Official Solicitor to act as Mr Y's litigation friend in the proceedings but, rather than adjourning the case for a hearing in the Court of Protection as the Official Solicitor sought, he ordered that the final hearing be expedited and listed before O'Farrell J in the Queen's Bench Division. O'Farrell J refused the Official Solicitor's renewed application for the case to be transferred to the Court of Protection; in her view, there was no common law principle or human rights law requirement that all cases concerning the withdrawal of CANH from a person who lacks capacity had to be sanctioned by the court.[125] O'Farrell J granted permission to appeal directly to the Supreme Court. In the intervening period Mr Y died from acute respiratory sepsis, but the Supreme Court determined that the appeal should go ahead because of the general importance of the issues raised by the case.

The Official Solicitor argued that both the common law and the ECHR, specifically Articles 2 (right to life), 6 (right to a fair trial), 8 (right to respect for private and family life), and 14 (prohibition of discrimination) imposed a universal requirement to obtain court approval prior to the withdrawal of CANH. It was submitted that only by requiring judicial scrutiny in every such case can human life and dignity be properly safeguarded. In a unanimous decision, however, Lady Black found that there is no requirement under the common law or human rights law to bring the matter before the court if:

(1) the clinicians have followed the MCA 2005 and good medical practice;

(2) there is no dispute among the clinicians and the family of the person who lacks capacity or others interested in his welfare that it is not in his best interests that he continues to receive that treatment; and

(3) no other doubts or concerns have been identified.

This applies to patients in PVS and MCS. Conversely, the Court found that if, at the end of the medical process, it is apparent that the way forward is finely balanced, or there is a difference of medical opinion, or a lack of agreement to a proposed course of action from those with an interest in the patient's welfare, then a court application can and should be made. This happened in the case of *Z v University Hospitals Plymouth NHS Trust*.[126] Following a heart attack and prolonged hypoxia, the prognosis for RS was, at best, progress to being in a minimally conscious state at the lower end of the spectrum. His extended yet largely estranged Roman Catholic family opposed a treatment withdrawal decision, with which clinicians and the patient's wife were in agreement. Treatment was withdrawn and

---

[124] For commentary on the implications of this decision, see Richard Huxtable, 'Dying Too Soon or Living too Long? Withdrawing Treatment from Patients with Prolonged Disorders of Consciousness after *Re Y*' (2019) 20(1) BMC Medical Ethics 91.

[125] *NHS Trust v Y* [2017] EWHC 2866 (QB).   [126] [2021] EWCA Civ 22.

restarted three times during the appeals process, which was based on the requisite new expert evidence presented on his diagnosis, but which was found to have been obtained in an underhand way. In following *Bland*, the best interests test, and the provisions of the MCA 2005, it was deemed that treatment should be withdrawn.

Another example of this conflict between clinicians and family members came in the case of *Cambridge University Hospitals NHS Foundation Trust v AH*.[127] The four daughters and sister of AH did not want life-sustaining treatment withdrawn. AH suffered a range of debilitating conditions as a result of her Covid-19 infection, which left her dependent on tube feeding and mechanical ventilation, as well as being paralysed below her neck and unable to speak. She was able to communicate using her eyes and head—though with decreasing reliability, and confounded by involuntary movements—and demonstrated signs of distress, mainly when her medical and comfort needs required to be met. Expert evidence was accepted that her continued decline was inevitable, despite family members alleging 'signs of improvement'[128] as AH was able to recognise them. Though there was some disagreement as the trial progressed, clinicians agreed that her 'behaviours are consistent with either MCS- or MCS+'.[129] Again the court assessed best interests with reference to the MCA 2005 and followed the approach of Lady Hale in *Aintree* on balancing a presumption in favour of life, against the broadly envisioned interests of the particular patient, including her religious beliefs and what choice she may have made (she had agreed to ventilation on initial admission and when she had capacity to do so). In Dr B's evidence, 'AH is self-aware and experiences the world'.[130] As far as decision-making was concerned, the court found that, 'She simply would not be able to weigh up or even retain the relevant considerations involved in the nuanced and complex decision as to whether her treatment should be continued, or not.'[131] Family members felt AH would want to remain on mechanical ventilation, but the court agreed with the official solicitor that against the considerable distress she was in, this was unlikely to be the case. The compelling medical evidence on the futility of continued treatment led Mrs Justice Theis to grant the declaration sought by the Trust for treatment to be withdrawn.

17.6 ADVANCE DECISIONS TO REFUSE TREATMENT

Treatment may also be withdrawn from a patient where they have made an Advance Decision (AD)[132] to refuse it. There is, of course, no reason why one should not make an advance decision to accept treatment in any circumstances; however, it would not be binding on healthcare workers per *Burke,* as discussed. What constituted a valid AD was undefined prior to the MCA 2005. Section 24 of that Act now states:

1. 'Advance decision' means a decision made by a person after he has reached 18 and when he has capacity to do so, that if—

    a. at a later time and in such circumstances as he may specify, a specified treatment is proposed to be carried out or continued by a person providing health care for him, and

    b. at that time he lacks capacity to consent to the carrying out or continuation of the treatment, the specified treatment is not to be carried out or continued.

---

[127] [2021] EWCOP 64.   [128] ibid. [46], [56], et seq.   [129] ibid. [42].   [130] ibid. [30].

[131] ibid. [87].

[132] The words 'advance directive' were generally applied in respect of the common law; the 2005 Act, however, uses the term 'advance decision'.

The MCA 2005 does not say how the decision is to be expressed. However, prior to the passing of the Act, it was held in *HE v A Hospital NHS Trust*[133] that it was not necessary for an AD to be in writing in order for it to be valid. The Act confirms that revocation or alteration of any such decision can occur other than by written means. This is subject to refusal not being likely to result in death; if that is likely to be the case, the AD must be in writing and witnessed.[134]

An AD is invalid if the patient has, subsequently, created a lasting power of attorney in favour of someone else to give or refuse consent to the specified treatment. More controversially, it is invalid if the patient has 'done anything' that is clearly inconsistent with the AD remaining their fixed decision. Moreover, an AD is not applicable if the treatment is not that *specified* in the decision nor if there are reasonable grounds for believing that 'circumstances exist' which the patient did not anticipate at the time the decision was made. Therefore, a number of uncertainties exist that are sufficient to allow healthcare professionals to ignore the AD or, indeed, to act to the contrary.

This is important because, while some doctors may welcome the opportunity to avoid making difficult *professional* decisions in what may prove to be a complex ethical situation, others will see the AD as an interference with their clinical consciences and, in particular, with the medico-legal presumption as to the priority afforded to the preservation of life.[135] The temptation to circumvent the decision may, therefore, be strong. For example, in *W v M*,[136] the Court held it was in best interests of a patient with MCS to continue ANH despite considerable evidence from her family that she would not wish to continue with 'this burdensome life with a lack of dignity'. The problem for M was that she had not completed a formal, written AD. Accordingly, it fell to the court to consider her overall best interests. It held that all cases of withdrawal of ANH from minimally conscious patients or those in PVS must come to court. Any prior statements short of the criteria for an advance decision are merely informal and the court will decide the outcome on a balance sheet assessment. The preservation of life carried great weight. In this case, M had some positive experiences and it was accordingly determined not to be in her best interests to withdraw care. This raises the serious question of how far a patient must go in expressing their wishes to have them respected, and particularly it raises the serious issue of whether anything short of an AD in accordance with sections 24–26 of the MCA 2005 can be more than 'informal'.

Similarly, in *An NHS Trust v D*,[137] the patient suffered irreparable brain damage and the question arose about the cessation of ANH. This was rejected despite the existence of a signed letter which included, inter alia, the very clear statement: 'I refuse any medical treatment of an invasive nature (including but not restrictive to placing a feeding tube in my stomach) if said procedure is only for the purpose of extending a reduced quality of life.' However, this still did not meet the requirements under the MCA 2005, as it had not been witnessed and there was not a specific statement that the decision should apply to the specific treatment. In the end, the judge preferred the preservation of life.

---

[133] [2003] 2 FLR 408.   [134] MCA 2005, s 25(5) and (6).

[135] For detailed analysis, see Sabine Michalowski, 'Advance Refusals of Life-Sustaining Medical Treatment: The Relativity of an Absolute Right' (2005) 68(6) MLR 958.

[136] [2011] EWHC 2443 (Fam). Applied in *St George's Healthcare NHS Trust v P* [2015] EWCOP 42, in which—on the facts—the treatment was held to be not overly burdensome and evidence of the patient's values and beliefs prior to loss of capacity pointed towards continuation of treatment.

[137] [2012] EWHC 885 (COP).

The validity of the AD will also turn on whether the patient had capacity to make it at the relevant time.[138] In *Nottinghamshire Healthcare NHS Trust v RC*,[139] a Jehovah's Witness suffered from personality disorders which caused him to self-harm. He signed an AD stating that no blood transfusions should be administered to him in any circumstances. The formal requirements for executing an advance decision under the MCA 2005 were found to be satisfied and the patient had capacity at the time it was made. Mostyn J therefore upheld his right to refuse a blood transfusion (notwithstanding that it would technically be possible to administer it if it was treatment for his personality disorder under mental health legislation; see Chapter 10). It was held that the duty to save life was subservient to the right to sovereignty over one's own body. When all legal formalities are satisfied and the patient's wishes and beliefs are clear and constant, then ADs will be respected.

In *Lancashire and South Cumbria NHS Foundation Trust v Q*,[140] the Trust sought a declaration as to whether an AD refusing treatment, made by the patient Q, was valid or whether at the time of creating the document, Q lacked capacity. Mr Justice Hayden found that no party had sought to suggest that the ADRT was invalid for any technical reason. The issue of capacity at the time of the AD would stand or fall with the issue of current capacity. Ultimately, Mr Justice Hayden concluded that to whatever extent Q may have exhibited low self-esteem and worthlessness, it was not evident to such a degree as to prevent patients lacking capacity from decision-making on this issue.

Despite the general principle that when all legal formalities are satisfied and the patient's wishes and beliefs are clear and constant, ADs will be respected, a doctor may nevertheless make simple errors—in both a positive and negative sense—as to the validity of the patient's decision.[141] It is one thing to say that 'doubt over the continuing validity of an advance directive must be resolved in favour of life unless clear and convincing evidence is offered to the contrary.'[142] However, this must be balanced against the principle enshrined in section 1 of the MCA 2005 that a patient is presumed to have capacity unless the contrary is established. Moreover, the doctor is in double jeopardy as to error. They are liable to an action in battery should they mistakenly conclude that the patient lacked capacity at the time an AD was initiated; by contrast, a failure to treat may be regarded as negligent should that failure be based on an unreasonably mistaken belief that a directive was valid. Michalowski has suggested that:

> A mistaken assumption that the patient was incompetent when making the advance directive and that his/her refusal was therefore not valid should accordingly only provide a defence in a battery action if the mistake was based on reasonable grounds.[143]

In a particularly useful analysis of the jurisprudence, Maclean has argued that:

> In deciding whether to accept a refusal of treatment, the courts will assess the patient's competence on the basis of the *outcome* of the decision that he or she has made.[144] [Emphasis added.]

---

[138] See also *A Local Authority v E (anorexia nervosa)* [2012] EWHC 1639 (COP), discussed in Chapter 10. Here the court held that an advance decision by an anorexic patient to prevent people feeding her was invalid on grounds of incapacity.

[139] [2014] EWCOP 1317.   [140] [2022] EWCOP 6.

[141] The importance of his or her assessment of the validity of the decision is apparent from the protective terms of s 26(2) and (3).

[142] *Re T (adult: refusal of treatment)* [1993] Fam 95, [112] (Lord Donaldson).

[143] Sabine Michalowski, 'Trial and Error at the End of Life: No Harm Done' (2007) 27(2) Oxford Journal of Legal Studies 257, 261.

[144] Alasdair Maclean, 'Advance Directives and the Rocky Waters of Anticipatory Decision-Making' (2008) 16(1) Medical Law Review 1, 6.

McLean goes on to suggest that, rather than protecting the patient's precedent autonomy, the MCA 2005 is open to criticism for the resulting 'vulnerability of advance directives' and that it (the Act) 'provides patients with a trump that only works when healthcare professionals and/or the courts are comfortable with the patient's decision'.[145] Case law might offer some support for this view. An important point that is made about practice, however, is that even if an AD is deemed to be invalid or inapplicable, 'healthcare professionals must consider the advance decision as part of their assessment of the person's best interests if they have reasonable grounds to think it is a true expression of the person's wishes'.[146]

However, some of this case law seems to suggest that expressions of autonomy carry no more weight than any other factor being weighed in the balance. In many ways this goes against the foundational tenets of the MCA 2005, which are to give effect to the self-determination of patients as far as is possible. There are also serious practical implications for patients and families if the courts are moving to a position where only a properly executed AD will carry any real weight. Many people will simply not be aware of the formal criteria and might make very clear advance statements in the belief that they will be respected.[147]

17.7 THE POSITION IN SCOTLAND

17.7.1 A DIFFERENT JURISDICTION

The outcome of a case similar to *Bland* was awaited with some interest in Scotland, accentuated in part by some very real jurisdictional variations between the two countries. The difficulty of deciding what were, essentially, criminal matters in a civil court was common to both jurisdictions. The House of Lords, while being unanimously wary on the point,[148] was quite prepared to accept a fait accompli: 'This appeal', said Lord Mustill, 'has reached this House, and your Lordships must decide it'. There was, however, no certainty that such pragmatism would be available to the Scottish courts. On the other hand, the English court in *Bland* was undoubtedly hampered by the absence of any residual powers of *parens patriae* and the issue was in some doubt in Scotland. This, then, was the uncertain position when Scotland's first PVS case came to the Inner House of the Court of Session by way of *Law Hospital NHS Trust v Lord Advocate*,[149] in which authority was sought by relatives of a middle-aged woman in PVS (Mrs Johnstone), and by the hospital treating her, to discontinue feeding.

The Inner House confirmed that it was not competent to issue a declarator to the effect that a proposed course of action was or was not criminal—it could, however,

---

[145] ibid. [22]. In fact, Maclean goes on to infer, albeit indirectly, that the Scottish Act, which accords only presumptive weight to advance decisions, is to be preferred to the English Act which attempts to impose legal imperative.

[146] Mental Capacity Act Code of Practice (2007), para 9.45. For commentary, see Mary Donnelly, 'Best Interests, Patient Participation and the Mental Capacity Act 2005' (2009) 17(1) Medical Law Review 1.

[147] Raanan Gillon, 'Editorial: Sanctity of Life Has Gone Too Far' (2012) 345 BMJ e4637; Rob Heywood, 'Revisiting Advance Decision Making Under the Mental Capacity Act 2005: A Tale of Mixed Messages?' (2015) 23(1) Medical Law Review 81.

[148] See [1993] 1 All ER 821, [864]–[865], [876], [880], [886]–[887] (per Lord Goff, Lord Lowry, Lord Browne-Wilkinson, and Lord Mustill, respectively).

[149] *Law Hospital NHS Trust v Lord Advocate* 1996 SLT 848, (1996) 39 BMLR 166. The case was reported by Lord Cameron from the Outer House to the Inner House without any preliminary judgment.

authorise a declaration in the knowledge that it would not bar proceedings in the High Court but in the hope that it would, in practice, ensure that no prosecution was undertaken there.[150]

17.7.2 *PARENS PATRIAE* MAY BE HERE NOT THERE

In contrast to the position in England, the Inner House suggested that the *parens patriae* jurisdiction survived in Scotland, though did not set out its scope, or whether it should be restricted to those falling within the definitions equivalent to those in the Adults with Incapacity (Scotland) Act 2000. Even so, the court jurisdiction in *Law Hospital* does not rely on the existence of *parens patriae*, nor indeed on the alternative *nobile officium* of the Court of Session. Through its exercise of that jurisdiction, the court finding in *Law Hospital* has the effect that any authority given by the court would have the same effect in law as if consent had been given by the patient. In deciding on the withdrawal of treatment, the court could act on its own initiative and would do so in the future.

The Inner House considered the numerous rulings that had been reached in several common law jurisdictions as to the correct test for exercising the power of consent or refusal of treatment on behalf of persons who lack capacity. It concluded that acting in the patient's best interests is the common denominator. It followed that if, as in Mrs Johnstone's case, treatment could be of no benefit, then there were no longer any best interests to be served.[151] Accordingly, the Lord Ordinary was authorised to provide a declarator to the effect that removal of life-sustaining treatment from Mrs Johnstone would not be unlawful in respect of its civil law consequences.[152]

17.7.3 SIMILARITIES WITH *RE Y*?

The Lord President also remarked that nothing in his opinion was intended to suggest that an application must be made in every case where it is intended to withdraw treatment:

> The decision as to whether an application is necessary must rest in each case with those who will be responsible for carrying that intention into effect, having regard in particular ... to any statements of policy which may, in the light of this case, be issued by the Lord Advocate.[153]

At this point we run into some difficulties following a statement by the Lord Advocate[154] to the effect that the policy of the Crown Office will be that no criminal prosecution will follow a decision to withdraw feeding, but that this is subject to authority to do so having first been obtained by way of the civil law. This appears to pre-empt the direction by the Inner House.

---

[150] 1996 SLT 848 [855] (Lord President Hope).

[151] 1996 SLT 848, [859]; (1996) 39 BMLR 166, [182]–[184] (Lord Hope).

[152] It is clear that such a complex manoeuvre will be unnecessary in the future when the Inner House will use its *parens patriae* powers, but it was convenient to use it in the instant case. See *Law Hospital NHS Trust v Lord Advocate (No 2)* 1996 SLT 869; (1996) 39 BMLR 166 [197].

[153] 1996 SLT 848, [860]; (1996) 39 BMLR 166 [184].

[154] John Robertson, 'Policy on Right to Die Welcomed' (The Scotsman, 1996) p 1. See the First Division decision in *Law Hospital NHS Trust v Lord Advocate* 1996 SLT 848 [860].

However, the Lord Advocate did not say he *would* prosecute in any case that was not so authorised. He went on to say, admittedly in an unofficial ambience:

> In Scotland, a decision to withdraw treatment in any case cannot be *guaranteed* immunity from [prosecution] unless the withdrawal has first been authorised by the Court of Session.[155] [Emphasis added.]

And yet the majority judgment of Lord Hope indicated that an application to the court is not necessary 'in every case'.[156] Both the Lord President and the Lord Advocate of the time agreed that decisions could be made on medical grounds and independently of the courts—but neither gave any guidance as to when it would be either necessary or unnecessary to seek judicial approval. The latter concluded in his paper: 'it is for doctors and relatives involved in such tragic situations to decide which course of action they wish to adopt'.[157]

We would hope and expect that good common sense would prevail, but also suggest that not many doctors will be prepared to trust to chance that they have 'got it right'. It is reasonable to expect the criminal law to set out the boundaries of impermissible conduct in advance. Vagueness in criminal law offends the widely recognised principle of legal certainty, which requires that crimes should be clearly defined. As such, the indefensible situation has now arisen where the doctor may be required to second-guess the criminal law. Retention of the *parens patriae* jurisdiction is also suggestive of an emergent 'gulf' between Scots and English law,[158] where the former seems still wedded to *Bland*.

This common law position remains unchanged after the passing of the Adults with Incapacity (Scotland) Act 2000. The Act allows for the appointment of a welfare guardian to act on behalf of the patient considered incapacitous,[159] but it is determinedly not concerned with any form of 'negative treatment'; that is, treatment which results in the death of the patient. Indeed, the then Scottish Executive made it very clear that withdrawal or withholding decisions are outside the remit of the legislation.[160] However, it has been argued[161] that it will be impossible to maintain a clear distinction between positive and negative treatment decisions involving incapable adults, not least because the courts will invariably become involved in settling disputes as to the best thing to do under the Act: to treat or not to treat? Although the powers of a proxy decision-maker under section 50 do not include a 'right' to refuse as such, their 'right' to a second opinion challenging a medical decision to continue intervention, and ultimately the 'right' to appeal to the court, will necessarily mean that a jurisprudence relating to negative treatment will develop around this legislation. Although there have been no further cases on which to test this hypothesis, it is worth noting that the 'medical treatment' referred to in that part of the Act 'includes any procedure or treatment designed to safeguard or promote physical or mental health',[162] which suggests that withdrawal leading to death may not fall within its scope.

---

[155] Lord Mackay of Drumadoon, 'Decision on the Persistent Vegetative State: *Law Hospital*' (1996), paper presented at the Symposium on Medical Ethics and Legal Medicine, Royal College of Physicians and Surgeons of Glasgow, 26 April 1996.

[156] *Law Hospital NHS Trust* v *Lord Advocate* 1996 SLT 848 [860].

[157] Lord Mackay of Drumadoon (n 155).

[158] On this point, see Jonathan Brown and Sarah Christie, 'Pater Knows Best: Withdrawal of Medical Treatment from Infants in Scotland' (2020) 40(4) Oxford Journal of Legal Studies 699.

[159] And replaced the office of tutor dative which was abolished by s 80.

[160] Scottish Executive Policy Memorandum, 8 October 1999.

[161] Graeme Laurie and John K Mason (n 98).

[162] Adults with Incapacity (Scotland) Act 2000, s 47(4).

17.8 TREATMENT WITHDRAWAL IN PVS: EUTHANASIA BY ANOTHER NAME?

An alternative, controversial approach to the problem of the management of PVS and other cases involving ANH/CANH is to admit that the deliberate removal of sustenance from a patient is indistinguishable from euthanasia, where death is a foreseeable consequence of an act under the guise of an omission. This has the advantage of removing much of what must be regarded as paralogical argument. It would also involve a complete change of direction in the current jurisprudence—a change on which the courts would be extremely reluctant to embark without the support of the legislature. Nonetheless, we should not shrink from considering the proposition.[163]

The 'slippery slope' fears of the judiciary and of many ethicists are summed up by Lord Goff in *Bland*, who declined to allow active steps to bring about death in PVS patients because this would be to authorise euthanasia and, 'once euthanasia is recognised as lawful in these circumstances, it is difficult to see any logical basis for excluding it in others'.[164] We question this view. If the concept of substituted judgement is accepted, removal of sustenance from PVS patients equates, at most, to passive, voluntary euthanasia. This is already practised widely under one name or another. PVS cases occupy a unique niche in the spectrum of euthanasia. All higher brain function has been permanently lost; there is no awareness and no sensation. There is no alternative of palliative care because there are no senses to palliate—as Lord Goff put it, 'there is no weighing operation to be performed'. This has now been confirmed by the Supreme Court in *Aintree*, as discussed. Only the vestiges of the person remain as the breathing body. Put another way, the patient is truly 'dead to the world' and, once their close relatives have come to terms with the situation, it is futile to maintain that respiration.

All this depends upon the certainty of definition and diagnosis. Anthony Bland's and Mrs Johnstone's conditions were unequivocal and the House of Lords distinguished *Bland* from other 'quality of life' cases such as *Re J*.[165] The two cases have very different ratios. In the former, a wholly insensate patient was deemed to have no interest in continued treatment, which could be discontinued as being futile. In the latter, it was accepted that some benefit could be derived from treatment of a patient who was not insensate, but it was held that non-treatment was to be preferred when any supposed benefit was weighed against other considerations such as pain and suffering. *S*,[166] *Re D*,[167] *Re H*,[168] *Re G*,[169] and *NHS Trust v X*[170] in particular, demonstrate a shift in thinking from that adopted in *Bland*, and towards that involved in *Re J*. One wonders if this is not something of a move towards acceptance of active euthanasia. The cases provide the most impressive example to date of the willingness of the British courts to take 'quality of life' decisions and, in our view, represent a significant step in this area of law. The MCS cases reaffirm the fundamental importance of the sanctity of life and the role of the balance sheet approach. Equally, we have *W Healthcare NHS Trust v KH*,[171] where the Court of Appeal placed considerable weight on the impact of the dying process on the sentient patient: only intolerability of living would justify a course of action that would hasten death.

---

[163] Kristin Savell, 'A Jurisprudence of Ambivalence: Three Legal Fictions Concerning Death and Dying' (2011) 17(1) Cultural Studies Review 52.

[164] [1993] 1 All ER 821 [867].   [165] [1990] 3 All ER 930.

[166] *Swindon and Marlborough NHS Trust v S* [1995] 3 Med LR 84.   [167] (1997) 38 BMLR 1.

[168] (1997) 38 BMLR 11.   [169] (2001) 65 BMLR 6.   [170] [2006] Lloyd's Rep Med 29.

[171] [2004] EWCA Civ 1324.

In the end, all the cases discussed under the umbrella concept of PDOC represent variations on what is meant by 'best interests'. Our next question is whether the jump from 'no interests' to 'a balance of interests' is acceptable in the management of PDOC, or whether it represents a quantum leap onto the slippery slope of ending 'valueless lives'.

A particularly interesting variation is to be found in *An NHS Trust* v *J*,[172] which we have mentioned. The judicial decision was founded largely on the ground that the treatment option proposed could do J no harm. It has been suggested that in this case the 'best interests' test was converted to a 'not against the interests' test.[173] And yet the recent decisions by the Supreme Court in *Aintree* and *Re Y* firmly cemented the role of best interests as the central consideration at common law, human rights law, and under statute. This centres our attention on the presumption in favour of life and the idea that 'benefit' is an eternally context-specific notion to be assessed only from the patient's perspective.

We must keep in mind that all the post-*Bland* cases have been scrupulously examined and all were supported not only by respected medical opinion but also by the Official Solicitor. All the patients were existing in appalling conditions and we doubt that the failure of a single arbitrary clinical test should be allowed to distinguish them in any significant way. It is at least arguable that the near-vegetative state is a more horrifying condition than is PVS itself.[174] We have long held that the approach adopted by the courts in the seminal case of *Re J*[175] could properly be applied to the withdrawal of vital treatment from severely damaged adult patients. *Re J* and its allied cases went a long way to medicalising the whole approach to termination of treatment decisions, subject to the sensitive handling of close relatives.

As has now been affirmed by the Supreme Court in *Re Y*, the courts should be involved only in those cases in which there is dispute between or within the healthcare and family groups. Public acceptance of this approach will be greatly eased by an open acceptance by the medical profession of the futility of treatment of patients. This was the position advocated by the BMA in respect of patients with severe dementia or who have suffered catastrophic stroke,[176] and it has now been affirmed by the Supreme Court in *Re Y*.

Inevitably, one is reminded of the calls in the House of Lords and the Court of Session for parliamentary intervention. While this has its attractions, the proposal is not of unquestionable merit. To legislate for PVS alone would be to concentrate on its particular clinical status and to segregate it from the general euthanasia debate—which is as it should be.[177] Other advantages of legislation could be that the limits of PVS were statutorily determined[178] and that a clear framework could be devised within which doctors withdrawing treatment could be seen to be acting lawfully without the need for routine court approval. A line could therefore be drawn between unequivocal and doubtful cases and a barrier placed at the edge of any developing slippery slope.

On the other hand, legislation of this type could be seen as disadvantageous in being unduly restrictive. While withdrawal of support from the *Bland*-type patient would be permissible, non-treatment options might be barred in many cases of brain damage in which only minimal cognitive function remained. To many, this would represent the primary function of the legislation; to others, it might seem an unacceptable price to pay for

---

[172] [2006] EWHC 3152 (Fam).

[173] Penney Lewis, 'Withdrawal of Treatment From a Patient in a Permanent Vegetative State: Judicial Involvement and Innovative "Treatment"' (2007) 15(3) Medical Law Review 392.

[174] Ronald Cranford, 'Misdiagnosing the Persistent Vegetative State' (1996) 313 BMJ 5.

[175] *Re J (a minor) (wardship: medical treatment)* [1990] 3 All ER 930.   [176] BMA (n 41).

[177] John K Mason and Deirdre Mulligan, 'Euthanasia by Stages' (1996) 347(9004) The Lancet 810.

[178] Perhaps based on the guidelines of the Royal College of Physicians (n 25) and (n 27).

the loss of individual judgement. As we have already suggested, generalisations are difficult to apply in a medical context. It might, therefore, be thought preferable to introduce purely enabling legislation or to amend the provisions of the MCA 2005 now that the Supreme Court has considered its terms in the context of futile treatment. The same could apply analogically with the Adults with Incapacity (Scotland) Act 2000, which has had a stalled consultation process since 2018.[179]

The argument is one of long standing and is likely to continue. In the interim, we suggest that there is one step we could take towards recognising an equivalence of treatment withdrawal and euthanasia, without giving offence. In their anxiety to avoid conflating the final management of PVS with euthanasia, the courts in England and Wales, Scotland, and the Republic of Ireland have been at pains to emphasise that the cause of death in PVS cases is the original injury.[180] While it is true to say that this was the ultimate and proximate cause of death, given that the patient has survived for a minimum of a year, death must be the result of starvation—otherwise, there would be no death, and no cause of death. There would be no difficulty in certifying death as being due to:

(i)   inanition due to lawful removal of life support, due to

(ii)   severe brain damage, due to

(iii) cerebral hypoxia.

This concession to transparency would, we feel, actually help to defuse the emotionalism that surrounds the ultimate management of PVS and other patients with PDOC. It would also ensure that the mortality statistics are correctly maintained correctly, including the incidence statistics for such decisions.

17.9 CONCLUSION

This chapter has charted the changing role of the concept of futility from absolute medical benchmark through to its deployment in a range of tragic and complex legal cases. We have not only identified the importance of challenging any assumptions about what references to futility might mean but also witnessed the myriad ways in which the concept has found appeal. We have also seen parallel developments in the jurisprudence, involving an increasingly strong message that the deployment of best interests must be on a case-by-case basis, while at the same time we have observed the courts bringing diverse groups of cases into line under this rubric. A common message for medics, ethicists, and lawyers alike is that the loose use of 'futility' is no longer defensible. Law, ethics, and medical practice are increasingly aligned on the need for robust and careful reflection on what futility actually means in any given context and for each particular patient—a position that has been strengthened following confirmation that the court need not always be approached for its view on the matter.

---

[179] Scottish Government, 'Adults with Incapacity Reform' (2018) available at <https://consult.gov.scot/health-and-social-care/adults-with-incapacity-reform/> accessed 25 October 2022.

[180] Franklin Miller, Robert Truog, and Dan Brock, 'Moral Fictions and Medical Ethics' (2010) 24(9) Bioethics 453, argue that the distinction between euthanasia and withdrawal of treatment is based upon legal fictions motivated by moral reasons to uphold the view that physicians do not/should not bring about their patient's death.

FURTHER READING

1. Hazel Biggs, 'Taking Account of the Views of the Patient, but Only if the Clinician (and the Court) Agrees—*R (Burke)* v *General Medical Council*' (2007) 19(2) Child and Family Law Quarterly 225–238.

2. Daniel Wei Liang Wang, 'Withdrawing Treatment From Patients with Prolonged Disorders of Consciousness: The Wrong Answer is What The Wrong Question Begets' (2020) 46(8) Journal of Medical Ethics 561–562, and response by Charles Foster, 'Withdrawing Treatment from Patients with Prolonged Disorders of Consciousness: the Presumption in Favour of the Maintenance of Life is Legally Robust' (2021) 47(2) Journal of Medical Ethics 119–120.

3. Richard Huxtable, 'Dying Too Soon or Living Too Long? Withdrawing Treatment from Patients with Prolonged Disorders of Consciousness after *Re Y*' (2019) 20 BMC Medical Ethics 91 (1–11).

4. Kristin Savell, 'A Jurisprudence of Ambivalence: Three Legal Fictions Concerning Death and Dying' (2011) 17(1) Cultural Studies Review 52–80.

5. Ian Wise, 'Withdrawal and Withholding of Medical Treatment for Patients Lacking Capacity who are in Critical Condition—Reflections on the Judgment of the Supreme Court in *Aintree University Hospitals NHS Foundation Trust v James*' (2014) 82(4) The Medico-Legal Journal 144–154.

18

EUTHANASIA AND ASSISTED SUICIDE

18.1 INTRODUCTION

Assisted death and euthanasia remain among the most hotly debated topics in medico-legal practice and scholarship, driven in large part by constant judicial and legislative activity. They also give rise to a confusion of definition, and a pattern has developed that admits two distinct forms. The *Oxford English Dictionary* definition is: 'a gentle and easy death, the bringing about of this action or omission which uses "assisted dying" as a means of relief from suffering, could be a form of euthanasia'. The *Concise OED*, however, offers: 'the painless killing of a patient suffering from an incurable disease or in an irreversible coma'.[1] Introducing the dual concepts of intention and activity clearly restricts the definition to correspond to 'mercy killing'. There are alternative specific descriptive terms for all other forms of 'assisted dying'. Though widely used and therefore relevant,[2] we believe that generalisations such as 'passive euthanasia' are contradictions in terms, which confuse the issue and are better avoided.

In this chapter, we discuss the subject only in relation to the adult patient, because unlike the infant, the adult may be able to express their wishes on the quality of their own life. Those responsible for their management will have a background of previous abilities and aspirations from which to measure the extent of any shortfall.

Antipathy to the premature termination of life can be based on fundamental and deeply held convictions which have a variety of roots, most particularly religious ones.[3] This sanctity is reflected in the human rights debate, where the right to life is embodied in Article 2 of the European Convention on Human Rights (ECHR): 'everyone's right to life shall be protected by law'. The European courts' interpretation has been that this does *not* include a right to death at one's choosing.[4] There is a strong public interest in protecting the interests of the vulnerable,[5] of whom those suffering

---

[1] The use of the word 'patient' does not limit the actor to the subject's medical attendant.

[2] For a reflection on different sides of the debate, see Emily Jackson and John Keown, *Debating Euthanasia* (OUP 2011). For a view on the scope of doctor's rights, see Julian Savulescu and Udo Schuklenk, 'Doctors Have No Right to Refuse Medical Assistance in Dying, Abortion or Contraception' (2017) 31(3) Bioethics 162. On the ethical arguments see Craig Paterson, *Assisted Suicide and Euthanasia: A Natural Law Ethics Approach* (Routledge 2017).

[3] Andriy Danyliv and Clayton O'Neill, 'Attitudes Towards Legalising Physician Provided Euthanasia in Britain: The Role of Religion Over Time' (2015) 128 Social Science and Medicine 52.

[4] See *Pretty* v *UK* (2002) 35 EHRR 1, [40].

[5] Now recognised in the Safeguarding Vulnerable Groups Act 2006. For a discussion of the developing notion of the 'vulnerable' autonomous person at common law, see Graeme Laurie and John K Mason, 'Trust or Contract: How Far Does the Contemporary Doctor–Patient Relationship Protect and Promote Autonomy?' in Pamela Ferguson and Graeme Laurie (eds.), *Inspiring a Medico-Legal Revolution: Essays in Honour of Sheila McLean* (Ashgate Publishing 2015).

from extreme disability or intense pain form a quintessential group. A growing number of jurisdictions allow for lawful assistance to achieve their own suicide. They do so on essentially constitutional grounds—that criminal prohibitions run contrary to an embedded human rights charter.

18.2 A CLASSIFICATION OF ASSISTED DYING

Here we will use the term 'assisted dying' deliberately to emphasise that we regard euthanasia as a far narrower concept than is often implied in the use of the term, despite common usage including all forms of assisted dying under that umbrella. 'Euthanasia' can be considered from the patient's point of view and divided into voluntary, non-voluntary, and involuntary categories, depending on whether the patient seeks death, is unable to express an opinion, or is ignored in the decision-making process. Alternatively, one can consider whether the actor who helps to bring about death takes an active or passive role, or whether death is brought about by act or through omission. The term 'active voluntary euthanasia', therefore, identifies a doctor who is 'active' in the process and a patient who is compliant in the act. Even so, we still need to add the nuances embedded in the patient's position: they may or may not have capacity,[6] with or without prior expressed wishes; they may be terminally or incurably but non-fatally ill. In the same way, the actor may be involved at any point from counselling to perpetration. We have attempted to illustrate this mosaic in **Figure 18.1**, which is structured on the degree of cooperation by the patient.[7]

18.3 HEALTH CARERS AS A DISTINCT GROUP

To act with the *intention* of ending a person's life in the absence of either a personal or proxy consent to do so ought, prima facie, to attract the attention of the criminal law. Motive, however, is irrelevant in the criminal jurisdictions of the UK, and the English Court of Appeal[8] and the Supreme Court[9] have made it clear that 'mercy killing' remains murder. Because this book is concerned with *medical* law and ethics,[10] we confine ourselves to assisted death in the context of the doctor–patient relationship. Health carers are conceptually isolated because while prosecutory compassion towards the caring relative may be justified as legal pragmatism, a professional relationship forecloses an emotional bond. It also both opens up the whole field of what constitutes good medical practice, and reintroduces us to the concept of the 'slippery slope' that we considered in the previous chapter—that is, acceptance of an exception to the moral norm will inevitably

---

[6] On the interface between suicide, mental disorder, and best interests, see Genevra Richardson, 'Mental Capacity in the Shadow of Suicide: What Can the Law Do?' (2013) 9(1) International Journal of Law in Context 87.

[7] A basic problem with our plan is that it is cylindrical, yet difficult to illustrate on the page—i.e. decisions as to discontinuance of medical support can be made in respect of patients both having and lacking capacity.

[8] *R v Inglis* [2011] 1 WLR 1110 [50] (Judge CJ): 'A belief that he or she was acting out of mercy . . . does not and cannot constitute any defence to the charge of murder'. For critical commentary, see David Thomas and Andrew Ashworth, 'Sentencing: Murder—Mercy Killing' (2011) 3 Criminal Law Review 243.

[9] *Nicklinson* v *Ministry of Justice* [2014] UKSC 38, [17].

[10] Though an interesting article questions whether end of life decisions are properly located in medical law: John Coggon, 'Assisted Dying and the Context of Debate: "Medical Law" v "End-of-Life Law"' (2010) 18(4) Medical Law Review 541.

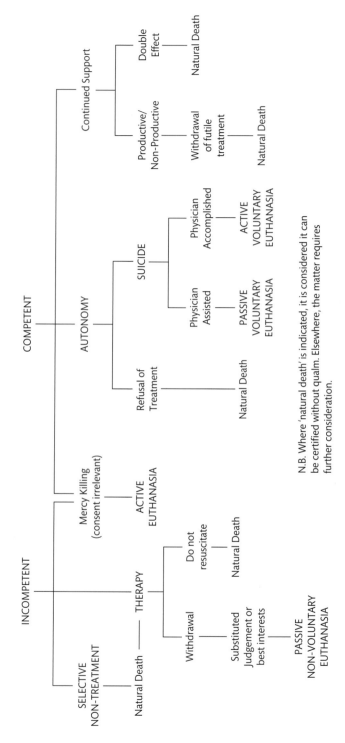

Figure 18.1 Ending life—a suggested outline

lead to further erosion of the modified norm. There is thus an incremental continuum between the typical cases of Dr Moor, who treated his dying patient by way of an easeful death; Dr Adams, who extended this to a number of elderly patients who were in pain but not dying; and Dr Shipman, who included perhaps hundreds of such patients. This potential movement pervades the whole topic of assistance in dying.

Criminal cases are rarely reported unless they demonstrate some specific point of law. It remains surprising how few relevant trials of doctors[11] there have been, despite many having claimed to have taken part in some form of premature termination of life, and a significant minority being prepared to do so.[12] The majority have been accused of no more than using therapeutic drugs in overdose. All the relevant verdicts have indicated the reluctance of British juries to convict a medical practitioner of a serious crime when the charge arises from what they see as the doctor's considered medical judgement.

As a GP, Dr Moor had admitted in the course of a public debate to having used painkillers to bring about the easy deaths of patients. He was charged with the murder of a terminally ill patient, having injected him with a lethal dose of diamorphine. The judge left the jury in no doubt as to his own view of the matter, by referring to Dr Moor's 'excellent character', and considering it an irony that, 'a doctor who goes out of his way to care for [the deceased] ends up facing the charge that he does.'[13] The jury acquitted Dr Moor within an hour.

Dr Adams' seminal case[14] was different because the patient was among several who were incurably but not terminally ill. It is thought that he treated her with increasing doses of opiates. Following her death, he was tried and acquitted of her murder. In summing up, Devlin J said: 'The doctor is entitled to relieve pain and suffering even if the measures he takes may incidentally shorten life.' This clear direction left the jury in little doubt, where 'incidental' obviously meant 'non-intentional'. It is also an early example of the invocation of the ethical doctrine of double effect, which we discussed in the previous chapter.

Involuntary euthanasia performed by a doctor leaves them as guilty of unlawful killing as anyone else who deliberately takes human life. Dr Shipman was convicted in 2000 of murdering 15 patients—a serial killing which cast a long shadow over the UK medical profession.[15] The distinction from other doctors, who have risked prosecution to end what they see as the unbearable suffering of terminally ill patients, is that he killed patients for reasons which may have been connected with a pathological desire to exercise control over life and death. The case has been widely used as an argument against lifting the current strict prohibitions on the taking of life.[16] It also led to legislation designed to ensure that the death certification process is robust.[17]

---

[11] We are being deliberately selective here. Other healthcare professionals, such as care home nurses, may be much more akin to close relatives.

[12] See e.g. Christopher Zinn, 'A Third of Surgeons in New South Wales Admit to Euthanasia' (2001) 323 BMJ 1268, and more recently Julia Zenz, Michael Tryba, and Michael Zenz, 'Palliative Care Professionals' Willingness to Perform Euthanasia or Physician Assisted Suicide' (2015) 60 BMC Palliative Care 14. These instances are becoming less frequent as assisted suicide is legalised from one jurisdiction to another.

[13] Clare Dyer, 'British GP Cleared of Murder Charge' (1999) 318 BMJ 1306. For discussion, see Robert Gillon, 'When Doctors Might Kill Their Patients' (1999) 318 BMJ 1431.

[14] Unreported, see Henry Palmer, 'Dr Adams' Trial for Murder' [1957] Criminal Law Review 365.

[15] The final number of patients killed may never be known. The Inquiry, however, was exceptionally far ranging and resulted in six reports between 2002 and 2005. See Dame J Smith, *Shipman: The Final Report* (2005) available at <https://www.gov.uk/government/organisations/shipman-inquiry> accessed 03 November 2022.

[16] Herbert Kinnell, 'Serial Homicide by Doctors: Shipman in Perspective' (2000) 321 BMJ 1594. Note that that Lady Smith did not consider that proposed safeguards went far enough (see n 15): Clare Dyer, 'Reform of Death Certificate System Doesn't Go Far Enough, Says Judge' (2009) 338 BMJ 435.

[17] Certification of Death (Scotland) Act 2011 ASP 11; Health and Care Act 2022, c 31, s 169.

The critical distinction to be derived from this series of cases lies in whether it is possible to 'medicalise' the deaths. At one end, we have dying patients undergoing treatment for serious pain, which calls for relief. The courts have been consistently prepared to apply the doctrine of necessity in such circumstances.[18] Dr Shipman's patients, however, were in no more discomfort than that which merited a visit to the doctor's surgery, so it was impossible to medicalise their deaths through an opiate overdose. The jury had no difficulty regarding the case as one of multiple murder.

18.4 NON-VOLUNTARY TERMINATION OF LIFE

A person considered to lack capacity by virtue either of status or of disability is still a creature in being, and the same criminal law applies in their respect. A patient found to lack capacity who is considered a candidate for an easeful death will almost certainly be under medical care. Given their increasing ability to maintain life in adverse conditions, doctors will be forced into considering death as a desirable therapeutic option. It was, however, repeatedly stressed by the courts that *Bland*[19] was not concerned with euthanasia. Here we revisit that scenario from the proposition that death is in the patient's best interests and so can be pursued as good medical practice.

Bland forcibly reminds us that it is unlawful to kill a person through a positive action, regardless of one's intentions; termination of the life of a patient lacking capacity can be lawful only if it is both achieved by a failure to act and can be justified on a 'best interests' basis. What one regards as euthanasia and as medical care of the dying depends on whether one is speaking in legal, moral, or medical terms. It is also a function of personal preference or prejudice. In this respect, if death can be certified as being due to natural causes, it is not euthanasia. Even so, treatment can be withdrawn, or not undertaken, either because it is non-productive or because its continuance results in an unacceptable quality of life.[20]

That treatment would be non-productive is a matter of *medical* futility, as discussed in Chapter 17, and *Bland* remains a very particular case which cannot be extrapolated without good reason. Clearly the same principles will apply when the patient's quality of life is so poor that they are positively *disadvantaged* by its preservation.[21] In either case, we are in the realm of what is, in our view unhelpfully, often referred to as passive non-voluntary euthanasia.

In our view, 'pure' passive euthanasia should be limited as a term to those relatively rare management decisions involving non-voluntary patients who have retained some cortical activity but are unable to make competent decisions, and who are also not known to have previously expressed an unequivocal preference as to treatment in the prevailing conditions. In *Aintree University Hospitals NHS Foundation Trust* v *James and Others*[22] the Supreme Court considered the principles and difficulties encountered in the management

---

[18] Although Dr Adams' case was by no means clear-cut, Lord Devlin later voiced serious doubts as to the result: Patrick Devlin, *Easing the Passing: The Trial of Dr Bodkin Adams* (The Bodley Head 1985).

[19] *Airedale NHS Trust* v *Bland* [1993] 1 All ER 821 (HL), confirmed by the Supreme Court in *Nicklinson* (n 9) [18], [22]–[26].

[20] For a critical examination of the problems of classification of assisted death, see Andrew McGee, 'Ending the Life of the Act/Omission Dispute: Causation in Withholding and Withdrawing Life-Sustaining Measures' (2011) 31(3) Legal Studies 467.

[21] It is to be noted that a failure to provide treatment in the patient's best interests does not contravene the ECHR: *An NHS Trust* v *D* (2000) 55 BMLR 19; *NHS Trust A* v *M, NHS Trust B* v *H* [2001] Fam 348.

[22] [2013] UKSC 67.

of such cases after the Mental Capacity Act 2005.[23] The importance of preserving life was regarded as the defining premise for the management of such patients. The legal question is not whether it would be lawful to withhold treatment, but whether it would be in the patient's best interests to provide it. If it is not, then it is a priori lawful. The 'balance sheet' approach to the assessment of best interests[24] is now integral to UK jurisprudence; it forms the basis for reference to 'passive non-voluntary euthanasia'.

18.4.1 NON-TREATMENT AT THE END OF LIFE

There is a general consensus of legal and medical opinion that the doctor need not resort to heroic methods to prolong the life—or the dying—of their patient. Here, we contrast medically productive and non-productive treatments, in asking whether a particular treatment is doing the *condition* any good. Factors such as the physical and psychological pain involved in treatment, its claim on scarce resources, and the general prospects for the patient and their family may all be taken into account.[25] Non-productivity and medical futility have much in common as treatment standards, with similar arguments for and against their adoption. Along with disconnecting ventilation, or withdrawing artificial nutrition and hydration, these issues were considered in greater detail in the previous chapter under the discussion of withholding and withdrawing medical treatment.

18.5 PATIENTS WITH CAPACITY

18.5.1 ACTIVITY AND PASSIVITY IN ASSISTED DYING

Those concerned to legalise the termination of life on medical grounds have tended to concentrate on what was historically known as voluntary euthanasia. This implies both that the patient has capacity and that they specifically request that their life be ended. This is an expression of patient autonomy—a seminal proposition to which we will return later. Within this framework, a patient's wishes may be effected either actively or passively. This distinction—or whether there is, indeed, any true distinction—is one of the most hotly contested issues in the assisted dying debate, and one which can be addressed on either legal or moral grounds.

As to the latter, criticism of what is generally known as the act/omission distinction we considered in the previous chapter, has been intense and sustained for decades. Numerous philosophical commentators[26]—and occasionally judges[27]—have expressed disquiet over the drawing of a sharp distinction between act and omission for the purposes of attributing liability for the consequences. One reason for arguing against the distinction is that it tolerates inconsistency and may merge into moral cowardice. On this view, a doctor who

---

[23] An apposite example prior to the enactment of the Mental Capacity Act 2005 lies in *W Healthcare NHS Trust* v *H*, discussed in Chapter 17.

[24] See *An NHS Trust* v *MB* [2006] 2 FLR 319 and discussion of benefits and burdens in *Aintree*, (n 22).

[25] Considerations of cost and of the distribution of other resources cannot be ignored here, although they must be secondary to the well-being and the dignity of the patient. At least two speeches in *Bland* confirmed that resources might be a legitimate concern of the clinician: [1993] 1 All ER 821 at 879, 893 [140] (Lord Browne-Wilkinson and Lord Mustill).

[26] For a wide-ranging analysis, see Len Doyal, 'The Futility of Opposing the Legalisation of Non-Voluntary and Voluntary Euthanasia' in Sheila McLean (ed.), *First Do No Harm* (Routledge 2006).

[27] See e.g. Lord Mustill in *Bland* (n 19).

knows that their failure to treat will result in death should accept the same responsibility for that death as if they had brought it about through a positive act.[28] In spite of this, there remain grounds for making this distinction in relation to assistance in dying to alleviate suffering, even if its validity is rightly doubted in other fields. But how, then, can this be justified?

One response is to say that the distinction reflects a widely held moral intuition which, even if it involves inconsistency, allows for the practical conduct of day-to-day moral life. Morality, like the law, needs to be rooted in daily experience. Doctors who observe a DNAR order are entitled to the comfort of thinking they are not actually killing the patient. A sophisticated morality will recognise such ordinary human needs. As one commentator put it at the height of the debate: 'Our gut intuition tells us that there is a difference between active and passive euthanasia and we are not going to be browbeaten into changing our minds by mere logic'[29]—and it is not beyond the capacity of moral philosophy to support this: 'We cannot capture our moral judgments by appeal to argument alone . . . in the area of dying; intuitions and conceptions formed by actual experience must be given weight.'[30] A second possible response would be a consequentialist one. The act/omission distinction plays an important role in the preservation of a near-absolute prohibition of killing. The weakening of this prohibition could have the effect of blunting the respect which we accord to human life. The combination of these two approaches is sufficient to tip the scales in favour of retaining the distinction.[31]

The legal position is, at least in one sense, clear. We can return to *Bland*, per Lord Mustill:[32]

> The English criminal law . . . draws a sharp distinction between acts and omissions. If an act resulting in death is done without lawful excuse and with intent to kill it is murder. But an omission to act with the same result and with the same intent is in general no offence at all.

So far, so good, but Lord Mustill rightly went on to say:[33]

> There is one important general exception at common law, namely that a person may be criminally liable for the consequences of an omission if he stands in such a relation to the victim that he is under a duty to act.

The illogicality of this distinction has more recently been acknowledged by the Supreme Court, which at the same time offered a pragmatic justification:

> While Lord Goff, Lord Browne-Wilkinson and Lord Mustill were all concerned about the artificiality of such a sharp legal distinction between acts and omissions in this context, they also saw the need for a line to be drawn, and the need for the law in this sensitive area to be clear.[34]

---

[28] Strongly argued by Emily Jackson, 'Whose Death is it Anyway? Euthanasia and the Medical Profession' (2004) 57(1) Current Legal Problems 414.

[29] Thurstan Brewin, 'Voluntary Euthanasia' (1986) 1(8489) Lancet 1085. See also Daniel Sulmany, 'Killing and Allowing to Die: Another Look' (1998) 26(1) Journal of Law, Medicine & Ethics 55.

[30] Grant Gillett, 'Euthanasia, Letting Die and the Pause' (1988) 14(2) Journal of Medical Ethics 61. This attitude was challenged by Malcolm Parker, 'Moral Intuition, Good Deaths and Ordinary Medical Practitioners' (1990) 16(1) Journal of Medical Ethics 28.

[31] The contrary argument has been put succinctly in an editorial by Len Doyal and Lesley Doyal, 'Why Active Euthanasia and Physician Assisted Suicide Should be Legalised' (2001) 323 BMJ 1079.

[32] *Bland* (n 19) [890].   [33] ibid.   [34] *Nicklinson*, (n 9) [18], quoting their Lordships in *Bland*.

This clarity extends also to the doctor who fails to provide, or who withdraws, treatment from a patient under their care: they cannot hide behind the general cover that there is no legal duty to rescue in the jurisprudence of the UK. There must be a justifiable reason for inaction and there is no doubt that, in the case of the patient with capacity, this is determined—or dictated—by the patient's autonomy, however this is expressed. This raises the collateral problems of distinguishing refusal of treatment from suicide and, more importantly in the present context, between suicide and physician-assisted death.

18.6 DYING AS AN EXPRESSION OF PATIENT AUTONOMY

18.6.1 REFUSAL OF TREATMENT

We have discussed refusal of treatment already under the heading of 'consent'. Here, we need only point out the obvious: consent to, or refusal of, treatment is a matter for the patient alone and this holds true even in life or death situations. The doctor is now bound, both legally and professionally, to accept a refusal—provided, of course, that it is competently expressed. Indeed, the General Medical Council (GMC) recognises the advance refusal as legally binding.[35] The rationale for this is to be found in *Re T*, where Lord Donaldson stated:

> This appeal is not in truth about 'the right to die'. There is no suggestion that Miss T wants to die . . . This appeal is about the 'right to choose how to live'. This is quite different, even if the choice, when made, may make an early death more likely.[36]

Medical jurisprudence would do well to reflect on the extensive moral steps which are being taken when it accepts the cult of self-determination as its dominant principle.[37] Nonetheless, that caveat being admitted, respect for personal autonomy is now firmly established in the modern community ethos and is reflected legally in the offence of battery—the concept of (informed) refusal has now achieved the same standing as that of (informed) consent,[38] supported by common law,[39] and shored up by human rights.[40] The conflict between personal autonomy and the public interest in protecting vulnerable groups has been well illustrated, for example, in the cases of Mrs Pretty[41] and Mr Nicklinson. At the same time,

---

[35] GMC, 'Treatment and Care Towards the End of Life: Good Practice in Decision Making' (2022) para 68 available at <https://www.gmc-uk.org/ethical-guidance/ethical-guidance-for-doctors/treatment-and-care-towards-the-end-of-life> accessed 03 November 2022.

[36] *Re T (adult: refusal of medical treatment)* [1992] 4 All ER 649 (CA) [652]; see Mental Capacity Act 2005 and associated Code of Practice (2016).

[37] For a searching analysis, see Onora O'Neill, *Autonomy and Trust in Bioethics* (CUP 2002). On the rise of autonomy in the UK, see Graeme Laurie, 'The Autonomy of Others: Reflections on the Rise and Rise of Patient Choice in Contemporary Medical Law' in Sheila McLean (ed.), *First Do No Harm: Law, Ethics and Healthcare* (Routledge 2006).

[38] So argued by Elizabeth Wicks, 'The Right to Refuse Medical Treatment Under the European Convention on Human Rights' (2001) 9(1) Medical Law Review 17.

[39] *St George's Healthcare NHS Trust v S, R v Collins, ex parte S* [1998] 3 All ER 673 is a strong authority in the UK, although the case of *Ms B* is the most important in the present context.

[40] Schedule 1 to the Human Rights Act 1998. For a positive judicial statement, see *Pretty v United Kingdom* (2002) 66 BMLR 147 [63].

[41] For an easy appreciation of the varied views on the application of Art 8 to assisted dying, see the Court of Appeal in *R (Purdy) v DPP* [2009] EWCA 92 [32]–[46].

the principles involved, and the complex association between refusal of treatment and suicide, are perfectly illustrated in the case of *Ms B*.[42]

Ms B was suffering from progressive paralysis, was maintained by the use of a ventilator, had already effected an advance directive, and had repeatedly asked that she be disconnected from her machine. The clinicians refused, so she sought a declaration that the treatment she was being given was an unlawful trespass. Butler-Sloss LJ made it clear that the court was concerned solely with the patient's legal capacity to accept or refuse treatment, and she emphasised the importance of a competent patient's free choice by imposing nominal damages of £100 against the hospital for their unlawful trespass. And yet the frank admission by the responsible doctors that they could not bring themselves to take the step of withdrawing ventilation from a viable patient is a striking and significant aspect of the case. In the event, another hospital was found that was willing to do so.[43] Even so, there is now such a mass of legal and professional medical precedent that ensures refusal of treatment is compatible with the law. This case shows how difficult it can be to distinguish refusal of treatment from suicide or, more significantly, from assisted death.

The Advance Directive

Refusal of treatment is ongoing until it is rescinded,[44] and the situation can be seen as being even less straightforward when a patient seeks to refuse in advance and to prescribe the manner of their death in circumstances that are as yet unforeseen, let alone realised. We are then into the field of the advance directive, the essential feature of which being that it should have been expressed while competent. The status of the advance directive, or decision,[45] is rightly discussed at this point under the umbrella heading of the capable patient. In theory, the principle of the advance directive is simple, and is now enshrined in statute[46]—the individual executes a document expressing their wishes as to treatment of a specific condition in the event of being disabled from doing so if the condition arises in the future; the physician acts upon it when the occasion arises. While advance directives commonly express a refusal of treatment, they may express the wish that life-prolonging measures be maintained—though they cannot, of course, *require* that such treatment be given.[47] Looked at in this way, the advance directive becomes an aspect of the right to choose rather than the right to die. Nevertheless, it is only *refusal* that has binding legal significance and this note is confined to that aspect.

While the theory may be simple, practice has its complications which give rise to criticism. Aside from the alarming specificity required,[48] perhaps the main concern lies

---

[42] *Ms B v An NHS Hospital Trust* [2002] 2 All ER 449. A very similar case had been heard before but had received little attention: *Re AK (adult patient) (medical treatment: consent)* [2001] 1 FLR 129.

[43] Ms B died some four weeks later.

[44] Moreover, a refusal can take the form of a declaration of intention never to consent in the future: *Re C (adult: refusal of medical treatment)* [1994] 1 All ER 819. However, Munby J has held that any condition purporting to make an advance directive irrevocable is contrary to public policy and void: *HE v A Hospital NHS Trust* [2003] 2 FLR 408.

[45] Increasingly referred to as advance decisions—including within the Mental Capacity Act 2005. We believe 'directive' to be more descriptively accurate, but the two terms should be regarded as interchangeable.

[46] MCA 2005, ss 25–27. For an assessment of the implementation of these provisions, see Rob Heywood, 'Revisiting Advance Decision Making Under the Mental Capacity Act 2005: A Tale of Mixed Messages' (2015) 23(1) Medical Law Review 81.

[47] *R (Burke) v General Medical Council* (2005) 85 BMLR 1 (CA).

[48] On this point and the resulting case law, see Caroyln Johnston, 'Advance Decision Making – Rhetoric or Reality?' (2014) 34(3) Legal Studies 497; including *X Primary Care Trust v XB* [2012] EWHC 1390 (Fam), on whether an advance directive was intended to be time limited.

in the fact that it is extremely difficult to devise an intelligible document which will be unambiguous in all circumstances; who, for example, is to define words such as 'severe', 'advanced', or 'comparable gravity'? For example, in *Sheffield Teaching Hospitals NHS Foundation Trust* v *TH*,[49] the evidence did not support an argument that a valid advance decision was in place. Instead, the court took a holistic view of the patient's best interests, taking into account the repeated and strong wishes of the patient to refuse treatment. The result was a declaration that ongoing treatment should not occur save in the case of anti- biotic treatment of minor infections to maintain the patient's comfort. Importantly, the court made it clear that 'wishes' and 'best interests' are not to be conflated.

The Mental Capacity Act 2005 lays down conditions which do not make the drafting of the directive any easier; it will not have effect if:

a) the treatment in question is not the treatment specified in the advance decision;

b) any circumstances specified in the advance decision are absent; or

c) there are reasonable grounds for believing that circumstances exist which the per- son did not anticipate at the time of his advance decision and which would have affected his advance decision had he anticipated them.[50]

The decision must be recorded in writing, and witnessed, if it involves refusal of life- sustaining treatment.[51]

There is a worrying trend that failure to comply with these provisions can under- mine the role of the patient's prior wishes in end-of-life decisions, whereby the courts are increasingly relying on sanctity of life as the benchmark from which it is all the more difficult to depart. Equally importantly, there is likely to be persistent concern that the patient has, during the critical phase, changed their mind; Dworkin points out that the person who drafts a 'living will' and the incompetent who benefits from it are, effectively, different persons, and the one need not necessarily be empowered to speak for the other.[52]

Given these imponderables, the doctor's dilemma is summed up in the words of Lord Donaldson:

> what the doctors *cannot* do is to conclude that, if the patient still had the necessary capacity in the changed situation [he being now unable to communicate], he would have reversed his decision . . . what they *can* do is to consider whether at the time the decision was made it was intended by the patient to apply in the changed situation.[53]

From this it is clear that the concerned doctor cannot ignore an advance decision;[54] what they can do is to challenge its *validity*—and, in view of the subjective nature of much of sections 24–6, this is likely to be comparatively easy.[55] It has been suggested that, should

---

[49] [2014] EWCOP 4.   [50] Section 25(4).

[51] Note that the decision is binding on health carers in England and Wales but is only of evidentiary value in Scotland under the Adults with Incapacity (Scotland) Act 2000, s 1(4)(a).

[52] Ronald Dworkin, *Life's Dominion* (Alfred A. Knopf 1993).

[53] *Re T (adult: refusal of medical treatment)*, (n 36) [60].

[54] See *Re AK (adult patient) (medical treatment: consent)* [2001] 1 FLR 129. The case concerned a 19-year old man with motor neurone disease who wished nutrition and hydration to be discontinued two weeks after he lost all capacity to communicate. On the matter of a directive being binding, see Gianluca Montanari Vergallo, 'Advance Healthcare Directives: Binding or Informational Value?' (2020) 29(1) Cambridge Quarterly of Healthcare Ethics 98.

[55] Note also that withdrawal (as opposed to alteration) of an advance decision as to life-sustaining treat- ment need not be in writing (2005 Act, s 24(4)) which makes its discovery even more dependent on the enthusiasm of outsiders.

there be conflict as to the validity or scope of an advance directive, the wording of the Act is biased in favour of the preservation of life.[56] This is understandable to the extent that an error leading to death cannot be rectified while one resulting in survival can always be corrected by reversion to the status quo.[57] Be that as it may, the trend seems to be towards viewing the 2005 Act as the only way to express an advance refusal and as such risks undermining the all-important value of patient self-determination, especially if many patients are likely to be unfamiliar with its terms. The concerns about and objections to advance directives discussed persist as yet another example of the difficulties of attempting to generalise in an intensely private arena.[58] Guidance as to the format for recording advance decisions was provided in *X Primary Care Trust v XB*.[59] It included that procedures that follow the Code of Conduct should be in place to investigate any uncertainties, and the directive should have been discussed with a healthcare professional. As noted, the court queried whether a 'valid until' clause should be included as a matter of course since each care plan should be patient-specific.[60]

18.6.2 SUICIDE AND ASSISTED SUICIDE

If a patient is permitted to put their life at risk in a negative way by refusing treatment, it is logical to suppose that they should be entitled to do so in a positive way. Suicide is not a criminal offence in the UK,[61] nor is it, so far as we know, in any part of the developed world. Whether this implies a legal right to end one's life is debatable, but we are not here concerned with the morality of suicide per se. Our interest lies in the residual offence of counselling, procuring, aiding, and abetting suicide. This remains an offence in England and Wales by virtue of section 2(1) of the Suicide Act 1961, which seems to recognise a specific, stand-alone form of homicide.[62] Section 2(1) states:

> A person ('D') commits an offence if (a) D does an act capable of encouraging or assisting the suicide or attempted suicide of another person, and (b) D's act was intended to encourage or assist suicide or an attempt at suicide.

The section goes on to state that D may commit an offence under this section whether or not a suicide, or an attempt at suicide, occurs.

Parenthetically, there is some doubt as to whether an offence of abetting suicide exists in Scotland, where the Suicide Act never applied—it is difficult to imagine a common law offence of abetting an act which is not, itself, a crime.[63] Worryingly, no specific guidance has yet been published by the Crown Office and Procurator Fiscal Service (COPFS) in

---

[56] Based on the different wording of s 26(2) and (3): Sabine Michalowski, 'Advance refusals of life-sustaining medical treatment: the relativity of an absolute right' (2005) 68(6) Modern Law Review 958.

[57] For judicial support for this, albeit when there was also a question of mental disorder, see *Nottinghamshire Healthcare NHS Trust v RC* [2014] EWCOP 1317.

[58] For a helpful appraisal, see David Shaw, 'A Direct Advance on Advance Directives' (2012) 26(5) Bioethics 267.

[59] [2012] EWHC 1390 (Fam).

[60] See further, Carolyn Johnston, 'Advance Decision Making—Rhetoric or Reality?' (2014) 34(3) Legal Studies 497.

[61] Suicide Act 1961, s 1.

[62] The section is modified by the Coroners and Justice Act 2009, s 59, changes that are for clarification rather of significant substance.

[63] For further discussion, see Health and Sport Committee of the Scottish Parliament, *Stage 1 Report on Assisted Suicide (Scotland) Bill* (SP Paper 712 6th Report, Session 4, 2015), paras 18–27.

Scotland.[64] That said, in *Ross v Lord Advocate*,[65] Lord Carloway found that prosecution will depend on the nature of the act:

> The criminal law in relation to assisted suicide in Scotland is clear. It is not a crime 'to assist' another to commit suicide. However, if a person does something which he knows will cause the death of another person, he will be guilty of homicide if his act is the immediate and direct cause of the person's death.

In any event, there are many uncertainties in relation to the conjoined matter of culpability and liability of the agent, who will often be a relative, but may potentially be a physician. The would-be suicide will be anxious to determine the least painful and most effective way of dying, but may be hampered by ignorance, or by physical incapability. We isolate this very specific situation under the heading of progressive neuromuscular disease, in which the would-be suicide may need some form of aid, and a doctor may firmly believe death to be in their patient's best interests. The law as it stands leads to a professional, moral, and/or legal impasse—as much of the recent judicial activity suggests.

18.6.3 SEEKING ADVICE ON A SECTION 2(1) APPLICATION

Direct Intervention: Taking the Fatal Action

Much of the modern jurisprudence under section 2(1) relates to patients seeking advice or clarification from the Public Prosecution Service as to whether it will proceed with charges against a loved one who assists in securing what the patient views as a dignified and timely death in the face of a degenerative and incapacitating disease (often neuro-muscular disease (NMD)).

The first significant case is *R (Pretty) v DPP*,[66] which was ultimately heard in the European Court of Human Rights (ECtHR). Often referred to—wrongly in our view—as active voluntary euthanasia, Mrs Pretty, who suffered from Motor Neurone Disease (MND) and was just able to communicate, sought the assurance of the Director of Public Prosecutions (DPP) that he would not bring charges against her husband under section 2(1) if he took steps to end her life at her own request but by an unspecified method.[67] The DPP declined to give this assurance, saying that it was improper to decline in advance to prosecute a breach of the criminal law.[68] This refusal was challenged by Pretty, by way of judicial review, on the ground that the decision infringed rights protected under the Human Rights Act 1998.

Pretty based her claim on five Articles in the ECHR: Article 2 (right to life); Article 3 (prohibition of torture and cruel and degrading treatment); Article 8 (right to respect for private life); Article 9 (right to freedom of thought, conscience, and religion); and Article 14 (prohibition of discrimination). Although the Court was clearly sympathetic to her plight, none of these Articles was deemed to be grounds on which to base a right

---

[64] The absence of clear and transparent guidance was challenged at judicial review in the reclaim motion in *Ross v Lord Advocate* [2016] CSIH 12, in which it was found that the lack of such clear guidance did not interfere with the petitioners' Art 8 rights. *Cf.* Catherine O'Sullivan, 'Mens Rea, Motive and Assisted Suicide: Does the DPP's Policy Go Too Far?' (2015) 35(1) Legal Studies 96.

[65] ibid. (*Ross*).   [66] (2002) 63 BMLR 1 (HL).

[67] Pretty could never have accomplished her suicide alone, and the option of assisted suicide was never available. In effect, her application could have included anything up to and including a proleptic amnesty for murder, an undertaking the DPP could never have given.

[68] It was also constitutionally impossible—Lord Bingham in the House of Lords drew attention to the Bill of Rights 1688, which denies the Crown and its servants any power to alter laws without the consent of Parliament.

to assistance with suicide. The Court rejected the argument that Article 2 created a right to self-determination in relation to life and death, holding that the right was clearly concerned with preventing the unjustified taking of life. The appellant's argument in respect of Article 3 was that there was an obligation on the part of the state to provide assistance in the prevention of suffering—a positive rather than a negative duty. This was rejected by the Court, which held that the state in this case was not in breach of its duty to prevent the infliction of suffering—Pretty's suffering resulted from a disease rather than from the act of any person.

In hindsight, the only Article which merited serious consideration was Article 8. However, the House of Lords did not consider a prohibition of assistance in suicide to engage autonomy for the purposes of that Article. The right of autonomy protected was the right to exercise autonomy while living one's life, and, as pointed out by Lord Bingham, there was nothing in the Article to suggest that it has any bearing on the choice to live no longer. This narrow interpretation is open to criticism in that the concept of autonomy, as it is generally understood, includes decisions about dying.[69] Dying is a part of life and it is difficult to imagine how at least some decisions about the nature of one's death could be seen to have nothing to do with the exercise of self-determination.[70] On appeal, the European Court appreciated the force of this argument, holding that Article 8 is indeed engaged by these decisions.[71] And so it fell to the UK to justify its legal position, and to the Court to consider both the interference and the justification under Article 8(2), which lists a number of exceptions that could be regarded as 'necessary in a democratic society'. In the event, the ECtHR agreed with the House of Lords in finding that the 'blanket' application of section 2(1) infringed none of the five Articles considered. In particular, Article 2 imposed a duty on the state to protect life and there was no implication that this created a right to die;[72] the prohibition of assisted suicide was accepted as necessary and not disproportionate to the need to protect the state's vulnerable citizens (Article 8); and that to distinguish between those who could and those who physically could not commit suicide—and, thus, to avoid any supposed discrimination against the latter contrary to Article 14—would be to undermine the protection of life that the 1961 Act was designed to safeguard.

Both the House of Lords and the ECtHR appreciated, and were influenced by, the fear that permitting assisted dying would open the door to abuse of the sick and the elderly. This attitude was summed up well by Lord Bingham when quoting with approval the conclusions of the House of Lords Select Committee on Medical Ethics:

> The message which society sends to vulnerable and disadvantaged people should not, however obliquely, encourage them to seek death, but should assure them of our care and support in life.[73]

---

[69] On this aspect of the case see Hazel Biggs, 'A Pretty Fine Line: Death, Autonomy and Letting it B' (2003) 11(3) Feminist Legal Studies 291, who maintained that *Pretty* and *Mrs B* are on a par; Dame Brenda Hale, 'A Pretty Pass: When is There a Right to Die?' (2003) 32(1) Common Law World Review 1.

[70] See Rosalind English, 'No Rights to Last Rites' (2001) 151(7012) New Law Journal 1844; Antje Pedain, 'The Human Rights Dimension of the Diane Pretty Case' (2003) 62(1) Cambridge Law Journal 181.

[71] *Pretty* (n 4).

[72] Parenthetically, the Supreme Court of Ireland has also held that a right to life does not imply a 'right to die' under the Irish Constitution: *Fleming v Ireland and Others* [2013] IESC 19. The Court did point out that this would not preclude the Irish Parliament (*Oireachtas*) from legislating on assisted suicide so long as it took account of the constitutional obligation of the state to protect the right to life. In June 2022, a Special Oireachtas committee was set up to examine assisted dying. It followed a poll that indicated a two-thirds support for assisted dying among the Irish electorate: Beau Donnelly, 'Special Oireachtas Committee to Examine Assisted Dying' *The Times* (05 July 2022) available at <https://www.thetimes.co.uk/article/special-oireachtas-committee-to-examine-assisted-dying-ws8r322hp> accessed 03 November 2022.

[73] *Pretty*, (n 4), [42] (Lord Bingham).

One of the main criticisms of *Pretty* is that it could be held that the interests of the individual are being sacrificed in order to establish an important social policy; it is arguable that it is morally unacceptable to allow this, as it could be seen as a clear infringement of the individual's basic human rights. Trenchant legal criticism was also levelled at the Suicide Act itself,[74] particularly at section 2(4)—'no proceedings shall be instituted for an offence under this section except by or with the consent of the Director of Public Prosecutions'. Professor Tur discussed the meaning of this and pointed out that either it can be definitional—that is, there is no crime in the absence of the DPP's consent—or it is dispensing—that is, it is always a crime but the DPP can dispense with prosecution in suitable cases. The judges in Pretty's case assumed the latter—as, we suspect, would most people. However, since the circumstances can only be assessed *after* the event, a dispensation is likely to lead to inconsistency and uncertainty—which is something the law should avoid.

Pretty was effectively seeking to legalise euthanasia—or, as we have seen, murder. The decision against her went unchallenged, as might well be expected, until a further high-profile case was heard in 2012.[75] Mr Nicklinson was in the disastrous state of the 'locked in syndrome'; he was totally paralysed but, nevertheless, retained his cognitive faculties, being able to communicate through sophisticated software by blinking his eyes. His case differed from that of Pretty insofar as his plea was limited to a declaration that it would not be unlawful, on the grounds of necessity, for his doctor to terminate his life. In short, he was asking for what, in our terminology, passes for physician-accomplished suicide—a process which is close to euthanasia but which is, at the same time, to be distinguished from physician-assisted suicide. Charles J, noting that the status of necessity as a potential defence against a charge of murder or assisting suicide was unclear, allowed the case to go to judicial review in that the Human Rights Act 1998 (and in particular ECHR Article 8) was arguably engaged.

The Divisional Court predictably refused the application.[76] The grounds were several and covered a wide number of issues. In summary, it was determined, first, that any change in the law on euthanasia was a matter for Parliament; second that euthanasia was equivalent to murder and there was no defence available on the basis of lack of causation, lack of intention or quasi-self-defence—the Court was unwilling to entertain a defence of necessity which should be employed with great caution; and, third, while Article 8 of the ECHR was certainly engaged in death decisions, a considerable margin of appreciation was available and a blanket ban on assisted death was not incompatible with the Article.[77] Nicklinson died from unassociated natural causes a week after the ruling. Despite this, his family was given leave to appeal.

Nicklinson v Ministry of Justice, heard before a bench of nine at the Supreme Court, is a complex amalgam of appeals and cross-appeals arising from the fact that Nicklinson had not been alone in his original arguments about the legality of assisted suicide, and because the DPP was implicated by the Court of Appeal ruling to the effect that she was required to clarify (yet further) her prosecution policy on assisted suicide. The DPP cross-appealed against this last point and the Nicklinson family continued to argue for the illegality of the 1961 Act. They were co-joined by Lamb, who also argued that the law should

---

[74] Richard Tur, 'Legislative Technique and Human Rights: The Sad Case of Assisted Suicide' [2003] Criminal Law Review 3.

[75] *Nicklinson* (n 9).

[76] Ibid.; *R (on the application of AM v DPP and Others)* (2012) 127 BMLR 107. AM's action was basically a combination of that brought by Pretty with unknown persons substituted for her husband and Purdy. It was rejected as requiring more of the DPP than was in the officer's power.

[77] Quoting *Haas v Switzerland* (2011) 53 EHRR 33 (repeated in *Koch v Germany* (2013) 56 EHRR 6 [52]; *Gross v Switzerland* (2014) 58 EHRR 7 [59]).

be changed to allow him assistance in dying, and by an appellant known as Martin, who was arguing for clearer DPP policy guidelines. On this last point the Supreme Court declined to rule that the DPP should amend her policy, and her appeal was accordingly successful. The law requires that any such policy be clear and transparent, but it would be inappropriate for the courts to dictate its terms.[78] In something of an aside, however, the Court noted that in evidence it had transpired that the current terms of the policy did not fully reflect the DPP's views. She was accordingly invited to reflect on the terms and to amend them accordingly, without any order being made to this effect. This judicial sleight of hand might also be seen to typify the majority's opinion of the appellants' arguments with respect to section 2 of the Suicide Act 1961.

In sum, these can be subsumed under the umbrella of a human rights challenge to the effect that the 'blanket ban' nature of the statutory provisions took the UK outside of its margin of appreciation under the ECHR. While the majority of the Court rejected this argument, it took the opportunity to point out the significant interference with Article 8 rights that the law represented. Moreover, it called into question the defensibility of the UK's position with respect to the robustness of the arguments for maintaining the status quo. Most significantly, it signalled that a court would be justified in making a declaration of incompatibility with the ECHR, albeit that it was not minded to do so at this time. Rather, Parliament was to be 'given the opportunity' to consider the position in light of this ruling.[79] Only Lord Kerr and the President, Lady Hale, were minded to make the declaration in the instant appeal, while Lord Clarke and Lord Sumption would intervene only if Parliament chose not to debate the issue. This remarkable 'non-decision' is as clear a message as possible for a UK court to send the legislature that circumstances must change, and we discuss the subsequent parliamentary events going forward. Nonetheless, we are compelled to comment on the unsatisfactory cat-and-mouse nature of these developments.[80] The institutions of the state are failing their citizens in not grasping the moral nettle on this issue, and are coming perilously close to an abrogation of constitutional responsibility.

An appeal to Strasbourg was inevitable, and the decision in *Nicklinson and Lamb* v *the United Kingdom* was rendered in July 2015.[81] Nicklinson failed (again) because he failed to show new substantive issues since *Pretty*, and because his argument was asking too much of the courts within the constitutional order; Lamb failed to exhaust domestic remedies relative to the particular basis of the appeal. Martin sought judicial review of GMC guidance, arguing that it breached his human rights in failing to provide him with sufficient advice in how to take his own life.[82]

The initial *Nicklinson* decision had been described as 'the death of humanity',[83] but the outcome of the appeals process should have catalysed parliamentary action, and indeed many forays into the field were initiated. However, the prohibition on assisting a suicide remains in place, and was most recently considered in *R (Conway)* v *The Secretary of State for Justice (Rev 1)*,[84] wherein the Court reaffirmed that section 2 is necessary to

[78] Interestingly, evidence from the DPP revealed only one (successful) prosecution under s 2 of the 1961 Act; moreover, no person had been prosecuted who provided assistance to the 498 people from the UK who had used the services of the Swiss Dignitas clinic in the period from 1998 to 2021 (16% of all users), see Dignitas, 'What Does Dignitas Offer' (2022) available at <http://www.dignitas.ch> accessed 03 November 2022.
[79] A point repeated at paras 113, 116, 118, 190, 197, and 204.
[80] For other comments, see Elizabeth Wicks, 'The Supreme Court Judgment in Nicklinson: One Step Forward on Assisted Dying: Two Steps Back on Human Rights' (2015) 23(1) Medical Law Review 144.
[81] [2015] ECHR 709 (Fourth Section).
[82] Martin's application was dismissed in *R (AM)* v *General Medical Council* [2015] EWHC 2096 (Admin).
[83] Seamus Burns, 'The Death of Humanity?' (2012) 162(7529) New Law Journal 1146.
[84] [2017] EWHC 2447 (Admin).

protect the weak and vulnerable, and opined that Parliament is entitled to maintain a clear bright-line rule which forbids people from providing assistance.

Indirect Intervention: Suicide and Medical Tourism[85]

Assisting a suicide will be unlawful under the Suicide Act 1961, section 2(1) only if it is conducted on a basis of immediacy and intent—the impersonal distribution of advice or information will not attract legal sanction.[86] In the circumstances envisaged here, however, the relationship will, more probably, be intimate and clearly distinguishable as such. There is now unfettered movement in search of medical interventions throughout the European Union (EU) and there is, of course, no reason why a person should not make their private arrangements for medical care in any part of the Union,[87] or indeed in the rest of the world. Such arrangements may include seeking assistance with suicide which is now legally available in a number of jurisdictions. As a result, an ongoing issue has arisen in the shape of providing assistance to the suicide-seeker in making travel arrangements and the like; this becomes particularly acute when EU citizens claim access to cross-border healthcare services because such claims cut into sensitive policy fields of Member States.[88]

The lawfulness of associating assisted travel with assisted dying was first tested as a specific issue in *Re Z (Local Authority: Duty)*,[89] in which a local authority sought to continue an interim injunction preventing a husband from taking his wife to Switzerland so that she might avail herself of the assisted suicide procedures available in that country. Z was suffering from cerebellar ataxia, an incurable and irreversible condition that left her physically incapable of fending for herself. The local authority had initially sought the injunction both to protect Z as someone it saw as vulnerable, and to deter Mr Z, who was, in its opinion, committing a criminal offence. At the substantive hearing, Hedley J refused the request. He held that the powers and responsibilities of an authority in such cases were to investigate and to protect individuals lacking capacity and/or those subject to undue influence. Any suspicion of criminality should be reported to the appropriate authorities; given that the criminal prosecution service had been informed, and that Z was deemed to have capacity, the authority's duties were exhausted. He further stated that the case 'afforded no basis for trying to ascertain the court's views about the rights or wrongs of suicide, assisted or otherwise'. The legal point was simply that adults with capacity are entitled to make their own decisions, and that they—and those who assist them—bear the responsibility for any decisions so taken. Thus, Z's case, while interesting to the private lawyer, gave us very little insight into the relevant medical law.[90]

This aspect of section 2(4) was ultimately addressed in a very similar and now infamous action by Ms Purdy who was concerned for the legal position of her husband

---

[85] See generally Daniel Sperling, *Suicide Tourism: Understanding the Legal, Philosophical, and Socio-Political Dimensions* (OUP 2019).

[86] *Attorney-General* v *Able* [1984] 1 All ER 277.

[87] *Luisi and Carbone* v *Ministero del Tesero* [1984] ECR 377. The full consequences of Brexit on this unfettered movement are yet to be determined, though it is possible to find examples in the press of Britons travelling to Dignitas in Switzerland, as recently as 2020. See e.g. Charlotte Fenton, 'The Day We Took Dad to Dignitas – and Why We're Campaigning for Assisted Dying to be Legalised in the UK' (iNews 10 July 2020) available at < https://inews.co.uk/news/long-reads/dignitas-assisted-dying-suicide-huntingtons-disease-terminal-illness-386063> accessed 03 November 2022.

[88] See further Niamh Nic Shuibhne, 'Margins of Appreciation: National Values, Fundamental Rights and EC Free Movement Law' (2009) 3(2) European Law Review 230.

[89] [2005] 1 FLR 740.

[90] For a brief analysis, see Bala Mahendra, 'Assisted Suicide: The Law Upheld' (2004) 154(7156) New Law Journal 1848.

should he accompany her to a jurisdiction where she could be lawfully assisted to die.[91] In effect, Purdy sought to fill the vacuum left by the evasive result of *Re Z*. Essentially, Purdy argued that the Act engaged her rights under Article 8(1) of the ECHR but that the state's licence to derogate from that Article 'in accordance with the law' under Article 8(2) could not apply in the absence of a specific public policy as to when the DPP would or would not exercise his discretion as to prosecution. The Divisional Court followed the House of Lords' ruling in *Pretty* that Article 8 was, effectively, unconcerned in cases of assisted suicide. However, even if that had not been the case, the Court held that the general provisions of administrative law and the guidance given to Crown Prosecutors in the Code of Practice under the Prosecution of Offenders Act 1985 were sufficiently clear to satisfy the requirement that the DPP, in using his discretion, was acting 'in accordance with the law'. An appeal to the Court of Appeal was rejected on essentially the same grounds.[92]

Purdy's case was, therefore, a matter of administrative law but with direct impact on medical law as a matter of transparency of policies impacting on individual autonomy.[93] There was no gainsaying the fact that many persons had previously left the UK for suicide in Switzerland, and none of their fellow travellers had been prosecuted. The DPP, therefore, took the opportunity to clarify the law in this area by reference to one of these.[94] In brief, he concluded that, even though there might be sufficient evidence on which to mount a prosecution in such cases—including, in particular, evidence of help to travel to a receptive clinic—there were, equally, times when it would not be in the public interest to do so. The conditions which militated against prosecution in the case under consideration included the facts that the abettors, in this case, the dead boy's parents, had not attempted to influence him to commit suicide, there was evidence of his intention to commit suicide were he able to do so, the action taken by the family was at the more remote end of the possible spectrum of assistance, and their son's death, rather than offering any benefit to the potential accused, actually caused them profound distress. The DPP was adamant that cases will differ on their facts and that a generalisation is impossible; what his statement did, however, was to outline an envelope of conditions within which prosecution will *not* proceed—which seemed to be as helpful a contribution to the debate as was possible in the circumstances. It is also noteworthy that the Lord Chief Justice made it as clear as he could that the courts would be less than enthusiastic in their response were a prosecution to be mounted in conditions such as those envisaged in *Purdy*.[95]

Purdy proceeded to the House of Lords (as it then was), where the main thrust of the opinion was to direct the DPP to formulate an offence-specific policy identifying the factors to be taken into consideration in deciding whether to prosecute in circumstances such as those exemplified by Purdy's condition[96]—which, in view of the action already taken, was scarcely a seismic contribution to the assisted-dying debate. The decision did, however, include two results that are of general significance. First, it confirmed that

---

[91] *R (Purdy)* v *DPP* [2008] EWHC 2565.   [92] [2009] EWCA Civ 92.

[93] For a brief analysis, see John K Mason, 'Unalike as Two Peas: *R (on the application of Purdy)* v *DPP*' (2009) 13 Edinburgh Law Review 298.

[94] Keir Starmer, 'Decision on Prosecution—The Death by Suicide of Daniel James' (09 December 2008) Crown Prosecution Service.

[95] *Purdy* (n 91) [80].

[96] *R (Purdy)* v *DPP* [2009] UKHL 45 [56] (Lord Hope). For the current DPP policy, see Crown Prosecution Service, *Policy for Prosecutors in Respect of* Cases of *Encouraging or Assisting Suicide* (2014) available at <https://www.cps.gov.uk/legal-guidance/suicide-policy-prosecutors-respect-cases-encouraging-or-assisting-suicide> accessed 03 September 2022.

Article 8 of the ECHR *is* engaged in decisions related to death and to assisted dying; indeed, the whole tenor of the debate points to the logic of legislating in the field by way of human rights rather than the criminal law.[97] Second, it made clear that, as a matter of human rights, we are entitled to clarity in the application of the law—a matter which may have far-reaching consequences in other areas where discretion can be exercised.

Despite itself declining to interfere with the content of the DPP's policy, the decision in *Purdy* opened rather than closed the book on judicial involvement in public policies in this field. An objection to its contribution is found in the comments in *Nicklinson* to the following effect:

> The purpose of the DPP publishing a code or policy is not to enable those who wish to commit a crime to know in advance whether they will get away with it. It is to ensure that, as far as is possible in practice and appropriate in principle, the DPP's policy is publicly available so that everyone knows what it is, and can see whether it is being applied consistently.[98]

In any event, most would surely agree that it would be undesirable, indeed unacceptable, to give carte blanche to the self-appointed 'mercy killer',[99] and it has been pointed out that any proposal for relaxing section 2(1) would have to accept that only help provided by medically qualified persons could be lawful.[100] This suggests that legitimising physician-assisted suicide might be an acceptable halfway house.

18.6.4 PHYSICIAN-ASSISTED SUICIDE

The classic case of physician-assisted suicide (PAS) involves the doctor in no more than providing the means of ending life—most commonly by the provision or prescription of the necessary drugs. The patient themselves will complete the act, which can then properly be described as an act of suicide, albeit assisted. Given this scenario, the doctor is the passive agent in the assisted-dying relationship. We regard it as essential to the euthanasia debate to accept that PAS is what it says—suicide, not homicide. This concept is important in that it contrasts vividly with the situation in which the patient physically cannot, or prefers not to, perform this final task and in which the doctor, in person and on request, administers the *coup de grâce*; we are, then, in the realm of physician-accomplished suicide or active voluntary euthanasia as has been discussed earlier—this is arguably of a different legal ambience.

The difficulty is that such distinctions will not always be so simple. Take, for example, the doctor who responds to a request to disconnect the ventilator in a case of progressive neurological disease—is this to be classed as refusal of treatment by the patient or as assisted suicide or even as physician-accomplished suicide? And what of the paralysed patient who wishes to die but is receiving no treatment that can be refused—is the ending of that life a matter of assisting suicide or of active euthanasia? Or, what is the position of

---

[97] In which case, Art 8(2) also has effect, and is significant, in Scotland despite the differences in the law on suicide. For discussion, see Sheila McLean, Carla Connelly, and John K Mason, 'Purdy in Scotland: We Hear, But Should We Listen?' [2009] 121(4) Juridical Review 265.

[98] *Nicklinson* (n 9) [141].

[99] Lord Falconer withdrew a proposed amendment to the Coroners and Justice Bill, which would have legitimised assisted suicide by way of assisted travel in the light of the *Purdy* decision.

[100] Dan Morris, 'Assisted Suicide Under the European Convention on Human Rights: A Critique' (2003) 1 European Human Rights Law Review 65.

the doctor who performs the venepuncture and then holds the syringe while the patient presses the plunger?[101] Hard as one may try to represent them, there are no bright dividing lines between refusal of treatment, suicide, assisted suicide, physician accomplished suicide, and euthanasia. Yet, clearly, there *are* distinctions to be made even if these be intuitive. Thus, we have Lord Donaldson saying:

> On other occasions, however, the difference may be obvious. In respect of assisted suicide and euthanasia, for example, it is not difficult to see a practical difference between the classic ploy of 'leaving the pills' and undertaking a lethal injection—and it is this sort of comparison that most people have in mind when addressing the subject.[102]

Again, we have the Court in the US case of *Vacco* v *Quill*:[103]

> [The] distinction between assisting suicide and withdrawing life-sustaining treatment in hopeless cases is logical, widely recognized and endorsed by the medical profession and by legal tradition,

and we only wish it *were* always so. The dilemma is, however, particularly well expressed in the specific context of the management of progressive neurological disease—a matter which is further characterised as unique in that, in the majority of cases, recourse to the ploy of 'double effect' is not an available management option.

Progressive (or Incurable) Neurological Disease

Insofar as the right of the competent adult to refuse life-saving treatment is now universally established and that the legal right to control one's body has found expression in the decriminalising of suicide, it is but a short step to hold that to refuse assistance in dying to a person who is incapable of ending their own life is an affront to that person's rights of autonomy, dignity, and freedom from torturous and degrading treatment or conditions.[104] It is important, though, to isolate two separate issues. One is the right to reject treatment, even if one is incapable of physically resisting the imposition of treatment. The second is more controversial and involves an attempt to assert a legal right to assistance in suicide.[105]

The *general* right to refuse treatment was discussed in detail previously. Here, we focus on that right when applied to the extreme examples of progressive or incurable

---

[101] These examples are taken from John K Mason and David Myers, 'Physician Assisted Suicide: A Second View from Mid-Atlantic' (1999) 28(3) Anglo-American Law Review 265, in which the comparative Anglo-American scene at the time is discussed in detail.

[102] See Larry Churchill and Nancy King, 'Physician Assisted Suicide, Euthanasia, or Withdrawal of Treatment' (1997) 315 BMJ 137; and more recently David Orentlicher, 'The Alleged Distinction Between Euthanasia and the Withdrawal of Life-Sustaining Treatment: Conceptually Incoherent and Impossible to Maintain' (2012) 1998(3) University of Illinois Law Review 837.

[103] 117 S Ct 2293 (1997).

[104] The issue was first raised in the UK in *Linsell*, in which a patient in the terminal stages of MND sought a declaration that her doctor would not be prosecuted if he administered potentially lethal doses of analgesics when her condition deteriorated. The patient withdrew her application when she heard that a substantial body of medical opinion had endorsed her doctor's planned palliative management regime, which meant that no ruling was required. See HC Deb 20 November 1997, col 720.

[105] For a meta-analysis of patient views, see Anke Erdmann et al., 'The Wish to Die and Hastening Death in Amyotrophic Lateral Sclerosis: A Scoping Review' (2021) 11(3) BMJ Supportive and Palliative Care 271. See also Kelly Fahrner-Scott et al., 'Embedded Palliative Care for Amyotrophic Lateral Sclerosis: A Pilot Program and Lessons Learned' (2022) 12(1) Neurology Clinical Practice 68.

neurological disease.[106] Its application in these circumstances was first upheld in the very significant Canadian decision in *Nancy B v Hôtel-Dieu de Québec*.[107] Nancy suffered from the Guillain-Barré syndrome. She existed by virtue of a ventilator, which she sought to be disconnected. She was supported in this by her family and the hospital. In making the required order, Dufour J called upon the Civil Code of Lower Canada (as it then was), which stated:

> Art 19.1 No person may be made to undergo care of any nature whether for examination, specimen taking, removal of tissue treatment or any other act, except with his consent,

and concluded that this encompassed ventilation. Nancy saw this as 'the slavery of a machine', which she could not herself disconnect. With the help of a third party, the disease would be allowed to take it natural course.

As a result of the order, the person responsible for the actual cessation of treatment would not violate the criminal law. At the same time, however, the judge ruled that not only would it not be homicide, it would also not amount to suicide or assisted suicide.

Nancy B was followed in England by the equally important case of *Ms B v An NHS Hospital Trust*, which we have already considered. It need only be reiterated here to drive home the lesson that the competent adult may reject treatment even if it will result in death. But, as we have already discussed, the case also vividly demonstrates the limitation of *doctors'* autonomy that is imposed by the doctrine.

There is, of course, also abundant evidence that removal of life support mechanisms at the request of the patient may well be obligatory in the US. Thus, in *Re Kathleen Farrell*,[108] an MND case, not only was a request for disconnection from the ventilator agreed, but the right to professional assistance during the agonal phase was upheld. An equally emphatic case arose in California, where the healthcare team was instructed to provide full facilities in order to ease the patient's dying.[109] It is thus clear that the US jurisdictions recognise a practical as well as a theoretical distinction between refusal of treatment and assisted suicide.[110]

The second issue—that of whether there is a legal right to assistance with suicide in the case of a person who cannot exercise their discretion—was considered initially and extensively by the Supreme Court of Canada in *Rodriguez v A-G of British Columbia*.[111] The arguments in Rodriguez's case, which concerned the setting up of a mechanism she could use to end her life should she become paralysed as a result of MND, were, in the main, based on Canadian constitutional law and the possible conflicts between the Canadian Charter of Rights and Freedoms and the Criminal Code; issues which have become relevant to UK law since the passage of the Human Rights Act 1998. It was held by a majority of 5:4 that, while the patient's autonomy was at stake, the deprivation of rights consequent on the refusal of such a request was not contrary to the principles of fundamental justice, which required a fair balance to be struck between the interests of the state and those of the individual; neither was

---

[106] The distinction is more than pedantic. Progressive disease (Pretty) will ultimately kill the patient; those with incurable disease (Nicklinson, Lamb, and Martin) may be kept alive for years. The medico-legal management of the two is not interchangeable. It has been reported that Nicklinson eventually refused food in an effort to end his own life: BBC News, 'Right-to-Die Man Tony Nicklinson Dead After Refusing Food' (BBC 22 August 2012) available at <http://www.bbc.co.uk/news/uk-england-19341722> accessed 03 November 2022.

[107] (1992) 86 DLR (4th) 385; (1992) 15 BMLR 95.   [108] 529 A 2d 404 (NJ, 1987).

[109] *Bouvia v Superior Court of Los Angeles County* 179 Cal App 3d 1127 (1986).

[110] See *Vacco v Quill* (n 103).   [111] *Rodriguez v A-G of British Columbia* (1993) 50 BMLR 1.

the liberty and security of the person compromised—one reason being that the provisions in section 241 of the Criminal Code prohibiting assisted suicide were there as a *protection* for the terminally ill who were particularly vulnerable as to their lives and their will to live.[112] This has strong flavours of the ECtHR ruling in *Pretty*.

However, the more recent decision of the Canadian Supreme Court in *Carter v Canada (Attorney General)* signifies a very different stance.[113] After being diagnosed with a fatal neurodegenerative disease in 2009, T brought this case challenging the constitutionality of the Criminal Code; she was joined by, among others, two parties who had accompanied their mother to Switzerland to complete her own assisted suicide.

In a landmark decision, the Supreme Court unanimously held that the existing legal prohibition of assisted suicide in section 14 of the Criminal Code unjustifiably infringed on citizens' Charter Rights—notably, section 7 'life, liberty, and security of the person'. Accordingly, the criminal provisions are of 'no force or effect' in prohibiting PAS for a competent adult so long as two criteria are satisfied: (i) the person validly consents to termination of their life, and (ii) they are suffering from a 'grievous and irremediable medical condition (including an illness, disease or disability) that causes enduring suffering that is intolerable to the individual in the circumstances of their condition'.[114] Given the historic nature of the ruling, the Court suspended its declaration for 12 months to allow the federal and provincial governments to respond, should they wish to do so.

This momentous decision is notable in many respects. First, note the *volte face* of the Supreme Court with respect to the relative weight to be given to individual autonomy as opposed to public protectionism. The current Court's concern was that total prohibition of PAS 'catches people outside this class [vulnerable persons]' and 'sweeps conduct into its ambit that is unrelated to the law's objective'.[115] In other words, this was 'grossly disproportionate', particularly relative to a dearth of evidence that vulnerable persons are disproportionately affected in countries where PAS already exists. Second, note the terms in which the ruling is couched: 'grievous and irremediable'; 'suffering that is intolerable'. This does not make terminal illness a threshold for qualification, and it is at odds with how much of the debate is conducted elsewhere. Finally, the Court felt entitled to revisit *Rodriguez*, and to invite the lower court to do so, for what is—to all extents and purposes—a fundamental shift in social circumstances. These shifts are both ideological and empirical. On the facts presented, for example, the trial court had found 'no evidence from permissive jurisdictions that people with disabilities are at heightened risk of accessing physician-assisted dying'; 'no evidence of inordinate impact on socially vulnerable populations in the permissive jurisdictions', and 'no compelling evidence that a permissive regime in Canada would result in a "practical slippery slope"'.[116] All of this was accepted by the Supreme Court and the baton was thus passed to Parliament, which adopted Bill C-14 (Medical Assistance in Dying).[117]

Many will posit that the developments in Canada are themselves a clear manifestation of the 'slippery slope' phenomenon, but we see it as a logical result—once you accept

---

[112] ibid. [410] (Sopinka J).   [113] [2015] SCC 5.   [114] ibid. [68], [127], [147].
[115] ibid. [86].   [116] ibid. [107].

[117] SC 2016 c. 3. For comment on the preceding case, see Stephanie Palmer, '"The Choice is Cruel": Assisted Suicide and the Charter of Rights in Canada' (2015) 74(2) Cambridge Law Journal 191; Amir Attaran, 'Unanimity on Death with Dignity—Legalizing Physician-Assisted Dying in Canada' (2015) 372 New England Journal of Medicine 2080. For comment on the subsequent legislation, see Harvey Chochinov and Catherine Frazee, 'Finding a Balance: Canada's Law on Medical Assistance in Dying' (2016) 388(10044) The Lancet 543; Ross Upshur, 'Unresolved Issues in Canada's Law on Physician-Assisted Dying' (2016) 388(10044) The Lancet 545; Aaron Trachtenberg and Braden Manns, 'Cost Analysis of Medical Assistance in Dying in Canada' (2017) 189(3) Canadian Medical Association Journal E101; Diane Kelsall, 'Physicians are not Solely Responsible for Ensuring Access to Medical Assistance in Dying' (2018) 190(7) Canadian Medical Association Journal E181.

physician assisted suicide, you *must* accept physician-accomplished suicide in cases of neuromuscular incapacity. You would also need to accept the possibility of changes to the eligibility criteria and safeguards in place.

Staying with the Canadian example, we would have in mind Bill C-7, which received Royal Assent in March 2021. It followed the 2019 Superior Court of Québec ruling in *Truchon* v *Canada* (AG),[118] which found 'reasonable foreseeability of natural death' to be unconstitutional as an eligibility criterion for medical assistance in dying. The Parliamentary Review that followed Bill C-7 was carried out by the Special Joint Committee on Medical Assistance in Dying. In February 2023, the Committee published its Second Report. Its Recommendations included that the Government of Canada should undertake consultations with minors on assisted dying, which should include 'minors with terminal illnesses, minors with disabilities, minors in the child welfare system and Indigenous minors, within five years of the tabling of this report' (Recommendation 14). It also Recommended that, 'the parents or guardians of a mature minor [should be] consulted in the course of the assessment process for MAID, but that the will of a minor who is found to have the requisite decision-making capacity ultimately take priority' (Recommendation 19). The Canadian situation exemplifies the fact that there is an ongoing appetite to consider expansion of eligibility criteria for medical assistance in dying—a policy we have seen played out in Belgium and the Netherlands.

The constitutional basis on which the Canadian law was changed following *Rodriguez* and *Carter*, has been mirrored in Germany and Italy, on the basis of rights akin to Article 8 ECHR, which annulled parts of the Criminal Code akin to section 2(1) of the Suicide Act 1961. There we see the sort of judicial activism unknown to the UK judiciary, in declaring an incompatibility and suggesting ways in which that may be remedied by the legislature.

In Germany, in 2020 the Federal Constitutional Court ruled on a case against a German- and Swiss-based association offering assisted suicide.[119] The court found that para 217 of the Criminal Code, banning assisted suicide, infringed Article 2(1) of the German Basic Law that supported a right of personality, including the right to self-determined death. Assistance could include provision of lethal medication, but not its administration. Crucially, however, the right is not subject to 'substantive criteria', such as diagnosis with a fatal disease.

A similar though less liberal outcome followed the *Cappato* case in Italy,[120] where Marco Cappato helped a Fabiano Antoniani travel to Switzerland to end his life, after the latter had been paralysed in a car accident. The court found that Article 580 of the Criminal Code, criminalising assisted suicide, was unconstitutional in that it infringed a 2017 Precedent that allowed the autonomous refusal of life-saving treatment. On that basis, the Constitutional Court found that it followed that a person is not forbidden from ending their life with the assistance of a third party, but not including a medical practitioner. The court went on to set out eligibility criteria, including on capacity, information disclosure, consent, irreversible pathology and intolerable suffering, as well as prior approval by an ethics committee. The class of 'suicide aspirants' was limited by confining the judgment to those kept alive artificially. In both the German and the Italian cases, the courts passed responsibility to the legislature to deal with the constitutional incompatibility.

---

[118] *Truchon c. Procureur général du Canada* (2019) QCCS 3792.

[119] See Budesverfassungsgericht, 'Criminalisation of Assisted Suicide Services Unconstitutional' (26 February 2020) available at <https://www.bundesverfassungsgericht.de/SharedDocs/Pressemitteilungen/EN/2020/bvg20-012.html> accessed 03 November 2022.

[120] Constitutional Court Decision No. 242 of November 22, 2019. See also Margherita Carotti, 'The Italian Constitutional Court and the Lawmaker: the 'Cappato case (Order no. 207/2018)' (Bachelor's Degree Thesis, LUISS 2019).

For patients in the UK who find themselves in the difficult circumstances such as those that affected Pretty and Purdy, [121] who clearly require some assistance in dying, the constitutional argument may be the only viable one to raise. And it may yet succeed, if we recall the interchange between Lady Hale and Lord Neuberger in *Nicklinson*, where the former considered the law to be incompatible with ECHR rights, by admitting no exceptions.

As Lord Kerr said in agreement with the rest of the bench in *Nicklinson*, 'this court has the constitutional authority to issue a declaration of incompatibility'.[122] This is a constitutional step that UK courts have so far shied away from, although Lady Hale did indicate in *Nicklinson* that she would be prepared to declare section 2(1) of the Suicide Act 1961 incompatible with Article 8 ECHR. Were that to happen, we would refer to the guiding 'steer' of Lady Hale in that case, which refers to that narrow class of degenerative neuro-muscular conditions referred to in this chapter: 'It would not be beyond the wit of a legal system to devise a process for identifying those people, those few people, who should be allowed help to end their own lives.'[123] She suggested the eligibility criteria should be capacity, lack of undue influence in reaching a free decision, in full knowledge of available options and consequences, and—crucially—the inability to carry out the decision without help.

These arguments remain for the time being legally hypothetical, and we leave it to one side and concentrate on the scenario that is generally accepted as representing euthanasia.

18.6.5 THE DOCTOR AS THE AGENT OF DEATH

Thus far, we have been at least moderately successful in finding alternative ideations to those commonly used in association with assisted dying, and in so doing have been able to subsume these within recognised medical jurisprudential bounds. That is because the management of dying is an integral part of medical practice. Such recourse is, however, scarcely available when the patient's request is not so much 'help me with my dying' but, rather 'help me to escape an intolerable life'—and that is the essence of voluntary euthanasia. We have, then, entered a new legal arena in that we have introduced an element of criminality to the doctor's role, and insofar as consent is no defence against the offence of inflicting severe injury. These were, in fact, precisely the two legal issues that had to be addressed by the Supreme Court of Canada in *Carter*. They remain an obstacle in most other jurisdictions, and the matter therefore remains that of the relationship between euthanasia and murder. This was unequivocally restated in *Bland*:

> that 'mercy killing' by active means is murder . . . has never so far as I know been doubted. The fact that the doctor's motives are kindly will for some, although not for all, transform the moral quality of his act, but this makes no difference in law. It is intent to kill or cause grievous bodily harm which constitutes the mens rea of murder, and the reason why the intent was formed makes no difference at all.[124]

---

[121] Remembering, of course, that the UK's attitude to neurological disease is established in *Pretty, Purdy*, and *Nicklinson*, which we discussed in detail earlier.

[122] *R (Nicklinson and Another)* v *Ministry of Justice* [2014] UKSC 38, [326]. For a more detailed discussion, see Murray Earle, '"Only Time Will Tell" – Escape from the Medically Assisted Suicide Spiral', in Edward Dove and Niamh Nic Shuibhne (eds.), *Law and Legacy in Medical Jurisprudence: Essays in Honour of Graeme Laurie* (CUP 2022).

[123] *Nicklinson* (n 9) [314].   [124] *Airedale* (n 19) [890] (Lord Mustill).

Even so, instinct—most appositely, instinct as demonstrated by jury verdicts—tells us that there is a further distinction to be made between assistance performed in response to terminal illness as opposed to the management of chronic, non-fatal illness, on which the case law is illustrative.

Homicide or Humanity?

The previous scenario was the problem when Dr Cox was charged with the attempted murder of Mrs Boyes, his patient of 13 years.[125] Boyes' rheumatoid arthritis was not, of itself, a fatal condition, but it caused intense pain and distress leading her to express a wish to die; she was, indeed, already categorised as 'not for resuscitation'.[126] At trial, it was admitted that Dr Cox injected her with two ampoules of potassium chloride, which is known to be potently cardiotoxic but, at the same time, is a substance having no analgesic value—and this is one factor which distinguished Dr Cox's case.[127] The issue at trial was, therefore, reduced to that of intent—did Dr Cox *intend* to kill his patient,[128] or did he hope to grant her a short pain-free period during the process of dying? As Ognall J put it at the outset of his summing-up:

> If he injected her with potassium chloride with the primary purpose of killing her, of hastening her death, he is guilty of the offence charged.[129]

And later:

> If a doctor genuinely believes that a certain course is beneficial to his patient, either therapeutically or analgesically, then even though he recognises that that course carries with it a risk to life, he is fully entitled, nonetheless, to pursue it. If in those circumstances the patient dies, nobody could possibly suggest that in that situation the doctor was guilty of murder or attempted murder.[130]

So, what distinguished Dr Cox from Dr Moor, Dr Martin, and Dr Munro?[131] Obviously, we can never know the precise reason for a jury verdict, but we can extract some factors which they may have found important—even if only subliminally. First, Mrs Boyes was incurably but not terminally ill. It is interesting that very few of the vast majority of sporadic attempts to legalise 'euthanasia' in the UK has attempted to go beyond the confines of terminal disease (compare now the Canadian position).[132] There may well be an intuitive distinction to be made on a 'sanctity of life' basis.[133] Second, Dr Cox injected a

---

[125] *R v Cox* (1992) 12 BMLR 38. Dr Cox was charged with attempted murder, presumably because Boyes had been cremated before her death was regarded as suspicious. Any arguments as to the cause of death would, therefore, have been speculative.

[126] See Chapter 17 of this book.

[127] Another trial concerned with voluntary euthanasia by way of injection of potassium chloride and lignocaine was aborted when the prosecution offered no evidence: *R v Lodwig* (1990) The Times, 16 March.

[128] Whether it was 'an act of mercy' was a matter only for the judge in sentencing, motive being irrelevant to the jury.

[129] *R v Cox* (n 125) [39].   [130] ibid. [41].

[131] For a particularly helpful review of Dr Munro's case and its comparison with that of Dr Cox, see James Goodman, 'The Case of *Dr Munro*: Are There Lessons to be Learnt?' (2010) 18(4) Medical Law Review 564.

[132] *Cf.* the Assisted Suicide (Scotland) Bill 2013, which included eligibility criteria relating to condition either 'terminal' or 'life-shortening', and Lord Falconer's Assisted Dying Bill 2014, which defined 'terminally ill' as 'an inevitably progressive condition which cannot be reversed by treatment' and 'as a consequence the person is reasonably expected to die within six months'. This last definition was also at the heart of the Rob Marris Private Member's Assisted Dying Bill introduced in June 2015.

[133] Although, logically, one might ask why one's life expectancy should affect one's relief from 'intolerable' suffering.

non-therapeutic substance and it is reasonable to assume that, while public opinion in the UK will give great latitude to the medical profession in its fight against suffering, it is not yet prepared to accept the use of a substance which has no analgesic effect and is known to be lethal when injected in concentrated form. Third, and as a direct result of this, he was unable to plead 'double effect' or necessity.

Dr Cox's case contained all the necessary elements of the classic murder case: intention to bring about death, direct action precipitating that death, and the absence of any defence or excuse based on the medical use of the drug. Even so, sympathy for Dr Cox was widespread.[134] No immediate custodial sentence was imposed; the GMC was content to admonish him on the grounds that, although his actions had fallen short of the high standards which the medical profession must uphold, he clearly acted in good faith; and the responsible regional health authority offered continued employment subject only to certain restrictions.[135] We believe that the jury decision was certainly right in law[136] but that such public dissatisfaction ultimately stems from distrust of the law's determination to dissociate motive from intent when faced with unlawful killing[137]—Dr Cox was certainly not a murderer as the word is commonly interpreted.[138]

Jackson summarised some of the resultant anomalies in a particularly powerful article.[139] She pointed out that the absolute prohibition of physician accomplished active euthanasia is in direct contradiction to the current movement towards the interests of the individual patient as the driving force in medicine; she concluded that the only logical reason for prohibiting doctors from complying with their patients' requests for euthanasia lies in the protection of an abstract idea as to the proper role of the medical profession[140]—and this she saw as being deeply anachronistic. Nonetheless, for reasons which appear elsewhere in this chapter, we cannot accept that individual doctors and their patients should be given free rein in this field absent specific legislation—the ghost of Dr Shipman lingers on. Moreover, any such legislation must, itself, be subject to the closest of scrutiny and subject to review.

---

[134] It had been reported that 11% of doctors in the US who were closely associated with relevant cases had received requests for a lethal injection and 4.7% had complied with the request at least once: Diane Meier et al., 'A National Survey of Physician-Assisted Suicide and Euthanasia in the United States' (1998) 338(17) New England Journal of Medicine 1193. See also Ruaidhri McCormack, Margaret Clifford, and Marian Conroy, 'Attitudes of UK Doctors Towards Euthanasia and Physician-Assisted Suicide: A Systematic Literature Review' (2012) 26 Palliative Medicine 23, and reports of 20% of US physicians having received such requests: Ezekiel Emanuel et al., 'Attitudes and Practices of Euthanasia and Physician-Assisted Suicide in the United States, Canada, and Europe' (2016) 316(1) Journal of the American Medical Association 79.

[135] Clare Dyer, 'GMC Tempers Justice with Mercy in Cox Case' (1992) 305 BMJ 1311.

[136] And that, therefore, Dr Adams' acquittal was dubious. Note, also, that, once motive is removed from the equation, Dr Cox's and Dr Shipman's cases are legally compatible.

[137] This view is central to the persuasive argument in Kenneth Boyd, 'Euthanasia: Back to the Future' in John Keown (ed.), Euthanasia Examined (CUP 1995).

[138] The French courts have also battled with cases similar to that of Dr Cox—the general impression being they will go to some lengths to avoid criminalising physician-accomplished euthanasia, though coming close with terminal sedation: see Ruth Horn, 'The "French Exception": The Right to Continuous Deep Sedation at the End of Life' (2018) 44(3) Journal of Medical Ethics 204. A proposed Bill legalising assisted suicide for those with a terminal disease was blocked in the French Parliament in 2011.

[139] Emily Jackson, 'Whose Death is it Anyway? Euthanasia and the Medical Profession' (2004) 57(1) Current Legal Problems 415.

[140] A case can be made for hiving off a 'duty' to provide euthanasia to specialists in the care of the terminally ill. See Hugh McLachlan, 'Assisted Suicide and the Killing of People? Maybe: Physician-assisted suicide and the Killing of Patients? No' (2010) 36(5) Journal of Medical Ethics 306.

Assistance or Accomplishment?

We have already mentioned the logical difficulty in maintaining a distinction between physician-assisted and physician-accomplished suicide in relation to the management of a progressive NMD. Much the same problem arises in the more common context of managing terminal malignant disease where, again, one has to balance the logical consequential association of the two concepts against the practical fear of the 'slippery slope'. Using the traditional terminology, one can identify a clear cascade from passive voluntary euthanasia (PAS) through active voluntary euthanasia (physician-accomplished suicide) to active non-voluntary—or true—euthanasia. At the time of writing, debate in the UK at the parliamentary levels has been confined to the legalisation of the first of these, and the chances of legislation which legalises the last being accepted in the UK remain remote. Indeed, it was concern about involvement of healthcare professionals in such processes that led the proponents of the (failed) Scottish Assisted Suicide Bill to put forward a new role of 'licensed facilitator' rather than morally implicate members of the medical professions.[141] Opposition might be very much less were it possible to legislate for PAS alone— an electorate that could not accept the doctor as an executioner might be less hostile to a doctor who could be regarded as a friend when one was in need. This view may be possible under the terms of the Assisted Dying Bill in the House of Lords (2021–22), which is forthright in stressing that the final act must be that of the patient, however assisted that person is by a 'health professional'[142].

The problem is, then, in two parts—first, is there any moral difference between physician-assisted and physician-accomplished suicide by which to justify the rigid legal distinction, and second, if there is, is it possible to legislate so as to accommodate the former without incorporating the latter and thereby further compromising our obligations to the vulnerable.

We will return to the problem of legislation later. As to the moral position, there is some evidence that, whatever their reasons, both doctors and the public will accept that there is a distinction to be made. In a major survey undertaken in Scotland over 20 years ago, McLean and Britton found that, given a change in the law, 43% of doctors across the UK would opt for the legalisation of PAS—defined as the patient's action leading to their own death. A similar proportion of the public (42%) would be in favour if the doctor performs the final act.[143] It is difficult to avoid the conclusion that, in this very sensitive situation, most people would wish to pass the ultimate responsibility to others.

The results obtained from public opinion polls are always subject to varied interpretation—indeed, the public itself can appear confused.[144] Thus, in McLean and Britton's survey, 67% thought that human beings should have the right to choose when to die (with 20% opposed) but only 55% (with 30% opposed) agreed that PAS should be legalised in Great Britain.[145] What is consistent, however, is a clear majority support for assisted dying. There is also a general trend showing an increase in that support, which is in line with an

---

[141] See the report of the Health and Sport Committee, (n 63) paras 232–256.

[142] Baroness Meacher's Assisted Dying Bill [HL] Clause 4(4). The same is true of the proposed Bill in Scotland, judging by the 2021 Consultation Document launched by Liam McArthur MSP.

[143] Sheila McLean and Andrea Britton, *Sometimes a Small Victory* (Institute of Law and Ethics in Medicine, University of Glasgow 1996).

[144] For example, see House of Lords Select Committee on the Assisted Dying for the Terminally Ill Bill, *Assisted Dying for the Terminally Ill Bill—First Report* (2005) ch 6 (Public Opinion).

[145] McLean and Britton (n 143). It was stated in *Compassion in Dying v State of Washington* 79 Fed 3d 790 (1996) that US opinion polls show majorities of between 64% and 73% in favour of PAS.

international trend to legislate in those terms. It is interesting to track that support along with successive Bills in UK legislatures.

A 2015 briefing on the Assisted Suicide (Scotland) Bill brought together evidence from a range of surveys, noting:

> [A] 2012 British Social Attitudes Survey, 80% of those with a disability supported a change in the law to allow a doctor to end the life of a person with a painful incurable disease if they requested it. This was slightly lower than for respondents without a disability (81%).[146] However, a more recent survey for SCOPE found that 62% of disabled people were worried that a change in the law to permit assisted suicide would put pressure on people with a disability to end their lives prematurely. 55% also believed that the current legal status of assisted suicide protects vulnerable people from pressure to end their lives.

The 2021 consultation on the Proposed Assisted Dying for Terminally Ill Adults (Scotland) Bill referred to the 2015 statistics, and went on to note that, 'Support [2019] is balanced across political affiliation, gender, age and social status. Recent polling on this issue shows that 87% of the Scottish public back the introduction of an assisted dying law', and that 'Polling has also shown that 88% of Scots living with a disability support assisted dying as a choice for terminally ill people.'[147]

At the time of Lord Falconer's Assisted Dying for the Terminally Ill Bill in 2005, the Select Committee First Report referred to a steady increase in approval rates for medical assistance in their death. This applied to a range of circumstances, including intolerable and incurable disease conditions. Approval rates rose from 75% to 82%.[148]

Like Liam MacArthur in the Scottish Parliament, in 2021 Baroness Meacher introduced the Assisted Dying Bill in the House of Lords. It had its second reading in October 2021. On public support, the House of Lords Library said:

> In August 2021, YouGov conducted a poll on public views of assisted dying in the UK for those with a terminal illness. 73% of those polled supported some form of doctor-assisted death for those with terminal illnesses. 50% supported similar measures for those suffering from a painful but not terminal illness. A separate 2019 poll of over 5,000 adults found that 84% supported some form of assisted dying proposals. This was an increase of two percentage points from the same poll conducted in 2015.[149]

A similar pattern can be observed in the views of medical practitioners. The Royal College of General Practitioners surveyed its members in 2013 with the result that a strong majority favoured continued opposition to a change in the law (77%, being 234 people), while a further 18% supported a move to a position of 'neutrality' and only 5% were in favour of a change in the law.[150] In 2020, 47% felt 'The RCGP should oppose a change in the law on assisted dying', 40% supported a change in the law, and 11% supported neutrality. While this appears to demonstrate a shift in opinion, the RCGP also noted that the differing methodologies meant accurate comparison is not possible.

---

[146] Assisted Suicide (Scotland) Bill. SPICe Briefing 15/02, 8 January 2015 p 18.

[147] Consultation p. 12, citing Populus 2019, Dignity in Dying Scotland fieldwork 11–24 March 2019.

[148] House of Lords Select Committee on the Assisted Dying for the Terminally Ill Bill, *Assisted Dying for the Terminally Ill Bill—First Report* (2005), para. 218. These statistics should be approached with caution, considering the detailed breakdown in the report.

[149] House of Lords, 'Briefing on the Assisted Dying Bill [HL]' (08 October 2021) available at <https://lordslibrary.parliament.uk/assisted-dying-bill-hl/> accessed 03 November 2022.

[150] See RCGP, 'Assisted Dying RCGP's 2020 Decision' (2020) available at <https://www.rcgp.org.uk/policy/rcgp-policy-areas/assisted-dying> accessed 03 November 2022.

The BMA, for its part, has demonstrated a clearer institutional shift, albeit from an unflinching opposition to legal reform,[151] to the adoption of a neutral stance. This neutrality was reflected in a survey of its members, with 50% supporting allowing prescription of lethal self-administered medication, and 47% in opposition. There was clearer support from palliative physician (76%) than those working in intensive care (45%) or emergency medicine (47%).[152]

The GMC has taken note of its members' concerns not to leave patients feeling abandoned at the end of life, and has issued guidance accordingly, while remaining opposed to a change in the law, and supporting a presumption in favour of life.[153] In contrast, organisations such as the Campaign for Dignity in Dying have reported an 84% of support from polled members of the public with respect to the introduction of a law on assisted dying for terminally ill adults.[154]

Whatever one is to make of these figures, it is interesting to note that the majority of Western anglophone medical 'establishments'—as represented by their national associations—remain ambivalent on the issues.[155] Nor, one feels, should moral questions be determined on the basis of straw polls.[156] The fact that a majority believes that something is right does not *make it* morally right; those who argue that public (or, indeed, professional) acceptance of PAS justifies its legalisation might consider whether, say, consistency requires them to support the morality of the death penalty in communities in which it is widely endorsed. In the legislative context it is worth bearing in mind that it is the poll of voting Members of Parliament that remains determinative, and that has shown little change over almost three decades of activity in the UK legislatures.

Ultimately, there may be strong pragmatic reasons for the view that the medical profession simply should not involve itself in actions which confuse its role. In this respect, the classic words of Capron still merit preservation:

> I never want to have to wonder whether the physician coming into my hospital room is wearing the white coat (or the green scrubs) of a healer, concerned only to relieve my pain and restore me to health, or the black hood of the executioner. Trust between patient and physician is simply too important and too fragile to be subjected to this unnecessary strain.[157]

On the other hand, in 2015 Dignity in Dying cited a Populus poll to the effect that of 5,000 members of the public, 87% felt a change in the law 'would either have increased

[151] See Jacky Davis, 'Most UK Doctors Support Assisted Dying, A New Poll Shows: The BMA's Opposition Does Not Represent Members' (2018) 360 BMJ online k301.

[152] The full results were published in October 2020 at BMA, 'Physician-Assisted Dying' (2020) available at <https://www.bma.org.uk/advice-and-support/ethics/end-of-life/physician-assisted-dying> accessed 03 November 2022.

[153] See GMC, 'Treatment and Care Towards the End of Life: Good Practice in Decision Making' (2010); GMC, 'When a Patient Seeks Advice or Information about Assistance to Die' (2013); and GMC, 'Treatment and Care Towards the End of Life: Good Practice in Decision Making' (2022).

[154] Campaign for Dignity in Dying, available at <https://www.dignityindying.org.uk/assisted-dying/public-opinion/> accessed 15 January 2023.

[155] Richard McMurray et al., 'Decisions Near the End of Life' (1992) 267(16) JAMA 2229; Charles-Gene McDaniel, 'US Doctors Reaffirm Opposition to Euthanasia' (1996) 313 BMJ 11.

[156] This was largely the view of the House of Lords Select Committee on the 2004 Bill, House of Lords Select Committee, *Assisted Dying for the Terminally Ill Bill—First Report* (2005).

[157] Alexander Capron, 'Legal and Ethical Problems in Decisions for Death' (1986) 14(3–4) Law, Medicine and Healthcare 141.

trust in doctors or that it would make no difference to the doctor-patient relationship',[158] while only 12% said that it would impact negatively. This contrasts with the BMA quali-tative study of the same year,[159] which found a balance of positive and negative views from members of the public on the possible effects on the doctor-patient relationship were assisted suicide to become legally permissible. The impact would be dependent on a range of factors such as the decision not being made by doctors, and the safeguards in place—that we consider later in this chapter with respect to legislative attempts.

This concern over trust has been the subject of close scrutiny. Emanuel and colleagues found in their survey of cancer patients and members of the public in general that 19% of the former and 26.5% of the latter would change doctors if their doctor spoke to them about euthanasia or PAS.[160] Trust is, however, only one of many considerations which are exposed in Capron's comment. In addition, there are the familiar issues of coercion and abuse, both of which may serve to render decisions to end life less than fully voluntary, as, indeed, may confusion. While the courts have traditionally expressed concerns about potential coercion of the vulnerable patient, we must consider, too, the moral or legal coercion of a system that puts the medical professions at the heart of assisted dying. It is to a consideration of the practical aspects of these practices that we now turn, first learning lessons from jurisdictions that have grasped the proverbial nettle.

18.7 ASSISTED DYING IN PRACTICE

18.7.1 THE DUTCH AND CONTINENTAL EUROPEAN EXPERIENCE

The focal area for much debate still lies in the Netherlands,[161] where medically prac-tised assisted dying became lawful in November 2000. This ended the previous legal situation under which euthanasia and assisted suicide were illegal,[162] but doctors who accelerated their patients' deaths would not be prosecuted provided they complied with certain requirements. These have now been consolidated in the Termination of Life on Request and Assisted Suicide (Review Procedures) Act 2001, which amends Article 293 of the Dutch Penal Code. Article 293(1) states that a person who terminates the life of another person at that other person's express and earnest request is liable to a term of

---

[158] Campaign for Dignity in Dying, 'Patients Would Trust Doctors More if Assisted Dying was Legal' (01 June 2015) available at <https://www.dignityindying.org.uk/news/patients-trust-doctors-assisted-dying/> accessed 03 November 2022.

[159] BMA, 'End-of-life Care and Physician-Assisted Dying: Public Dialogue Research' (2015), p 55 et seq.

[160] Emanuel et al. (n 134).

[161] Much of our authority for what follows derived initially from Julia Nicol, Marisa Tiedeman, and Dominique Valiquet, *Euthanasia and Assisted Suicide: International Experiences* (Library of Parliament 2008); Penney Lewis and Isra Black, 'The Effectiveness of Legal Safeguards in Jurisdictions that Allow Assisted Dying' (2012) 2016(35) KCL Law School Research Paper No. available at <https://ssrn.com/abstract=2824513> accessed 03 November 2022; Nicole Steck et al., 'Euthanasia and Assisted Suicide in Selected European Countries and US States: Systematic Literature Review' (2013) 51(10) Medical Care 938. Further updates may be found at The Globe Post, 'Euthanasia: Where It's Legal in Europe' (2021) available at <https://theglobepost.com/2021/04/07/where-is-euthanasia-legal-europe/> accessed 03 November 2022 and Euronews, 'Euthanasia in Europe: Where is Assisted Dying Lgeal' (2022) available at <https://www.euronews.com/2019/09/25/where-in-europe-is-assisted-dying-legal-> accessed 03 November 2022.

[162] Understood as the deliberate termination of a patient's life by a physician acting on the patient's request; the Dutch Act does not differentiate between the two.

imprisonment of not more than twelve years or a fine. Article 293(2) stipulates that this offence shall not be punishable if it has been committed by a physician who has met the requirements of due care and who informs the municipal autopsist of this.

The concept of due care is defined in Article 2 of the 2001 Act, which states that the physician must:

(a) be satisfied that the patient's request is voluntary and carefully considered;

(b) be satisfied that the patient's suffering was unbearable, and that there was no prospect of improvement;

(c) have informed the patient about his or her situation and prospects;

(d) have come to the conclusion, together with the patient, that there is no reasonable alternative in light of the patient's condition;

(e) have consulted at least one other independent physician who must have seen the patient and provided a written opinion on the requirements of due care referred to in (a) to (d); and

(f) have terminated the patient's life or assisted with suicide with due medical care and attention.

This is essentially a codification of the due care conditions which had evolved in the jurisprudence, starting with *Re Schoonheim*,[163] and they are further fleshed out by the Regional Review Committees (RRC), which review all cases.[164] For example, they have identified that there must be a sufficient physician-patient relationship to allow the physician to form a judgment concerning the requirements of due care, and have interpreted criterion (f) as requiring the use of the appropriate method, substance and dosage as recommended by professional guidelines, and the attending with the patient until death occurs. The requirement for an independent consultation is often now satisfied by consultations with specialised physicians participating in the SCEN (Support and Consultation Regarding Euthanasia in the Netherlands) Project. These physicians are available to advise doctors who are faced with a request for physician-assisted death, and to act as independent consultants under the Act. A non-binding best practices protocol has been implemented among SCEN physicians. Several Supreme Court cases have also offered guidance. In *Re Chabot*,[165] the Court confirmed that mental as well as physical suffering can justify assisted dying, warning, however, that the physician must be 'extremely cautious'. In *Re Brongersma*,[166] the Court held that neither the previous rules nor the 2001 Act covered 'tired of life' situations; physicians must limit themselves to requests for assisted dying from patients suffering from a medically classifiable physical or psychiatric sickness or disorder.

Controversially, the 2001 Act provides for euthanasia on what in UK jurisdictions are known as competent minors:[167] children aged between 12 and 16 who are deemed to have

---

[163] 27 November 1984, NJ 1985 No. 106 (Supreme Court).

[164] Specifically, a physician must report an assisted death to the Medical Examiner using a prescribed form indicating that he has complied with the due care criteria. The ME conducts an examination of the deceased patient to ascertain the completeness and accuracy of the physician's report, and then notifies the relevant RRC, of which there are five, each comprising an uneven number of members, including a physician, a legal expert, and an ethicist. The RRC determines whether the incident is within the limits of the Dutch Act, or should be referred to the criminal authorities. The conclusions of the RRCs are published online, and the RRCs additionally issue a joint annual report.

[165] 21 June 1994, NJ 1994 No. 65627 (Supreme Court).

[166] 24 December 2002, NJ 2003 No. 16721 (Supreme Court).   [167] Arts 2(3) and (4).

a 'reasonable understanding' of their interests may give consent to euthanasia, provided that their decision is agreed to by their parents, and children aged 16 and 17 may opt for euthanasia, but this may only be carried out if the parents (or those exercising parental authority) have been involved in the decision. The 2001 Act also allows for prior consent, thus recognising the validity of advance decisions. A written declaration of this nature has the effect of a concrete request for euthanasia which may be exercised when the patient is no longer capable of expressing their will. One consequence of this is that a patient who does not have the capacity to object, but who may, in fact, not now want to die, could be killed by a doctor who, possessing an earlier written authorisation, decides that it would be better for the patient to do so.

The scale of the practice of euthanasia in the Netherlands is disputed, although most studies suggest that it is extensive.[168] While there was a marked drop in absolute numbers and in the proportion of deaths (1.8%) in 2005, the figures rose again by 2010, and again by 2015,[169] with an 8% rise in and 2017,[170] reaching a record in absolute numbers in 2020.[171] This should be seen in light of an expansion of the Dutch provisions to include children aged 12–16, with parental consent being mandatory, and the Dutch government proposing its authorisation for children under aged 12.[172]

Although the doubts as to the reporting integrity of physicians seemed, at one time, to have been largely dispelled (about 80% of cases were reported in 2005 as compared with 54% in 2001),[173] there is still a strong element of subjectivity in reporting, which makes analysis of the figures both difficult, and an ongoing phenomenon. This is in part due to under-reporting, and in part due to differences in data collection methods.[174] It is also worth noting the figures are for both euthanasia and assisted suicide combined. This leads us back to the infamous practical slippery slope which, in effect, postulates that you cannot legislate for limited euthanasia because it will be impossible to prevent people breaching the rules.[175]

---

[168] This high incidence might, in itself, give rise to concern. The House of Lords, for example, estimated that, if the Dutch model were to be implemented in Britain, it could lead to 13,000 deaths a year. This is to be compared with 650 deaths per year if the Oregon model, below, were adopted: House of Lords Select Committee on the Assisted Dying for the Terminally Ill Bill, *Assisted Dying for the Terminally Ill Bill—First Report* (2005), para 243.

[169] For a reporting and analysis of the statistics, see A Stef Groenewoud et al., 'Euthanasia in the Netherlands: a Claims Data Cross-Sectional Study of Geographical Variation' (2020) BMJ Supportive & Palliative Care available at <https://pubmed.ncbi.nlm.nih.gov/33446488/> accessed 03 November 2022.

[170] NOS News, 'Opnieuw Meer Meldingen Van Euthanasie' (7 March 2018) available at <https://nos.nl/artikel/2221012-opnieuw-meer-meldingen-van-euthanasie> accessed 03 November 2022.

[171] Right to Life News, 'Netherlands had Record Number of Euthanasia Procedures in 2020' (21 May 2021) available at <https://righttolife.org.uk/news/netherlands-had-record-number-of-euthanasia-procedures-in-2020> accessed 03 November 2022.

[172] BBC, 'Netherlands Backs Euthanasia for Terminally Ill Children Under 12' (14 October 2020) available at <https://www.bbc.co.uk/news/world-europe-54538288> accessed 03 November 2022. This proposal was renewed in June 2022, by the Health Minister, Ernst Kuipers. Note the law in Belgium has allowed euthanasia regardless of age, but conditional, since 2014, by amending the 2002 Euthanasia Act.

[173] Paul van der Maas et al., 'Euthanasia, Physician-Assisted Suicide, and Other Medical Practices Involving the End of Life in the Netherlands, 1990–1995' (1996) 335(22) New England Journal of Medicine 1699.

[174] Robert Preston, 'Death on Demand? An Analysis of Physician-Administered Euthanasia in The Netherlands' (2018) 125(1) British Medical Bulletin 145.

[175] Stephen Smith, 'Evidence for the Practical Slippery Slope in the Debate on Physician-Assisted Suicide and Euthanasia' (2005) 13(1) Medical Law Review 17.

There are certainly indications that there is a slippery slope in the Netherlands. The 2017 review suggests a general climb in deaths per 1,000 due to euthanasia.[176] In our view, this is better seen as an example of its logical format which warns us that, if a logical case can be made for a movement from position A1 to position A2, then the same logic can, and will, enable us to move from position A2 to A3.[177] Indeed, opponents of the Netherlands model have consistently expressed concern that the grounds for its exercise will inevitably become more trivial until what matters is not the grounds for wanting to die, but the want itself.[178] Such concerns do not appear ill-founded when one reads that a Dutch psychiatrist was found to be medically justified in assisting the suicide of a physically healthy woman who was depressed,[179] or legally justified in ending the life of a patient with Alzheimer's disease, where the law remained unclear on seeking the views of someone no longer mentally competent.[180] This is precisely the situation foreseen by those who oppose legalising the termination of life and, for example, the Dutch Commission for the Acceptability of Life Terminating Action having recommended that, in some circumstances, the life of a patient suffering from severe dementia without serious physical symptoms might be terminated with or without their having executed an advance directive on the point.[181]

Whether this is a cause for concern depends, of course, on whether one believes the resulting position to be morally less acceptable than the original. The slippery slope is a subjective concept and we admit that we are among those who fear its influence in the context of voluntary euthanasia. There are, of course, those who would deny the very existence of such slopes,[182] and we ourselves would not accept the proposition that, once a decision of doubtful morality has been taken, the erection of a slippery slope is *inevitable*. We would rather see the analogy as a descending lift which stops at various landings. Using this model, we are no longer slipping but, rather, getting off at, and standing on, new platforms each of which represents a new moral threshold from which to assess the next call for an incremental shift—and this is what is happening. We suggest that the Dutch experience should be taken as an object lesson rather than as a paradigm.[183]

A major difficulty in assessing the Dutch experience lies in definition, and this probably derives from their use of the term 'medical decisions concerning the end

---

[176] Dutch Government, 'Report on the Third Evaluation of the Dutch Euthanasia Law' (2017) available at <https://publicaties.zonmw.nl/fileadmin/zonmw/documenten/Kwaliteit_van_zorg/Evaluatie_Regelgeving/Derde_evaluatie_Wtl.pdf> accessed 07 November 2022.

[177] For discussion of the distinction between slippery slopes, see Stephen Smith, 'Fallacies of the Logical Slippery Slope in the Debate on Physician-Assisted Suicide and Euthanasia' (2005) 13(2) Medical Law Review 234.

[178] Concern becomes even more real when one reads Tony Sheldon, 'Dutch Euthanasia Law Should Apply to Patients "Suffering Through Living" Report Says' (2005) 330(7482) BMJ 61. For an example of the pressures, see Suzanne Ost and Alexandra Mullock, 'Pushing the Boundaries of Lawful Assisted Dying in the Netherlands: Existential Suffering and Lay Assistance' (2011) 18(2) European Journal of Healthcare Law 163.

[179] 'Mercy-killing doctor freed' *The Scotsman* (22 April 1993) p 8. See also Tony Sheldon, 'Dutch Approve Euthanasia for a Patient with Alzheimer's Disease' (2005) 330 BMJ 1041.

[180] BBC News, 'Dutch Euthanasia Case: Doctor Acted in Interest of Patient, Court Rules' (11 September 2019) available at <https://www.bbc.co.uk/news/world-europe-49660525> accessed 04 November 2022.

[181] Henk Hellema, 'Dutch Doctors Support Life Termination in Dementia' (1993) 306(6889) BMJ 1364.

[182] See David Enoch, 'Once You Start Using Slippery Slope Arguments, You're on a Very Slippery Slope' (2001) 21(4) Oxford Journal of Legal Studies 629; Robin Downie, et al., *Healthy Respect: Ethics in Health Care* (2nd edn, OUP 2001).

[183] See John Griffiths, Heleen Weyers, Maurice Adams, *Euthanasia and Law in Europe* (Hart 2008); Lewis and Black (n 161).

of life' (MDEL).[184] MDEL includes a wide spectrum of activity ranging from manifest euthanasia, through the concept of 'double effect',[185] to the most controversial, and hard to unravel, group involving termination of life without an explicit request. Griffiths extrapolated the available data to suggest that, on these grounds, an MDEL is the immediate cause of death in more than half the deaths in the Netherlands due to chronic disease.[186]

The pioneering legislation in the Netherlands did not immediately lead to a large number of other jurisdictions following suit.[187] Nevertheless, it has now spread to the other members of Benelux.[188] Belgium adopted the Act on Euthanasia 2002, another Act which reflected what was happening in practice.[189] Curiously, the Act made no mention of PAS, leaving that practice in legal limbo[190]—the probability is that it is subsumed under the doubtful umbrella of euthanasia. The Grand Duchy of Luxembourg followed suit in 2008—albeit only after narrowly escaping a constitutional crisis in so doing. The Benelux countries have now introduced measures which standardise the use of advance directives, but have retained individual regulation of euthanasia; surprisingly, there is no suggestion of introducing residency requirements for availability.[191]

One of the biggest controversies to arise has been the acceptance into law of euthanasia for minors in Belgium (although note the existing provisions in the Netherlands), and the euthanasia of a dementia patient who never requested the service.[192] On the former, the significant difference is that Belgium imposes no cut-off age limit (while the Dutch rule is 12 years of age). The criteria to qualify in Belgium require that the child be terminally ill, in unbearable pain, make repeated requests, and be assessed by two doctors and a psychiatrist or psychologist. Their legal representatives must also consent. To many, both of these developments will be a step too far, especially given the potential coercion that severe suffering can bring (in the case of the former) and the inability to consent in (in the case of the latter).[193] To others, it is but a logical extension of

---

[184] Griffiths (ibid.) suggests that this would be better expressed as 'medical procedures that shorten life'.

[185] Which we have discussed at length.

[186] See also, Mette Rurup et al., 'The First Five Years of Euthanasia Legislation in Belgium and the Netherlands: Description and Comparison of Cases' (2012) 26(1) Palliative Medicine 43.

[187] For debate on the ambivalence of opinion in the Council of Europe see John Keown, 'Mr Marty's Muddle: A Superficial and Selective Case for Euthanasia in Europe' (2006) 32(1) Journal of Medical Ethics 29; and the associated commentary by Guy Widdershaven at 34.

[188] A whole issue of the European Journal of Health Law is devoted to the specific issue of PAS: Graeme Laurie, 'Physician Assisted Suicide in Europe: Some Lessons and Trends' (2005) 12(1) European Journal of Health Law 5.

[189] In 2000, it was revealed that the incidence of euthanasia in the Flemish-speaking part of the country was similar to that revealed in the earlier Netherlands studies: Luc Deliens et al., 'End of Life Decisions in Medical Practice in Flanders, Belgium: A Nationwide Survey' (2000) 356(9244) Lancet 1806.

[190] Herman Nys, 'Physician Assisted Suicide in Belgian law' (2005) 12(1) European Journal of Health Law 39.

[191] World Federation of Right to Die Societies, 'BeNeLux Parliament's Resolutions on Euthanasia and Advance Directives' (30 April 2012) available at <https://wfrtds.org/benelux-parliaments-resolutions-on-euthanasia-and-advance-directives/> accessed 04 November 2022.

[192] For more on the latter, see CBC, 'Euthanasia Dispute in Belgium: When do Doctors Cross a Line?' (16 February 2018) available at <https://www.cbc.ca/news/health/euthanasia-dispute-belgium-demen-tia-1.4538785> accessed 03 November 2022.

[193] Andrew Siegel, Dominic Sisti, and Arthur Caplan, 'Pediatric Euthanasia in Belgium: Disturbing Developments' (2014) 311(19) Journal of American Medical Association 1963.

recognising autonomy in human beings and/or to addressing their suffering according to their own will, stated or presumed.[194]

Assisted suicide was decriminalised in Switzerland in 1942 (Article 115 of the Swiss Penal Code).[195] The essential element of the law is the motive of the assisting person; there is no criminality provided that the assistance is a selfless act—that is, without personal motive.[196] This provision is not directed only to the medical profession. The position of the 'mercy killer' is, however, different because direct assistance to die in these circumstances remains liable to prosecution in the absence of a genuine 'suicide'. The overall result is that what was once a trickle of terminally ill patients in search of an 'easy death' into Switzerland from more conservative countries has now become something of a stream that may grow substantially in future years if other jurisdictions maintain their status quo.[197] It has been reported by Dignitas, for example, that between 1998 and 2013, the clinic assisted 244 Britons to die. The organisation Dignity in Dying has estimated this is the equivalent of one Briton using the service every two weeks.[198]

18.7.2 THE CHANGING LANDSCAPE IN NORTH AMERICA

We have argued that there *are* good moral and practical grounds for dissociating PAS from euthanasia—indeed, we will suggest later that it may be the solution to a social dilemma—and there is legislative precedent for so doing. Having seen an initiative designed to decriminalise active voluntary euthanasia fail in California,[199] Oregon introduced its Death with Dignity Act (DWDA) in 1994, which concerned assisted suicide only, and it was adopted in 1997.[200] Under the Oregon Act, it is lawful for a doctor to prescribe a lethal dosage of a drug for a patient who wishes to end their life, but not to involve themself in the suicidal act. The patient must make the request voluntarily and must be competent and be suffering from a terminal illness. Critics of the law have pointed out

[194] Luc Bovens, 'Child Euthanasia: Should we Just Not Talk About it?' (2015) 41(8) Journal of Medical Ethics 630.

[195] Olivier Guillod and Aline Schmidt, 'Assisted Suicide Under Swiss Law' (2005) 12(1) European Journal of Health Law 23. It is to be noted that voluntary euthanasia is still unlawful although there is no minimum penalty for killing on compassionate grounds. For a review of the Swiss situation, see Samuel Fischer et al., 'Suicide Assisted by Two Swiss Right-to-Die Organisations' (2008) 34(11) Journal of Medical Ethics 810. For empirical determinants suggesting gender disparity and increased access dependent on social circumstances, see Nicole Steck et al., 'Suicide Assisted by Right-to-Die Associations: a population based cohort study' (2014) 43(2) International Journal of Epidemiology 614.

[196] This even extends, theoretically, to assistance borne out of indifference; i.e. when the party assisting the suicide has neither a selfish nor a selfless motive.

[197] Note that, while active euthanasia is covered in Benelux, only assisted suicide is lawful in Switzerland. For a comparison with the German position, see Kathrin Becker-Schwarze, 'Legal Restrictions of Physician Assisted Suicide' (2005) 12(1) European Journal of Health Law 9. And between the Netherlands and Oregon: Francis Pakes, 'The Legalization of Euthanasia and Assisted Suicide: A Tale of Two Cities' (2005) 33(2) International Journal of the Sociology of Law 71.

[198] Scottish Parliament Information Centre, *SPICe Briefing: Assisted Suicide (Scotland) Bill* (2015), p 15.

[199] A further Act—the Compassionate Choices Act 2005 (AB 654)—failed in the Judiciary Committee. It was, however, revived in 2007, passed the Judiciary Committee, but was then put on hold. The End of Life Option Act came into effect in 2016. It provides for terminally ill adults to receive a prescription to terminate their lives. California's End of Life Act came into effect on 1 January 2022.

[200] The US Supreme Court has decreed that statutes which prohibit assisted suicide—which were in force in 34 states—are not unconstitutional; the arguments are, however, essentially based on US constitutional law and have very little relevance outside the U.S.: *Vacco* v *Quill* 521 US 793 (1997); *Washington* v *Glucksberg* 117 S Ct 2258 (1997).

that it empowers the physician to determine matters such as competence and voluntariness, and it has been suggested that it naively accepts medical reassurances of compliance with the requirements.[201] The fact that Oregon's Medicaid Plan, which provides medical cover for indigent patients, will pay for PAS while excluding several other treatments is of particular interest.

A number of challenges were mounted following the passage of the Act, including the introduction into Congress of the proposed Pain Relief Promotion Act 1999, which would have directly banned the use of controlled drugs to end life, even where it was legal under assisted-suicide legislation.[202] The failure of this Bill did not deter the US Government from further attempts to prevent assisted suicide through the use of drug administration regulations but, ultimately, the Supreme Court found the actions of the Attorney General to be unconstitutional and upheld the validity of the Oregon Act.[203]

As something of an envoi to the Oregon position, it is worth noting how often and with what success the Act has been used. In 1998, there were 24 prescription recipients and 16 DWDA deaths. Both numbers rose steadily to 2017, in which there were 218 prescription recipients and 143 DWDA deaths, implicating 92 (attending) physicians. Interestingly, the pattern of prescription recipients to deaths has remained fairly static over the 20 years of the Act's operation, possibly suggesting that the receipt of the prescription itself might restore a degree of dignity and control to people's lives without the need to follow through on the final act. A 2021 data summary published by the Oregon Health Department indicated that, 'As of January 21, 2022, 238 people had died in 2021 from ingesting the prescribed medications',[204] though 383 prescriptions were received in 2021, written by 133 physicians[205] (down from 142 the previous year). That was a 25% increase on the previous year. With steady increases in those seeking to end their lives, has come a concomitant increase in attending physicians. Most prescriptions were for those who were older, white, better educated, in hospice care, diagnosed with cancer, and who died at home.[206] Of further patient characteristics, the 2021 Data Summary reported that, 'As in previous years, the three most frequently reported end-of-life concerns were loss of autonomy (93%), decreasing ability to participate in activities that made life enjoyable (92%), and loss of dignity (68%).'[207]

It is undeniable that the number of deaths has risen steadily from year to year, and there has only been one known Oregonian failure (a man who woke up three days after taking his drug).[208] In some instances a prescription was issued, and the patient outlived their prognosis. There has however been some suggestion that—as in the case of the Dutch experience—it is difficult to maintain strict objectivity in statistical analysis that depends

[201] Susan Martyn and Henry Bourguignon, 'Now is the Moment to Reflect: Two Years of Experience with Oregon's Physician-Assisted Suicide Law' (2000) 8(1) Elder Law Journal 1.

[202] David Orentlicher and Arthur Caplan, 'The Pain Relief Promotion Act of 1999' (2000) 283(2) Journal of American Medical Association 255.

[203] *Gonzales* v *Oregon* 546 US 243 (2006), affirming *Oregon* v *Ashcroft* 368 F 3d 1118 (2004; 9th Circuit CA).

[204] Oregon Death With Dignity Act, 2021 Data Summary, Public Health Division. 2022. Executive Summary.

[205] ibid., p.5 and 7.

[206] ibid., interestingly, neurological disease accounted for only 15% (8% the previous year) of deaths, and heart disease just 11% (12% in 2020).

[207] ibid., p. 7.

[208] Don Colburn, 'Fewer Turn to Assisted Suicide' (The Oregonian, 11 March 2005). But the dangers associated with 'undercover' PAS (in Australia) are stressed in Roger Magnusson, 'Euthanasia: Above Ground, Below Ground' (2004) 30(5) Journal of Medical Ethics 441. The author argues that legalising PAS may be a safer option than prohibition.

upon self-reporting.[209] On the other hand, we must take into account that the DWDA requires the Oregon Health Authority to collect the very statistical information referred to previously, and to publish an annual report. In the end, individual readers must judge the significance of the figures for themselves.[210]

It may be significant that a number of other US states have followed Oregon. Having once rejected the proposition, the state of Washington implemented legal provisions in much the same terms as Oregon and by a very similar majority (59:41).[211] A major feature of both Acts is that depression must be excluded as an influence on choice before a person can be lawfully assisted to die. It seems to us to be arguable that a person would not wish to die *unless* they were depressed, and the distinguishing diagnosis must be difficult to make.[212] Other states to implement laws include Montana, which made the step through a court mandate,[213] Vermont, the District of Columbia, Colorado, and Hawaii.[214] Of course, we have already noted the Canadian Medical Assistance in Dying Act 2015, and the province of Québec has adopted the End-of-Life Care Act 2014.[215]

In all of the jurisdictions, medical practitioners play a central role. With the exception of Switzerland, they must determine a person's capacity and eligibility under the law, ensure that any consent is valid, and be present at the time of death (although this is not so in Oregon). Even in Switzerland, doctors are implicated because only they can prescribe the necessary legal substances.[216] They also have in common a central concern for the exercise of autonomous power at the end of life while, at the same time, distancing themselves from approving suicide.[217] Nonetheless, it seems clear that the movement towards legalising assisted dying is gaining momentum on a global scale while, at the same time, opposition remains fierce. As a result, and apparently against the European trend, there is no move in the UK to extend assistance in dying beyond assistance in suicide—and there are very good reasons why we should clearly define this particular Rubicon as marking the boundary between what is lawful and what is not.

[209] Wendy Hiscox, 'Physician-Assisted Suicide in Oregon: The "Death with Dignity" Data' (2007) 8(3) Medical Law International 197. The author also draws attention to the strong influence which professional organisations will have on the implementation of statutes.

[210] For reference to data trends, see Sílvia Merina et al., 'Trends in Hastened Death Decision Criteria: A Review of Official Reports' (2022) 126(7) Health Policy 643. For reference to further critiques of the quality of data, see Abbi Hobbs and Devyani Gajjar, 'Assisted Dying' (POSTbrief, 26 September 2022) available at <https://post.parliament.uk/research-briefings/post-pb-0047/> accessed 04 November 2022, p 28.

[211] Washington Death with Dignity Act, Ch. 70.245. For a brief description, see Clare Dyer, 'Washington State Legalises Physician Assisted Suicide' (2008) 337(7679) BMJ 1133. The closeness of the judicial and political differences has been a feature of the US debate as a whole.

[212] See Linda Ganzini, Elizabeth Goy, and Steven Dobscha, 'Prevalence of Depression and Anxiety in Patients Requesting Physicians' Aid in Dying: Cross Sectional Survey' (2008) 337 BMJ 1682; Thomas Szasz, 'Diagnoses are not Diseases' (1991) 338(8782–8783) Lancet 1574.

[213] See *Baxter* v *Montana* (2009) P 3d WL5155363 (Mont SC).

[214] See the Vermont Patient Choice and Control at End of Life Act 2013, Ch. 13, the DC Death with Dignity Act 2015, L21–0182, the Colorado End-of-Life Options Act 2016, and the Hawaii Relating to Health Act, HB2739. Note that California introduced the End of Life Options Act 2016, which was overturned in 2018, but came into effect in 2022 as the End of Life Act.

[215] Ch. S32.0001. For more, see Québec, *Rights of a person at the end of life* (Government of Québec 2016), available at <https://publications.msss.gouv.qc.ca/msss/en/document-001601/> accessed 04 November 2022.

[216] For discussion and challenge on these matters see *Haas* v *Switzerland* (2011) 23 EHRR 53.

[217] Here, note Washington's Death with Dignity Act, which insists that actions taken in accordance with the Act 'do not for any purpose, constitute suicide, assisted suicide, mercy killing or homicide under the law'.

18.7.3 THE POSITION IN THE UK[218]

As we have already intimated, the euthanasia debate will not go away and is still alive in the UK. In England and Wales, Lord Falconer introduced his Assisted Dying Bill in the House of Lords (2014); it received a second reading after ten hours of debate, and was debated a further two days in Committee before the 2014–15 Session ended. Rob Marris MP tabled the Assisted Dying (No 2) Bill in the House of Commons (2015); it was debated for over four hours and rejected (330–118). Lord Falconer introduced another Assisted Dying Bill in the House of Lords (2015); it never came up for debate. Lord Hayward introduced an Assisted Dying Bill in the House of Lords (2016), but Parliament was dissolved before it got a second reading.

Lord Falconer's Oregon-model Bill has come and gone between editions of this book. Most recently it failed for want of parliamentary time, but it has been resurrected more or less wholesale by a Private Member's Bills brought first by Rob Marris MP, and most recently by Baroness Meacher in the House of Lords.

The Marris Bill failed to achieve the status of law, but successive debates did lead to the unanimous vote in the House of Lords on an amendment brought by Lord Pannick to require judicial confirmation in the High Court that a terminally ill person has reached 'a voluntary, clear, settled and informed' decision. This might be seen to be akin to the judicial oversight of withdrawal/withholding decisions with respect to patients with severe disorders of consciousness (see Chapter 17).

Like its predecessor Bill, Baroness Meacher's Assisted Dying Bill wrote Lord Pannick's amendment into clause 1. Additional so-called 'safeguards' in the Bill include that the person applying for assistance is aged over 18, has capacity to make the decision, and has been resident in the jurisdiction for more than one year. Terminal illness is defined as an irreversible progressive condition that is reasonably expected to lead to death within six months. The applicant's capacity and 'settled intention', and the existence of such a condition, would need to be countersigned by two qualified medical practitioners. Assistance in dying would take the form of a prescription with medicines or supply of a device, with which a person will be able to end their own life. The Bill provided for conscientious objection by medical practitioners, and would have amended the Suicide Act 1961 to disapply section 2 to a person providing assistance under what would become the Assisted Dying Act. The Bill proceeded no further than its second reading after the end of the 2021–22 parliamentary session.

Attention to these matters has also been strong in Scotland in recent years. After a failed Oregon-type consultation in 2005, Margo MacDonald MSP formulated an End of Life Choices (Scotland) Bill,[219] which sought to legalise active euthanasia while coming close to de-medicalising the process. After its rejection by the Scottish Parliament,[220] Ms MacDonald secured sufficient votes in September 2012 to permit her to reintroduce a Bill in Holyrood in 2013 as the Assisted Suicide (Scotland) Bill, which following her death was taken up by Patrick Harvey MSP. The Bill purported to offer lawful assistance to persons with 'an illness or progressive condition that is terminal *or life-shortening*', which potentially opened the scope of the putative law considerably. It would not be as narrow as the English counterpart nor, indeed, like Oregon on which much inspiration had been drawn. In a major departure from other medically based models,[221] the Bill proposed a

---

[218] For a discussion on why successive Bills have failed, and the lack of judicial activism on the issue in the UK, see Earle (n 122).

[219] The Bill was later renamed the End of Life Assistance (Scotland) Bill.

[220] For analysis, see Graeme Laurie and John K Mason, 'Assisted Dying or Euthanasia? Comments on the End of Life Assistance (Scotland) Bill' (2010) 14(3) Edinburgh Law Review 493.

[221] For an assessment of the role of various actors, see Adam McCann, 'Comparing the Law and Governance of Assisted Dying in Four European Nations' (2015) 2(1) European Journal of Comparative Law and Governance 37.

role for 'Licensed Facilitators', for 'practical assistance', and to be present at the suicide. Two doctors would still have been required to certify capacity and the eligibility criteria, but would be far more removed from the final act. The Bill fell before the Scottish Parliament on 27 May 2015, but not before robust consideration by the Health and Sport Committee.[222] The supporting documentation is an excellent resource for those interested in the moral and political nuances of this field.[223]

Most recently, in September 2021 Liam MacArthur MSP launched a Consultation on a Proposed Assisted Dying for Terminally Ill Adults (Scotland) Bill. In October 2022, he won the right to introduce the Bill, which is expected in 2023. What is of interest here is the proposal to effectively equate terminal and unbearable by using the definition of 'terminal' in the Social Security (Scotland) Act 2018. This removed a time limit and referred simply to a person being 'unable to recover' from the progressive disease diagnosed by a registered medical practitioner. Other proposed safeguards would be broadly similar to those in Baroness Meacher's Bill.

What has not yet happened in UK jurisdictions is an escape from an assisted suicide spiral, in which the courts deem change to be a matter for Parliament, and yet Parliament fails to enact the change favoured by a number of other European jurisdictions, and to do so on the basis of a right to private and family life.[224] In our view, any change to the current position in UK jurisdictions will likely be through the legislature, but ushered in through a court ruling, following Lady Hale's lead in *Nicklinson* and declaring section 2(1) of the Suicide Act 1961 to run contrary to Article 8 of the European Convention on Human Rights, that is being in effect unconstitutional.[225]

18.8 CONCLUSION

Whatever the future may hold for medical-led assisted dying in the UK, it is certain that changes will come about only as a result of extensive argument and with little chance of consensus. One wonders, then, is legislation needed and, if it is, does it have to be as complex and meticulous as recent efforts? It will be clear that, throughout this discussion, we have tended to the view that there is little need for legislation in respect of the incurably or terminally ill adult patient; the great majority of life or death decisions can be—and are—based on good medical practice which is contained by relatively clear legal and moral guidelines; when put to the test, the euthanasia calculus needs to be enlisted only in the cases of 'mercy killing' and physician-assisted or physician-accomplished suicide. We doubt if there is serious, extensive support for the first of these in the UK. The movement in favour of formally legalising voluntary euthanasia and PAS is, however, strong, and the autonomy-based arguments advanced by its supporters merit a response. As will be apparent from our discussion, we believe that there are persuasive reasons for rejecting the legalisation of voluntary euthanasia, not the least of these being the extent to which the policy of euthanasia in the Netherlands has been adequately policed and progressively more widely interpreted. The uncertainty of the common law has been used

---

[222] Health and Sport Committee of the Scottish Parliament (n 63). It is interesting to note in passing that the Committee decided not to make any particular recommendation to Parliament.

[223] For a summary of that Scottish Bill and how it fits in the assisted dying landscape as of January 2015, see Scottish Parliament Information Centre (n 198).

[224] For an in-depth discussion of the German and Italian judicial use of constitutional rights analogous to Art 8 ECHR to declare unconstitutional a part of the Criminal Code analogous to s 2 of the Suicide Act 1961, see Earle (n 122).

[225] This view is supported by the extent to which the judgment in *Nicklinson* was referred to in parliamentary debates on Lord Falconer's 2015 Bill.

as a justification for change in the law, and although this has been clarified greatly in cases such as *Pretty*, *Ms B*, and *Purdy*, the most recent decision by the Supreme Court in *Nicklinson* is the clearest possible message that the courts support further clarity but remain reluctant to take this upon themselves. And yet, the example of the Supreme Court of Canada shows a boldness and subtlety of spirit that is able to avoid blanket categories of lawful/unlawful or autonomous/vulnerable as the means by which to police and promote the needs of a very wide range of citizens in our society. Even if most of the medical circumstances that people experience at the ends of their lives are not clearly covered by most of the law, there remain a few—but no less important—groups of people for whom this is not true. The law and its institutions are required to deliver justice also to these citizens.

For us, the key concerns are those of 'which groups' and 'which professionals' are to benefit from, or be implicated in, any legal change. It might well be argued that it is illogical, in principle, to restrict any proposal to terminal disease; we must, however, bow to pragmatism when facing the challenges of drafting a proposal that has any chance of seeing the light of day. Equally, legal reform need not be revolutionary and completed overnight. Initial eligibility could be given to the terminally ill on the understanding that any legislation would be kept under rigorous review—both as to whether it was being abused and as to whether it should be extended in the name of fairness. It is essential to accommodate the management of what is the burning question of the present-day debate—that is, the patient with intractable neuromuscular disease as exemplified by Mrs Pretty and Mr Nicklinson, lest we risk allowing our judicial system to be driven purely by pragmatism at the expense of core principles and values. Indeed, a case can be made out for advocating an independent legislative approach to such cases. As for professionals, we find much merit in the Scottish concept of the 'licensed facilitator', coupled with a robust legally recognised conscience clause. No one, not least a medical professional, should be required to take any part in the cessation of the life of another person. Equally, the ethical imperative of 'First, do no harm' can reasonably be interpreted by many as assisting in the ultimate relief of suffering for those who have chosen this for themselves.

FURTHER READING

1. Emily Jackson and John Keown, *Debating Euthanasia* (OUP 2011).

2. Andrew McGee, 'Ending the Life of the Act/Omission Dispute: Causation in Withholding and Withdrawing Life-Sustaining Measures' (2011) 31(3) Legal Studies 467.

3. Gianluca Montanari Vergallo, 'Advance Healthcare Directives: Binding or Informational Value?' (2020) 29(1) Cambridge Quarterly of Healthcare Ethics 98.

4. Murray Earle, '"Only Time Will Tell" – Escape from the Medically Assisted Suicide Spiral', in Edward Dove and Niamh Nic Shuibhne (eds.), *Law and Legacy in Medical Jurisprudence: Essays in Honour of Graeme Laurie* (CUP 2022).

5. Stephen Smith, 'Evidence for the Practical Slippery Slope in the Debate on Physician-Assisted Suicide and Euthanasia' (2005) 13(1) Medical Law Review 17.

6. Sílvia Merina et al., 'Trends in Hastened Death Decision Criteria: A Review of Official Reports' (2022) 126(7) Health Policy 643.

INDEX